MOSBY'S®
TEXTBOOK FOR
Medication
Assistants

Second Edition

MOSBY'S®
TEXTBOOK FOR
Medication Assistants

Karen Anderson, MSN, RN

Adjunct Faculty and Externship Coordinator
San Diego State University, School of Nursing
San Diego, California

ELSEVIER

Elsevier
3251 Riverport Lane
St. Louis, Missouri 63043

MOSBY'S® TEXTBOOK FOR MEDICATION ASSISTANTS,
SECOND EDITION

ISBN: 978-0-323-79050-5

Notice

Practitioners and researchers must always rely on their own experience and knowledge in evaluating and using any information, methods, compounds or experiments described herein. Because of rapid advances in the medical sciences, in particular, independent verification of diagnoses and drug dosages should be made. To the fullest extent of the law, no responsibility is assumed by Elsevier, authors, editors or contributors for any injury and/or damage to persons or property as a matter of products liability, negligence or otherwise, or from any use or operation of any methods, products, instructions, or ideas contained in the material herein.

Previous edition copyrighted 2009.

Library of Congress Control Number: 2021946162

Content Strategist: Nancy O'Brien/Kelly Skelton
Content Development Specialist: Dominque McPherson/Andrae Akeh
Director, Content Development: Ellen M. Wurm-Cutter
Publishing Services Manager: Shereen Jameel
Senior Project Manager: Karthikeyan Murthy
Design Direction: Amy Buxton

Printed in India

Last digit is the print number: 9 8 7 6 5 4 3

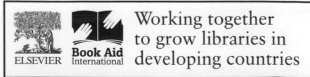

To my beautiful son, Ian Anderson, for constantly reminding me that there is so much good in this world. You inspire me to be a better mother, a better friend, and a better nurse. Your heart is filled with love and hope, and dreams and kindness. You are untainted by the world that surrounds us. May we all live and love as you do.

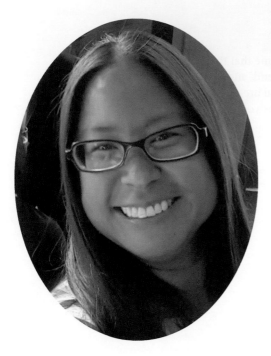

Karen V. Anderson received her Bachelor of Science in Nursing from the University of Texas at Austin and her Master of Science in Nursing Education from Kaplan University. She started her career as a nursing assistant and became a staff nurse on a medical/surgical and telemetry unit after passing the NCLEX. She was a travel nurse for 8 years and worked in 4 states, 8 cities, and 10 different hospitals. Through her travels, she ended up in San Diego, California, where she discovered her love for nursing education. Her career also includes experience as a charge nurse, resource nurse, simulation champion, assistant dean, and director. She worked as a camp nurse for two years and also as an elementary school nurse for two years.

Currently, Karen teaches nursing at San Diego State University. She has held positions as a medical/surgical clinical instructor, Nursing Externship Coordinator, and RN-BSN Health Assessment lab instructor. Her latest roles include Clinical Placement Coordinator and Nurse Simulationist. She serves as adjunct faculty at West Coast University, where she teaches Issues and Trends in Nursing online. She works per diem for Healthcare Training Associates as a skills evaluator for the nursing assistant certification (CNA) exam in California. Karen has contributed to several nursing textbooks, including: *deWit's Fundamental Concepts and Skills for Nursing*, 5th and 6th editions, by Patricia Williams; *Basic Geriatric Nursing*, 7th and 8th editions, by Patricia Williams; and *Saunders Q & A Review for the NCLEX-PN Examination*, 5th edition, by Linda Silvestri.

REVIEWERS

Susan Farah, RN, MOI Instructor
Assistant Director of Nursing, Infection Preventionist, Nurse Practice Educator
Bradford Square Rehabilitation Center
Frankfort, Kentucky

Abimbola Farinde, PhD, PharmD
Professor
College of Business
Columbia Southern University
Orange Beach, Alabama

Cindy George, RN, BSN
Program Administrator
Education
Phoenix, Arizona

James Graves, PharmD
University of Missouri Health Center
Columbia, Missouri

Tammy Inman, RN
Program Coordinator, Primary Instructor
Cliff Park High School
Springfield, Ohio

Fran Johnson, RN, BSN
Registered Nurse
Nursing Education, Health
Moore Norman Technology Center—SP Campus
Oklahoma City, Oklahoma

Kelly Kathleen Parker, RN-BSN, MA
Director of Health Career Education
CNA/MA Training
Nashville Health Career Center
832 Wedgewood Ave.
Nashville, Tennessee

Wendy Marlene Pickard, RN, BS, ONC
Course Coordinator
Health Professions Institute
Austin Community College
Austin, Texas

Carolyn Spano, MS Nursing Education, RN
Clinical Development Director
Haven Health Group
Gilbert, Arizona

Cassellen J. Springer RDA, CPC-A, MBA
Allied Health Director
Emergency Medical Training Professionals, Inc.
Lexington, Kentucky

Carol Mar Guess Williams, RN, BSN, MSN, FNP
Program Director
Nursing Entry Level
Pima Community College
Tucson, Arizona

Kristen K. Woods, RN, MN
Nursing Assistant and Medication Assistant Program Coordinator
Maricopa Nursing
Gateway Community College
Phoenix, Arizona

ACKNOWLEDGMENTS

I could not have written this 2nd edition of *Mosby's Textbook for Medication Assistants* without the dedication, guidance, and recommendations of the following people:

- The reviewers who provided their expertise and feedback that helped shape this revision
- Nancy O'Brien, Senior Content Strategist, for her patience, kindness, and expertise in guiding me through this process. She answered numerous emails and took many of my calls in order to help me navigate this project.
- Kelly Skelton, Content Strategist, for stepping in midstream and offering unending guidance and expertise all the way to the end.
- Dominque McPherson, Content Development Specialist, for skillfully reviewing my manuscript and providing support throughout this project. Andrae Akeh, Content Development Specialist, for also coming in partway through this project and providing support all the way to the end.
- Amy Buxton, Designer, for the beautifully artistry that incorporates shapes and colors that make me smile.
- Karthikeyan Murthy, Production Manager, for his patience and motivation. It's been a pleasure working with such a hard-working professional.

I also want to thank Patricia Williams for recommending me to Nancy O'Brien to take on this project. Patricia has invited me to contribute to several of her LVN/LPN textbooks. She now thinks my writing is worthy of this project. Thank you, Patricia, for believing in me! Thank you, Nancy, for taking a chance on me!

NEW TO THIS EDITION

- This edition includes updated figures, illustrations, tables and drug information in each of the drug-related chapters.
- An entire chapter dedicated to infection control and prevention was added. Included in the chapter are procedures vital to stopping the spread of infection, such as hand washing and donning and removing Personal Protective Equipment (PPE). Covid-19 is discussed along with pandemics and epidemics. The importance of vaccinations is discussed.
- Disease information was updated and simplified, making it easier to understand how and when drugs are used to treat different diseases.
- Review questions were added or updated to reflect new information added to the chapters.

The use of MA-Cs in a variety of healthcare settings has risen significantly in many states, increasing the need for an updated textbook. Information and curricula from several states were reviewed along with the curriculum by the National Council of State Boards of Nursing (NCSBN). Like the nursing assistant role, states vary regarding curricula, program length, range of functions, title, and so on.

Mosby's Textbook for Medication Assistants, 2nd edition follows the NCSBN's "Medication Assistant-Certified (MA-C) Model Curriculum." With NCSBN approval, the term *medication assistant-certified (MA-C)* is used when referring to medication assistants and nursing assistive personnel with similar titles.

This textbook is designed to serve the teaching and learning needs of instructors and students focused on the MA-C role. It is a valuable resource for competency test review and a reference for the MA-C who seeks to learn or review additional information about drugs and giving them safely.

ORGANIZATIONAL STRATEGIES

The role of the MA-C is based on the foundational knowledge and skills gained from becoming a certified nursing assistant. The values and principles of the CNA should also be reflected in the MA-C. Those values and principles include:
- Patients and residents are persons who have inherent dignity and value. They have basic needs and protected rights.
- Federal and state laws—directly and indirectly—define the roles, range of functions, and limitations of the MA-C role.
- MA-C roles and functions vary among states and agencies.
- The MA-C role has legal and ethical aspects.
- Limits on MA-C functions and role depend on effective delegation by a licensed nurse. *Delegation Guidelines* are integrated throughout the book as appropriate.
- Safety is a critical need for the person and MA-C.
- Infection control and prevention are critical needs for the person and MA-C.
- Understanding body structure and function is an essential aspect of safety.
- The nursing process is the basis for safe medication administration. The MA-C assists the nurse with and has a valuable role in the nursing process.

Learning about medications and how to safely give them inherently presents teaching and learning challenges. Therefore, additional strategies are employed to foster a user-friendly format for teaching and learning.
- An appropriate reading level is necessary to facilitate the learning process. Because of generic and trade names and the nature of pharmacology, the reading level is approximately that of the eighth grade.
- "Drug," rather than "medication," is used for reading ease and simplification.

- With safety as an ultimate goal, the *Six Rights of Drug Administration* are stressed in text and in the procedures focused on various routes of drug administration.
- Parenteral dose forms—intradermal, subcutaneous, intramuscular, and intravenous—are NOT included in this book.
- Adult dosages are the focus of this text. Pediatric dosages are not included. Even if a drug has no pediatric use, phrases such as "adult dosages" and "initial adult dosage" are used throughout the book for safety purposes.
- The MA-C is an assistant to the nurse. He or she, at all times, functions under the direction and supervision of a licensed nurse. The MA-C does not function independently and does not make patient or resident care decisions. The nursing process serves as the framework for presenting drug information.
- The person's safety and comfort are central to the MA-C role. *Promoting Safety and Comfort* boxes are integrated throughout the book as appropriate.
- Body structure and function and common health problems are integrated into the drug-related chapters.
- A template is used to present classes of drugs and specific drug information. The template includes a description of the drug's action, uses, and goals of therapy followed by "Assisting With the Nursing Process" for that drug class or drug:
  - Assessment—the observations to report and record
  - Planning—dose forms
  - Implementation—dosages and when and how to give the drug
  - Evaluation—side effects to report and record

FEATURES AND DESIGN

Besides content issues, attention also is given to the book's features and designs. The following features and design elements make the book more readable and user-friendly (see Student Preface, pp. xi-xiv):
- **Objectives**—list the learning objectives for the chapter.
- **Procedures**—a list of the procedures in the chapter follows the list of objectives.
- **Key Terms with definitions**—are at the beginning of each chapter.
- **Key Abbreviations**—for quick reference, the abbreviations used in the chapter are listed in the chapter-opening section. Some are used, but not defined, in the chapter. Examples include mg, mL, g, mcg, and MAR. Defined in earlier chapters, they are included for reference purposes in the "Key Abbreviations" lists.
- **Boxes and tables**—list principles, guidelines, signs and symptoms, nursing measures, and drug information. They are an efficient way for instructors to highlight content and they are useful study guides for students.
- **Procedure boxes divided into Quality of Life, Pre-Procedure, Procedure, and Post-Procedure steps**—Each procedure section has a subtitle. *Quality of Life, Pre-Procedure,*

Procedure, and *Post-Procedure* steps are included to show the procedure as a whole and reinforce learning. The *Quality of Life* section in the procedure boxes reminds the student of six fundamental courtesies:

- Knock before entering the room.
- Address the person by name.
- Introduce yourself by name and title.
- Explain the procedure to the person before beginning and during the procedure.
- Protect the person's rights during the procedure.
- Handle the person gently during the procedure.

- **Illustrations**—the book contains numerous full-color photographs and line art.
- **Key terms in blue, bold print**—are included throughout the text. The definition is presented in narrative in the text.
- **Focus on Communication boxes**—suggest what to say and questions to ask when interacting with patients, residents, and the nursing team.
- **Delegation Guidelines**—are associated with procedures and drug classes. They focus on the information needed from the nurse and the care plan about critical aspects of the procedure and the observations to report and record. Step 1 in the procedures refers the student to the appropriate *Delegation Guidelines.*
- **Promoting Safety and Comfort boxes**—focus the student's attention on the need to be safe and cautious and promote comfort when giving drugs. "Safety" and "Comfort" subtitles are used. Step 1 in the procedures refers the student to the appropriate *Promoting Safety and Comfort* boxes.
- **Focus on Older Persons boxes**—provide age-specific information about giving drugs to older persons.
- **Review Questions**—are found at the end of each chapter. The goal is to provide the student with a mechanism to review the chapter content. The questions are not intended to be test questions. They are structured to allow a thorough review of the content. The answers to the review questions are found on the Evolve Resources site: http://evolve.elsevier.com/Anderson/medasst/.

Because of the ever-changing pharmacology arena, the final manuscript for this textbook was reviewed by James Graves, PharmD.

This book was designed for you. It was designed to help you learn and to prepare for the certification exam. The book is a useful resource as you gain experience and expand your knowledge.

This preface provides some study guidelines and helps you use the book. When given a reading assignment, do you read from the first page to the last page without stopping? How much do you remember? You will learn more if you use a study system. A useful study system has these steps:

- Survey or preview
- Question
- Read and record
- Recite and review

SURVEY OR PREVIEW

Before you start a reading assignment, preview or survey the assignment. This gives you an idea of what the assignment covers. It also helps you recall what you already know about the subject. Carefully look over the assignment. Preview the chapter title, headings, subheadings, and terms or ideas in bold print or italics. Also survey the objectives, key terms, boxes, and review questions at the end of the chapter. Previewing only takes a few minutes. Remember, previewing helps you become familiar with the material.

QUESTION

After previewing, form questions to answer while you read. Questions should relate to what might be asked on a test or how the information applies to giving care. Use the title, headings, and subheadings to form questions. Avoid questions that have one-word answers. Questions that begin with what, how, or why are helpful. While reading, you may find that a question does not help you study. If so, just change the question. Remember, questioning sets a purpose for reading—changing a question only makes this step more useful.

READ AND RECORD

Reading is the next step. Reading is more productive after determining what you already know and what you need to learn.

Read to find answers to your questions. The purpose of reading is to:

- Gain new information
- Connect new information to what you know already

Break the assignment into smaller parts and answer your questions as you read each part. Also, mark important information (underline, highlight, or make notes). Underlining and highlighting remind you of what you need to learn. Go back and review the marked parts later. Making notes results in more immediate learning. To make notes, write down important information in the margins or in a notebook. Use words and statements to jog your memory about the material.

Work with the information to best remember what you read. Organize information into a study guide. Study guides have many forms. Diagrams or charts show relationships or steps in a process. Note taking in outline format is also very useful. The following is a sample outline.

1. Main heading
   a. Second level
   b. Second level
      i. Third level
      ii. Third level
2. Main heading

RECITE AND REVIEW

Finally, recite and review. Use your notes and study guides. Answer the questions you formed earlier. Also answer other questions that came up when reading and answering the "Review Questions" at the end of each chapter. Answer all questions out loud (recite).

Reviewing is more about when to study rather than what to study. You already determined what to study during the preview, question, and reading steps. The best times to review are right after the first study session, one week later, and before a quiz or test.

This book was also designed to help you study. Special design features are described on the next pages.

We hope you enjoy learning and your work. You and your work are important. You and the care you give make a difference in the person's life!

11

Oral, Sublingual, and Buccal Drugs

OBJECTIVES

- Define the key terms and key abbreviations used in this chapter.
- Identify solid and liquid oral dose forms.
- Explain how to use the equipment for giving oral dose forms.
- Know the equivalents for household, apothecary, and metric measurements.
- Explain how to give oral, sublingual, and buccal drugs.
- Perform the procedures described in this chapter.

PROCEDURES

- Giving an Oral Drug—Solid Form
- Giving an Oral Drug—Liquid Form

KEY TERMS

buccal Inside the cheek (*bucco*)
capsule A gelatin container that holds a drug in a dry powder or liquid form
elixir A clear liquid made up of a drug dissolved in alcohol and water
emulsion An oral dose form containing small droplets of water-in-oil or oil-in-water
lavage Washing out the stomach
lozenge A flat disk containing a medicinal agent with a flavored base; troche
medicine cup A plastic container with measurement scales
medicine dropper A small glass or plastic tube with a hollow rubber ball at one end

meniscus The lowest point of liquid in a medicine cup.
soufflé cup A small paper or plastic cup used for solid drug forms
sublingual Under (*sub*) the tongue (*lingual*)
suspension A liquid containing solid drug particles
syringe A plastic measuring device with three parts—tip, barrel, and plunger
syrup An oral dose form containing a drug dissolved in sugar
tablet A dried, powdered drug compressed into a small disk
troche See "lozenge"

KEY ABBREVIATIONS

GI   Gastrointestinal
ISMP   Institute for Safe Medication Practices

ODT   Orally disintegrating tablets
PO   By mouth (per os)

Oral drugs are given by mouth—the *oral route*. Drugs are given directly into the gastrointestinal (GI) tract. The oral route is commonly used for giving drugs and offers the following advantages:
- Most drugs have oral dose forms.
- Oral drugs are easy to administer.
- Most people can swallow oral drugs easily.
- The procedure is noninvasive, meaning:
  - The skin is not pierced as for an injection.
  - Nothing is inserted into a body opening (e.g., vagina, rectum).
- The drug can be retrieved from the stomach to lessen adverse drug events. If necessary, an orogastric or nasogastric tube is inserted to wash out (lavage) the stomach.

However, oral drugs do have their share of problems and limitations:
- They have the slowest rate of absorption and onset of action.
- Some may harm or discolor the teeth.

- Some may have an unpleasant taste or smell.
- Some may cause nausea.
- They cannot be given if the person:
  - Is vomiting
  - Has gastric or intestinal suction
  - Is at risk for aspiration
  - Is unconscious or comatose
  - Cannot swallow

An order for an oral drug is written as one of the following:
- PO—per os (*per* means *by*; *os* means *mouth*)
- By mouth
- Orally

See p. 122 for sublingual and buccal drugs.
See *Promoting Safety and Comfort: Oral Drugs.*

116

Objectives tell what is presented in the chapter.

Procedures: a list of the procedures in the chapter follows the list of objectives.

Key Terms are the important words and phrases in the chapter. Definitions are given for each term. The key terms introduce you to the chapter content. They are also a useful study guide.

Key Abbreviations are a quick reference to the abbreviations used in the chapter. They are listed after the "Key Terms."

---

150   CHAPTER 15   Drugs Affecting the Nervous System

BOX 15-1   Clinical Uses of Drugs Affecting the Autonomic Nervous System

Angina. Angina (*pain*) is chest pain that occurs when the heart needs more oxygen. Chest pain may be described as a tightness, pressure, squeezing, or burning in the chest. The person may appear pale, feel faint, and perspire. Nausea, fatigue, weakness, and difficulty breathing may occur. Some persons complain of "gas" or indigestion.
Aortic stenosis. The left ventricle is enlarged. There is constriction or narrowing (*stenosis*) in the aortic valve.
Arrhythmia. An abnormal heart rhythm.
Asthma. The airway becomes inflamed and narrow, making it difficult for the person to breathe. Extra mucus is produced. Wheezing and coughing are common. The chest may feel tight. Symptoms are mild to severe and are usually triggered by allergies.
Biliary colic. Smooth muscle pain associated with the passing of stones through the bile ducts.
Bronchospasm. Smooth muscles of the lungs contract. The airway narrows and becomes blocked. Coughing and wheezing may occur. See "Asthma."
Emphysema. A lung disease. Oxygen and carbon dioxide exchange cannot occur in affected alveoli. The person has shortness of breath and a cough. Sputum may contain pus. Fatigue is common. The person uses extra effort to breathe in and out, and the body does not get enough oxygen. Breathing is easier when the person sits upright and slightly forward.
Enuresis. Urinary incontinence in bed at night.
Heart failure. Heart failure or congestive heart failure occurs when the heart is weakened and cannot pump normally. Blood backs up and tissue congestion occurs.
Hypertension. In a person with hypertension (*high blood pressure*), the resting blood pressure is too high. The systolic pressure is 130 mm Hg (millimeters of mercury) or higher (*hyper*), or the diastolic pressure is 80 mm Hg or higher. Such measurements must occur several times for accurate diagnosis. Narrowed blood vessels are a common cause; the heart pumps with more force to move blood through narrowed vessels.
Hypotension. The systolic blood pressure is below (*hypo*) 90 mm Hg and the diastolic pressure is below 60 mm Hg.
Indigestion. A vague feeling of discomfort above the stomach after eating. Fullness, heartburn, bloating, and nausea are common symptoms.

Irritable bowel syndrome. This disorder may come and go. Nerves that control muscles in the GI tract are too active and the GI tract becomes sensitive to food, feces, gas, and stress. The person experiences abdominal pain, bloating, and constipation or diarrhea.
Migraine. A recurring vascular headache resulting in an intense pulsing or throbbing pain in one area of the head. During a migraine, the person may be sensitive to light and sound. They may experience nausea and vomiting.
Myasthenia gravis. Means *grave muscle weakness.* It is a neuromuscular disease in which the affected person experiences weakness of the skeletal muscles. Muscle weakness increases during activity and improves with rest. Muscles that control the eye and eyelid movement, facial expression, chewing, talking, and swallowing are commonly involved. Muscles that control breathing and movement in the neck, arms, and legs may be affected.
Myocardial infarction (MI). *Myocardial* refers to the heart muscle. *Infarction* means tissue death. When MI occurs, part of the heart muscle dies. Sudden cardiac death (*sudden cardiac arrest*) can occur. Blood flow to the heart muscle is suddenly blocked, and the person may have severe chest pain, usually on the left side. The pain is often described as crushing, stabbing, or squeezing. Pain or numbness in one or both arms, the back, neck, jaw, or stomach may occur. Other signs and symptoms may include indigestion, dyspnea, nausea, dizziness, perspiration, and cold, clammy skin.
Mydriasis. Dilation of the pupil of the eye.
Parkinson's disease. The area of the brain that controls muscle movement is affected.
Peptic ulcer. A sore in the lining of the esophagus, stomach, or duodenum of the small intestine.
Pylorospasm. A spasm of the pyloric sphincter in the stomach.
Tremors. Quivering movements resulting from involuntary contraction and relaxation of skeletal muscles.
Urethral colic. Sharp pain caused by obstruction or smooth muscle spasm of the urethra.
Ventricular dysrhythmia. An abnormal heart rhythm occurring in the heart's ventricles.

TABLE 15-1   Adrenergic Agents

Generic Name	Brand Name	Dose Forms	Clinical Use	Adult Oral Dose
albuterol	Proventil, Ventolin	Aerosol: 90 mcg per puff Tablets: 2, 4 mg Syrup: 2 mg/5 mL Tablets: extended-release 4, 8 mg	Asthma, emphysema	PO: 2-4 mg three to four times daily Inhale: two inhalations q4-6h
ephedrine		Capsules: 25 mg	Nasal decongestant, hypotension	25-50 mg q3-4h
metaproterenol	Alupent	Aerosol: 0.65 mg/puff	Bronchospasm	See manufacturer's recommendations
phenylephrine	Neo-Synephrine	Ophthalmic drops: 2.5%, 10% Nasal solutions: 0.25%, 0.5%, 1% Tablets: 10 mg Syrup: 2.5 mg/5 mL	Shock, hypotension, nasal decongestant, ophthalmic vasoconstrictor, mydriatic	PO: 10-20 mg q4-6h PRIN Nasal: 2-3 drops or sprays in each nostril q4h; use for less than 3 days Eyes: 1-2 drops two to three times daily
terbutaline	Brethine, Bricanyl	Tablets: 2.5, 5 mg	Emphysema, asthma, premature labor	5 mg q6h

Modified from Willihnganz M: Clayton's Basic Pharmacology for Nurses, ed 18, St Louis, 2020, Elsevier.

Boxes and tables contain important rules, principles, guidelines, signs and symptoms, nursing measures, and drug information in a list format. They identify important information and are useful study guides.

Procedures are written in a step-by-step format. They are divided into Quality of Life, Pre-Procedure, Procedure, and Post-Procedure sections for studying ease. The Quality of Life section lists six simple courtesies that show respect for the person.

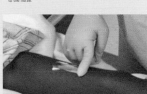

CHAPTER 12 Topical Drugs 127

APPLYING A CREAM, LOTION, OINTMENT, AND POWDER

Quality of Life

Remember to:
- Knock before entering the person's room.
- Address the person by name.
- Introduce yourself by name and title.
- Explain the procedure to the person before and during the procedure.
- Protect the person's rights during the procedure.
- Handle the person gently during the procedure.

Pre-procedure

1. Follow *Delegation Guidelines: Applying Creams, Lotions, Ointments, and Powders.* See *Promoting Safety and Comfort: Applying Creams, Lotions, Ointments, and Powders.*
2. Check the most recent drug order and compare to the medication profile. Focus on the 6 Rights of Drug Administration (Chapter 10).
3. Check with the nurse if you have any questions.
4. Perform hand hygiene.
5. Collect necessary items:
   - Soap or other cleansing agent
   - Washcloth and towel
   - Wash basin with warm water
   - Gauze squares or cotton balls
   - Sterile tongue blade
   - Sterile cotton-tipped applicator
   - Gloves
   - MAR

Procedure

6. Read the order on the MAR.
7. Select the right drug from the drug cart/system.
8. Compare the drug order on the MAR against the pharmacy label on the drug container. **(First safety check.)** Review the 6 Rights of Drug Administration (Chapter 10).
9. Check the drug container for an expiration date and bring the drug to the person's bedside.
10. Provide for privacy.
11. Identify the person by checking the ID bracelet against the MAR. Make sure you use at least two identifiers according to agency policy. Call the person by name. Follow agency policy if using a barcode scanner.
12. Put on gloves.
13. Position the person to expose the application site; then, expose the site.
14. Clean and dry the application site.
15. Observe the application site.
16. Remove and discard gloves. Perform hand hygiene. Put on new, clean gloves.
17. Compare the drug order on the MAR against the pharmacy label on the drug container. **(Second safety check.)** Review the 6 Rights of Drug Administration (Chapter 10).
18. Shake the lotion thoroughly.
19. Open the container and place the lid or cap upside down on a clean surface. For an ointment or cream:
    a. *From a jar:* use a tongue blade to remove the ordered amount.
    b. *From a tube:* squeeze the ordered amount onto a tongue blade or cotton-tipped applicator.
20. Close the container. Compare the drug order on the MAR against the pharmacy label on the drug container. **(Third safety check.)** Review the 6 Rights of Drug Administration (Chapter 10).

21. Apply the topical dose form:
    a. Lotion:
       (1) Hold the bottle in your non-dominant hand with the label in the palm of your hand. This prevents the contents from smearing the label during pouring.
       (2) Pour some lotion onto a cotton ball or gauze square. Do not let any part of the container touch the cotton ball.
       (3) Gently but firmly dab the lotion onto the skin. Do not rub.
       (4) Repeat steps 21 a (1)–(3) with a new cotton ball or gauze square until the area is covered.
    b. Cream or ointment:
       (1) Transfer the cream or ointment from the tongue blade or cotton-tipped applicator to your gloved hand or index finger (if necessary).
       (2) Apply the agent to the skin with the tongue blade, cotton-tipped applicator, or your gloved hand or finger (Fig. 12-1).
       (3) Apply the agent in a thin layer in the direction of hair growth. Use firm, gentle strokes.
    c. Powder:
       (1) Apply in a thin, even layer with your gloved hand.
       (2) Smooth over the area for even coverage.
23. Return the container to the drug cart/system.

Post-procedure

24. Discard the used supplies or unit-dose packages.
25. Follow agency policy for soiled linen.
26. While wearing gloves, empty and clean the wash basin. Return it and other supplies to their proper location.
27. Remove the gloves and perform hand hygiene.
28. Provide for comfort and complete a safety check before leaving the room. (See the inside back cover of this book.)
29. Unscreen the person.
30. Record the *right documentation* on the MAR:
    - The date, time, drug name, dosage, and route of administration
    - The application site
    - Your name or initials
31. Report and record any specific patient or resident observations or concerns to the nurse.

Fig. 12-1 A cream is applied with a gloved index finger. (Courtesy Rick Brady, from Lilley LL and others: *Pharmacology and the nursing process,* ed 5, St Louis, 2007, Mosby.)

CHAPTER 11 Oral, Sublingual, and Buccal Drugs 117

PROMOTING SAFETY AND COMFORT

Oral Drugs

Safety

If a drug order is written as "per os," check with the nurse before giving the drug. The Institute for Safe Medication Practices (ISMP) lists "per os" as an error-prone abbreviation. This is because "os" can be mistaken for OS—oculus sinister—which means *left eye.* OS also is an error-prone abbreviation.

ORAL DOSE FORMS

Oral drugs come in the following dose forms:
- *Capsule.* A capsule is a small, cylindrical gelatin container that holds a drug in a dry powder or liquid form. This form is used for drugs that have an unpleasant odor or taste. You can identify a drug by the size, color, and shape, as well as the manufacturer's symbol on the capsule (Fig. 11-1). *Timed-release* or *sustained-release capsules* contain granules (Fig. 11-2). The granules dissolve at different rates and, over a period of time, there is a continuous release of the drug. Fewer doses are needed per day; usually every 12 or 24 hours.
- *Tablets.* A tablet is a dried, powdered drug compressed into a small disk.
  - *Scored* tablets are grooved for use in dividing the dose (Fig. 11-3, *A*).
  - *Layered* tablets have layers (Fig. 11-3, *B*). More than one drug is given at the same time.
  - *Enteric-coated* tablets have a special coating (Fig. 11-3, *C*) that prevents the tablet from dissolving in the stomach. The tablet dissolves in the small intestine. It should not be crushed or chewed.
  - *Caplets* are tablets shaped in the form of a capsule.
  - *Orally disintegrating tablets* (ODT) are placed under the tongue and dissolve rapidly (usually within seconds). They are used for rapid onset of action, meaning the drug starts working very quickly.
- *Sublingual Film or Strips.* A film or strip placed under the tongue that dissolves quickly. No additional liquid is needed to take a drug in this form. The drug dissolves quickly upon

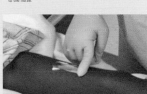

Fig. 11-3 *A,* Scored tablet. *B,* Layered tablet. *C,* Enteric-coated tablet.

Fig. 11-4 Lozenge. (From Edmunds MW: *Introduction to clinical pharmacology,* ed 5, St Louis, 2006, Mosby.)

contact with a wet surface (e.g., the tongue). This is especially useful for people who have trouble swallowing.
- *Lozenges.* A lozenge (troche) is a flat disk containing a medicinal agent with a flavored base (Fig. 11-4). The base is a hard or soft sugar candy. Lozenges are held or sucked in the mouth to slowly dissolve; the ingredients of the lozenge are released slowly.
- *Elixirs.* An elixir is a clear liquid made up of a drug dissolved in alcohol and water. A flavor is added to improve the taste.
- *Emulsions.* An emulsion contains small droplets of water-in-oil or oil-in-water. This form is used to mask bitter tastes or to increase the ability to dissolve.
- *Suspensions.* A suspension is a liquid containing solid drug particles. Before giving a suspension, shake the bottle well to thoroughly mix the particles. Many oral liquid antacids and liquid antibiotics are suspensions.
- *Syrups.* A syrup contains drugs dissolved in a sugar solution. The sugar helps mask the drug's bitter taste. Syrups are most commonly used for children.

See *Focus on Communication: Oral Dose Forms.*

FOCUS ON COMMUNICATION

Oral Dose Forms

Use terms that patients and residents can understand. Capsules and tablets are commonly called "pills" and lozenges are commonly called "cough drops." A person is more likely to understand "it's time to take your pills" than "it's time to take your capsules (or tablets)." You may also say, "it's time for your medicine."

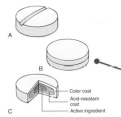

Fig. 11-1 Capsules.

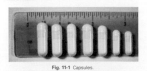

Fig. 11-2 Timed-release capsule.

Color illustrations and photographs visually present key ideas, concepts, or procedure steps. They help you apply and remember the written material.

Bold, blue type is used to highlight the key terms in the text. You again see the key term and read its definition. This helps reinforce your learning.

Focus on Communication boxes suggest what to say and questions to ask when interacting with patients, residents, and the nursing team.

---

126 CHAPTER 12 Topical Drugs

BOX 12-1 Rules for Applying Creams, Lotions, Ointments, and Powders

- Perform hand hygiene before and after application.
- Follow the 6 Rights of Medication Administration (Chapter 10).
- Follow Standard Precautions.
- Follow isolation precautions as ordered (Chapter 6).
- Wear gloves.
- Do not let the dose form touch your skin.
- Provide for privacy.
- Position the person to expose the application site. Avoid unnecessary exposure.
- Clean and dry the skin as directed by the nurse before applying a dose form. Soap and water are typically used if the person's skin condition allows. Make sure previous applications are thoroughly removed.
- Observe the skin. Report and record your observations. See *Delegation Guidelines: Applying Creams, Lotions, Ointments, and Powders.*
- See *Promoting Safety and Comfort: Applying Creams, Lotions, Ointments, and Powders.*
- Shake lotions thoroughly. The lotion should have a uniform color throughout.
- Apply the dose form to clean, dry skin.
- Apply the correct amount. Use a sterile tongue blade or sterile cotton-tipped applicator to remove the dose from a jar. If applying the drug by gloved hand or finger, use the tongue blade or cotton-tipped applicator to transfer the dose to your hand or finger.
- Do not let the drug container touch the person's skin.
- Cover the site with gauze or other covering as directed by the nurse, care plan, and MAR. Ointments and creams may stain or soil garments and linens.
- See procedure: *Applying Nitroglycerin Ointment, p. 128-129.*

Applying Creams, Lotions, Ointments, and Powders

Each topical dose form is applied differently. Lotions are dabbed on the skin with gauze or a cotton ball. Use a tongue blade, cotton-tipped applicator, or a gloved hand or finger to apply ointments and creams. Powders are applied in a thin, even layer. To safely apply a topical dose form, follow the rules in Box 12-1. Also practice medication safety (Chapter 10). To apply a nitroglycerin ointment, see p. 128-129.

See *Focus on Older Persons: Applying Creams, Lotions, Ointments, and Powders.*

See *Delegation Guidelines: Applying Creams, Lotions, Ointments, and Powders.*

See *Promoting Safety and Comfort: Applying Creams, Lotions, Ointments, and Powders.*

FOCUS ON OLDER PERSONS

Applying Creams, Lotions, Ointments, and Powders

Increasingly dry skin occurs with aging. Long-term use of soap also dries the skin. Dry skin is easily damaged. Thorough rinsing is needed when using soap. If necessary, the nurse and care plan may direct you to use a different cleansing agent.

DELEGATION GUIDELINES

Applying Creams, Lotions, Ointments, and Powders

Before applying a topical dose form, you need the following information from the nurse, care plan, and MAR:
- Whether or not isolation precautions are required. If yes:
  - What type of precaution.
  - What personal protective equipment is needed.
  - Special measures for cleaning and drying the skin.
  - What cleansing agent to use.
  - The exact site of application.
- What to use to apply the drug (e.g., tongue blade, cotton-tipped applicator, or gloved hand or finger).
- Whether or not you need to cover the application. If yes, how to cover the application site (e.g., gauze, see-through dressing and tape, and so on).

- What observations to report and record:
  - Color of the skin
  - Locations and descriptions of rashes
  - Dry skin
  - Bruises or open skin areas
  - Pale or reddened areas, particularly over bony parts
  - Blisters
  - Drainage or bleeding from wounds or body openings
  - Skin temperature
  - Complaints of pain or discomfort
  - When observations should be reported
  - Which specific patient or resident concerns to immediately report

PROMOTING SAFETY AND COMFORT

Applying Creams, Lotions, Ointments, and Powders

Safety

Use caution when applying powder; accidentally inhaling powder can irritate the airway and lungs. Do not shake or sprinkle powder onto the person's skin. To safely apply powder:
- Turn away from the person.
- Sprinkle a small amount of powder onto your hands or a cloth.
- Apply the powder in a thin layer.
- Make sure powder does not get on the floor; powder is slippery and may cause falls.

Comfort

A skin area is exposed to apply topical dose forms. Provide for privacy. Screen the person and close all doors and window coverings (e.g., drapes, shades, blinds, and shutters). Avoid unnecessary exposure; expose only the needed area.

The person may have a rash or skin lesion. Skin disorders may be contagious; the person knows the disease can be spread to others. As a result, self-esteem may suffer. Be sure to treat the person with dignity and respect.

Focus on Older Persons boxes provide age-specific information about giving drugs to older persons.

Delegation Guidelines boxes describe what information you need from the nurse and care plan before giving a drug. They also tell you what information to report and record.

Promoting Safety and Comfort boxes focus your attention on the need to be safe and cautious and promote comfort when giving drugs.

CHAPTER 22 Drugs Used to Treat Angina, Peripheral Vascular Disease, and Heart Failure 223

REVIEW QUESTIONS

Circle the BEST answer.

1. Nitrates relieve angina by:
   a. dilating the coronary arteries
   b. lowering the heart rate
   c. lowering blood pressure
   d. increasing oxygen use
2. Which is the *most* common side effect from nitrates?
   a. dizziness
   b. flushing
   c. fainting
   d. headache
3. Tell the nurse at once after the person takes:
   a. 1 dose of sublingual nitroglycerin
   b. 2 doses of sublingual nitroglycerin
   c. 3 doses of sublingual nitroglycerin
   d. 4 doses of sublingual nitroglycerin
4. Sustained-released nitroglycerin tablets are taken:
   a. in the morning before breakfast
   b. on an empty stomach every 8 to 12 hours
   c. with meals
   d. at bedtime
5. The application sites for transdermal disks are rotated:
   a. daily
   b. every 8 hours
   c. every other day
   d. weekly
6. A transdermal nitroglycerin disk is dislodged. What should you do?
   a. Remove the disk and apply a new one.
   b. Reapply the disk.
   c. Leave the disk as is until the next ordered dose.
   d. Tape the disk in place.
7. Beta blockers are used to treat angina because they:
   a. dilate coronary arteries
   b. reduce oxygen demands
   c. raise blood pressure
   d. prevent the clumping of platelets
8. Before giving a beta blocker for angina, you need to measure the person's:
   a. weight
   b. intake and output
   c. blood pressure in the supine and standing positions
   d. apical pulse for 30 seconds
9. Calcium channel blockers are used in the treatment of angina. They do all the following, *except*:
   a. decrease myocardial oxygen demand
   b. dilate the coronary arteries
   c. dilate peripheral vessels
   d. prevent the clumping of platelets
10. ACE inhibitors are used to prevent:
    a. CAD
    b. PVD
    c. MI
    d. peripheral vascular disease

11. Before giving a drug for peripheral vascular disease, you should ask the person:
    a. to void
    b. to rate their pain
    c. if you may take the apical pulse for 1 minute
    d. what application site they prefer
12. Besides dilating blood vessels, ACE inhibitors prevent:
    a. peripheral vascular disease
    b. blood clots
    c. atherosclerosis
    d. vasodilation
13. Intermittent claudication occurs with:
    a. deep vein thrombosis
    b. arteriosclerosis obliterans
    c. Raynaud's disease
    d. heart failure
14. Pentoxifylline is used to treat intermittent claudication. The drug:
    a. prevents the clumping of red blood cells and platelets
    b. reduces oxygen needs
    c. dilates blood vessels
    d. constricts blood vessels
15. A person taking pentoxifylline complains of chest pain and shortness of breath. What should you do?
    a. Tell the nurse at once.
    b. Have the person take a nitroglycerin tablet.
    c. Measure blood pressure in the supine and standing positions.
    d. Have the person rest.
16. A platelet aggregation inhibitor prevents:
    a. platelet production
    b. platelets from clumping
    c. the destruction of platelets
    d. platelets from splitting
17. Heart failure can be treated with the following drug classes, *except*:
    a. nitrates
    b. ACE inhibitors
    c. beta blockers
    d. ARBs
18. Digoxin (Lanoxin) is used in the treatment of heart failure. It:
    a. prevents vasoconstriction
    b. promotes sodium excretion
    c. increases the force of heart muscle contraction
    d. decreases blood flow to the kidneys
19. The maintenance dose of digoxin (Lanoxin) is usually:
    a. 0.125 to 0.25 mg daily
    b. 0.25 to 0.5 mg daily
    c. 1.25 to 2.5 mg daily
    d. 2.5 to 5 mg daily

Review Questions are useful study guides. They help you to review what you have learned. They can also be used when studying for a test or competency evaluation. The answers to the review questions are found on the Evolve Resources site: http://evolve.elsevier.com/Anderson/medasst/

CONTENTS

The Medication Assistant

OBJECTIVES

- Define the key terms and key abbreviations used in this chapter.
- Describe nurse practice acts.
- Identify the reasons for denying, revoking, or suspending a license or certification.
- Describe the standards for nursing assistants.
- Describe how regulatory agencies are responsible for nursing assistants.
- Explain how to maintain professional boundaries.
- Explain how to become a medication assistant-certified.
- Identify where medication assistants-certified can work.
- Explain the importance of a job description for medication assistants-certified.
- Explain the role and range of functions for medication assistants-certified.
- Identify what medication assistants-certified can and cannot do.

KEY TERMS

boundary crossing A brief act or behavior outside of the helpful zone

boundary signs Acts, behaviors, or thoughts that warn of a boundary crossing or violation

boundary violation An act or behavior that meets your needs, not the person's

drug A chemical substance that has an effect on a living organism

medication A drug used to prevent and treat disease; medicine

medication assistant-certified (MA-C) Nursing assistants who are allowed by state law to give drugs

medicine See "medication"

nursing assistants Individuals employed to give direct hands-on care and perform delegated nursing care tasks under the supervision of a licensed nurse

nurse practice act The law that regulates nursing practice in a state

professional boundaries Those which separate helpful behaviors from behaviors that are not helpful

professional sexual misconduct An act, behavior, or comment that is sexual in nature and occurs within the scope of employment

standard of care Refers to the skills, care, and judgment required by nursing assistants under similar conditions

KEY ABBREVIATIONS

CNA Certified nursing assistant or or certified nurse aide
CPR Cardiopulmonary resuscitation
EMT Emergency medical technician
GED General education diploma
IM Intramuscular
IV Intravenous
LNA Licensed nursing assistant
LPN Licensed practical nurse
LVN Licensed vocational nurse

MA-C Medication assistant-certified
MAR Medication administration record
NATCEP Nursing Assistant Training and Competency Evaluation Program
NCSBN National Council of State Boards of Nursing
OBRA Omnibus Budget Reconciliation Act of 1987
PRN, prn As needed
RN Registered nurse
RNA Registered nurse aide

Nursing assistants are individuals employed to give direct hands-on care and perform delegated nursing care tasks under the supervision of a licensed nurse. Licensed nurses are registered nurses (RNs) and licensed practical nurses (LPNs)/licensed vocational nurses (LVNs). Nursing assistants assist nurses in giving care. State laws determine what nursing assistants can do. In some states, they can give (administer) certain types of drugs. Drugs are chemical substances that have an effect on living organisms. Medications or medicines are those drugs used to prevent and treat disease.

Nursing assistants who are allowed by state law to give drugs are called medication assistants-certified (MA-C). Some states use other titles. *Medication aide, certified medication aide,* and *certified medication technician* are examples. MA-C is used in this book. MA-Cs:

- Are certified nursing assistants or certified nurse aides (CNAs). Some states use the terms *licensed nursing assistant*

(LNA) and *registered nurse aide* (RNA). CNA is used in this book.
- Have additional education and training as required by state law.
- Have passed the required certification tests.
- May give prescribed drugs within the limits defined by state law.
- Are supervised by licensed nurses.

STATE LAWS AND AGENCIES

Each state has a nurse practice act. The law regulates nursing practice in that state. It does so to protect the public's welfare and safety. A nurse practice act:
- Defines RN and LPN/LVN.
- Describes the scope of practice for RNs and LPNs/LVNs.
- Describes education and licensing requirements for RNs and LPNs/LVNs.
- Protects the public from persons practicing nursing without a license. Persons who do not meet the state's requirements cannot perform nursing functions.

The law allows for denying, revoking, and suspending licenses and certifications covered under the law. The purpose for doing so is to protect the public from unsafe nursing personnel. Reasons include:
- Being convicted of a crime in any state
- Selling or distributing drugs
- Using the person's drugs for oneself
- Placing a person in danger from the overuse of alcohol or drugs
- Demonstrating grossly negligent nursing practice
- Being convicted of abusing or neglecting children or older persons
- Violating a nurse practice act and its rules and regulations
- Demonstrating incompetent behaviors
- Aiding or assisting another person to violate a nurse practice act and its rules and regulations
- Making medical diagnoses
- Prescribing drugs and treatments

Nursing Assistants

A state's nurse practice act is used to decide what nursing assistants can do. Some nurse practice acts also regulate CNA and MA-C roles, functions, education, and certification requirements. In other states, there are separate laws for nursing assistants.

Legal and advisory opinions about nursing assistants are based on the state's nurse practice act. So are any state laws about their roles and functions. If you do something beyond the legal limits of your role, you could be practicing nursing without a license. This creates serious legal problems for you, your employer, and the nurse supervising your work.

The Omnibus Budget Reconciliation Act of 1987 (OBRA) is a federal that applies to all 50 states. OBRA sets minimum requirements for nursing assistant training and evaluation. Each state must have a Nursing Assistant Training and Competency

Evaluation Program (NATCEP). Once you have passed the state's education and competency evaluation program for nursing assistants, you will earn the title of certified nursing assistant or certified nurse aide (CNA). Some states license or register nursing assistants. They are LNAs or RNAs.

After you become a CNA, you must pass the state's education and competency evaluation program for medication assistants in order to become an MA-C. Titles vary among states. The National Council of State Boards of Nursing (NCSBN) uses the title medication assistant-certified (MA-C).

Nursing assistants must be able to function with reasonable skill and safety. Like nurses, they can have their certification, license, or registration denied, revoked, or suspended. The NCSBN lists these reasons for doing so:
- Drug or substance abuse or dependency.
- Abandoning a patient or resident.
- Abusing a patient or resident.
- Fraud or deceit. Examples include:
  - Filing false personal information
  - Providing false information when applying for certification—initial, reinstatement, or renewal
- Neglecting a patient or resident.
- Violating professional boundaries (p. 3).
- Giving unsafe care.
- Performing acts beyond the CNA or MA-C role.
- Misappropriating (stealing, theft) or misusing property.
- Obtaining money or property from a patient or resident. Doing so through fraud, falsely representing oneself, or through force are examples.
- Having been convicted of a crime. Examples include murder, assault, kidnapping, rape or sexual assault, robbery, sexual crimes involving children, criminal mistreatment of children or a vulnerable adult, drug trafficking, embezzlement (to take a person's property for one's own use), theft, and arson (starting fires).
- Failing to abide by the expectations of CNAs and MA-Cs. (Box 1-1).
- Putting patients and residents at risk for harm.
- Violating the privacy of a patient or resident.
- Failing to maintain the confidentiality of patient or resident information.

Regulatory Agencies

Each state has a *state board of nursing* or similar agency. The board is created and given powers by the state's nurse practice act. The board protects the public's health, safety, and welfare. It does so by regulating nursing education and nursing practice. In many states, the board of nursing also regulates the education and practice of nursing assistants. In others, a different state agency has that responsibility. A Department of Public Health is an example.

The regulatory agency responsible for nursing assistants:
- Makes sure that standards of care are met. Standard of care refers to the skills, care, and judgment required by nursing assistants under similar conditions.
- Makes sure that they are competent.

BOX 1-1 CNA and MA-C Expectations

Whether a CNA or MA-C, always remember to:
- Only perform tasks you are trained to do and follow the nurse's directions. Always follow state laws and rules that regulate your practice.
- Only perform appropriate tasks that have been delegated by the nurse. Communicate with the nurse if issues occur.
- Let the nurse know why you've completed the delegated task. Communicate with the nurse if the person's status changes.
- Participate in training opportunities in order to remain competent in performing tasks assigned to you.
- Ask the nurse to explain their expectations, especially when unclear.
- Function as a member of the healthcare team and provide care based on the care plan.
- Respect healthcare team members.
- Accept responsibility for your behavior and actions while working with the nurse and helping residents.
- Respect the rights, concerns, decisions, and dignity of residents and others.
- Perform safety measures to ensure residents, others, and self are protected.
- Observe residents as directed by the nurse and assist in identifying their needs.
- Respect other people's property and belongings.
- Protect confidential information and respect the privacy of residents, family members, and others.

- Approves individuals for initial certification, reinstatement, and certification renewal.
- Approves educational programs for nursing assistants.
- Investigates complaints about a CNA or MA-C violating a law.
- Takes disciplinary action if a CNA or MA-C violated a law. Possible actions include:
  - Denying, suspending, or revoking certification.
  - Filing a letter of concern. This is done when the regulatory agency does not have enough evidence to take other action.
  - Noting on the certification and registry that there is a complaint against the CNA or MA-C.
  - Referring criminal violations to a law enforcement agency.
  - Imposing a fine.
- Maintains a state registry for nursing assistants.

PROFESSIONAL BOUNDARIES

A *boundary* limits or separates something. For example, a fence forms a boundary. It tells you to stay within or on the side of the fenced area. As a nursing assistant, you help patients, residents, and families. Therefore, you enter into a helping relationship with them. The helping relationship has professional boundaries.

Professional boundaries separate helpful behaviors from behaviors that are not helpful (Fig. 1-1). The boundaries create a helpful zone. If your behaviors are outside of the helpful zone, you are over-involved with the person or under-involved. Boundary crossings, boundary violations, or professional sexual misconduct can occur.

PROFESSIONAL BOUNDARIES

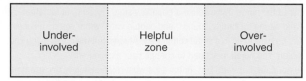

Fig. 1-1 Professional Boundaries. (Modified and redrawn from the National Council of State Boards of Nursing, Inc., *A Nurse's Guide to Professional Boundaries,* 2018, Chicago, IL.)

A boundary crossing is a brief act or behavior outside of the helpful zone. The act or behavior may be thoughtless or something you did not mean to do. Or it could be on purpose if it meets the person's needs. For example, you give a crying patient a hug. The hug meets the person's needs at that time. If you give the hug to meet your needs, the act is wrong. Also, it is wrong to hug the person every time you see him or her.

A boundary violation is an act or behavior that meets your needs, not the person's. The act or behavior is unethical. It violates the standards in Box 1-1. The person could be harmed. Boundary violations include:
- Abuse.
- Giving a lot of personal information about yourself. You tell a person about your personal relationships or problems.
- Keeping secrets with the person.

Professional sexual misconduct is an act, behavior, or comment that is sexual in nature and occurs within the scope of employment. It is sexual misconduct even if the person consents or makes the first move.

Some boundary violations and some professional sexual misconduct also are crimes. To maintain professional boundaries, follow the rules in Box 1-2. Be alert to boundary signs. Boundary signs are acts, behaviors, or thoughts that warn of a boundary crossing or violation (Box 1-3).

Some patients, residents, and families want to thank the staff for the care given. Sometimes they send thank you cards and letters. Sometimes they offer gifts—candy, cookies, money, gift cards, flowers, and so on. Accepting gifts is a boundary violation. When offered a gift, you can say:
- "Thank you so much for thinking of me. It's very kind of you. However, it is against agency policy to accept gifts of any kind. I do appreciate your offer."
- "Thank you for wanting me to have the flowers your friend sent. They are lovely. However, staff cannot receive gifts because it is against agency policy. Let me help you find a way to take them home."

BECOMING AN MA-C

MA-C training involves classroom learning and clinical experiences. This includes practicing and demonstrating required skills. Giving oral drugs, applying ointments to the skin, and applying eye drops are examples. The training program length and number of hours vary by state.

BOX 1-2 Rules for Maintaining Professional Boundaries

- Follow the standards listed in Box 1-1.
- Talk to the nurse if you sense a boundary sign, crossing, or violation.
- Avoid caring for family, friends, and people with whom you do business. This may be hard to do in a small community. Always tell the nurse if you know the person. The nurse may need to change your assignment.
- Do not date, flirt with, kiss, or have a sexual relationship with current patients or residents. The same applies to family members of current patients or residents.
- Do not make sexual comments or jokes.
- Do not use offensive language.
- Do not discuss your sexual relationships with patients, residents, or their families.
- Do not say or write things that could suggest a romantic or sexual relationship with a patient, resident, or family member.
- Use touch correctly. Do not touch or handle sexual and genital areas except when necessary to give care. Such areas include the breasts, nipples, perineum, buttocks, and anus.
- Do not accept gifts, loans, money, credit cards, or other valuables from a patient, resident, or family member.
- Do not give gifts, loans, money, credit cards, or other valuables to a patient, resident, or family member.
- Do not borrow from a patient, resident, or family member. This includes money, personal items, and transportation.
- Maintain a professional relationship at all times. Do not develop any personal relationship or friendship with the person or family member.
- Do not visit or spend extra time with a person that is not part of your assignment.
- Do not share personal or financial information with a person or family member.
- Do not help a person or family member with his or her finances.
- Ask these questions before you date or marry a person whom you cared for. Be aware of the risk for sexual misconduct.
  - How long ago did you assist with the person's care?
  - Was the person's care short-term or long-term?
  - What kind and how much information do you have about the person? How will that information affect your relationship with the person?
  - Will the person need more care in the future?
  - Does dating or marrying the person place the person at risk for harm?

BOX 1-3 Boundary Signs

- You think about the person when you are not at work.
- You organize your work and provide other care around the person's needs.
- You spend free time with the person. You visit with the person during breaks, during mealtimes, when off duty, and so on.
- You trade assignments with other staff so you can provide the person's care.
- You give more care or attention to the person at the expense of other patients and residents.
- You believe that you are the only person who understands the person and his or her needs.
- The person gives you gifts or money.
- You give the person gifts or money.
- You share information about yourself with the person.
- You talk about your work situation with the person.
- You flirt with the person.
- You make comments that have a sexual message.
- You tell the person "off-color" jokes.
- You notice more touch between you and the person.
- You use foul, vulgar, or offensive language when talking to the person.
- You and the person have secrets.
- You choose the person's side when he or she disagrees with other staff or the family.
- You select what you report and record. You do not give complete information.
- You do not like questions about the care you give or your relationship with the person.
- You change how you dress or your appearance when you will work with the person.
- You receive gifts from the person after he or she leaves the agency.
- You have contact with the person after he or she leaves the agency.

Eligibility Requirements

To become an MA-C, you need to take a state-approved training program. But first you must meet program entrance requirements. Most states require that you:

- Be at least 18 years old.
- Have a high school diploma or general education diploma (GED).
- Read, write, spell, speak, and understand English.
- Be a CNA.
- Have worked as a CNA. The length of time worked varies among states—90 days to 1 year. Six months is common.
- Be competent in basic math skills.
- Have cardiopulmonary resuscitation (CPR) certification.

Certification and Registry Requirements

MA-C certification and registry requirements vary by state. Generally, they involve:

- Successfully completing a state-approved training program—classroom training, demonstrating required skills, and clinical experience
- Passing a competency evaluation—written test and skills test
- Completing an application form
- Paying required application fees
- Submitting fingerprint information
  Certification can be denied for the reasons listed on p. 2.

Certification Renewal

MA-Cs must renew their certification every year or every two years as required by state law. Each state has renewal requirements.

Generally, an MA-C must provide the following to the regulatory agency:

- A completed renewal application.
- The required fee.
- A verified statement about any felony convictions:
  - Since initial certification.
  - Since last certification renewal.
- Evidence of continuing education. The number of required hours varies by state.
- Evidence of having worked as an MA-C or CNA during the renewal period. The number of required hours varies by state.
- Other state requirements.

WORK SETTINGS

Before accepting a job, you must know where MA-Cs are allowed to work in your state. MA-Cs usually work in agencies that employ licensed nurses. They include:

- Hospitals
- Long-term care facilities (nursing homes, nursing centers)
- Prisons and other correctional facilities
- Assisted living residences
- Centers for persons who are developmentally disabled
- Home health agencies
  States may allow MA-Cs to work in settings without a licensed nurse. Such settings include:
- Child day care centers
- Adult day care centers
- Private homes when supervised by the patient or his or her caregiver
- Schools
- Foster family homes
- Group homes

JOB DESCRIPTION

Your job description is a document describing what the agency expects you to do. It also states educational requirements.

Always obtain a written job description when you apply for a job. Ask questions about it during your job interview. Before accepting a job as an MA-C, make sure it includes giving drugs. Tell the employer about administration methods and routes that you did not learn. Also advise the employer of drugs that you cannot give for moral or religious reasons. Clearly understand what is expected before taking a job. Do not take a job that requires you to:

- Act beyond the legal limits of your role
- Function beyond your training limits
- Perform acts that are against your morals or religion

Your training prepares you to give drugs in certain ways. The agency may not let you do everything you learned. Other agencies want you to do things that you did not learn. Use your job description to discuss such issues with your supervisor.

No one can force you to do something beyond the legal limits of your role. Sometimes jobs are threatened for refusing to follow a nurse's orders. Often staff obey out of fear. That is why you must understand your role and functions.

RESPONSIBILITES AND PRACTICE LIMITS

To protect persons from harm, you must understand what you can do, what you cannot do, and the legal limits of your role. In some states, this is called *scope of practice*. You may also hear it called *range of functions*.

Your role as an MA-C is to give drugs. When working in an agency—hospital, nursing center, or other health care facility— *you should not have a patient care or resident care assignment.* You should not be assisting persons with hygiene, elimination, moving and transfers, comfort, or other nursing care measures. You must not be distracted or taken away from your role of giving drugs. If you are assisting one person in a private home, you can assist the person with his or her other needs.

MA-C functions and responsibilities vary among states and agencies. Before giving a drug, make sure that:

- Your state allows MA-Cs to do so.
- It is in your job description.
- You have the necessary education and training.
- A nurse is available to answer questions and to supervise you.

Box 1-4 describes the Responsibilites and Practice Limits of the MA-C. Since laws differ from one state to the next, you must know what you can do in the state in which you are working. For example, you move from Oregon to Texas. You must learn the laws and rules in Texas. Or you might work in two states. For example, you work in agencies in Kansas and Oklahoma. You must know the laws and rules of both states.

Some MA-Cs are also emergency medical technicians (EMTs). EMTs give emergency care outside of health care settings *("in the field")*. EMTs work under the direction of doctors in hospital emergency departments. State laws and rules for EMTs and MA-Cs differ. For example, Joan Woods is an EMT for a fire department. When off duty, she is an MA-C at Deer Valley Nursing Center. Her state allows EMTs to start IV lines and give IV drugs in the field. However, MA-Cs do not start IV lines or give IV drugs. Ms. Woods cannot start IV lines or give IV drugs when working as an MA-C.

The situation is similar for persons who were medics or corpsmen in military service. When working as MA-Cs, medics and corpsmen must follow their state laws and rules for MA-Cs. As with EMTs, the ability to do something does not give the right to do so in all settings.

State laws and rules limit MA-C functions. Your job description reflects those laws and rules. An agency can further limit what you can do. So can a nurse based on the person's needs. However, no agency or nurse can expand your range of functions beyond what is allowed by your state's laws and rules.

BOX 1-4   Responsibilities and Practice Limits of the MA-C

Responsibilities of the MA-C

As an MA-C, your responsibilities include:

Giving:
- Drugs under the supervision of a licensed nurse and following state laws and rules
- Drugs following the Six Rights of Drug Administration (Chapter 10)
- Drugs "as needed" (PRN/prn) to a person as specified by the nurse
- Drugs prescribed by the doctor using the medication administration record (MAR)

Reporting to the nurse at once:
- Signs and symptoms that appear life-threatening
- Side effects and adverse reactions
- Events that appear life-threatening
- Drugs that you observed to have no effect or undesirable effects on the person
- Drugs that have no effect or undesirable effects as reported by the person

Performing delegated procedures such as:
- Vital signs—temperature, pulse, respirations, blood pressure, and pain
- Weight and height
- Intake and output
- Blood glucose

Reporting and recording:
- Findings of tasks delegated by the nurse
- Drugs given following agency policy and procedures
- Drug errors or suspected drugs errors

Preventing drug errors and following agency policies and procedures

Practice Limits of the MA-C

Do not do the following, unless allowed by your state law:
- Do not give a drug if the person must first be assessed. Only licensed nurses assess.
- Do not give a drug if the person is not stable and their nursing needs are changing.
- Do not give the first dose of a newly ordered drug.
- Do not give a drug until a licensed nurse is available to monitor the person's progress.
- Do not give a drug until a licensed nurse is available to monitor how the drug affects the person.
- Do not give a drug that must be injected into the person's body by needle or other means: intramuscular (IM); subcutaneous; intradermal; intravenous (IV).
- Do not make decisions about as needed (PRN, prn) drugs.
- Do not make decisions about withholding (not giving) a drug.
- Do not make calls to doctors or accept orders from doctors or other health professionals authorized by state law to prescribe drugs.
- Do not calculate a dosage or convert from one system of measurement to another to determine the correct dosage. (Chapter 10 and Appendix A).
- Do not regulate IV fluids.
- Do not program insulin pumps.

■ REVIEW QUESTIONS

Circle the BEST answer.

1. Nursing assistants can give drugs only if:
   a. the person's condition is stable
   b. a licensed nurse is in the agency
   c. it is part of the CNA job description
   d. allowed by state law

2. You are an MA-C working in a nursing center. You are supervised by:
   a. a licensed nurse
   b. a CNA
   c. the person needing the drug
   d. the doctor who ordered the drug

3. The purpose of a nurse practice act is to:
   a. protect the public's welfare and safety
   b. deny, suspend, or revoke nursing licenses
   c. investigate complaints about CNAs or MA-Cs violating a law
   d. determine what nursing assistants can do

4. Medication assistants are certified after:
   a. becoming a CNA
   b. passing the state-required education and competency evaluation
   c. meeting the requirements of the National Council of State Boards of Nursing
   d. working 1 year as a CNA

5. You are an MA-C. You can have your certification revoked for the following reasons *except:*
   a. drug abuse
   b. deciding to give a drug without the nurse's consent
   c. taking telephone orders from a doctor
   d. refusing to give the first dose of a newly ordered drug

6. You are an MA-C. You can have your certification revoked for the following reasons *except:*
   a. taking a person's drugs for your own use
   b. assessing a person's need for a drug
   c. violating a person's privacy
   d. refusing to accept a verbal order from a doctor

7. You are not sure if you should give a certain drug. What should you do?
   a. Ask the patient or resident.
   b. Ask the nurse.
   c. Give the drug.
   d. Report the error.

8. Which agency can deny, revoke, or suspend an MA-C's certification?
   a. The state board of nursing.
   b. The state regulatory agency responsible for MA-Cs.
   c. The National Council of State Boards of Nursing.
   d. The agency in which the MA-C is employed.

9. On your days off, you call the agency to check on a patient. This is a:
   a. professional boundary
   b. boundary crossing
   c. boundary violation
   d. boundary sign
10. To maintain professional boundaries, your behaviors must:
    a. help the person
    b. meet your needs
    c. be biased
    d. show that you care
11. A patient asks you out to dinner. You accept. This is a:
    a. professional boundary
    b. boundary crossing
    c. boundary violation
    d. boundary sign
12. You accept a "thank you" gift from a patient. This is a:
    a. professional boundary
    b. boundary crossing
    c. boundary violation
    d. boundary sign
13. To renew your MA-C certification, you will likely need:
    a. proof of continuing education hours
    b. to take another written exam
    c. to take another skills test
    d. a physical examination

14. You give a person a drug for pain relief. Later the person continues to complain of pain. What should you do?
    a. Give the same drug again.
    b. Tell the nurse at once.
    c. Offer other comfort measures.
    d. Tell the person to give the drug more time to take effect.
15. MA-Cs can:
    a. give oral drugs
    b. give IV drugs
    c. give IM drugs
    d. program insulin pumps

Circle T if the statement is true. Circle F if the statement is false.
16. T F Some states allow MA-Cs to work in settings that do not employ a licensed nurse.
17. T F You are a CNA and an MA-C. Your agency's job description for nursing assistants does not include giving drugs. Because you are an MA-C, you can still give drugs as directed by the nurse.
18. T F You are an MA-C. A nurse tells you to give a drug that requires using a needle. You can give the drug.
19. T F State law allows you to give a certain drug. A nurse or an agency can make you give the drug.
20. T F You are assigned to give drugs and the personal care for 8 residents. Resident care is part of your role as an MA-C.

Answers to these questions can be found on the Evolve Resources site: http://evolve.elsevier.com/Anderson/medasst/

2

Delegation

OBJECTIVES

- Define the key terms and key abbreviations used in this chapter.
- Describe the delegation process.
- Explain your role in the delegation process.

- Explain how to accept or refuse a delegated task.
- Describe the MA-C's role in the medication administration process.
- Explain what nurses can and cannot delegate to MA-Cs.

KEY TERMS

accountable Being responsible for one's actions and the actions of others who performed the delegated tasks; answering questions about and explaining one's actions and the actions of others

delegate To authorize another person to perform a nursing task in a certain situation

nursing task Nursing care or a nursing function, procedure, activity, or work that does not require an RN's or LPN's/LVN's professional knowledge or judgment

KEY ABBREVIATIONS

CNA Certified nursing assistant or certified nurse aide
LPN Licensed practical nurse
LVN Licensed vocational nurse
MA-C Medication assistant-certified

mg Milligram
NCSBN National Council of State Boards of Nursing
PRN As needed
RN Registered nurse

Licensed nurses supervise your work. You perform nursing tasks related to the person's care. A **nursing task** is the nursing care or a nursing function, procedure, activity, or work that does not require an RN's or LPN's/LVN's professional knowledge or judgment. If allowed by state law, giving certain drugs is a nursing task that can be delegated to MA-Cs.

MA-C functions and responsibilities vary among states and agencies. Before you give any drug, make sure that:
- Your state allows you to do so
- The task is in your job description
- You have the necessary education and training
- A nurse is available to answer questions and to supervise you

DELEGATION PRINCIPLES

Delegate means to authorize another person to perform a nursing task in a certain situation. The person must be competent to perform a task in the given situation. For example, you know how to give oral drugs. However, Mr. Jones has developed a swallowing problem. The nurse wants to assess whether he has a problem swallowing drugs. You do not assess. Therefore, the nurse gives the oral drugs.

Who Can Delegate

RNs can delegate nursing tasks to LPNs/LVNs and CNAs and MA-Cs. In some states, LPNs/LVNs can delegate tasks to CNAs and MA-Cs. RNs and LPNs/LVNs can only delegate tasks within their scope of practice. And they can only delegate tasks that are in the CNA's or MA-C's job description.

Delegation decisions must protect the person's health and safety. The delegating nurse is legally accountable for the nursing task. **Accountable** means to be responsible for one's actions and the actions of others who performed the delegated tasks. It also involves answering questions about and explaining one's actions and the actions of others.

The delegating nurse must make sure that the task was completed safely and correctly. If the RN delegates, the RN is responsible for the delegated task. If the LPN/LVN delegates, the LPN/LVN is responsible for the delegated task. The RN also supervises LPNs/LVNs. Therefore, the RN is legally accountable for the tasks that LPNs/LVNs delegate to CNAs and MA-Cs. The RN is accountable for all nursing care.

CNAs and MA-Cs cannot delegate. You cannot delegate any task to other nursing assistants or to any other worker. You can ask someone to help you. But you cannot ask or tell someone to do your work.

Delegation Process

To make delegation decisions, the nurse follows a process. The person's needs, the nursing task, and the staff member doing the task must fit. The nurse can decide *to delegate* the task to you. Or the nurse can decide *not to delegate* the task. The person's needs and the task may require a nurse's knowledge, judgment, and skill. You may be asked to assist.

Do not get offended or angry if you cannot perform a task that is usually delegated to you. The nurse decides what is best for the person at the time. That decision is also best for you at that time. You should not do something that requires a nurse's judgment. For example, you always give Mrs. Doyle her oral drugs. Now she is weak and refusing her drugs. The nurse wants to assess her behaviors while she is refusing her drugs. The nurse decides to give the drugs. At this time Mrs. Doyle needs the nurse's judgment and knowledge.

The person's circumstances are central factors in delegation decisions. Delegation decisions must result in the best care for the person. A nurse risks a person's health and safety with poor delegation decisions. Also, the nurse may face serious legal problems. If you perform a task that places the person at risk, you can also face serious legal problems.

The National Council of State Boards of Nursing (NCSBN) describes the delegation process in four steps.

Step 1—Assess and Plan. Step 1 is done by the nurse. To safely delegate, the nurse needs to understand the person's needs. And the nurse needs to know your knowledge, skills, and job description.

When assessing the person's needs, the nurse answers these questions:

- What is the nature of the person's needs? How complex are the needs? How can they vary? How urgent are the care needs?
- What are the most important long-term needs? What are the most important short-term needs?
- How much judgment is needed to meet the person's needs and give care?
- How predictable is the person's health status? How does the person respond to health care?
- What kind of problems might arise from the needed nursing task? How severe might the problems be?
- What actions are needed if a problem arises? How complex are those actions?
- What kind of emergencies or incidents might arise? How likely are they to occur?
- How involved is the person in health care decisions? How involved is the family?
- How will delegating the nursing task help the person? What are the risks to the person?

To assess your knowledge and skills, the nurse answers these questions:

- What knowledge and skills are needed to safely perform the nursing task?
- What is your role in the agency? What is in your job description?
- What are the conditions under which the nursing task will be performed?

- What is expected after the nursing task is performed?
- What problems can arise from the nursing task? What problems might the person develop during the nursing task?

The nurse then decides whether it is safe to delegate the nursing task. It must be safe for the person and safe for you. If delegation is deemed unsafe, the nurse stops the delegation process. If delegation is safe for the person and you, the nurse moves to step 2.

Step 2—Communication. This step involves the nurse and you. The nurse must provide clear and complete directions about:

- How to perform and complete the task
- What observations to report and record
- When to report observations
- What specific patient and resident concerns to report at once
- Priorities for nursing tasks
- What to do if the person's condition or needs change

The nurse needs to make sure that you understand the directions. The nurse asks you questions to make sure you understand. He or she may ask you to explain what you are going to do. You should not be annoyed or insulted by the nurse's questions. He or she must make sure that safe care is given. This protects the person and you.

Before performing a delegated nursing task, you must have the opportunity to discuss the task with the nurse. Make sure that you:

- Ask questions about the delegated task.
- Ask questions about what you are expected to do.
- Tell the nurse if you have not done the task before. Also tell the nurse if you have not done it often.
- Ask for needed training or supervision.
- Restate what is expected of you.
- Restate what specific patient or resident concerns to report to the nurse and when.
- Explain how and when you will report your progress in completing the task.
- Know how to contact the nurse if there is an emergency.
- Know what the nurse wants you to do if there is an emergency.

After completing a delegated task, you must report and record the care given. You also report and record your observations. See Chapter 4.

Step 3—Surveillance and Supervision. *Surveillance* means to keep a close watch over someone or something. *Supervise* means to oversee, direct, or manage. In this step, the nurse observes the care you give. The nurse has to make sure that you complete the task correctly. The nurse also observes the person's condition and response to your care. How often the nurse makes observations depends on:

- The person's health status and needs.
- Whether the person's condition is stable or unstable.
- Whether the nurse can predict the person's responses and risk to care.
- The setting where the nursing task occurs.
- The resources and support available.
- Whether the nursing task is simple or complex.

The nurse must follow up on any problems or concerns. For example, the nurse must take action if you did not complete the nursing task in a timely manner. The nurse also must take action if the nursing task did not meet expectations. An unexpected change in the person's condition is also cause for the nurse to act.

The nurse must be alert for signs and symptoms that signal a possible change in the person's condition. With your help, the nurse can take action before the person's condition changes in a major way.

Sometimes problems arise in completing a nursing task. By supervising you, the nurse can detect and solve problems early. This helps you complete the task safely and on time.

After you complete the task, the nurse may review and discuss what happened with you. This helps you learn. If a similar situation happens in the future, you have ideas about how to adjust.

Step 4—Evaluation and Feedback. This step is done by the nurse. *Evaluate* means to judge. The nurse decides whether the delegation was successful. The nurse answers these questions:

- Was the nursing task done correctly?
- Did the person respond to the nursing task as expected?
- Was the outcome (the result) as desired? Was the result good or bad?
- Was communication between you and the nurse timely and effective?
- What went well? What were the problems?
- Does the care plan need to change (Chapter 4)? Or can the plan stay the same?
- Did the nursing task present ways for the nurse or you to learn?
- Did the nurse give you the right feedback? *Feedback* means to respond. The nurse tells you what you did correctly. If you did something wrong, the nurse tells you that too. Feedback is another way in which you can learn and improve the care you give.
- Did the nurse thank you for completing the nursing task?

The Five Rights of Delegation

The NCSBN's *The Five Rights of Delegation* is another way to view the delegation process. In using the "five rights," the nurse answers the questions listed in the four steps described above. *The Five Rights of Delegation* are:

- *The right task.* Can the task be delegated? Is the nurse allowed to delegate the task? Is the task in your job description?
- *The right circumstances.* What are the person's physical, mental, emotional, and spiritual needs at this time?
- *The right person.* Do you have the training and experience to safely perform the task for this person?
- *The right directions and communication.* The nurse must give clear directions. The nurse tells you what to do and when to do it. The nurse tells you what observations to make and when to report back. The nurse allows questions and helps you set priorities.
- *The right supervision and evaluation.* The nurse guides, directs, and evaluates the care you give. The nurse demonstrates tasks as necessary and is available to answer questions. The less experience you have with a task, the more supervision you need. Complex tasks require more supervision than do basic tasks. Also, the person's circumstances affect how much supervision you need. The nurse assesses how the task affected the person and how well you performed the task. The

nurse tells you what you did well and how to improve your work. This helps you learn and give better care.

Your Role in Delegation

You perform delegated nursing tasks for or on *a person*. You must protect the person from harm. You have two choices when a task is delegated to you. You either *agree* or *refuse* to do the task. Use *The Five Rights of Delegation* in Box 2-1.

Accepting a Task. When you agree to perform a task, you are responsible for your own actions. What you do or fail to do can harm the person. *You must complete the task safely.* Ask for help when you are unsure or have questions about a task. Report to the nurse what you did and the observations you made.

Refusing a Task. You have the right to say "no." Sometimes refusing to follow the nurse's directions is your right and duty. You should refuse to perform a task when:

- The task is beyond the legal limits of your role.
- The task is not in your job description.
- You were not prepared to perform the task.
- The task could harm the person.
- The person's condition has changed.
- You do not know how to use the supplies or equipment.
- Directions are not ethical or legal.
- Directions are against agency policies.
- Directions are unclear or incomplete.
- A nurse is not available for supervision.

BOX 2-1 The Five Rights of Delegation for Nursing Assistants

The Right Task
- Does your state allow you to perform the task?
- Were you trained to do the task?
- Do you have experience performing the task?
- Is the task in your job description?

The Right Circumstances
- Do you have experience performing the task given the person's condition and needs?
- Do you understand the purposes of the task for the person?
- Can you perform the task safely under the current circumstances?
- Do you have the equipment and supplies to safely complete the task?
- Do you know how to use the equipment and supplies?

The Right Person
- Are you comfortable performing the task?
- Do you have concerns about performing the task?
- Do you understand what the nurse expects?

The Right Directions And Communication
- Did the nurse give clear directions and instructions?
- Did you review the task with the nurse?
- Do you understand what the nurse expects?

The Right Supervision
- Is a nurse available to answer questions?
- Is a nurse available if the person's condition changes or if problems occur?

Modified from the National Council of State Boards of Nursing, Inc. and American Nurses Association, *National Guidelines for Nursing Delegation: The five rights of delegation*, 2019, Chicago, IL.

Use common sense. This protects you and the person. Ask yourself whether what you are doing is safe for the person.

Never ignore an order or a request to do something. Tell the nurse about your concerns. If the task is within the legal limits of your role and in your job description, the nurse can help increase your comfort with the task. The nurse can:

- Answer your questions
- Demonstrate the task
- Show you how to use supplies and equipment
- Help you as needed
- Observe you performing the task
- Check on you often
- Arrange for needed training

Do not refuse a task because you do not like it or do not want to do it. You must have sound reasons. Otherwise, you place the person at risk for harm. You also could lose your job.

DELEGATING TO MA-Cs

The actual task of giving certain drugs may not require a nurse's judgment. Therefore, nurses can delegate to MA-Cs the task of giving such drugs. However, *the nurse cannot delegate the nursing actions and judgments needed before and after a drug is given.*

Fig. 2-1 shows the MA-C's place and role in the entire process of medication administration. The MA-C's role is to give the drug. It is one step in the process. The nurse cannot delegate any other step in the process shown in Fig. 2-1. Those steps involve:

- Assessing the person's need for a drug
- Determining the need for PRN drugs
- Assessing and evaluating side effects
- Recognizing allergic reactions
- Assessing and evaluating immediate desired effects
- Assessing and evaluating effects that are unusual and not expected
- Recognizing when continued use of the drug may be harmful
- Recognizing when the person no longer needs the drug
- Anticipating effects which may rapidly affect the person's life or well-being
- Making judgments and decisions about what actions to take if the person's life or well-being is threatened

Sometimes a drug dosage needs to be converted or calculated before the drug is given. For example, the doctor orders 500 mg (milligrams) of a drug. Each tablet contains 250 mg. A calculation shows to give two tablets. Some states do not allow MA-Cs to convert or calculate drug dosages. The nurse cannot delegate that task in those states. Other states allow MA-Cs to do simple conversions and calculations. Converting and calculating dosages are described in Appendix A.

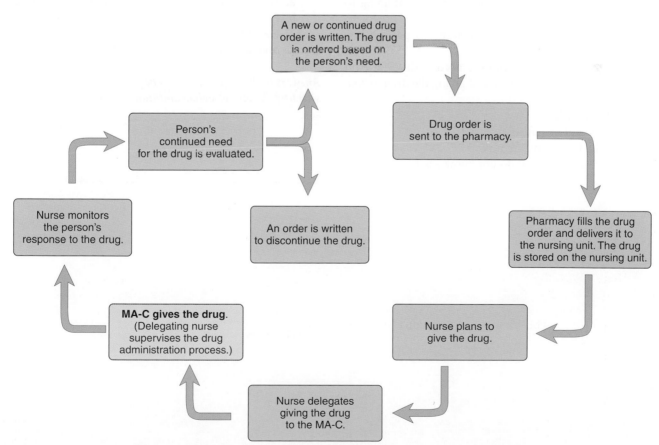

Fig. 2-1 The MA-C's Place and Role in the Medication Administration Process.

REVIEW QUESTIONS

Circle the BEST answer.

1. You are responsible for:
   a. supervising other nursing assistants
   b. delegation decisions
   c. completing delegated nursing assistant tasks safely
   d. nursing tasks

2. You are asked to give a drug. Your state does not allow MA-Cs to give that drug. Which is *true*?
   a. If a nurse delegated the task, there is no legal problem.
   b. You could be practicing nursing without a license.
   c. You can give the drug if giving drugs is in your job description.
   d. If you give the drug safely, there is no legal problem.

3. A nurse delegates giving drugs to you. Which is *false*?
   a. Nurses can delegate to you the responsibility of giving drugs.
   b. The delegation decision must be safe for the person.
   c. The delegated task must be in your job description.
   d. The delegating nurse is responsible for making sure the drugs were given safely.

4. Giving certain drugs is in your job description. Which is *false*?
   a. The nurse must delegate the task to you.
   b. The nurse can delegate the task if the person's circumstances are right.
   c. You must have the necessary education and training to complete the task.
   d. You must have clear directions before you perform the task.

5. The nurse decided that Mr. Monroe needs a drug for pain relief. The nurse delegates the task of giving the drug to you. You must:
   a. complete the task
   b. decide to accept or refuse the task
   c. delegate the task if you are busy
   d. ignore the request if you do not know what to do

6. The nurse asks you to give a drug. You can refuse to perform a task for these reasons *except*:
   a. the task is beyond the legal limits of your role
   b. the task is not in your job description
   c. you do not like the task
   d. a nurse is not available to supervise you

7. You decide to refuse the task of giving a certain drug. What should you do?
   a. Delegate the task to a CNA.
   b. Communicate your concerns to the nurse.
   c. Ignore the request.
   d. Talk to the director of nursing.

8. Mr. Monroe complains of pain. He asks for a pain-relief drug. What should you do?
   a. Assess his complaint of pain.
   b. Tell the nurse.
   c. Call the doctor.
   d. Give the drug.

9. As an MA-C, what is your role in the medication administration process?
   a. Sending drug orders to the pharmacy.
   b. Receiving filled drug orders from the pharmacy.
   c. Giving drugs as delegated by the nurse.
   d. Monitoring the person's response to the drug.

10. Which of the following can the nurse delegate to you?
    a. Determining whether a person needs a PRN drug.
    b. Evaluating side effects and allergic reactions.
    c. Deciding when a drug is no longer needed.
    d. Making and reporting observations.

Answers to these questions can be found on the Evolve Resources site: http://evolve.elsevier.com/Anderson/medasst/

3

Ethics and Laws

- Define the key terms and key abbreviations used in this chapter.
- Describe ethical conduct.
- Describe the rules of conduct for MA-Cs.
- Explain the rights of hospital patients and nursing center residents.
- Identify two types of advance directives.
- Explain the Federal Food, Drug, and Cosmetic Act.
- Explain the Comprehensive Drug Abuse Prevention and Control Act.
- Explain how unintentional torts, intentional torts, and crimes differ.
- Explain why possessing a controlled substance is a crime.
- Describe elder, child, and domestic abuse.

KEY TERMS

abuse The intentional mistreatment or harm of another person

advance directive A document stating a person's wishes about health care when that person cannot make his or her own decisions

assault Intentionally attempting or threatening to touch a person's body without the person's consent

battery Touching a person's body without his or her consent

civil law Laws concerned with relationships between people

crime An act that violates a criminal law

criminal law Laws concerned with offenses against the public and society in general

defamation Injuring a person's name and reputation by making false statements to a third person

ethics Knowledge of what is right conduct and wrong conduct

false imprisonment Unlawful restraint or restriction of a person's freedom of movement

fraud Saying or doing something to trick, fool, or deceive a person

invasion of privacy Violating a person's right not to have his or her name, photo, or private affairs exposed or made public without giving consent

law A rule of conduct made by a government body

libel Making false statements in print, in writing, or through pictures or drawings

malpractice Negligence by a professional person

misappropriation To dishonestly, unfairly, or wrongly take for one's own use

neglect Failure to provide the person with the goods or services needed to avoid physical harm, mental anguish, or mental illness

negligence An unintentional wrong in which a person did not act in a reasonable and careful manner and a person or the person's property was harmed

protected health information Identifying information and information about the person's health care that is maintained or sent in any form (paper, electronic, oral)

slander Making false statements orally

tort A wrong committed against a person or the person's property

vulnerable adult A person 18 years old or older who has a disability or condition that makes him or her at risk to be wounded, attacked, or damaged

KEY ABBREVIATIONS

AHA American Hospital Association
DEA Drug Enforcement Administration
DNR Do not resuscitate
FDA Food and Drug Administration
HIPAA Health Insurance Portability and Accountability Act of 1996

MA-C Medication assistant-certified
OBRA Omnibus Budget Reconciliation Act of 1987
OTC Over-the-counter
POLST Physician Orders for Life-Sustaining Treatment

Nurse practice acts, your training and job description, and safe delegation serve to protect patients and residents from harm (Chapter 2). Protecting them from harm also involves a complex set of rules and standards of conduct. They form the ethical and legal aspects of care.

ETHICAL ASPECTS

Ethics is knowledge of what is right conduct and wrong conduct. Morals are involved. It also deals with choices or judgments about what should or should not be done. An ethical

---

BOX 3-1   Code of Conduct for Nursing Assistive Personnel

- Respect each person as an individual.
- Know the limits of your role and knowledge.
- Perform only those tasks that are within the legal limits of your role.
- Perform only those tasks that you have been prepared to do.
- Perform no act that will cause the person harm.
- Take a drug only when prescribed and ordered by a doctor.
- Carry out the directions and instructions of the nurse to your best possible ability.
- Follow the agency's policies and procedures.
- Complete each task safely.
- Be loyal to your employer and co-workers.
- Act as a responsible citizen at all times.
- Keep the person's information confidential.
- Protect the person's privacy.
- Protect the person's property.
- Consider the person's needs to be more important than your own.
- Report errors and incidents at once.
- Be accountable for your actions.

Courtesy of American Hospital Association, 2003.

---

person behaves and acts in the right way. He or she does not cause a person harm.

Ethical behavior also involves not being *prejudiced* or *biased*. To be prejudiced or biased means to make judgments and have views before knowing the facts. Judgments and views usually are based on one's values and standards. They are based on the person's culture, religion, education, and experiences. Do not judge the person by your values and standards. Do not avoid persons whose standards and values differ from your own.

Ethical problems involve making choices. You must decide what is the right thing to do. The rules of conduct for nursing assistive personnel can guide your thinking and behavior (Box 3-1). Also see "Professional Boundaries" in Chapter 1.

THE PERSON'S RIGHTS

In April 2003, the American Hospital Association (AHA) issued *The Patient Care Partnership: Understanding Expectations, Rights, and Responsibilities* (Box 3-2). The document explains the person's rights and expectations during hospital stays. The relationship among the doctor, the health team, and the patient is stressed.

Nursing center residents have rights as United States citizens. They also have rights under the Omnibus Budget and Reconciliation Act of 1987 (OBRA). OBRA is a federal law. It applies to all 50 states. Nursing centers must provide care in a manner and in a setting that maintains or improves each person's quality of life, health, and safety. Resident rights are a major part of OBRA (Box 3-3).

ADVANCE DIRECTIVES

The Patient Self-Determination Act and OBRA give persons the right to accept or refuse medical treatment. They also give the right to make advance directives. An advance directive is a document stating a person's wishes about health care when that person cannot make his or her own decisions. Advance directives usually forbid certain care if there is no hope of recovery. Living wills and durable power of attorney for health care are common advance directives.

Living Will

A *living will* is a document about measures that support or maintain life when death is likely. Tube feedings, ventilators, and cardiopulmonary resuscitation are examples. A living will may instruct doctors:

- Not to start measures that prolong dying
- To remove measures that prolong dying

Durable Power of Attorney

Durable power of attorney for health care also is an advance directive. It gives the power to make health care decisions to another person. Usually this is a family member, friend, or lawyer. When a person cannot make health care decisions, the person with durable power of attorney can do so.

Do Not Resuscitate

Doctors often write *do not resuscitate (DNR)* or *no code* orders for terminally ill persons. This means that the person will not be resuscitated. The person is allowed to die with peace and dignity. The orders are written after consulting with the person and family. The family and doctor make the decision if the person is not mentally able to. Some advance directives address resuscitation.

Physician Orders for Life-Sustaining Treatment

The Physician Orders for Life-Sustaining Treatment (POLST) form is a doctor's order sheet that is recognized in most states. It is part of a person's medical record that says which life-sustaining treatments should be performed and which should not. A POLST form is a medical order for the specific medical treatments you want during a medical emergency. It follows the person when transferred from one facility to the next. For example, it goes with the person when they leave a care center for the hospital. In some states, the information is stored in a computerized database so the person's health care wishes can be communicated to other health care team members.

You may not agree with care and resuscitation decisions. However, you must follow the person's or family's wishes and the doctor's orders. These may be against your personal, religious, and cultural values. If so, discuss the matter with the nurse. An assignment change may be needed.

Quality of care cannot be less because of the person's advance directives. Health care agencies must inform all persons of the right to advance directives on admission. This information is in writing. The medical record must document whether the person has made them.

FEDERAL DRUG LAWS

Ethics is about what you should or should not do. Laws tell you what you can and cannot do. A law is a rule of conduct made by a government body. The U.S. Congress and state legislatures make laws. Enforced by the government, laws protect the public welfare. The intent of federal drug laws is to make drugs as safe as possible for patients, residents, and anyone who uses drugs. The laws also ensure that the drug does what is claims to do. The goal is safe and effective drug use.

BOX 3-2   The Patient Care Partnership

Understanding Expectations, Rights, and Responsibilities
What to expect during your hospital stay:
- high-quality hospital care
- a clean and safe environment
- involvement in your care
- protection of your privacy
- help when leaving the hospital
- help with your billing claims

When you need hospital care, your doctor and the nurses and other professionals at our hospital are committed to working with you and your family to meet your healthcare needs. Our dedicated doctors and staff serve the community in all its ethnic, religious, and economic diversity. Our goal is for you and your family to have the same care and attention we would want for our families and ourselves.

The sections that follow explain some of the basics about how you can expect to be treated during your hospital stay. They also cover what we need from you to care for you better. If you have questions at any time, please ask them. Unasked or unanswered questions can add to the stress of being in the hospital. Your comfort and confidence in your care are important to us.

What to Expect During Your Hospital Stay
High-Quality Hospital Care
Our first priority is to provide you the care you need, when you need it, with skill, compassion, and respect. Tell your caregivers if you have concerns about your care or if you have pain. You have the right to know the identity of doctors, nurses, and others involved in your care, and you have the right to know when they are students, residents, or other trainees.

A Clean and Safe Environment
Our hospital works hard to keep you safe. We use special policies and procedures to avoid mistakes in your care and keep you free from abuse or neglect. If anything unexpected and significant happens during your hospital stay, you will be told what happened, and any resulting changes in your care will be discussed with you.

Involvement in Your Care
You and your doctor often make decisions about your care before you go to the hospital. Other times, especially in emergencies, those decisions are made during your hospital stay. When decision making takes place, it should include the following:

Discussing Your Medical Condition and Information About Medically Appropriate Treatment Choices
To make informed decisions with your doctor, you need to understand:
- the benefits and risks of each treatment;
- whether your treatment is experimental or part of a research study;
- what you can reasonably expect from your treatment and any long-term effects it might have on your quality of life;
- what you and your family will need to do after you leave the hospital;
- the financial consequences of using uncovered services or out-of-network providers.

Please tell your caregivers if you need more information about treatment choices.

Discussing Your Treatment Plan
When you enter the hospital, you sign a general consent to treatment. In some cases, such as surgery or experimental treatment, you may be asked to confirm in writing that you understand what is planned and agree to it. This process protects your right to consent to or refuse a treatment. Your doctor will explain the medical consequences of refusing recommended treatment. It also protects your right to decide if you want to participate in a research study.

Getting Information From You
Your caregivers need complete and correct information about your health and coverage so that they can make good decisions about your care. That includes the following:
- past illnesses, surgeries, or hospital stays
- past allergic reactions
- any medicines or dietary supplements (such as vitamins and herbs) that you are taking
- any network or admission requirements under your health plan

Understanding Your Healthcare Goals and Values
You may have healthcare goals and values or spiritual beliefs that are important to your well-being. They will be taken into account as much as possible throughout your hospital stay. Make sure your doctor, your family, and your care team members know your wishes.

Understanding Who Should Make Decisions When You Cannot
If you have signed a healthcare power of attorney stating who should speak for you if you become unable to make healthcare decisions for yourself, or a living will or advance directive that states your wishes about end-of-life care, give copies to your doctor, your family, and your care team. If you or your family members need help making difficult decisions, counselors, chaplains, and others are available to help.

Protection of Your Privacy
We respect the confidentiality of your relationship with your doctor and other caregivers and the sensitive information about your health and healthcare that is part of that relationship. State and federal laws and hospital operating policies protect the privacy of your medical information. You will receive a Notice of Privacy Practices that describes the ways in which we use, disclose, and safeguard patient information and that explains how you can obtain a copy of information from our records about your care.

Preparing You and Your Family for When You Leave the Hospital
Your doctor works with hospital staff and professionals in your community. You and your family also play an important role in your care. The success of your treatment often depends on your efforts to follow medication, diet, and therapy plans. Your family may need to help care for you at home.

You can expect us to help you identify sources of follow-up care and to let you know if our hospital has a financial interest in any referrals. As long as you agree that we can share information about your care with them, we will coordinate our activities with your caregivers outside the hospital. You can also expect to receive information and, where possible, training about the self-care you will need when you go home.

Help With Your Bill and Filing Insurance Claims
Our staff will file claims for you with healthcare insurers or other programs, such as Medicare and Medicaid. They also will help your doctor with needed documentation. Hospital bills and insurance coverage are often confusing. If you have questions about your bill, contact our business office. If you need help understanding your insurance coverage or health plan, start with your insurance company or health benefits manager. If you do not have health coverage, we will try to help you and your family find financial help or make other arrangements. We need your help in collecting needed information and other requirements to obtain coverage or assistance.

While you are here, you will receive more detailed notices about some of the rights you have as a hospital patient and how to exercise them. We are always interested in improving. If you have questions, comments, or concerns, please contact: (relevant department here).

BOX 3-3   Resident's Rights

The Right to Information

- The person has a copy of resident's rights as well as the facility rules and regulations.
- The person has access to all of his or her records—medical record, contracts, incident reports, and financial records.
- The person receives information about his or her total health condition. Information is given in language the person can understand. Interpreters are used as needed. Sign language or other aids are used for those with hearing losses. Assistance will be provided if a sensory impairment exists.
- The person receives information about his or her doctor. This includes the doctor's name and specialty and how to contact the doctor.
- Be informed of all changes in medical condition.
- Be informed of a change in rooms or roommates.

The Right to Refuse Treatment and Participate in One's Own Care

- The person must consent to treatment or to take part in research. If a person does not give consent or refuses treatment, it cannot be given. This includes refusing drugs. If a person refuses a certain treatment, the center must provide all other services.
- Advance directives are part of the right to refuse treatment. They include living wills or instructions about life support.
- Receive good, honest, and thoughtful care.
- Residents have the right not to have body movements restricted. This includes physical and chemical restraints.

The Right to Privacy and Confidentiality

- Privacy is maintained during treatment and care of one's personal needs, including using the bathroom.
- Only staff directly involved in care and treatments are present. The person must give consent for others to be present.
- Privacy is maintained when visiting with others and for phone calls.
- Mail is sent, received, and opened without others interfering. No one can open mail the person sends or receives without his or her consent.
- Information about the person's care, treatment, and condition is kept confidential. So are medical, personal, and financial records.

The Right to Make Independent Choices

- Residents can choose their own doctors.
- Residents manage their own financial affairs.
- Residents take part in planning and deciding about their care and treatment. They can choose activities, schedules, and care based on their preferences.
- Residents can choose friends and visitors inside and outside the center. They can visit with friends, relatives, organizations, or individuals providing health, social, legal, or other services. They can also refuse visitors.
- Residents can form and take part in resident and family groups. Groups can discuss concerns and suggest center improvements. They also can plan activities.

- Residents can take part in social, cultural, religious, and community events, inside and outside the nursing center. They have the right to help in getting to and from events of their choice.

The Right to Disputes and Grievances

- Residents can voice concerns, questions, and complaints about treatment or care to the ombudsman program or state survey and certification agency.
- The person cannot be punished in any way for voicing the dispute or grievance.
- Residents must be provided the address and telephone number of the state ombudsman and state survey agency.
- Representatives from the state survey agency and ombudsman programs can visit the resident.

The Rights During Transfers and Discharges

- Residents may remain in the nursing facility unless a transfer or discharge:
  - is necessary to meet the resident's welfare.
  - is appropriate because the resident's health has improved, and he or she no longer requires nursing home care.
  - is needed to protect the health and safety of other residents or staff.
  - is required because the resident has failed, after reasonable notice, to pay the facility charge for an item or service provided at the resident's request.
- Residents will receive 30-day notice of transfer or discharge which includes the reason, effective date, location to which the resident is transferred or discharged, the right to appeal, and the name, address, and telephone number of the state long-term care ombudsman.
- Residents have the right to safe transfer or discharge through sufficient preparation by the nursing home.

The Right to Dignity, Respect, and Freedom

- Residents have the right to be treated with consideration, respect, and dignity and spoken to in a polite and courteous manner.
- Residents can keep and use personal items. This includes clothing and some furnishings. Items are labeled with the person's name.
- The center must protect the resident's property and investigate reports of lost, stolen, or damaged items. Police help is sometimes needed.
- Residents must be free from verbal, sexual, physical, or mental abuse and involuntary seclusion (p. 19). Involuntary seclusion is:
  - Separating a person from others against his or her will
  - Keeping the person confined to a certain area
  - Keeping the person away from his or her room without consent
- Nursing centers must investigate suspected or reported cases of abuse.
- Nursing centers cannot employ persons who were convicted of abusing, neglecting, or mistreating others.
- Restraints are not used for staff convenience or to discipline a person.
- Nursing centers must care for residents in a manner that promotes dignity and self-esteem. It must also promote physical, psychological, and mental well-being.
- The nursing center's environment must promote quality of life. It must be clean, safe, and as home-like as possible.

Federal Food, Drug, and Cosmetic Act of 1938

The Federal Food, Drug, and Cosmetic Act of 1938 requires the Food and Drug Administration (FDA) to:

- Determine the safety and effectiveness of drugs before marketing
- Ensure that manufacturers meet labeling requirements
- Ensure that advertising standards are met when manufacturers market drugs

Manufacturers must submit new drug applications to the FDA. The FDA reviews safety studies before approving a drug for sale.

The law was strengthened by the *Durham-Humphrey Amendment of 1951.* The amendment requires that drugs that that cannot be used safely without professional supervision be dispensed only by prescription. For example, drugs that are toxic, are habit-forming, or are known to have harmful effects require a prescription. All other drugs can be sold over-the-counter (OTC).

The *Kefauver-Harris Amendment* was passed in 1962. It requires that a drug be proven both safe and effective before it is approved for sale.

BOX 3-4 Schedules of Controlled Substances

SCHEDULE I DRUGS
- High potential for abuse.
- No currently accepted medical use in the United States.
- Lack accepted safety for use under medical supervision.
- Examples—lysergic acid diethylamide (LSD), marijuana, peyote, heroin, "ecstasy"

SCHEDULE II DRUGS
- High potential for abuse.
- Have an accepted medical use in the United States.
- May lead to severe psychological or physical dependence.
- Examples—hydrocodone, cocaine, methamphetamine, methadone, hydromorphone (Dilaudid), meperidine (Demerol), oxycodone (OxyContin), morphine, fentanyl, Dexedrine, Adderall, and Ritalin

SCHEDULE III DRUGS
- High potential for abuse. Less potential than Schedule I and II drugs.
- Have an accepted medical use in the United States.
- May lead to moderate or low physical dependence. May lead to high psychological dependence.

- Examples—Tylenol with codeine, ketamine, anabolic steroids, testosterone, buprenorphine (Suboxone), and benzphetamine (Didrex)

SCHEDULE IV DRUGS
- Low potential for abuse. Less potential than those in Schedule III.
- Have an accepted medical use in the United States.
- May lead to limited physical or psychological dependence.
- Examples—alprazolam (Xanax), carisoprodol (Soma), clonazepam (Klonopin), clorazepate (Tranxene), diazepam (Valium), lorazepam (Ativan), midazolam (Versed), temazepam (Restoril), and triazolam (Halcion)

SCHEDULE V DRUGS
- Low potential for abuse. Less potential than those in Schedule IV.
- Have an accepted medical use in the United States.
- Have limited potential for physical or psychological dependence.
- A prescription may not be required.
- Examples—Lomotil, Robitussin A-C, Lyrica, and Phenergan with codeine

---

Comprehensive Drug Abuse Prevention and Control Act of 1970

The Comprehensive Drug Abuse Prevention and Control Act of 1970 serves to control the manufacturing, distributing, and dispensing of drugs that require control because they are highly addictive. It is commonly called the *Controlled Substance Act*. A *controlled substance* is a drug or chemical substance whose possession and use are controlled by law. The Drug Enforcement Administration (DEA) enforces this law. The DEA gathers intelligence, trains, and conducts research about dangerous drugs and drug abuse.

The Act has five classifications or *schedules* of controlled substances (Box 3-4). How a drug is scheduled depends on:
- The degree of control
- Required record-keeping
- Required order forms
- Other regulations

All drugs in Schedules II, III, and IV require a prescription. So do some drugs in Schedule V. The pharmacist must have the prescriber's approval before refilling a prescription.

Prescriptions must contain:
- The prescriber's name, address, and DEA registration number
- The prescriber's signature
- The name and address of the patient or resident
- The date of issue

When a Schedule II drug is given, the person giving the drug must record the following information:
- The name of the person receiving the drug
- The date and time the drug was given
- The drug given
- The dosage given

TORTS AND CRIMES

Civil laws are concerned with relationships between people. Examples of civil laws are those that involve contracts and nursing practice. A person found guilty of breaking a civil law usually has to pay a sum of money to the injured person.

Criminal laws are concerned with offenses against the public and society in general. An act that violates a criminal law is called a crime. A person found guilty of a crime is fined or sent to prison.

You are legally responsible *(liable)* for your own actions. The nurse is liable as your supervisor. However, you are not relieved of personal liability. Remember, sometimes refusing to follow the nurse's directions is your right and duty (Chapter 2).

Torts

Tort comes from the French word meaning *wrong*. Torts are part of civil law. A tort is a wrong committed against a person or the person's property. Torts may be unintentional, meaning that harm was not intended. Some torts are intentional, meaning that harm was intended.

Unintentional Torts. Negligence is an unintentional wrong. The negligent person did not act in a reasonable and careful manner. As a result, a person or the person's property was harmed. The person causing the harm did not intend or mean to cause harm. The person failed to do what a reasonable and careful person would have done. Or he or she did what a reasonable and careful person would not have done. The negligent person may have to pay damages (a sum of money) to the one injured.

Malpractice is negligence by a professional person. A person has professional status because of training and the service provided. Nurses, doctors, and pharmacists are examples.

What you do or do not do can lead to a lawsuit if harm results to the person or property of another. *Standard of care* refers to skills, care, and judgments required by a health team member under similar conditions (Chapter 1). Standards of care come from:
- Laws, including nurse practice acts
- Textbooks
- Agency policies and procedures
- Manufacturer instructions for equipment and supplies
- Job descriptions
- Approval and accrediting agency standards

- Standards and guidelines issued by government agencies

As an MA-C, the following actions could lead to charges of negligence:

- You give a drug to the wrong person.
- You give the wrong drug.
- You give the wrong dosage.
- You give a drug the wrong way.
- You give a drug at the wrong time.
- You do not give an ordered drug.

Intentional Torts. Intentional torts are acts meant to be harmful. The act is done knowingly. Intentional torts include the following:

- **Defamation** is injuring a person's name and reputation by making false statements to a third person. **Libel** is making false statements in print, in writing, or through pictures or drawings. **Slander** is making false statements orally.
- **False imprisonment** is the unlawful restraint or restriction of a person's freedom of movement.
- **Invasion of privacy** is violating a person's right not to have his or her name, photo, or private affairs exposed or made public without giving consent. The Health Insurance Portability and Accountability Act of 1996 (HIPAA) protects the privacy and security of a person's health information. **Protected health information** refers to identifying information and information about the person's health care that is maintained or sent in any form (paper, electronic, oral). Failure to comply with HIPAA rules can result in fines, penalties, and criminal action including jail time. Follow agency policies and procedures. Direct any questions about the person or the person's care to the nurse. Box 3-5 lists ways to protect the person's privacy.
- **Fraud** is saying or doing something to trick, fool, or deceive a person. The act is fraud if it does or could cause harm to a person or the person's property.

Crimes

Murder, robbery, rape, kidnapping, and abuse are crimes. So is possession of a controlled substance. Assault and battery may result in both civil and criminal charges.

Assault and Battery. Assault is intentionally attempting or threatening to touch a person's body without the person's consent. The person fears bodily harm.

BOX 3-5 **Protecting the Right to Privacy**

- Keep all information about the person confidential.
- Cover the person when he or she is being moved in hallways.
- Screen the person. Close the privacy curtain and the door when giving care. Also, close window coverings.
- Expose only the body part involved in care or a procedure.
- Do not discuss the person or the person's treatment with anyone except the nurse supervising your work. "Shop talk" is a common cause of invasion of privacy. ("Shop talk" is jargon or subject matter related to your work.)
- Ask visitors to leave the room when care is given.
- Do not open the person's mail.
- Allow the person to visit with others in private.
- Allow the person to use the phone in private.
- Follow agency policies and procedures required to protect privacy. This includes those related to computer use.
- Never share information about a patient or resident on social media.
- Never post pictures of patients or residents on social media.

Battery is touching a person's body without his or her consent. Consent is the important factor in assault and battery. The person must consent to any procedure, treatment, or other act that involves touching the body. The person has the right to withdraw consent at any time.

Protect yourself from being accused of assault and battery. Explain to the person what is to be done and get the person's consent. Consent may be verbal—"yes" or "okay." Or it can be a gesture—a nod, turning over for a back rub, or holding out an arm so you can take a pulse.

Possession of Controlled Substances. Federal and state laws make the possession of controlled substances without a prescription a crime. Nurses give controlled substances only under the direction of a licensed health care provider.

Nurses can have controlled substances in their possession if:

- The nurse is giving a controlled substance to a person under a doctor's order.
- The nurse is a patient for whom a doctor has prescribed a controlled substance.
- The nurse is the official custodian of a limited supply of controlled substances on a nursing unit in an agency.

A controlled substance may be ordered for a person but not used. The drug must be returned to where it was obtained, such as the doctor or pharmacy.

Violating or failing to comply with the Controlled Substance Act can result in a fine, a prison term, or both. State laws vary about MA-Cs giving Schedule II drugs. So do MA-C job descriptions. You must know what your state and agency allow you to do.

REPORTING ABUSE

Abuse is the intentional mistreatment or harm of another person. Abuse is a crime. It can occur at home or in a health care agency. Abuse has one or more of these elements:

- Willful causing of injury
- Unreasonable confinement
- Intimidation (to make afraid with threats of force or violence)
- Punishment
- Depriving the person of the goods or services needed for physical, mental, or psychosocial well-being

Abuse causes physical harm, pain, or mental anguish. Protection against abuse extends to persons in a coma. The abuser is usually a family member or caregiver—spouse, partner, adult child, and others. The abuser can be a friend, neighbor, landlord, or other person. Both men and women are abusers. Both men and women are abused.

State laws, accrediting agencies, and OBRA do not allow agencies to employ persons who were convicted of abuse, neglect, or mistreatment. Before hiring, the agency must thoroughly check the applicant's work history. All references are checked. Efforts must be made to find out about any criminal records.

The agency also checks nursing assistive personnel registries for findings of abuse, neglect, or mistreatment. It also is checked for misusing or stealing a person's property.

Vulnerable Adults

Vulnerable comes from the Latin word *vulnerare*, which means *to wound*. **Vulnerable adults** are persons 18 years old or older who have disabilities or conditions that make them at risk to be wounded, attacked, or damaged. They have problems caring for or protecting themselves due to:

- A mental, emotional, physical, or developmental disability
- Brain damage
- Changes from aging

All patients and residents, regardless of age, are considered vulnerable. Older persons and children are at risk for abuse.

Elder Abuse

Elder abuse is any knowing, intentional, or negligent act by a caregiver or any other person to an older adult. The act causes harm or serious risk of harm. Nursing assistive personnel can lose their certification, license, or registration because of elder abuse. Elder abuse can take these forms:

- *Physical abuse.* This involves inflicting, or threatening to inflict, pain or injury. Grabbing, hitting, slapping, kicking, pinching, hair-pulling, or beating are examples. It also includes *corporal punishment*—punishment inflicted directly on the body. Beatings, lashings, and whippings are examples. Depriving the person of a basic need also is physical abuse.
- *Neglect.* Failure to provide the person with the goods or services needed to avoid physical harm, mental anguish, or mental illness is called **neglect.** This includes failure to provide health care or treatment, food, clothing, hygiene, shelter, or other needs. In health care, neglect includes but is not limited to:
  - Leaving the person lying or sitting in urine or feces
  - Keeping persons alone in their rooms or other areas
  - Failing to answer call lights
- *Verbal abuse.* Using oral or written words or statements that speak badly of, sneer at, criticize, or condemn the person is called verbal abuse. It includes unkind gestures.
- *Involuntary seclusion.* This involves confining the person to a certain area. People have been locked in closets, basements, attics, and other spaces.
- *Financial exploitation or misappropriation.* To *exploit* means to use unjustly. **Misappropriation** means to dishonestly, unfairly, or wrongly take for one's own use. The older person's resources (money, property, assets) are misused by another person. Or the resources are used for the other person's profit or benefit. The person's money is stolen or used by another person. It is also misusing a person's property.
- *Emotional or mental abuse.* This involves inflicting mental pain, anguish, or distress through verbal or nonverbal acts. Humiliation, harassment, ridicule, and threats of punishment are examples. It includes being deprived of needs such as food, clothing, care, a home, or a place to sleep.
- *Sexual abuse.* The person is harassed about sex or is attacked sexually. The person may be forced to perform sexual acts out of fear of punishment or physical harm.
- *Abandonment. Abandon* means to leave or desert someone. The person is deserted by someone who is responsible for his or her care.

There are many signs of elder abuse. The abused person may show only some of the signs in Box 3-6.

Federal and state laws require the reporting of elder abuse. The Elder Justice Act became law in 2010. It explains how suspected abuse should be reported. The law states that if a center

BOX 3-6 Signs of Elder Abuse

- Living conditions are unsafe, unclean, or inadequate.
- Personal hygiene is lacking. The person is not clean. Clothes are dirty.
- Weight loss—there are signs of poor nutrition and inadequate fluid intake.
- Assistive devices are missing or broken—eyeglasses, hearing aids, dentures, cane, walker.
- Medical needs are not met.
- Frequent injuries—conditions behind the injuries are strange or seem impossible.
- Old and new injuries—bruises, pressure marks, welts, scars, fractures, and punctures.
- Complaints of pain or itching in the genital area.
- Bleeding and bruising around the breasts or in the genital area.
- Burns on the feet, hands, buttocks, or other parts of the body. Cigarettes and cigars cause small circle-like burns.
- Pressure ulcers or contractures.
- The person seems very quiet or withdrawn.
- Unexplained withdrawal from normal activities.
- The person seems fearful, anxious, or agitated.
- Sudden change in alertness.
- Depression.
- Sudden changes in finances.
- The person does not seem to want to talk or answer questions.
- The person is restrained. Or the person is locked in a certain area for long periods.
- The person cannot reach toilet facilities, food, water, and other needed items.
- Private conversations are not allowed. The caregiver is present during all conversations.
- Strained or tense relationships with a caregiver.
- Frequent arguments with a caregiver.
- The person seems anxious to please the caregiver.
- Drugs are not taken properly. Drugs are not bought. Or too much or too little of the drug is taken.
- Visits to the emergency room may be frequent.
- The person may change doctors often. Some people do not have a doctor.

receives federal funding, they can be fined if suspected abuse is not reported immediately. The law also states that a person who reports suspected abuse cannot be punished by the center. You may suspect abuse. If so, discuss the matter and your observations with the nurse. Give as many details as possible. The nurse contacts health team members as needed.

The nurse also contacts community agencies that investigate elder abuse. They act at once if the problem is life-threatening. Sometimes the help of police or the courts is necessary.

Child Abuse and Neglect

Child abuse and neglect is the intentional harm or mistreatment of a child younger than 18 years old. It involves the following:

- Any recent act or failure to act on the part of a parent or caregiver.
- The act or failure to act results in death, serious physical or emotional harm, sexual abuse, or exploitation.
- The act or failure to act presents a likely or immediate risk for harm.

The abuser usually is a household member—a parent, a parent's partner, a brother or sister, or a nanny. Usually an abuser is someone the family knows. Just like with elder abuse, the abuser can be a friend, neighbor, landlord, or other person.

Types of Child Abuse and Neglect. Child abuse and neglect can take different forms. Often more than one type is present.

- *Physical abuse* is injuring the child on purpose. It can cause bruising, fractures, or death. Physical abuse includes striking, kicking, burning, biting, shaking, punching, or beating the child. Any action that injures the child is physical abuse.
- *Neglect* is failing to provide for a child's basic needs. Neglect generally includes the following categories:
  - *Physical neglect* is failure to provide necessary food, shelter, or supervision.
  - *Medical neglect* is failure to provide necessary medical or mental health treatment. (If the treatment is against a religious belief, this is not considered medical neglect.)
  - *Educational neglect* is failure to educate a child or attend to special education needs.
  - *Emotional neglect* is not meeting a child's emotional needs. Allowing a child to use drugs or alcohol is also emotional abuse.
- *Sexual abuse* is using, persuading, or forcing a child to engage in sexual contact, activity, or behavior. It can take many forms and does not need to include physical contact between the abuser and the child.
  - *Rape or sexual assault*—forced sexual acts with a person against his or her will.
  - *Molestation*—sexual advances toward a child. It includes kissing, touching, or fondling sexual areas. The abuser may kiss, touch, or fondle the child. Or the child is forced to kiss, touch, or fondle the abuser.
  - *Incest*—sexual activity between family members. The abuser may be a parent, stepparent, brother or sister, stepbrother or stepsister, aunt or uncle, cousin, or grandparent.
  - *Child pornography*—taking pictures or videotaping a child involved in sexual acts.

- *Child prostitution*—forcing a child to engage in sexual activity for money. Usually the child is forced to have many sexual partners.
- *Emotional abuse* is injuring the child mentally or his or her sense of self-worth. The abuser may constantly criticize, threaten, or reject the child. Emotional abuse also includes withholding love, support, or guidance. The child has changes in behavior, emotional responses, thinking, reasoning, learning, and so on. The child may show anxiety, depression, withdrawal, or aggressive behaviors.
- *Parental substance abuse* is part of child abuse and neglect in some states. It is harmful to children of any age to be exposed to illegal drug activity in their homes or environment.
- *Substance abuse* involves:
  - Making a controlled substance in the presence of a child
  - Making a controlled substance on the premises occupied by a child
  - Allowing a child to be present where there are chemicals or equipment used to make or store a controlled substance
  - Selling, distributing, or giving drugs or alcohol to a child
  - Using a controlled substance that impairs a caregiver's ability to adequately care for a child
  - Exposing a child to equipment and supplies for using, selling, or distributing drugs
  - Exposing a child to other drug-related activities
- *Abandonment* is when a parent's identity or whereabouts are unknown. The child is left by the parent in circumstances where the child suffers serious harm. Or the parent fails to maintain contact with the child or provide support for the child.

Box 3-7 lists some of the signs and symptoms of child abuse and neglect. You must be alert for any unexplained changes in the

---

BOX 3-7 Signs and Symptoms of Child Abuse and Neglect

Physical Abuse
- Bruises or welts on the face (eyes, lips, mouth, cheeks), back, buttocks, abdomen, chest, and inner thighs.
- The injury matches the shape of the object causing the welt may be seen. The shape may be of a belt, belt buckle, wooden spoon, chain, clothes hanger, rope, or other object.
- Burns and scalds on the feet, hands, back, buttocks, or other body parts.
- Intentional burns leave a pattern from the item causing the burn: cigarettes, irons, curling irons, ropes, stove burners, and radiators are examples.
- In scalds, the area put in hot liquid is clearly marked. For example, a scald to the hand looks like a glove. A scald to the foot looks like a sock.
- Fractures of the nose, skull, arms, or legs.
- Bite marks.
- Injuries that do not match the explanation.

Neglect
- Fails to gain weight
- Wants to eat large amounts of food
- Steals food
- Is dirty or has a severe body odor
- Lacks the correct clothing for the weather
- Abuses alcohol or drugs
- States that no one is home

Sexual Abuse
- Bleeding, cuts, and bruises of the genitalia, anus, breasts, or mouth
- Stains or blood on underclothing
- Painful urination
- Signs and symptoms of urinary tract infection
- Vaginal discharge
- Genital pain and/or odor
- Difficulty walking or sitting
- Pregnancy or sexually transmitted infection
- Fearful behaviors—nightmares, depression, unusual fears, attempts to run away
- Sexual behavior that does not fit with one's age
- Attaches very quickly to strangers or new adults

Emotional Abuse
- Sudden changes in self-confidence
- Delay in emotional or physical development
- Depression or suicidal thoughts
- Headaches
- Stomachaches
- Abnormal fears
- Nightmares
- Attempts to run away

child's body or behavior. Child and parent behaviors may signal that something is wrong. The child may be quiet and withdrawn. He or she may fear adults. Sometimes children are afraid to go home. Sudden behavior changes are common in sexual abuse. Bed-wetting, thumb-sucking, loss of appetite, poor grades, and running away from home are examples. Some children attempt suicide.

Parents give different stories about what happened. Injuries are blamed on play accidents or other children. Frequent emergency room visits are common.

Child abuse is complex. Many more behaviors, signs, and symptoms are present than are discussed here. The health team must be alert for signs and symptoms of child abuse. All states require the reporting of suspected child abuse. However, someone should not be falsely accused.

If you suspect child abuse, share your concerns with the nurse. Give as much detail as you can. The nurse contacts health team members and child protection agencies as needed.

Domestic Abuse

Domestic abuse—also called domestic violence, intimate partner abuse, partner abuse, and spousal abuse—occurs in relationships. One partner has power and control over the other. Such power and control occur through abuse where the abuser prevents a partner from doing what they wish or forces them to behave in a way they don't want. Domestic abuse causes fear and harm. Abuse may be physical, sexual, emotional/verbal, economic, or social. Usually more than one type of abuse is present.

*   *Physical abuse*—unwanted punching, slapping, grabbing, choking, poking, biting, pulling hair, twisting arms, or kicking. It may involve burns and weapons. Withholding food or sleep is also abuse. Death is a constant threat.
*   *Sexual abuse*—unwanted sexual contact. Withholding sex from the victim as a control mechanism is also considered abuse.
*   *Emotional/verbal abuse*—unkind and hurtful remarks and name-calling. They make the person feel unwhole, unattractive, and without value.
    *   *Digital abuse*—the use of technologies such as texting and social networking to bully, harass, stalk, or intimidate a partner. Often this behavior is a form of verbal or emotional abuse perpetrated online.
*   *Economic abuse*—controlling money. Having or not having a job is controlled by the abuser. So are paychecks, money gifts from family and friends, and money for household expenses (food, clothing).
*   *Social abuse*—controlling friendships and other relationships. The abuser controls phone calls, car use, leaving the home, and visits with family and friends. Trapping a partner in their home and isolating them from friends and family is abuse.

Patients and residents can suffer from domestic abuse. For example, one partner slaps the other during a visit. Or a spouse uses another spouse's money for their own benefit rather than buying her husband's blood pressure medication.

Domestic abuse is a safety issue. Like child and elder abuse, domestic abuse is complex. The victim often hides the abuse. He or she may protect the abusive partner. State laws vary about reporting domestic abuse. It is the ethical duty of the health team to give information about safety and community resources. If you suspect domestic abuse, share your concerns with the nurse. The nurse gathers information to help the person.

REVIEW QUESTIONS

Circle the BEST answer.

1. Ethics is:
   a. making judgments before you have the facts
   b. knowledge of what is right and wrong conduct
   c. a behavior that meets your needs, not the person's
   d. skills, care, and judgments required of a health team member

2. Which of the following is ethical behavior?
   a. sharing information about a patient with your family
   b. accepting gifts from a resident's family
   c. reporting errors
   d. calling your family before answering a signal light

3. A person has made an advance directive. The person wants measures removed that prolong dying. What should you do about the drugs ordered?
   a. Discuss the drug orders with the nurse.
   b. Withhold the drugs.
   c. Give the drugs as needed.
   d. Return the drugs to the pharmacy.

4. Which advanced directive follows the person from the care center to the hospital?
   a. living will
   b. do not resuscitate
   c. Physician Orders for Life-Sustaining Treatment
   d. durable power of attorney

5. The Federal Food, Drug, and Cosmetic Act requires the following, *except:*
   a. that a drug is safe before it is marketed
   b. that manufacturers meet labeling requirements
   c. that advertising standards are met
   d. that drugs fit into one of the five drug classifications

6. What is another name for the Comprehensive Drug Abuse Prevention and Control Act?
   a. the Federal Food, Drug, and Cosmetic Act
   b. the Patient Self-Determination Act
   c. the Controlled Substance Act
   d. the Omnibus Budget Reconciliation Act

7. A prescription must contain the following, *except:*
   a. the cost of the drug
   b. the prescriber's DEA registration number
   c. the name of the patient or resident
   d. the date the prescription was issued
8. Which has no medical use in the United States?
   a. Schedule I drugs
   b. Schedule II drugs
   c. Schedule III drugs
   d. Schedule IV drugs
9. Which is *not* a crime?
   a. abuse
   b. murder
   c. negligence
   d. robbery
10. These statements are about negligence. Which is *true?*
    a. It is an intentional tort.
    b. The negligent person acted in a reasonable manner.
    c. Harm was caused to a person or a person's property.
    d. A prison term is likely.
11. Threatening to touch the person's body without the person's consent is:
    a. assault
    b. battery
    c. defamation
    d. false imprisonment
12. Restraining a person's freedom of movement is:
    a. assault
    b. battery
    c. defamation
    d. false imprisonment
13. Photos of a patient are shown to others without their consent. This is:
    a. battery
    b. fraud
    c. invasion of privacy
    d. malpractice
14. A person asks if you are a nurse. You answer "yes." This is:
    a. negligence
    b. fraud
    c. libel
    d. slander
15. Who is at risk for being wounded, attacked, or damaged?
    a. children
    b. older adults
    c. persons with disabilities
    d. all patients and residents
16. You scold an older person for refusing to take ordered drugs. This is:
    a. physical abuse
    b. neglect
    c. emotional abuse
    d. verbal abuse
17. Which is *not* part of the Elder Justice Act?
    a. An elder person has rights to privacy and to make their own health care decisions.

    b. If a center receives federal funding, they can be fined if suspected abuse is not reported immediately.
    c. It explains how suspected abuse should be reported.
    d. A person who reports suspected abuse cannot be punished by the center.
18. A child is deprived of food, clothing, and shelter. This is:
    a. abuse
    b. physical neglect
    c. abandonment
    d. emotional abuse
19. A child has a black eye, bruises on her face, and bite marks on her arms. These are signs of:
    a. physical abuse
    b. sexual abuse
    c. neglect
    d. substance abuse
20. A child complains of painful urination and has blood on their underclothing. These are signs of:
    a. physical abuse
    b. sexual abuse
    c. neglect
    d. substance abuse
21. You notice a child has a delay in their emotional development and appears depressed. These are signs of:
    a. physical abuse
    b. emotional abuse
    c. neglect
    d. substance abuse
22. These statements are about domestic abuse. Which is *true?*
    a. It always involves physical harm.
    b. It always involves violence.
    c. One partner has control over the other partner.
    d. Only one type of abuse is usually present.
23. You suspect a person was abused. What should you do?
    a. Tell the family.
    b. Call the police.
    c. Tell the nurse.
    d. Ask the person about the abuse.

Circle T if the statement is true. Circle F if the statement is false.

24 T F   An older person's money is taken and misused by another person. This is an example of misappropriation.
25 T F   All Schedule V drugs require a prescription.
26 T F   Possessing a controlled substance without a valid prescription is a crime.
27 T F   Withholding sex from a person as a control mechanism is considered sexual abuse.
28 T F   The use of technologies such as texting and social networking to bully, harass, stalk, or intimidate a partner is a form of verbal or emotional abuse perpetrated online.

Answers to these questions can be found on the Evolve Resources site: http://evolve.elsevier.com/Anderson/medasst/

4

Assisting With the Nursing Process

OBJECTIVES

- Define the key terms and key abbreviations used in this chapter.
- Explain the purpose of the nursing process.
- Describe the steps of the nursing process
- Explain your role in each step of the nursing process.
- Explain the difference between objective data and subjective data.
- Identify the observations that you need to report to the nurse.
- Explain how to measure vital signs, weight and height, and blood glucose.
- Explain how to communicate with the nursing team.
- Explain how to accurately report and record vital signs, weight and height, blood glucose, and other patient data.
- Perform the procedures described in this chapter.

PROCEDURES

- Taking a Temperature
- Taking a Pulse
- Counting Respirations
- Measuring Blood Pressure
- Measuring Weight and Height
- Measuring Blood Glucose

KEY TERMS

assessment Collecting information about the person; a step in the nursing process

end-of-shift report A report that the nurse gives at the end of the shift to the oncoming shift

evaluation To measure whether goals in the planning step were met; a step in the nursing process

implementation To perform or carry out nursing measures in the care plan; a step in the nursing process

medical diagnosis The identification of a disease or condition by a doctor

nursing care plan A written guide about the person's care; care plan

nursing diagnosis Describes a health problem that can be treated by nursing measures; a step in the nursing process

nursing intervention An action or measure taken by the nursing team to help the person reach a goal; nursing measure, nursing action

nursing process The method nurses use to plan and deliver nursing care; its five steps are assessment, nursing diagnosis, planning, implementation, and evaluation

objective data Information that is seen, heard, felt, or smelled by an observer; signs

observation Using the senses of sight, hearing, touch, and smell to collect information

planning Setting priorities and goals; a step in the nursing process

signs See "objective data"

subjective data Things a person tells you about that you cannot observe through your senses; symptoms

symptoms See "subjective data"

vital signs Temperature, pulse, respirations, blood pressure, and pain

KEY ABBREVIATIONS

BP Blood pressure
C Celsius; centigrade
F Fahrenheit
ft Feet
Hg Mercury
HR heart rate
in Inch
IV Intravenous
kg Kilograms

lb Pound
MDS Minimum Data Set
mm Millimeter
mm Hg Millimeters of mercury
OASIS Outcome and Assessment Information Set
OBRA Omnibus Budget Reconciliation Act of 1987
OSHA Occupational Safety and Health Administration
RR Respiratory rate

Nurses communicate with each other about the person's strengths, problems, needs, and care. This information is shared through the nursing process. The **nursing process** is the method nurses use to plan and deliver nursing care. It has five steps:

- Assessment
- Nursing diagnosis
- Planning
- Implementation
- Evaluation

THE NURSING PROCESS

The nursing process is a tool used to identify a person's nursing needs. The tool helps the nurse create a plan that helps meet those needs. Good communication is needed between the person and the nursing team.

Each step is important. If done in order with good communication, nursing care is organized and has purpose. All nursing team members work toward the same goals. The person feels safe and secure with consistent care.

The nursing process is ongoing and revolves around the patient or person. New information is gathered, and the person's needs may change. However, the steps remain the same. You will see the continuous and overlapping nature of the nursing process as each step is explained (Fig. 4-1).

Assessment

Assessment involves collecting information about the person. Nurses use many sources, such as the person's health and drug

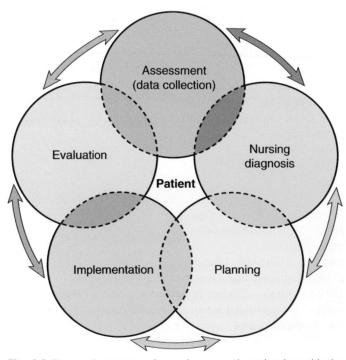

Fig. 4-1 The nursing process is continuous and overlapping with the patient's needs at the center.

history. The drug history includes drugs used currently—prescription drugs, over-the-counter drugs, herbal products, and street drugs. Drug allergies also are part of the drug history. The health and drug histories tell about current and past health problems.

The family's health history is important. Many diseases are genetic. That is, the risk for certain diseases is inherited from parents. For example, a mother had breast cancer. Her daughters are at risk.

Information from the doctor is reviewed. So are test results and past medical records.

An RN assesses the person's body systems and mental status. You assist the nurse with assessment by reporting and recording what you observe about the person.

Observation is using the senses of sight, hearing, touch, and smell to collect information:

- You *see* how the person lies, sits, or walks. You see flushed or pale skin. You see red and swollen body areas.
- You *listen* to the person breathe, talk, and cough. You use a stethoscope to listen to the heartbeat and to measure blood pressure.
- Through *touch,* you feel whether the skin is hot or cold or moist or dry. You use touch to take the person's pulse.
- *Smell* is used to detect body, wound, and breath odors. You also smell odors from urine and bowel movements.

Objective data (signs) are seen, heard, felt, or smelled by an observer. You can feel a pulse. You can see urine. You cannot feel or see the person's pain, fear, or nausea. **Subjective data (symptoms)** are things a person tells you about that you cannot observe through your senses. For example, the person says: "Whenever I take this drug, I feel sick to my stomach."

Box 4-1 lists the basic observations you need to make and report to the nurse. Box 4-2, lists the observations that you must report at once. You also measure vital signs, height, and weight. In some states and agencies, you measure blood glucose (p. 38). Make notes of your observations and measurements. Use them when reporting and recording (pp. 41).

The assessment step never ends. New information is collected with every patient or resident contact. New observations are made. The person shares more information. Often the family adds more information.

See Focus on Older Persons: Assessment.

Nursing Diagnosis

The RN uses assessment information to make a nursing diagnosis. A **nursing diagnosis** describes a health problem that can be treated by nursing interventions (or nursing measures). Some nursing diagnoses associated with drug therapy are listed in Box 4-3. The problem may exist or develop. Nursing diagnoses can relate to the desired (therapeutic) effects of drugs. They also can relate to the side effects of drugs. For example: *Risk for Injury related to side effects of confusion, disorientation, dizziness, and light-headedness.* (p. 26)

BOX 4-1 BASIC OBSERVATIONS

Ability to Respond
- Is the person easy or hard to wake up?
- Can the person give his or her name, the time, and location when asked?
- Does the person identify others correctly?
- Does the person answer questions correctly?
- Does the person speak clearly?
- Are instructions followed correctly?
- Is the person calm, restless, or excited?
- Is the person conversing, quiet, or talking a lot?

Movement
- Can the person squeeze your fingers with each hand?
- Can the person move their arms and legs?
- Are the person's movements shaky or jerky?
- Does the person complain of stiff or painful joints?

Pain or Discomfort
- Where is the pain located? (Ask the person to point to the pain.)
- Does the pain go anywhere else?
- How does the person rate the severity of the pain—mild, moderate, severe?
- How does the person rate the pain on a scale of 1 to 10 (Chapter 18)?
- When did the pain begin?
- What was the person doing when the pain began?
- How long does the pain last?
- How does the person describe the pain?
  - Sharp
  - Severe
  - Knife-like
  - Dull
  - Burning
  - Aching
  - Comes and goes
  - Depends on position
- Was a pain-relief drug given?
- Did the pain-relief drug relieve the pain? Is the pain still present?
- Is the person able to sleep and rest?
- What is the position of comfort?

Skin
- Is the skin pale or flushed?
- Is the skin cool, warm, or hot?
- Is the skin moist or dry?
- What color are the lips and nail beds?
- Is the skin intact? Are there broken areas? If yes, where?
- Are sores or reddened areas present? If yes, where?
- Are bruises present? If yes, where?
- Does the person complain of itching? If yes, where?

Eyes, Ears, Nose, and Mouth
- Is there drainage from the eyes? What color is the drainage?
- Are the eyelids closed? Do they stay open?
- Are the eyes reddened?
- Does the person complain of spots, flashes, or blurring?
- Is the person sensitive to bright lights?
- Is there drainage from the ears? What color is the drainage?
- Can the person hear? Is repeating necessary? Are questions answered correctly?

- Is there drainage from the nose? What color is the drainage?
- Can the person breathe through the nose?
- Is there breath odor?
- Does the person complain of a bad taste in the mouth?
- Does the person complain of painful gums or teeth?
- Do the gums bleed with oral hygiene?

Respirations
- Do both sides of the person's chest rise and fall with respirations?
- Is breathing labored?
- Is breathing noisy?
- Does the person complain of pain or difficulty breathing?
- What is the amount and color of sputum?
- What is the frequency of the person's cough? Is it dry or productive?

Bowels and Bladder
- Does the person use the toilet, bedside commode, bedpan, or urinal?
- Is the person continent or incontinent?
- Is the abdomen firm or soft?
- Does the person complain of gas?
- What is the amount, color, and consistency of each bowel movement?
- What is the frequency of bowel movements?
- Can the person control bowel movements?
- Does the person have pain or difficulty urinating?
- What is the amount and color of urine?
- What is the frequency of urination?
- Is the urine clear or cloudy? Are there particles in the urine?
- Does urine have a foul smell?
- Can the person control the passage of urine?

Appetite
- Does the person like the food served?
- How much of the meal is eaten?
- What foods does the person like?
- Can the person chew food?
- What is the amount of fluid taken?
- What fluids does the person like?
- How often does the person drink fluids?
- Can the person swallow food and fluids?
- Does the person complain of nausea?
- What is the amount and color of the vomit?
- Does the person have hiccups?
- Is the person belching?
- Does the person cough when swallowing?

Activities of Daily Living
- Can the person perform personal care without help?
- Bathing?
- Brushing teeth?
- Combing and brushing hair?
- Shaving?
- Does the person feed himself or herself?
- Can the person walk?
- What amount and kind of help is needed?

Bleeding
- Is the person bleeding from any body part? If yes, where and how much?

BOX 4-2　Observations to Report at Once

- A change in the person's ability to respond
  - A responsive person is no longer responsive.
  - A non-responsive person is now responsive.
- A change in the person's mobility
  - The person cannot move a body part.
  - The person can now move a body part.
- Complaints of sudden, severe pain
- A sore or reddened area on the person's skin
- Complaints of a sudden change in vision
- Complaints of pain or difficulty breathing
- Abnormal respirations
- Complaints of or signs of difficulty swallowing
- Vomiting
- Bleeding
- Dizziness
- Diarrhea
- Vital signs outside their normal ranges

BOX 4-3　Brief List of Nursing Diagnoses Associated With Drug Therapy

- Activity Intolerance
- Acute Confusion
- Acute Pain
- Anxiety
- Chronic Confusion
- Chronic Pain
- Constipation
- Decreased Cardiac Output
- Diarrhea
- Fatigue
- Fluid Volume Deficit
- Fluid Volume Excess
- Grieving
- Imbalanced Nutrition
- Impaired Dressing and Grooming
- Impaired Gas Exchange
- Impaired Memory
- Impaired Physical Mobility
- Impaired Swallowing
- Impaired Tissue Integrity
- Impaired Urinary System Function
- Impaired Verbal Communication
- Ineffective Airway Clearance
- Ineffective Breathing Pattern
- Ineffective Coping
- Ineffective Tissue Perfusion
- Insomnia
- Knowledge Deficit
- Nausea
- Noncompliance
- Risk for Aspiration
- Risk for Falls
- Risk for Infection
- Risk for Injury
- Risk for Unstable Blood Glucose Level
- Risk for Violence
- Sexual Dysfunction

FOCUS ON OLDER PERSONS
Assessment

Long-Term Care

The Omnibus Budget Reconciliation Act of 1987 (OBRA) requires the Minimum Data Set (MDS) for nursing center residents. The MDS is an assessment and screening tool. The form is completed when the person is admitted to the center. It provides extensive information about the person. Examples include memory, communication, hearing and vision, physical function, and activities.

Your observations will help the nurse complete the MDS. Other members of the person's health care team also help complete the MDS. The RN responsible for the person's care makes sure the MDS is complete. The MDS is updated before each care conference. A new MDS is completed once a year and whenever a significant change occurs in the person's health status. An RN signs the MDS. A signed MDS means that it is complete and accurate.

Home Health

Medicare-certified home care agencies use the Outcome and Assessment Information Set (OASIS). It is used for adult home care patients. The OASIS is a tool used to collect assessment and observation information . It also helps with planning a person's care.

Nursing diagnoses and medical diagnoses are not the same. A **medical diagnosis** is the identification of a disease or condition by a doctor. Cancer, stroke, heart attack, infection, and diabetes are examples. Doctors order drugs, therapies, and surgery to cure or heal.

A person can have many nursing diagnoses. They deal with the total person—physical, emotional, social, and spiritual needs. They may change as assessment information changes. Or new nursing diagnoses are added.

Planning

The person, family, and health team help the RN plan care. **Planning** involves setting priorities and goals. Priorities relate to what is most important for the person. Goals are aimed at the person's highest level of well-being and function—physical, emotional, social, and spiritual. Goals promote health and prevent health problems. They also promote rehabilitation.

Nursing interventions are chosen after goals are set. An *intervention* is an action or measure. A **nursing intervention** is an action or measure taken by the nursing team to help the person reach a goal. *Nursing intervention, nursing action,* and *nursing measure* mean the same thing. A nursing intervention does not need a doctor's order. Nursing interventions related to drug therapy include:

- Taking actions that minimize the expected side effects. For example, a drug causes dry mouth. The care plan includes frequent oral hygiene.
- Reporting unexpected side effects such as those listed in Box 4-2.

Some nursing measures come from a doctor's order. For example, a doctor orders a pain-relief drug for Mrs. Lange. The nurse includes this order in the care plan.

The **nursing care plan (care plan)** is a written guide about the care a person should receive. It has the person's nursing diagnoses and goals. It also has the measures or actions needed in order to reach each goal. The care plan is a communication tool. Nursing staff use it to see what care to give. The care plan helps ensure that the nursing team members provide care that meets the person's needs.

Each agency has a care plan form. It is found in the medical record, on the Kardex, or on a computer.

The RN may conduct a care conference to share information and ideas about the person's care. During a care conference, the resident and family discuss the resident's care and needs. The purpose is to develop or revise the person's nursing care plan. Effective care is the goal. Nursing assistants usually take part in the conference.

The plan is carried out. It may change as the person's nursing diagnoses change.

Implementation

To *implement* means to perform or carry out. The **implementation** step is performing or carrying out the nursing measures included in the care plan. Care is given in this step.

Nursing care ranges from simple to complex. The nurse delegates nursing tasks that are within your legal limits and job description. The nurse may ask you to assist with complex measures.

You report the care given to the nurse. You record the care given in the person's medical record. Reporting and recording are done *after* giving care, not before. Also report and record your observations. Observing is part of assessment. New observations may change the nursing diagnoses. If so, care plan changes are made. To give correct care, you need to know about any changes in the care plan.

Evaluation

Evaluation means to measure. The **evaluation** step involves measuring whether the goals in the planning step were met. Progress is evaluated. Goals may be met, not met, or partially met. Assessment information is used for this step. Changes in nursing diagnoses, goals, and the care plan may result.

It is the RN's responsibility to evaluate the goals related to drug therapy. The RN will:
- Assess the person's response to the drug prescribed
- Observe for signs and symptoms of recurring illness
- Observe for signs and symptoms of adverse drug effects
- Determine the person's ability to receive information about their drugs
- Determine the person's ability to self-administer drugs
- Assess whether the person will comply with ordered drug therapies—take drugs as ordered, at the right time, in the right way

The nursing process never ends. Nurses constantly collect information about the person. Nursing diagnoses, goals, and the care plan may change as the person's needs change.

ASSISTING WITH ASSESSMENT

Vital signs, weight, and blood glucose are measurements used to assess and evaluate the person's response to drug therapy. Often a specific measurement is needed before giving a drug. For example, a person is to receive a drug that lowers the pulse. Before giving the drug, you take the person's pulse. If the pulse is too low, the nurse tells you not to give the drug.

Accurate measurements are essential. So are accurate reporting and recording.

Vital Signs

The **vital signs** of body function are:
- Temperature
- Pulse
- Respirations
- Blood pressure
- Pain (Chapter 18)

A person's vital signs vary within certain limits. They are affected by sleep, activity, eating, weather, noise, exercise, drugs, anger, fear, anxiety, pain, and illness.

Vital signs are part of the assessment step in the nursing process. They are measured to detect changes in normal body function. They tell about responses to treatment. They often signal life-threatening events.

The person should be at rest when vital signs are measured. Unless otherwise ordered, measure temperature, pulse, respirations, and blood pressure with the person lying or sitting. You should report the following vital signs immediately:
- Any vital sign that is changed from a prior measurement
- Vital signs above the normal range
- Vital signs below the normal range

You learned how to measure vital signs in your CNA training program. A basic review is provided here.

Body Temperature. *Body temperature* is the amount of heat in the body. It is a balance between the amount of heat produced and the amount lost by the body.

Thermometers are used to measure temperature. It is measured using the Fahrenheit (F) and centigrade or Celsius (C) scales. See Box 4-4 for temperature sites. See Table 4-1 for the normal ranges for each site.

Glass Thermometers. The glass thermometer is filled with a mercury-free mixture. When heated, the substance expands and rises in the tube. When cooled, the substance contracts and moves down the tube.

PROMOTING SAFETY AND COMFORT
Glass Thermometers

Safety

Mercury glass thermometers are no longer used today. Glass thermometers are now filled with a mercury-free mixture. Do not assume all glass thermometers are mercury-free. Some patients in home settings may still have mercury thermometers. Swallowed mercury can cause mercury poisoning. Therefore, the Occupational Safety and Health Administration (OSHA) recommends using mercury-free devices.

Glass thermometers break easily. Broken rectal thermometers can injure the rectum and colon. The person may bite down and break an oral thermometer. Cuts in the mouth are risks. Whenever possible, use an electronic thermometer instead of a glass thermometer.

If a mercury-glass thermometer breaks, tell the nurse at once. Mercury is a hazardous substance. Do not touch the mercury. Do not let the person do so. Follow agency procedures for handling hazardous materials.

Do the following to prevent infection, promote safety, and obtain an accurate measurement:
- Use the person's thermometer.
- Use a rectal thermometer only for rectal temperatures.
- Follow Standard Precautions and the Bloodborne Pathogen Standard (Chapter 6).

BOX 4-4   Temperature Sites

Oral Site
Oral temperatures are *not* taken if the person:
- Is an infant or child younger than 5 years of age
- Is unconscious
- Has had surgery or an injury to the face, neck, nose, or mouth
- Is receiving oxygen
- Breathes through the mouth
- Has a nasogastric tube
- Is delirious, restless, confused, or disoriented
- Is paralyzed on one side of the body
- Has a sore mouth
- Has a convulsive (seizure) disorder

Rectal Site
Rectal temperatures are taken when the oral site cannot be used. The modified left lateral recumbent position is used for a rectal temperature. It is the preferred site for infants and children younger than 3 years old.
Rectal temperatures are *not* taken if the person:
- Has diarrhea
- Has a rectal disorder or injury

- Has heart disease
- Had rectal surgery
- Is confused or agitated

Tympanic Membrane Site
The site has fewer microbes than the mouth or rectum. The risk of spreading infection is reduced. This site is *not* used if the person has:
- An ear disorder
- Ear drainage

Temporal Artery Site
Measures body temperature at the temporal artery in the forehead. The site is non-invasive.

Axillary (underarm) Site
Less reliable than the other sites. It is used when the other sites cannot be used.

Table 4-1   Normal Body Temperatures

Site	Baseline	Normal Range
Oral	98.6° F (37° C)	97.6° to 99.6° F (36.5° to 37.5° C)
Rectal	99.6° F (37.5° C)	98.6° to 100.6° F (37.0° to 38.1° C)
Tympanic membrane	98.6° F (37° C)	97.6° to 99.6° F (36.5° to 37.5° C)
Temporal artery	98.6° F (37° C)	97.6° to 99.6° F (36.5° to 37.5° C)
Axillary	97.6° F (36.5° C)	96.6° to 98.6° F (35.9° to 37.0° C)

Glass thermometers are reusable. Long- or slender-tip thermometers are used for oral and axillary temperatures (Fig. 4-2, A). So are thermometers with pear-shaped tips (Fig. 4-2, C). Rectal thermometers have stubby tips (Fig. 4-2, B). The stem of glass thermometers is color-coded:
- Blue—oral and axillary thermometers
- Red—rectal thermometers

See Promoting Safety and Comfort: Glass Thermometers.

Electronic Thermometers. Electronic thermometers are used for oral, rectal, and axillary temperatures (Fig. 4-3). The temperature is measured in a few seconds and is shown on the front of the device. Rectal temperatures typically require a separate rectal probe. Rectal probes are always colored red.

A disposable probe cover (sheath) protects the probe. The probe cover is discarded immediately after use. This helps prevent the spread of infection.

Tympanic Membrane Thermometers. Tympanic membrane thermometers measure temperature at the tympanic membrane in the ear (Fig. 4-4). The covered probe is inserted in the ear. The temperature is measured in 1 to 3 seconds.

These thermometers are comfortable. They are not invasive like rectal thermometers. The ear has fewer microbes than the mouth or rectum. There is less risk of spreading infection. Do not check a tympanic temperature if there is ear drainage or if the person complains of an earache.

Temporal Artery Thermometers. Body temperature is measured at the temporal artery (Fig. 4-5). The device is gently stroked across the forehead and temporal artery. The temperature of the

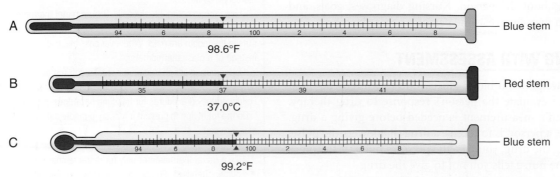

Fig. 4-2 Types of glass thermometers. **A,** The long or slender tip. **B,** The stubby tip (rectal thermometer). **C,** The pear-shaped tip.

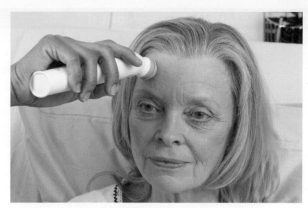

Fig. 4-5 Temporal artery thermometer.

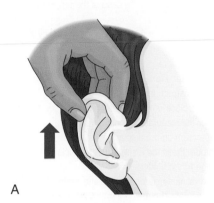

A

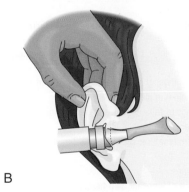

B

Fig. 4-3 The covered probe of the electronic thermometer is inserted under the tongue.

Fig. 4-4 Using a tympanic membrane thermometer. **A,** The ear is pulled up and back. **B,** The probe is inserted into the ear canal.

blood in the temporal artery is measured—the same temperature as the blood from the heart.

Body temperature is measured in 3 to 4 seconds. Follow the manufacturer's instructions for using, cleaning, and storing the device. Some devices have probe covers.

Taking Temperatures. The site used to measure body temperature depends on the person's condition. The equipment used depends on the site and what is used in your agency.

See *Delegation Guidelines: Taking Temperatures.*

See *Promoting Safety and Comfort: Taking Temperatures.*

DELEGATION GUIDELINES

Taking Temperatures

Before taking a person's temperature, you need this information from the nurse and the care plan:
- What site to use for each person—oral, rectal, axillary, tympanic membrane, or temporal artery
- What thermometer to use for each person—glass, electronic, or other type
- How long to leave a glass thermometer in place
- When to take temperatures
- Which persons are at risk for elevated temperatures
- What observations to report and record:
  - A temperature that is changed from a prior measurement
  - A temperature above or below the normal range for the site used
- When to report observations
- What specific patient or resident concerns to report at once

TAKING A TEMPERATURE

Quality of Life

Remember to:
- Knock before entering the person's room.
- Address the person by name.
- Introduce yourself by name and title.
- Explain the procedure to the person before starting and during the procedure.
- Protect the person's rights during the procedure.
- Handle the person gently during the procedure.

Pre-procedure

1. Follow *Delegation Guidelines: Taking Temperatures.* See *Promoting Safety and Comfort:*
   - *Glass Thermometers,* p. 27
   - *Taking Temperatures,* p. 31
2. For an *oral temperature,* ask the person not to eat, drink, smoke, or chew gum for at least 15 to 20 minutes or as required by agency policy.

TAKING A TEMPERATURE—cont'd

3. Perform hand hygiene.
4. Collect the following:
   - Thermometer—glass, electronic, tympanic membrane, or temporal artery
   - Probe and probe covers (if needed)
   - Plastic covers if used (glass thermometers)
   - Gloves
   - Toilet tissue (rectal temperature)
   - Water-soluble lubricant (rectal temperature)
   - Towel (axillary temperature)
5. Plug the oral or rectal probe into the electronic thermometer.
6. Identify the person. Check the ID bracelet against the assignment sheet. Also call the person by name.
7. Provide for privacy.

Procedure

8. Position the person for an oral, rectal, axillary, or tympanic membrane temperature.
9. Put on gloves if contact with blood, body fluids, secretions, or excretions is likely.
10. For a *glass thermometer:*
    a. Rinse the glass thermometer in cold water if it was soaking in a disinfectant. Dry it with tissues.
    b. Check for breaks, cracks, or chips.
    c. Shake down the thermometer below the lowest number. Hold the thermometer by the stem.
    d. Insert it into a plastic cover if used.
    e. Hold the probe in place for the time indicated depending on the site. Follow agency policy.
    f. Remove the glass thermometer.
    g. Use tissues to remove the plastic cover. Discard the cover and tissues. Wipe the thermometer with a tissue if no cover was used. Wipe from the stem to the bulb end. Discard the tissue.
    h. Read the thermometer.
       (1) Hold it at the stem. Bring it to eye level.
       (2) Turn it until you can see the numbers and the long and short lines.
       (3) Turn it back and forth slowly until you can see the silver or red line (Fig. 4-6).
       (4) Read the nearest degree (long line). For a Fahrenheit (F) thermometer, every other long line is an even degree from 94° to 108° F. For a centigrade thermometer, each long line means 1 degree.
       (5) Read the nearest tenth of a degree (short line). For a Fahrenheit thermometer, the short lines mean 0.2 (two-tenths) of a degree. For a centigrade thermometer, each short line means 0.1 (one-tenth) of a degree.
    i. Note the person's name, temperature, and temperature site on your notepad or assignment sheet.
    j. Shake down the glass thermometer.

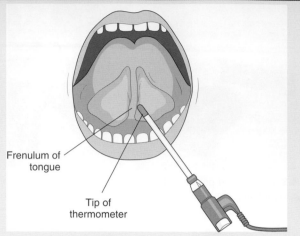

Frenulum of tongue

Tip of thermometer

Fig. 4-7 The thermometer is placed at the base of the tongue and to one side.

    k. Clean the glass thermometer according to agency policy. Return it to the holder.
11. For an *electronic thermometer:*
    a. Start the thermometer. Place a probe cover on the thermometer as per the manufacturer instructions.
    b. Hold the probe in place until you hear a tone or see the temperature displayed as per the manufacturer instructions.
    c. Read the temperature on the display.
    d. Remove the probe. Press the eject button to discard the cover.
    e. Return the probe to the holder.
    f. Note the person's name, temperature, and temperature site on your notepad or assignment sheet.
    g. Return the electronic thermometer to the charging unit.
12. For an *oral temperature:*
    a. Ask the person to open the mouth and raise the tongue.
    b. Place the covered probe at the base of the tongue and to one side. If using a glass thermometer, place the bulb end under the tongue and to one side (Fig. 4-7).
    c. Ask the person to lower the tongue and close the mouth around the thermometer to hold it in place.
    d. Ask the person not to talk. Remind the person not to bite down on a glass thermometer.
    e. Leave a glass thermometer in place for 2 to 3 minutes or as required by agency policy.
13. For a *rectal temperature:*
    a. Put a small amount of lubricant on a tissue.
    b. Lubricate the bulb end of the thermometer.
    c. Expose the anal area.
    d. Raise the upper buttock to expose the anus (Fig. 4-8).

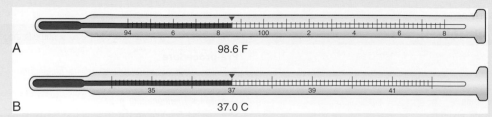

A   98.6 F

B   37.0 C

Fig. 4-6 A, A Fahrenheit thermometer. The temperature measurement is 98.6° F. **B,** Centigrade thermometer. The temperature measurement is 37.0° C.

TAKING A TEMPERATURE—cont'd

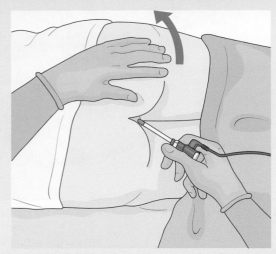

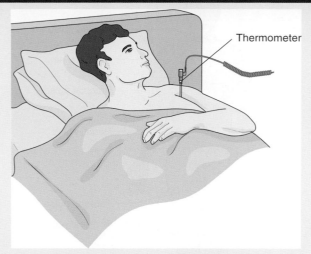

Thermometer

Fig. 4-8 The rectal temperature is taken with the person in modified left lateral recumbent position. The buttock is raised to expose the anus.

Fig. 4-9 The thermometer is held in place in the axilla by bringing the person's arm over the chest.

e. Insert the covered glass thermometer 1 inch into the rectum. Insert an electronic thermometer ½ inch into the rectum. Do not force the thermometer. Hold a glass thermometer in place for 2 minutes or as required by agency policy. Do not let go of it while it is in the rectum.

f. If using an electronic thermometer, hold the probe or thermometer in place until the temperature shows on the display.

g. Remove thermometer from rectum.

h. Wipe the anal area to remove excess lubricant and any feces. Discard used toilet tissue.

14. For an *axillary temperature:*

a. Help the person remove an arm from the gown. Do not expose the person.

b. Dry the axilla with the towel.

c. Place the covered probe in the axilla. For a glass thermometer, place the bulb end of the thermometer in the center of the axilla.

d. Place the person's arm over the chest to hold the thermometer in place (Fig. 4-9). You may need to hold the thermometer and the arm in place if they cannot help.

e. Leave a glass thermometer in place for 5 to 10 minutes or as required by agency policy.

f. Remove thermometer from axilla.

g. Help the person put the gown back on.

15. For a *tympanic membrane temperature:*

a. Ask the person to turn his or her head so the ear is in front of you.

b. Pull up and back on the ear to straighten the ear canal.

c. Insert the covered probe gently.

d. Hold the probe or thermometer in place until the temperature shows on the display.

16. For a *temporal artery temperature:*

a. Choose the side of the head that is exposed. Do not use the side covered by hair, a dressing, hat, or other covering. If the person was in the side-lying position, do not use the side that was on a pillow.

b. Place the thermometer at the side of forehead between the hairline and eyebrows.

c. Slide the thermometer across the forehead.

d. Read the temperature display.

17. Remove and discard gloves. Perform hand hygiene.

Post-procedure

18. Provide for comfort and complete a safety check before leaving the room. (See the inside back cover of this book.)

19. Unscreen the person.

20. Perform hand hygiene.

21. Report and record the temperature in Fahrenheit (F) or Celsius (C) as per agency policy. Note the temperature site when reporting and recording. Report an abnormal temperature to the nurse at once.

PROMOTING SAFETY AND COMFORT

Taking Temperatures

Safety

Thermometers are inserted into the mouth, rectum, axilla, and ear. Each area has many microbes. Some areas may contain blood. Therefore, each person has his or her own glass thermometer. It should be cleaned after every use. When using an electronic thermometer, a new probe cover is placed each time. This prevents the spread of microbes and infection.

When taking a rectal temperature, your gloved hands may come in contact with feces. If so, remove the gloves and perform hand hygiene. Then note the temperature on your notepad or assignment sheet. Put on clean gloves to complete the procedure.

Follow Standard Precautions and the Bloodborne Pathogen Standard (Chapter 6) when taking temperatures.

Comfort

Remove the thermometer in a timely manner. Do not leave it in place longer than needed. This affects the person's comfort. For example, an oral (glass) thermometer is left in place for 2 to 3 minutes. Do not leave it in place longer than that.

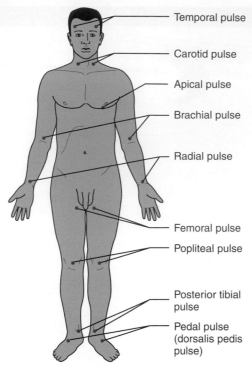

Fig. 4-10 The pulse sites.

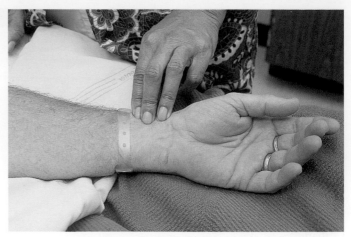

Fig. 4-11 The middle three fingers are used to take the radial pulse.

Pulse. The *pulse* is the beat of the heart felt at an artery as a wave of blood passes through the artery. A pulse is felt every time the heart beats.

The pulse sites are shown in Fig. 4-10. The radial pulse is used most often. It is easy to reach and find. You can take a radial pulse without disturbing or exposing the person.

The *pulse rate* is the number of heartbeats or pulses felt in 1 minute. This is also known as the *heart rate (HR)*. The pulse rate varies for each age group (Table 4-2). The adult pulse rate is between 60 and 100 beats per minute. A pulse rate of fewer than 60 or more than 100 is considered abnormal. Report abnormal pulse rates to the nurse at once.

* *Tachycardia* is a rapid *(tachy)* heart rate *(cardia)*. The heart rate is more than 100 beats per minute.
* *Bradycardia* is a slow *(brady)* heart rate *(cardia)*. The heart rate is fewer than 60 beats per minute.

The *rhythm* of the pulse should be regular. That is, pulses are felt in a pattern. The same time interval occurs between beats. An irregular pulse occurs when the beats are not evenly spaced or beats are skipped.

Force relates to pulse strength. A forceful pulse is easy to feel. It is described as *strong, full,* or *bounding.* Hard-to-feel pulses are described as *weak, thready,* or *feeble.*

Taking a Pulse. You will take radial, apical, and apical-radial pulses. You must accurately count, report, and record the pulse rate accurately.

* *Radial pulse.* The *radial pulse* is used for routine vital signs. Place the first 2 or 3 fingers of one hand against the radial artery. The radial artery is on the thumb side of the wrist (Fig. 4-11). Count the pulse for 30 seconds. Then multiply the number by 2. This gives the number of beats per minute. If the pulse is irregular, count it for 1 minute. In some agencies, all radial pulses are taken for 1 minute. Follow agency policy.
* *Apical pulse.* The *apical pulse* is on the left side of the chest slightly below the nipple (Fig. 4-12). Apical pulses are taken on persons who:
  * Have heart disease
  * Have irregular heart rhythms
  * Take drugs that affect the heart

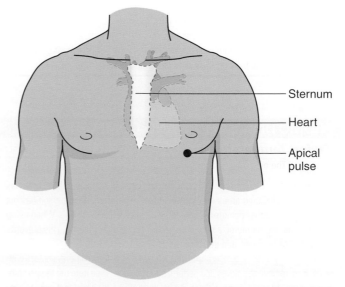

Fig. 4-12 The apical pulse is located 2 to 3 inches to the left of the sternum (breastbone) and below the left nipple.

Table 4-2	**Pulse Ranges by Age**
AGE	**PULSE RATE PER MINUTE**
Birth to 1 year	80–190
2 years	80–160
6 years	75–120
10 years	70–110
12 years and older	60–100

Count the apical pulse for 1 minute. The heartbeat normally sounds like a *lub-dub*. Count each *lub-dub* as one beat. Do not count the *lub* as one beat and the *dub* as another. The apical pulse is taken with a stethoscope.

• *Apical-radial pulse.* The apical and radial pulse rates should be equal. Sometimes heart contractions are not strong enough to create pulses in the radial artery. Then the radial pulse rate is less than the apical pulse rate. This may occur in people with heart disease. To see whether the apical and radial pulses are equal, two staff members are needed. One takes the radial pulse; the other takes the apical pulse. The *pulse deficit* is the difference between the apical and radial pulse rates. To obtain the pulse deficit, subtract the radial rate from the apical rate. (The apical pulse rate is never less than the radial pulse rate.)

See *Delegation Guidelines: Taking a Pulse.*
See *Promoting Safety and Comfort: Taking a Pulse.*

DELEGATION GUIDELINES
Taking a Pulse

Before taking a pulse, you need this information from the nurse and the care plan:
• What pulse to take for each person—radial, apical, or apical-radial
• When to take the pulse
• What other vital signs to measure
• How long to count the pulse—30 seconds or 1 minute
• Whether the nurse has concerns about certain patients or residents
• What observations to report and record:
  • The pulse site
  • The pulse rate—report a pulse rate fewer than 60 (bradycardia) or more than 100 beats (tachycardia) per minute at once
  • Pulse deficit for an apical-radial pulse
  • Whether the pulse is regular or irregular
  • Pulse force—strong, full, bounding, weak, thready, or feeble
• When to report the pulse rate
• What specific patient or resident concerns to report at once

TAKING A PULSE

QUALITY OF LIFE
Remember to:
• Knock before entering the person's room.
• Address the person by name.
• Introduce yourself by name and title.
• Explain the procedure to the person before starting and during the procedure.
• Protect the person's rights during the procedure.
• Handle the person gently during the procedure

PRE-PROCEDURE
1. Follow *Delegation Guidelines: Taking a Pulse.* See *Promoting Safety and Comfort: Taking a Pulse.*
2. Ask a nursing team member to help you take an apical-radial pulse.
3. Perform hand hygiene.
4. Collect a stethoscope and antiseptic wipes for an apical pulse or an apical-radial pulse.
5. Identify the person. Check the ID bracelet against the assignment sheet. Also call the person by name.
6. Provide for privacy.

PROCEDURE
7. Have the person sit or lie down.
8. For a *radial pulse:*
   a. Locate the radial pulse on the thumb side of the person's wrist. Use your first 2 or 3 middle fingers.
   b. Note whether the pulse is strong or weak and regular or irregular.
   c. Count the pulse for 30 seconds. Multiply the number of beats by 2. Or count the pulse for 1 minute if:
      • Directed by the nurse and care plan.
      • Required by agency policy.
      • The pulse was irregular.
      • Required for your state competency test.
9. For an *apical pulse:*
   a. Expose the nipple area of the left chest. Do not expose a woman's breasts.
   b. Clean the earpieces and diaphragm with the wipes.
   c. Warm the diaphragm in your palm.
   d. Place the earpieces in your ears.
   e. Find the apical pulse. Place the diaphragm 2 to 3 inches to the left of the breastbone and below the left nipple.

   f. Count the pulse for 1 minute. Note whether it is regular or irregular.
   g. Cover the person. Remove the earpieces.
10. For an *apical-radial pulse:*
   a. Follow steps 9 a–e.
   b. Your helper finds the radial pulse (Fig. 4-13).
   c. Give the signal to begin counting.
   d. You and your helper will count the pulse for 1 minute.
   e. Give the signal to stop counting.
   f. Subtract the radial pulse from the apical pulse for the pulse deficit.
   g. Note the force (ie. strong, weak, bounding, or thready) and the rhythm (ie. regular or irregular) of the pulse.
11. Note the person's name and pulse or heart rate (HR) on your notepad or assignment sheet. For an apical-radial pulse, note the apical and radial pulse rates and the pulse deficit.

POST-PROCEDURE
12. Provide for comfort and complete a safety check before leaving the room. (See the inside back cover of this book.)
13. Unscreen the person.
14. Clean the earpieces and diaphragm of the stethoscope with the wipes.
15. Return the stethoscope to its proper place.
16. Perform hand hygiene.
17. Report and record your observations. Record the pulse rate and note the site. Report an abnormal pulse rate to the nurse at once. For an apical-radial pulse, note:
   • The apical and radial pulse rates
   • The pulse deficit

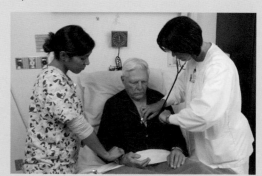

Fig. 4-13 Taking an apical-radial pulse. One worker takes the apical pulse. The other takes the radial pulse.

PROMOTING SAFETY AND COMFORT

Taking a Pulse

Safety	Comfort
Do not use your thumb to take a pulse. The thumb has a pulse. Use your first two or three fingers to take a pulse. You could mistake the pulse in your thumb for the person's pulse. Reporting and recording the wrong pulse rate can harm the person. Stethoscopes are in contact with many persons and staff. To prevent infection, wipe the earpieces and diaphragm with antiseptic wipes before and after use.	Stethoscope diaphragms tend to be cold. Warm the diaphragm in your hand before applying it to the person. Cold diaphragms can startle the person.

Respirations. *Respiration* means breathing air into (inhalation) and out of (exhalation) the lungs. Each respiration involves one inhalation and one exhalation. The chest rises during inhalation. It falls during exhalation.

The healthy adult has 12 to 20 respirations per minute. This is known as the *respiratory rate* (RR). Respirations are normally quiet, effortless, and regular. Both sides of the chest rise and fall equally.

Count respirations when the person is at rest. Position the person so you can see the chest rise and fall. People tend to change their breathing patterns when they know their respirations are being counted. Therefore, the person should not know that you are counting them.

Count respirations right after taking a pulse. Keep your fingers or stethoscope over the pulse site. (The person assumes you are taking the pulse.) To count respirations, watch the chest rise and fall. Count them for 30 seconds. Multiply the number by 2 for the number of respirations in 1 minute. If an abnormal pattern is noted, count the respirations for 1 minute.

In some agencies, respirations are counted for 1 minute. Follow agency policy.

See Delegation Guidelines: Respirations.

DELEGATION GUIDELINES

Respirations

Before counting respirations, you need this information from the nurse and the care plan:

- How long to count respirations for each person—30 seconds or 1 minute
- When to count respirations
- Whether the nurse has concerns about certain patients or residents
- What other vital signs to measure
- What observations to report and record:
  - The respiratory rate
  - Equality and depth of respirations
  - Whether the respirations were regular or irregular
  - Whether the person has pain or difficulty breathing
  - Any respiratory noises
  - An abnormal respiratory pattern
- When to report observations
- What specific patient or resident concerns to report at once

COUNTING RESPIRATIONS

PROCEDURE

1. Follow *Delegation Guidelines: Respirations.*
2. Keep your fingers or stethoscope over the pulse site.
3. Do not tell the person you are counting respirations.
4. Begin counting when the chest rises. Count each rise and fall of the chest as 1 respiration.
5. Note the following:
   - Whether respirations are regular
   - Whether both sides of the chest rise equally
   - The depth of respirations
   - Whether the person has any pain or difficulty breathing
   - An abnormal respiratory pattern
6. Count respirations for 30 seconds. Multiply the number by 2. Count respirations for 1 minute if:
   - Directed by the nurse and care plan.
   - Required by agency policy.
   - They are abnormal or irregular.
   - Required for your state competency test.
7. Note the person's name, respiratory rate (RR), and other observations on your notepad or assignment sheet.

POST-PROCEDURE

8. Provide for comfort and complete a safety check before leaving the room. (See the inside back cover of this book.)
9. Unscreen the person.
10. Perform hand hygiene.
11. Report and record the respiratory rate and your observations. Report abnormal respirations to the nurse at once.

Blood Pressure. *Blood pressure* (BP) is the amount of force exerted against the walls of an artery by the blood. BP is controlled by:

- The force of heart contractions
- The amount of blood pumped with each heartbeat
- How easily the blood flows through the bold vessels

The period of heart muscle contraction is called *systole.* The heart is pumping blood. The *systolic pressure* is the amount of force needed to pump blood out of the heart into the arterial circulation. It is the higher pressure.

The period of heart muscle relaxation is called *diastole.* The heart is at rest. The *diastolic pressure* is the pressure in the arteries when the heart is at rest. It is the lower pressure.

BOX 4-5 Guidelines for Measuring Blood Pressure

- Do not take blood pressure on an arm:
  - With an IV (intravenous) infusion
  - With a cast
  - With a dialysis access site
  - On the side of breast surgery
  - That is injured
- Ask the nurse if you're not sure which arm to use
- Let the person rest for 10 to 20 minutes before measuring blood pressure.
- Measure blood pressure with the person sitting or lying. Sometimes the doctor orders a blood pressure to be measured in the standing position.
- Apply the cuff to the bare upper arm. Clothing can affect the measurement.
- Make sure the cuff is snug. Loose cuffs can cause inaccurate readings.
- Use a larger cuff if the person is obese or has a large arm. Use a small cuff if the person has a very small arm. Ask the nurse which size to use.
- Place the diaphragm of the stethoscope firmly over the brachial artery. The entire diaphragm must have contact with the skin.
- Make sure the room is quiet. Talking, TV, radio, and sounds from the hallway can affect an accurate measurement.
- Have the manometer where you can clearly see it.
- Measure the systolic and diastolic pressures.
  - Expect to hear the first blood pressure sound at the point where you last felt the radial or brachial pulse. The first sound is the systolic pressure.
  - The point where the sound disappears is the diastolic pressure.
- Take the blood pressure again if you are not sure of an accurate measurement. Wait 30 to 60 seconds before repeating the measurement.
- Tell the nurse at once if you cannot hear the blood pressure.

BP is measured in millimeters (mm) of mercury (Hg). Box 4-5 lists the guidelines for measuring BP. The systolic pressure is recorded over the diastolic pressure. A systolic pressure of 120 mm Hg (millimeters of mercury) and a diastolic pressure of 80 mm Hg is written as 120/80 mm Hg.

Because it can vary so easily, BP has normal ranges:

- *Systolic pressure*—less than 120 mm Hg
- *Diastolic pressure*—less than 80 mm Hg

BP is normally measured in the brachial artery. You need a stethoscope and a sphygmomanometer to measure BP. The sphygmomanometer has a cuff and a measuring device called a manometer. The cuff is wrapped around the upper arm. Tubing connects the cuff to the manometer. Another tube connects the cuff to a small, handheld bulb. A valve on the bulb is turned so the cuff inflates as the bulb is squeezed. The inflated cuff causes pressure over the brachial artery. The valve is turned the other way to deflate the cuff. The stethoscope is used to listen to the sounds in the brachial artery as the cuff is deflated. BP is measured as the cuff is deflated.

With an electronic BP monitor, the cuff is also wrapped around the upper arm over the brachial artery. No stethoscope is needed. A button is pressed to inflate the cuff. The cuff deflates automatically. The BP is displayed. The wrist monitor works in the same way except the monitor is wrapped around the wrist. Follow the manufacturer's instructions on the proper use of this equipment.

See *Delegation Guidelines: Blood Pressure*.

See *Promoting Safety and Comfort: Blood Pressure*.

DELEGATION GUIDELINES
Measuring Blood Pressure

Before measuring BP, you need this information from the nurse and the care plan.

- When to measure BP
- Which arm to use
- The person's normal BP range
- Whether the nurse has concerns about certain patients or residents
- Whether the person needs to be lying down, sitting, or standing
- What size cuff to use—regular, child-sized, extra large, bariatric.
- What observations to report and record
- When to report the BP measurement
- What patient or resident concerns to report at once

PROMOTING SAFETY AND COMFORT
Blood Pressure

Safety

Some sphygmomanometers contain mercury. Mercury is a hazardous substance. OSHA recommends that health care agencies replace outdated sphygmomanometers with mercury-free devices. If using a mercury sphygmomanometer, handle the device carefully. If one breaks, call for the nurse at once. Do not touch the mercury. Do not let the person touch it. The agency must follow special procedures for handling all hazardous substances.

Comfort

Inflate the cuff only to the extent necessary (see procedure: *Measuring Blood Pressure*). The inflated cuff causes discomfort. The higher the inflation, the greater the discomfort.

MEASURING BLOOD PRESSURE

QUALITY OF LIFE

Remember to:

- Knock before entering the person's room.
- Address the person by name.
- Introduce yourself by name and title.
- Explain the procedure to the person before starting and during the procedure.
- Protect the person's rights during the procedure.
- Handle the person gently during the procedure.

PRE-PROCEDURE

1. Follow *Delegation Guidelines: Measuring Blood Pressure*. See *Promoting Safety and Comfort: Blood Pressure*
2. Perform hand hygiene.
3. Collect the following:
   - Sphygmomanometer
   - Stethoscope
   - Antiseptic wipes

MEASURING BLOOD PRESSURE—cont'd

4. Identify the person. Check the ID bracelet against the assignment sheet. Also call the person by name.
5. Provide for privacy.

PROCEDURE

6. Wipe the stethoscope earpieces and diaphragm with the wipes. Warm the diaphragm in your palm.
7. Have the person sit or lie down.
8. Position the person's arm level with the heart. The palm is up.
9. Stand no more than 3 feet away from the manometer.
10. Expose the upper arm.
11. Squeeze the cuff to expel any remaining air. Close the valve on the bulb.
12. Find the brachial artery at the inner aspect of the elbow. (The brachial artery is on the little finger side of the arm.) Use your fingertips.
13. Place the arrow on the cuff over the brachial artery (Fig. 4-14, *A*). Wrap the cuff around the upper arm at least 1 inch above the elbow. It should be even and snug.
14. *One-step method:*
    a. Place the stethoscope earpieces in your ears.
    b. Find the radial or brachial artery.

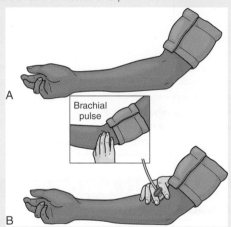

c. Inflate the cuff until you can no longer feel the pulse. Note this point.
d. Inflate the cuff 30 mm Hg beyond the point where you last felt the pulse.
15. *Two-step method:*
    a. Find the radial or brachial artery.
    b. Inflate the cuff until you can no longer feel the pulse. Note this point.
    c. Inflate the cuff 30 mm Hg beyond the point where you last felt the pulse.
    d. Deflate the cuff slowly. Note the point when you feel the pulse.
    e. Wait 30 seconds.
    f. Place the stethoscope earpieces in your ears.
    g. Inflate the cuff 30 mm Hg beyond the point where you felt the pulse return.
16. Place the diaphragm of the stethoscope over the brachial artery (Fig. 4-14, *B*). Do not place it under the cuff.
17. Deflate the cuff at an even rate of 2 to 4 millimeters per second. Turn the valve counterclockwise to deflate the cuff.
18. Note the point where you hear the first sound. This is the systolic reading. It is near the point where the radial pulse disappeared.
19. Continue to deflate the cuff. Note the point where the sound disappears. This is the diastolic reading.
20. Deflate the cuff completely. Remove it from the person's arm. Remove the stethoscope earpieces from your ears.
21. Note the person's name and BP on your notepad or assignment sheet.
22. Return the cuff to the case or wall holder.

POST-PROCEDURE

23. Provide for comfort and complete a safety check before leaving the room. (See the inside back cover of this book.)
24. Unscreen the person.
25. Clean the earpieces and diaphragm with the wipes.
26. Return the equipment to its proper place.
27. Perform hand hygiene.
28. Report and record the BP. Report an abnormal BP to the nurse at once.

Fig. 4-14 Measuring blood pressure. **A,** The cuff is over the brachial artery. **B,** The diaphragm of the stethoscope is over the brachial artery.

Measuring Weight and Height

Weight and height are measured on admission to the agency. The doctor uses the measurements to determine the dosages of some drugs. Then the person is weighed daily, weekly, or monthly. This is done to measure weight gain or loss.

A person's weight is measured in either pounds (lb) or kilograms (kg). The person's height is measured in feet (ft) and inches (in). Follow the agency's policy for recording height and weight.

When measuring weight and height, follow these guidelines:
- The person wears only a gown or pajamas. Clothes add weight. No footwear is worn. Footwear adds to the weight and height measurements.
- The person voids before being weighed. A full bladder adds weight.
- Weigh the person at the same time of day. Before breakfast is the best time. Food and fluids add weight.
- Use the same scale for daily, weekly, and monthly weights. Scales weigh differently.

- Balance the scale at zero (0) before weighing the person. For balance scales, move the weights to zero. A digital scale should read at zero.

See *Delegation Guidelines: Measuring Weight and Height.*

See *Promoting Safety and Comfort: Measuring Weight and Height.*

DELEGATION GUIDELINES
Measuring Weight and Height

Before measuring weight and height, you need this information from the nurse and the care plan:
- When to measure weight and height
- What scale to use
- Which unit of measure to record weight (lb or kg)
- When to report the measurements
- What specific patient or resident concerns to report at once

PROMOTING SAFETY AND COMFORT
Measuring Weight and Height

Safety

Follow the manufacturer's instructions when using chair, bed, wheelchair, or lift scales when measuring a person's weight. Also follow the agency's procedures. When measuring a person's height, follow the manufacturer's instructions on how to use the height rod. Practice safety measures to prevent falls.

Comfort

The person wears only a gown or pajamas for the weight measurement. Provide comfort by preventing chilling and drafts throughout the procedure.

MEASURING WEIGHT AND HEIGHT

QUALITY OF LIFE

Remember to:

- Knock before entering the person's room.
- Address the person by name.
- Introduce yourself by name and title.
- Explain the procedure to the person before starting and during the procedure.
- Protect the person's rights during the procedure.
- Handle the person gently during the procedure.

PRE-PROCEDURE

1. Follow *Delegation Guidelines: Measuring Weight and Height.* See *Promoting Safety and Comfort: Measuring Weight and Height.*
2. Ask the person to void.
3. Perform hand hygiene.
4. Identify the person. Check the ID bracelet against the assignment sheet. Also call the person by name.
5. Bring the scale and paper towels (for a standing scale) to the person's room or assist the person to the platform scale.
6. Provide for privacy.

PROCEDURE

7. Place the paper towels on the scale platform.
8. Move the weights to zero (0). The pointer is in the middle.
9. Be sure person is only wearing a gown or pajamas. Remove all other clothing and footwear. Assist as needed.
10. Help the person stand in the center of the scale. Arms are at the sides (Fig. 4-15A).
11. Move the weights until the balance pointer is in the middle (Fig. 4-15B).
12. Note the weight on your notepad or assignment sheet.
13. Ask the person to stand very straight.
14. Raise the height rod above the level of the person's head. Lower the height rod until it rests on top of the person's head (Fig. 4-16).
15. Note the height on your notepad or assignment sheet.
16. Raise the height rod. Help the person step off of the scale.
17. Help the person get dressed. Provide nonskid footwear if they will be up. Or help the person back to bed.
18. Lower the height rod. Adjust the weights to zero (0) if this is your agency's policy.
19. Discard the paper towels.

POST-PROCEDURE

20. Provide for comfort and complete a safety check before leaving the room. (See the inside back cover of this book.)
21. Unscreen the person.
22. Return the scale to its proper place.
23. Perform hand hygiene.
24. Report and record the person's weight and height.

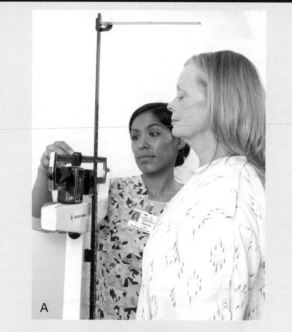

A

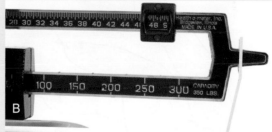

B

Fig. 4-15 A, The person is weighed. **B,** The weight is read when the balance pointer is in the middle.

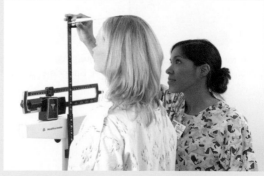

Fig. 4-16 Height is measured.

Blood Glucose Testing

Blood glucose testing is used for persons with diabetes. The doctor uses the results to regulate the person's drugs and diet. For the test, capillary blood is obtained through a skin puncture.

A drop of capillary blood is collected through a skin puncture. A fingertip is the most common site for skin punctures. These sites provide easy access and do not require clothing removal. The person feels a sharp pinch. Discomfort is brief.

Inspect the site carefully. Look for signs of trauma and skin breaks. Avoid sites that are swollen, bruised, cyanotic (bluish color), scarred, or calloused. Blood flow to these areas is poor. A *callus* is a thick, hardened area on the skin. Calluses often form over frequently used areas, such as the tips of the thumbs and index fingers. Therefore, the thumbs and index fingers are not good sites for skin punctures.

Do not use the center, fleshy part of the fingertip. The site has many nerve endings. A puncture at the site is painful. Use the side toward the tip of the fingertip on the middle or ring finger (Fig. 4-17).

A sterile lancet is used to puncture the skin (Fig. 4-18). A *lancet* is a short, pointed blade. The short blade punctures but does not cut the skin. The lancet is inside a protective cover. You do not touch the actual blade. All types of lancets are disposable. A lancet is discarded into the sharps container after use.

A glucometer (glucose meter) is used to measure blood glucose. A drop of blood is collected on a test strip (reagent strip) that has been inserted into the glucometer. The blood glucose result is shown on the monitor. Many different glucometers are available. The speed with which results are displayed varies with the manufacturer. Some take 1 minute. Others take 5 seconds or less.

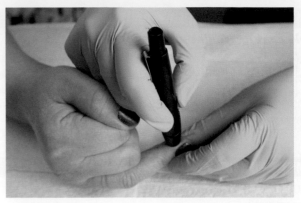

Fig. 4-18 A lancet is a device used to puncture the skin.

In agencies, glucose meters are tested daily for accuracy. The manufacturer has instructions for testing the device. There are many different kinds of glucometers. You will learn to use the device used in your agency. Always follow the manufacturer's instructions.

See *Delegation Guidelines: Blood Glucose Testing*.
See *Promoting Safety and Comfort: Blood Glucose Testing*.

DELEGATION GUIDELINES
Blood Glucose Testing

Many states and agencies allow nursing assistive personnel to test blood glucose. If the task is delegated to you, make sure that:
- Your state allows nursing assistive personnel to perform the procedure
- The procedure is in your job description
- You have the necessary training
- You know how to use the agency's equipment
- You review the procedure with a nurse
- The nurse is available to answer questions and to supervise you

If the above conditions are met, you need the following information from the nurse:
- Which sites you can use for the skin puncture
- Which sites to avoid for the skin puncture
- When to check to blood glucose—usually before meals
- What to report and record:
  - The time the blood glucose was checked
  - The blood glucose test results
  - The site used for the skin puncture
  - The amount of bleeding at the skin puncture site
  - Any signs of a *hematoma* (a swelling [oma] that contains blood [hemat])
  - How the person tolerated the procedure
  - Complaints of pain at the skin puncture site
  - Other observations or resident complaints
  - When to report observations and the blood glucose measurement
  - What specific patient or resident concerns to report at once

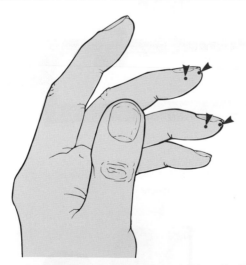

Fig. 4-17 Site for skin punctures. (From Bonewit-West, K., *Clinical Procedures for Medical Assistants,* 5th ed., Philadelphia, Saunders, 2000.)

BOX 4-6   Rules for Blood Glucose Testing

- Follow the manufacturer's instructions for the glucometer.
- Know how to use the equipment. Request any necessary training.
- Make sure the glucometer was tested for accuracy. Check the testing log.
- Enter a code or username if required by the agency.
- Scan the bar code on the bottle of test strips if needed.
- Check the color of test strips. Do not use them if they are discolored.

- Check the expiration date of the reagent strips. Do not use them if the date has passed.
- Follow the manufacturer's instructions for test times.
- Report the results to the nurse at once.
- Record the result following agency policy.

PROMOTING SAFETY AND COMFORT

Blood Glucose Testing

Safety

Accurate results are important. Inaccurate results can harm the person. Follow the rules in Box 4-6 when testing blood specimens for glucose.

Make sure you know how to use the equipment. Use only the type of test strip specified by the manufacturer. Otherwise you will get inaccurate results.

Contact with blood is likely. Follow Standard Precautions and the Bloodborne Pathogen Standard (Chapter 6). Disinfect the glucometer after checking a person's blood glucose. Follow the manufacturer's in-structions for the disinfectant used.

Comfort

The heel is used for skin punctures in infants younger than 1 and who are not yet walking. The third finger (ring finger) is used for children. See Fig. 4-19.

Older persons often have poor circulation in their fingers. To increase blood flow, apply a warm washcloth or wash the hands in warm water.

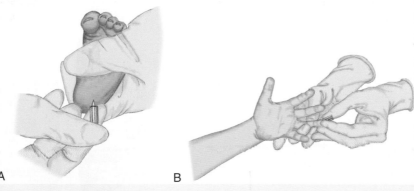

Fig. 4-19 A, Heel site is used for skin punctures in infants younger than 1. **B,** The third finger (ring finger) is used for skin punctures in children. (From James, S.R., Ashwill, J.W., Droske, S.C., *Nursing Care of Children: Principles and Practice,* 3rd ed., St. Louis, Saunders, 2007.)

MEASURING BLOOD GLUCOSE

Quality Of Life

Remember to:

- Knock before entering the person's room.
- Address the person by name.
- Introduce yourself by name and title.
- Explain the procedure to the person before starting and during the procedure.
- Protect the person's rights during the procedure.
- Handle the person gently during the procedure.

Pre-Procedure

1. Follow *Delegation Guidelines: Blood Glucose Testing.* See *Promoting Safety and Comfort: Blood Glucose Testing.*
2. Perform hand hygiene.
3. Collect the following supplies:
   - Sterile lancet
   - Antiseptic wipes
   - Gloves
   - 2 x 2 gauze squares
   - Glucometer
   - Test strips (Use the correct ones for the meter. Check the expiration date.)

- Paper towels
- Warm washcloth

4. Read the manufacturer's instructions for the lancet and glucometer.
5. Arrange your work area.
6. Identify the person. Check the ID bracelet against the assignment sheet. Also call the person by name.
7. Provide for privacy.

Procedure

8. Help the person to a comfortable position.
9. Put on the gloves.
10. Prepare the supplies:
    a. Open the antiseptic wipes.
    b. Prepare the lancet. Follow manufacturer's instructions.
    c. Turn on the glucometer.
    d. Follow the prompts on the screen. You may need to scan the patient's ID. Scan the bar code on the test strips or compare it to the one on the glucometer display.
    e. Remove a test strip from the bottle. Insert it into the glucometer (Fig. 4-20). Place the cap securely on the bottle.

MEASURING BLOOD GLUCOSE—cont'd

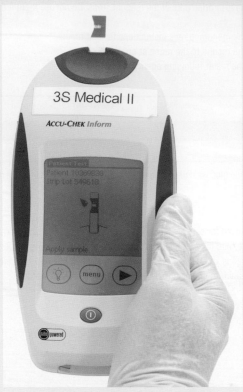

Fig. 4-20 A test strip in the glucometer.

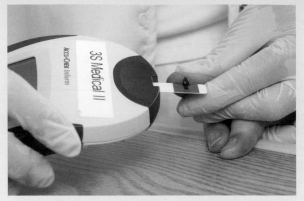

Fig. 4-21 A drop of blood is applied to the test strip.

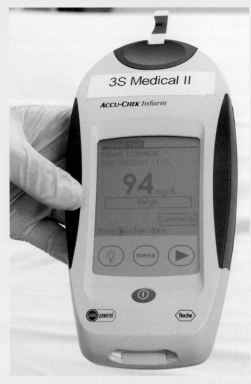

Fig. 4-22 The result is displayed on the glucometer.

11. Perform a skin puncture to obtain a drop of blood:
    a. Inspect the person's fingers. Select a skin puncture site.
    b. Warm the finger. Rub it gently or apply a warm washcloth.
    c. Massage the hand and finger toward the puncture site. This brings more blood to the site.
    d. Lower the finger below the person's waist. This increases blood flow to the site.
    e. Use your non-dominant hand to hold the finger with your thumb and forefinger.
    f. Clean the site with an antiseptic wipe. *Do not touch the site after cleaning.*
    g. Let the site dry. *Do not blow on it or fan it.*
    h. Place the lancet against the side of the finger or the top of the fingertip.
    i. Push the button on the lancet to puncture the skin. (Follow the manufacturer's instructions.)
    j. Apply gentle pressure below the puncture site. Wipe away the first blood drop using a 2 x 2 gauze square.
    k. Apply gentle pressure below the puncture site again. Let a large drop of blood form.

12. Collect and test the specimen. Follow the manufacturer's instructions and agency procedures for the glucometer used.
    a. Lightly touch the reagent strip to the blood drop (Fig. 4-21). Do not smear the blood.
    b. Use a gauze square to apply pressure to the puncture site until bleeding stops. If able, let the person apply pressure to the site.
    c. The glucometer will start timing automatically when the blood is applied. Wait the length of time required by the manufacturer.
    d. Read the result on the display (Fig. 4-22). Note the person's name and blood glucose on your notepad or assignment sheet. Tell the person the result.
    e. Turn off the glucose meter.

13. Discard the lancet into the sharps container.
14. Discard the gauze and test strip following agency policy.
15. Remove and discard the gloves. Perform hand hygiene.

POST-PROCEDURE

16. Provide for comfort and complete a safety check before leaving the room. (See the inside back cover of this book.)
17. Unscreen the person.
18. Disinfect the glucometer. Follow the manufacturer's instructions for the disinfectant used.
19. Return the glucometer to its proper place.
20. Perform hand hygiene.
21. Report and record the blood glucose result and your observations.

COMMUNICATION

Communication is when one person sends a message to another person who receives it and interprets it. Communication is essential for the successful use of the nursing process. Nursing team members must communicate effectively with one another. For good communication:

- Use words that mean the same thing to you and the receiver of the message. Avoid using words with more than one meaning.
- "Small," "moderate," and "large" mean different things to different people. Is small the size of a dime? Or is it the size of a quarter? In health care, different meanings can cause serious problems.
- Use familiar words. If you do not know what a word means, ask the nurse. It is acceptable to use a medical dictionary.
- Be brief and concise. Do not add unrelated or unnecessary information. Stay on the subject. Avoid wandering in thought. Do not get wordy.
- Give information in a logical and orderly manner. Organize your thoughts. Present them step-by-step.
- Give facts and be specific. The receiver should have a clear picture of what you are saying. You report a pulse rate of 110. It is more specific and factual than saying the "pulse is fast."

Communication Barriers

Communication barriers prevent the sending and receiving of messages. Communication fails. You must avoid these barriers when communicating with the nurse:

- Using unfamiliar language
- Cultural differences
- Changing the subject
- Giving your opinion
- Failing to listen

Reporting and Recording

The nursing team communicates by reporting and recording. *Reporting* is the oral account of care and observations. *Recording (charting, documentation)* is the written account of care and observations.

Reporting. You report care and observations to the nurse. When reporting, follow the rules in Box 4-7. Report to the nurse when:

- The nurse instructs you to do so.
- You leave the unit for meals, breaks, or other reasons.
- There is a change from normal or a change in the person's condition. This must be reported at once.
- Observations need to be shared during the end-of-shift report.

BOX 4-7   Rules for Reporting and Recording

Rules for Reporting

- Be prompt, thorough, and accurate.
- Give the person's name and room and bed number.
- Give the time your observations were made or the care was given. Use conventional time (AM or PM) or 24-hour clock time according to agency policy.
- Report only what you observed and did yourself.
- Report care measures that you expect the person to need. For example, the person may need the bedpan during your meal break.
- Report expected changes in the person's condition. For example, the person may be tired after lunch.
- Give reports as often as the person's condition requires. Or give them when the nurse asks you to.
- Report at once any changes from normal or changes in the person's condition.
- Use your written notes to give a specific, concise, and clear report.

Rules for Recording

General Rules

- Follow agency policies and procedures for recording. Ask for needed training.
- Include the date and time for every recording. Use conventional time (AM or PM) or 24-hour time according to agency policy.
- Use only agency-approved abbreviations.
- Use correct spelling, grammar, and punctuation.
- Do not use ditto marks.
- Sign or save all entries as required by agency policy.
- Check the name and identifying information on the chart. You must record on the correct chart.
- Record only what you observed and did yourself. Do not record for another person.
- Never chart a procedure, treatment, or care measure until after it is completed.
- Be accurate, concise, and factual. Do not record judgments or interpretations.
- Record in a logical manner and in sequence.
- Be descriptive. Avoid terms with more than one meaning.

- Use the person's exact words whenever possible. Use quotation marks ("...") to show a direct quote.
- Chart any changes from normal or changes in the person's condition. Also chart that you told the nurse (include the nurse's name), what you said, and the time you made the report.
- Do not omit information.
- Record safety measures. Examples include placing the call light within reach, assisting the person when up, or reminding a person not to get out of bed.

On Computer

- Log in using your username and password. Do not chart using another person's username.
- Check the time your entry is made. Make sure it is the right time.
- Check for accuracy. Review your entry before saving.
- Save your entries. Unsaved data will be lost.
- Follow the manufacturer's instructions for changing or uncharting a mistaken entry. Most electronic systems keep a record of an entry before a change was made. The first entry is still visible.
- Log off when done charting. This prevents others from charting under your username.

On Paper

- Make sure each form has the person's name and other identifying information.
- Always use ink. Use the ink color required by the agency.
- Make sure writing is readable and neat.
- Never erase or use correction fluid. Draw a line through the incorrect part. Date and initial the line. Write "mistaken entry" over it if this is agency policy. Then rewrite the part. Follow agency policy for correcting errors.
- Sign your entries. Include your name and title.
- Do not skip lines. Draw a line through the blank space of a partially completed line or to the end of the page. This prevents others from recording in a space with your signature.

From Kostelnick, C., *Mosby's Textbook for Long-Term Care Nursing Assistants*, 8th ed., St. Louis, Mosby, 2020.

- Box 4-7
- ***End-of Shift Report.*** The nurse gives a report at the end of the shift to the oncoming shift. This is called the **end-of-shift report** or change-of-shift report. The nurse reports about:
  - The care given
  - The care to give during other shifts
  - The person's current condition
  - Likely changes in the person's condition
  - In some agencies, the entire nursing team hears the end-of-shift report as they come on duty. In other agencies, only nurses hear the report. After the report, information is shared with nursing assistants.

Recording. When recording (documenting, charting) on the person's chart, you must communicate clearly and thoroughly. Follow the rules in Box 4-7. Anyone who reads your charting should know:

- What you observed
- What you did
- The person's response

The medication administration record is used to record what drugs were given and when. See Chapter 9.

Recording Time. The 24-hour clock (military time or international time) has four digits (Fig. 4-23). The first two digits are for the hours: 0100 = 1:00 AM; 1300 = 1:00 PM. The last two digits are for minutes: 0110 = 1:10 AM. The colons and AM and PM abbreviations are not used. The 24-hour clock always uses 4 digits.

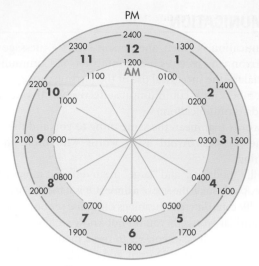

Fig. 4-23 The 24-hour clock.

For AM times from 1:00 AM to 9:00 AM, remove the colon and add 0 as the first digit: 7:45 AM = 0745. For PM times add 12 to the clock time. If it is 2:00 PM, add 12 and 2 for 1400. For 8:35 PM, add 12 and 835 for 2035.

Communication is better with the 24-hour clock. You must use AM and PM with conventional clock time. Someone may forget to use AM or PM. Or writing may be unclear. This means that the correct time is not communicated. Harm to the person could result.

REVIEW QUESTIONS

Circle the BEST answer.

1. Which is *not* a step in the nursing process?
   a. observation
   b. assessment
   c. planning
   d. implementation

2. The nursing process:
   a. involves guidelines for care plans
   b. is a care conference
   c. involves a health history and a drug history
   d. is the method nurses use to plan and deliver nursing care

3. What happens during assessment?
   a. Goals are set.
   b. Information is collected.
   c. Nursing measures are carried out.
   d. Progress is evaluated.

4. Which is a symptom?
   a. redness
   b. vomiting
   c. pain
   d. pulse rate of 78

5. Which is a sign?
   a. nausea
   b. headache
   c. dizziness
   d. dry skin

6. You gave a drug to a person. Which observation should you report at once?
   a. The person had a bowel movement.
   b. The person is not responding to you.
   c. The person's pulse is 80 beats per minute.
   d. The person complains of stiff, painful joints.

7. You gave a drug to a person. Which observation should you report at once?
   a. The person can no longer move a body part.
   b. The person answers questions correctly.
   c. The person has a breath odor.
   d. The person walked to the dining room.

8. Measures in the nursing care plan are carried out. This is:
   a. a nursing diagnosis
   b. planning
   c. implementation
   d. evaluation

9. Which statement is *true*?
   a. The nursing process is done without the person's input.
   b. You are responsible for the nursing process.
   c. The nursing process is used to communicate the person's care.
   d. Nursing process steps can be done in any order.

10. The nursing care plan is:
    a. written by the doctor
    b. a guide with measures to help the person
    c. the same for all persons
    d. the drugs ordered for the person

11. Which is a nursing diagnosis?
    a. cancer
    b. heart attack
    c. kidney failure
    d. acute pain
12. The nurse uses the following to evaluate the person's response to drug therapy, *except:*
    a. vital signs
    b. weight
    c. Minimum Data Set
    d. blood glucose
13. You are checking a rectal temperature. The following supplies are needed, *except:*
    a. a blue thermometer probe
    b. water-soluble lubricant
    c. a probe cover
    d. a red thermometer probe
14. A person has heart disease. You can measure temperature at the following sites *except*
    a. the oral site
    b. the rectal site
    c. the tympanic membrane site
    d. the temporal artery site
15. You take a person's pulse. Before giving a drug, which should you report to the nurse?
    a. a rate of 82 beats per minute
    b. a strong pulse
    c. an irregular pulse
    d. a pulse deficit of 0
16. Which respiratory rate is *not* normal for an adult?
    a. 12 respirations per minute
    b. 16 respirations per minute
    c. 20 respirations per minute
    d. 24 respirations per minute
17. When measuring vital signs, you count respirations:
    a. before taking the temperature
    b. before taking the pulse
    c. after taking the pulse
    d. after taking the blood pressure
18. Blood pressure is usually measured:
    a. in the radial artery
    b. in the brachial artery
    c. in the carotid artery
    d. at the apical pulse
19. Which blood pressure is *not* normal?
    a. 118/80 mm Hg
    b. 128/72 mm Hg
    c. 114/68 mm Hg
    d. 110/74 mm Hg

20. The diastolic blood pressure is:
    a. 30 mm Hg above where the pulse was last felt
    b. 30 mm Hg below where the pulse was last felt
    c. where the first sound is heard
    d. where the last sound is heard
21. When checking blood glucose, which is the best site for a skin puncture?
    a. the thumb
    b. the index finger
    c. the ring finger
    d. the little finger
22. Which is used to measure blood glucose?
    a. glucometer
    b. lancet
    c. reagent strip
    d. sphygmomanometer
23. You are measuring blood glucose. How long should you time the test?
    a. 30 seconds
    b. 1 minute
    c. 2 minutes
    d. as stated in the manufacturer's instructions
24. When should you record that you gave a person a drug?
    a. before giving the drug
    b. after giving the drug
    c. at the end of the shift
    d. when reporting to the nurse

Circle T if the statement is true. Circle F if the statement is false.

25. T   F   Drugs can affect a person's vital signs.
26. T   F   A person receives drugs for heart disease. When taking the pulse, you use the apical site.
27. T   F   You are checking a person's blood pressure using an electronic blood pressure machine. A stethoscope is needed.
28. T   F   You notice the test strips for testing blood glucose are discolored. It is okay to use them.
29. T   F   A drug is ordered for 1630 hours. You should give the drug at 4:30 PM.
30. T   F   You make a mistake when recording a drug. You can erase the error.

Answers to these questions can be found on the Evolve Resources site: http://evolve.elsevier.com/Anderson/medasst/

5

Body Structure and Function

OBJECTIVES

- Define the key terms and key abbreviations used in this chapter.
- Identify the basic structures of the cell.
- Explain how cells divide.

- Describe four types of tissue.
- Identify the structures of each body system.
- Identify the functions of each body system.

KEY TERMS

artery A blood vessel that carries blood away from the heart

capillary A tiny blood vessel; food, oxygen, and other substances pass from the capillaries into the cells

cell The basic unit of body structure

digestion The process of physically and chemically breaking down food so that it can be absorbed for use by the cells

hemoglobin The substance in red blood cells that carries oxygen and gives blood its color

hormone A chemical substance secreted by the endocrine glands into the bloodstream

immunity Protection against a disease or condition; the person will not get or be affected by the disease

menstruation The process in which the lining of the uterus breaks up and is discharged from the body through the vagina

metabolism The burning of food for heat and energy by the cells

organ Groups of tissues with the same function

peristalsis Involuntary muscle contractions in the digestive system that move food down the esophagus through the alimentary canal

respiration The process of supplying the cells with oxygen and removing carbon dioxide from them

system Organs that work together to perform special functions

tissue A group of cells with similar functions

vein A blood vessel that returns blood back to the heart

KEY ABBREVIATIONS

ACTH Adrenocorticotropic hormone
ADH Antidiuretic hormone
CNS Central nervous system
GH Growth hormone
GI Gastrointestinal

mL Milliliter
RBC Red blood cell
T4 Thyroid hormone; thyroxine
TSH Thyroid-stimulating hormone
WBC White blood cell

You help patients and residents meet basic needs. Their bodies do not work at peak levels because of illness, disease, or injury. Your care promotes comfort, healing, and recovery. You need to know the body's normal structure and function. It will help you understand signs, symptoms, and the reasons for drug therapy.

CELLS, TISSUES, AND ORGANS

The basic unit of body structure is the **cell.** Cells have the same basic structure. Function, size, and shape may differ. Cells are very small. You need a microscope to see them. Cells need food, water, and oxygen to live and function.

Fig. 5-1 shows the cell and its structures. The *cell membrane* is the outer covering. It encloses the cell and helps it hold its shape. The *nucleus* is the control center of the cell. It directs the

cell's activities. The nucleus is in the center of the cell. The *cytoplasm* surrounds the nucleus. Cytoplasm contains smaller structures that perform cell functions. *Protoplasm* means *living substance.* It refers to all structures, substances, and water within the cell. Protoplasm is a semi-liquid substance, much like an egg white.

Chromosomes are thread-like structures in the nucleus. Each cell has 46 chromosomes. Chromosomes contain *genes.* Genes control the traits children inherit from their parents. Height, eye color, and skin color are examples.

The nucleus controls cell reproduction. Cells reproduce by dividing in half. The process of cell division is called *mitosis.* It is needed for tissue growth and repair. During mitosis, the 46 chromosomes arrange themselves into 23 pairs. As the cell divides, the 23 pairs are pulled in half. The two new cells are identical. Each has 46 chromosomes (Fig. 5-2).

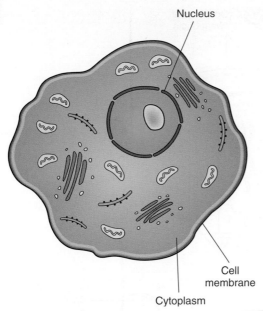

Fig. 5-1 Parts of a cell.

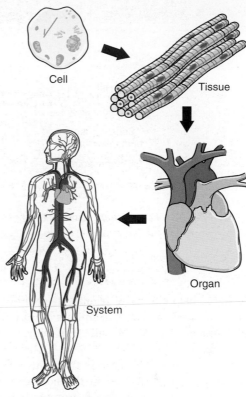

Fig. 5-3 Organization of the body.

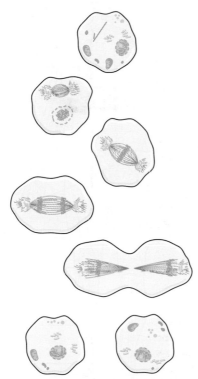

Fig. 5-2 Cell division.

Cells are the body's building blocks. Groups of cells with similar functions combine to form **tissues,** Examples of tissues include:

• *Epithelial tissue* covers internal and external body surfaces. Tissue lining the nose, mouth, respiratory tract, stomach, and intestines is epithelial tissue. So are the skin, hair, nails, and glands.

• *Connective tissue* anchors, connects, and supports other tissues. It is in every part of the body. Bones, tendons, ligaments, and cartilage are connective tissue. Blood is a form of connective tissue.

• *Muscle tissue* stretches and contracts to let the body move.

• *Nerve tissue* receives and carries impulses to the brain and back to body parts.

Groups of tissue with the same function form **organs.** An organ has one or more functions. Examples of organs are the heart, brain, liver, lungs, and kidneys. **Systems** are formed by organs that work together to perform special functions (Fig. 5-3).

THE INTEGUMENTARY SYSTEM

The *integumentary system,* or *skin,* is the largest system. *Integument* means *covering.* The skin covers the body. It has epithelial, connective, and nerve tissue. It also has oil glands and sweat glands. There are two skin layers (Fig. 5-4):

• The *epidermis* is the outer layer. It has living cells and dead cells. The dead cells were once deeper in the epidermis. They were pushed upward as the cells divided. Dead cells constantly flake off. They are replaced by living cells. Living cells also die and flake off. Living cells of the epidermis contain *pigment.* Pigment gives skin its color. The epidermis has no blood vessels and few nerve endings.

• The *dermis* is the inner layer. It is made up of connective tissue. Blood vessels, nerves, sweat glands, and oil glands are in the dermis. So are hair roots.

The epidermis and dermis are supported by *subcutaneous tissue.* The subcutaneous tissue is a thick layer of fat and connective tissue.

Oil glands, sweat glands, hair, and *nails* are skin appendages:

• Oil glands—lie near the hair shafts. They secrete an oily substance into the space near the hair shaft. Oil travels to the skin surface. This helps keep the hair and skin soft and shiny.

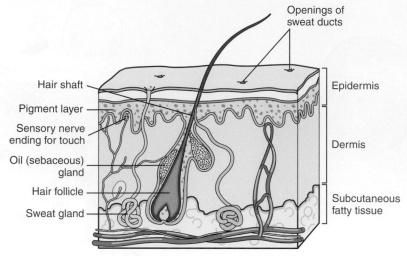

Fig. 5-4 Layers of the skin.

- Sweat glands—help the body regulate temperature. Sweat consists of water, salt, and a small amount of wastes. Sweat is secreted through pores in the skin. The body is cooled as sweat evaporates.
- Hair—covers the entire body, except the palms of the hands and the soles of the feet. Hair in the nose and ears and around the eyes protects these organs from dust, insects, and other foreign objects.
- Nails—protect the tips of the fingers and toes. Nails help fingers pick up and handle small objects.
  The skin has many functions:
- It is the body's protective covering.
- It prevents microorganisms and other substances from entering the body.
- It prevents excess amounts of water from leaving the body.
- It protects organs from injury.
- Nerve endings in the skin sense both pleasant and unpleasant stimulation. Nerve endings are over the entire body. They sense cold, pain, touch, and pressure to protect the body from injury.
- It helps regulate body temperature. Blood vessels dilate (widen) when temperature outside the body is high. More blood is brought to the body surface for cooling during evaporation. When blood vessels constrict (narrow), the body retains heat. This is because less blood reaches the skin.

THE MUSCULOSKELETAL SYSTEM

The musculoskeletal system provides the framework for the body. It lets the body move. This system also protects and gives the body shape.

Bones

The human body has 206 *bones* (Fig. 5-5). There are four types of bones:
- *Long bones* bear the body's weight. Leg bones are long bones.
- *Short bones* allow skill and ease in movement. Bones in the wrists, fingers, ankles, and toes are short bones.
- *Flat bones* protect the organs. They include the ribs, skull, pelvic bones, and shoulder blades.

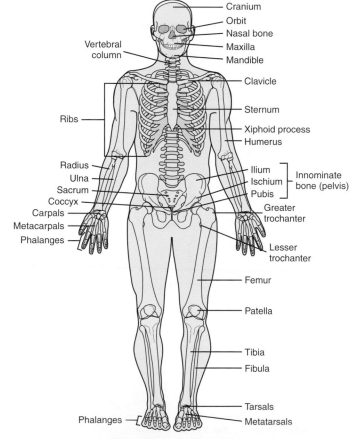

Fig. 5-5 Bones of the body.

- *Irregular bones* are the vertebrae in the spinal column. They allow various degrees of movement and flexibility.

Bones are hard, rigid structures. They are made up of living cells. They are covered by a membrane called *periosteum*. Periosteum contains blood vessels that supply bone cells with oxygen and food. Inside the hollow centers of the bones is a substance called *bone marrow*. Blood cells are formed in the bone marrow.

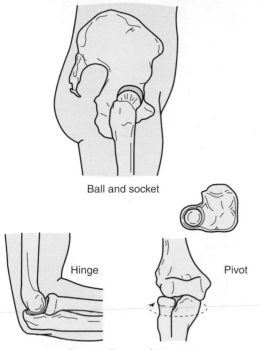

Fig. 5-6 Types of joints.

Ball and socket

Hinge

Pivot

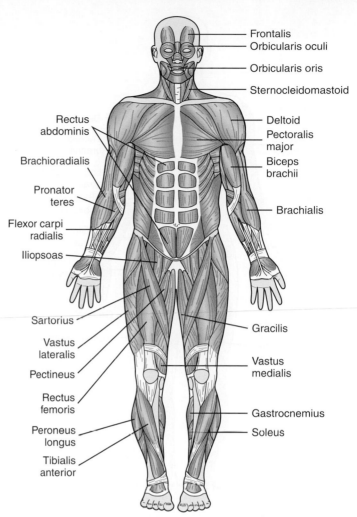

Fig. 5-7 Anterior view of the muscles of the body.

Joints

A *joint* is the point at which two or more bones meet. Joints allow movement. *Cartilage* is the connective tissue at the end of the long bones. It cushions the joint so that the bone ends do not rub together. The *synovial membrane* lines the joints. It secretes *synovial fluid.* Synovial fluid acts as a lubricant so the joint can move smoothly. Bones are held together at the joint by strong bands of connective tissue called *ligaments.*

There are three major types of joints (Fig. 5-6):

- A *ball-and-socket joint* allows movement in all directions. It is made up of the rounded end of one bone and the hollow end of another bone. The rounded end of one fits into the hollow end of the other. The joints of the hips and shoulders are ball-and-socket joints.
- A *hinge joint* allows movement in one direction. The elbow is a hinge joint.
- A *pivot joint* allows turning from side to side. A pivot joint connects the skull to the spine.

Muscles

The human body has more than 500 *muscles* (Fig. 5-7 and Fig. 5-8). Some are voluntary. Others are involuntary.

- *Voluntary muscles* can be consciously controlled. Muscles attached to bones *(skeletal muscles)* are voluntary. Arm muscles do not work unless you move your arm; likewise, for leg muscles. Skeletal muscles are *striated.* That is, they look striped or streaked.
- *Involuntary muscles* work automatically. You cannot control them. They control the action of the stomach, intestines, blood vessels, and other body organs. Involuntary muscles also are called *smooth muscles.* They look smooth, not streaked or striped.
- *Cardiac muscle* is in the heart. It is an involuntary muscle. However, it appears striated like skeletal muscle.

Muscles have three functions:

- Movement of body parts
- Maintenance of posture
- Production of body heat

Strong, tough connective tissues called *tendons* connect muscles to bones. When muscles contract (shorten), tendons at each end of the muscle cause the bone to move. The body has many tendons. See the Achilles tendon in Fig. 5-8. Some muscles constantly contract to maintain the body's posture. When muscles contract, they burn food for energy. Heat is produced. The more muscle activity, the greater the amount of heat produced. Shivering is how the body produces heat when exposed to cold. Shivering is from rapid, general muscle contractions.

THE NERVOUS SYSTEM

The nervous system controls, directs, and coordinates body functions. Its two main divisions are:

- The *central nervous system* (CNS). It consists of the brain and spinal cord (Fig. 5-9).
- The *peripheral nervous system.* It involves the *nerves* throughout the body (Fig. 5-10).

Nerves carry messages or impulses to and from the brain. Nerves connect to the spinal cord. They are easily damaged and

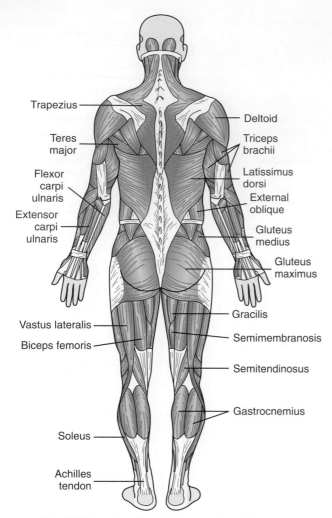

Fig. 5-8 Posterior view of the muscles of the body.

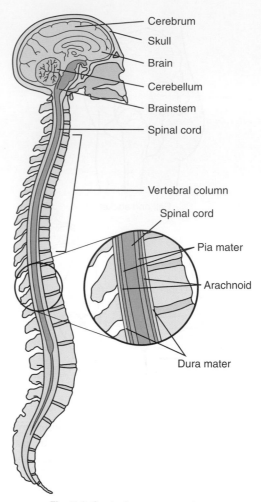

Fig. 5-9 Central nervous system.

take a long time to heal. Some nerve fibers have a protective covering called a *myelin sheath*. The myelin sheath also insulates the nerve fiber. Nerve fibers covered with myelin conduct impulses faster than those fibers without it.

The Central Nervous System

The *brain* and *spinal cord* make up the central nervous system. The brain is covered by the skull. The three main parts of the brain are the *cerebrum*, the *cerebellum*, and the *brainstem* (Fig. 5-11).

The cerebrum is the largest part of the brain. It is the center of thought and intelligence. The cerebrum is divided into two halves called the *right* and *left hemispheres*. The right hemisphere controls movement and activities on the body's left side. The left hemisphere controls the right side.

The outside of the cerebrum is called the *cerebral cortex*. It controls the highest functions of the brain. These include reasoning, memory, consciousness, speech, voluntary muscle movement, vision, hearing, sensation, and other activities.

The cerebellum regulates and coordinates body movements. It controls balance and the smooth movements of voluntary muscles. Injury to the cerebellum results in jerky movements, loss of coordination, and muscle weakness.

The brainstem connects the cerebrum to the spinal cord. The brainstem contains the *midbrain, pons,* and *medulla.* The midbrain and pons relay messages between the medulla and the cerebrum. The medulla is below the pons. The medulla controls heart rate, breathing, blood vessel size, swallowing, coughing, and vomiting. The brain connects to the spinal cord at the lower end of the medulla.

The spinal cord lies within the spinal column. The cord is 17 to 18 inches long. It contains pathways that conduct messages to and from the brain.

The brain and spinal cord are covered and protected by three layers of connective tissue called meninges:

- The outer layer lies next to the skull. It is a tough covering call the *dura mater.*
- The middle layer is the *arachnoid.*
- The inner layer is the *pia mater.*

The space between the middle layer (arachnoid) and inner layer (pia mater) is the *arachnoid space.* The space is filled with *cerebrospinal fluid.* It circulates around the brain and spinal cord. Cerebrospinal fluid protects the central nervous system. It cushions shocks that could easily injure brain and spinal cord structures.

The Peripheral Nervous System

The peripheral nervous system has 12 pairs of *cranial nerves* and 31 pairs of *spinal nerves.* Cranial nerves conduct impulses between the brain and the head, neck, chest, and abdomen.

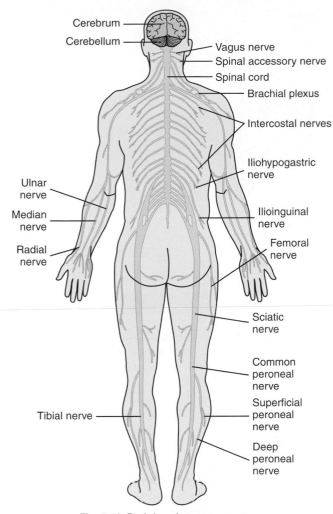

Fig. 5-10 Peripheral nervous system.

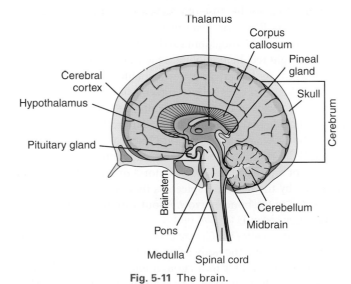

Fig. 5-11 The brain.

They conduct impulses for smell, vision, hearing, pain, touch, temperature, and pressure. They also conduct impulses for voluntary and involuntary muscles. Spinal nerves carry impulses from the skin, extremities, and the internal structures not supplied by cranial nerves.

Some peripheral nerves form the *autonomic nervous system.* This system controls involuntary muscles and certain body functions. The functions include the heartbeat, blood pressure, intestinal contractions, and glandular secretions. These functions occur automatically.

The autonomic nervous system is divided into the *sympathetic nervous system* and the *parasympathetic nervous system.* They balance each other. The sympathetic nervous system speeds up functions. The parasympathetic nervous system slows functions. When you are angry, scared, excited, or exercising, the sympathetic nervous system is stimulated. The parasympathetic nervous system is activated when you relax. It also is activated when the sympathetic system is stimulated for too long.

The Sense Organs

The five senses are *sight, hearing, taste, smell,* and *touch.* Receptors for taste are in the tongue. They are called *taste buds.* Receptors for smell are in the nose. Touch receptors are in the dermis, especially in the toes and fingertips.

The Eye. Receptors for vision are in the *eyes* (Fig. 5-12). The eye is easily injured. Bones of the skull, eyelids and eyelashes, and tears protect the eyes from injury. The eye has three layers:

- The *sclera,* the white of the eye, is the outer layer. It is made of tough connective tissue.
- The *choroid* is the second layer. Blood vessels, the *ciliary muscle,* and the *iris* make up the choroid. The iris gives the eye its color. The opening in the middle of the iris is the *pupil.* Pupil size varies with the amount of light entering the eye. The pupil constricts (narrows) in bright light. It dilates (widens) in dim or dark places.
- The *retina* is the inner layer. It has receptors for vision and the nerve fibers of the *optic nerve.*

Light enters the eye through the *cornea.* It is the transparent part of the outer layer that lies over the eye. Light rays pass to the *lens,* which lies behind the pupil. The light is then reflected to the retina. Light is carried to the brain by the optic nerve.

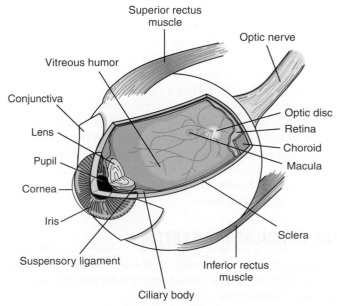

Fig. 5-12 The eye.

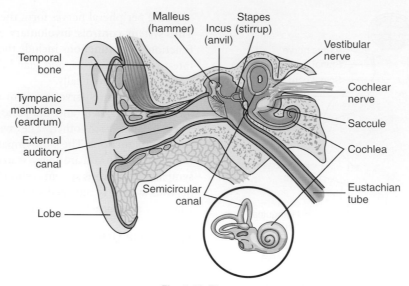

Fig. 5-13 The ear.

The *aqueous chamber* separates the cornea from the lens. The chamber is filled with a fluid called *aqueous humor.* The fluid helps the cornea keep its shape and position. The *vitreous humor* is behind the lens. It is a gelatin-like substance that supports the retina and maintains the eye's shape.

The Ear. The *ear* is a sense organ (Fig. 5-13). It functions in hearing and balance. It has three parts: the *external ear, middle ear,* and *inner ear.*

The external ear (outer part) is called the *pinna* or *auricle.* Sound waves are guided through the external ear into the *auditory canal.* Glands in the auditory canal secrete a waxy substance called *cerumen.* The auditory canal extends about 1 inch to the *eardrum.* The eardrum *(tympanic membrane)* separates the external and middle ear.

The middle ear is a small space. It contains the *eustachian tube* and three small bones called *ossicles.* The eustachian tube connects the middle ear and the throat. Air enters the eustachian tube so that there is equal pressure on both sides of the eardrum. The ossicles amplify sound received from the eardrum and transmit the sound to the inner ear. The three ossicles are:

- The *malleus.* It looks like a hammer.
- The *incus.* It looks like an anvil.
- The *stapes.* It is shaped like a stirrup.

The inner ear consists of *semicircular canals* and the *cochlea.* The cochlea looks like a snail shell. It contains fluid. The fluid carries sound waves from the middle ear to the *acoustic nerve.* The auditory nerve then carries the message to the brain.

The three semicircular canals are involved with balance. They sense the head's position and changes in position. They send messages to the brain.

THE CIRCULATORY SYSTEM

The circulatory system is made up of the *blood, heart,* and *blood vessels.* The heart pumps blood through the blood vessels. The circulatory system has many functions:

- Blood carries food, oxygen, and other substances to the cells.
- Blood removes waste products from cells.

- Blood and blood vessels help regulate body temperature. The blood carries heat from muscle activity to other body parts. Blood vessels in the skin dilate to cool the body. They constrict to retain heat.
- The system produces and carries cells that defend the body from microbes that cause disease.

The Blood

The blood consists of blood cells and *plasma.* Plasma is mostly water. It carries blood cells to other body cells. Plasma also carries substances that cells need to function. This includes food (proteins, fats, and carbohydrates), hormones (p. 56), and chemicals.

Red blood cells (RBCs) are called *erythrocytes.* They give blood its red color because of a substance in the cell called **hemoglobin.** As RBCs circulate through the lungs, hemoglobin picks up oxygen. Hemoglobin carries oxygen to the cells. When blood is bright red, hemoglobin in the RBCs is saturated (filled) with oxygen. As blood circulates through the body, oxygen is given to the cells. Cells release carbon dioxide (a waste product). It is picked up by the hemoglobin. RBCs saturated with carbon dioxide make the blood look dark red.

The body has about 25 trillion (25,000,000,000,000) RBCs. About 4½ to 5 million cells are in a cubic millimeter of blood (the size of a tiny drop). RBCs live for 3 or 4 months. They are destroyed by the liver and spleen as they wear out. New RBCs are formed in the bone marrow. About 1 million RBCs are produced every second.

White blood cells (WBCs) are called *leukocytes.* They have no color. They protect the body against infection. There are about 5,000 to 10,000 WBCs in a cubic millimeter of blood. At the first sign of infection, WBCs rush to the infection site. There they multiply rapidly. The number of WBCs increases when there is an infection. WBCs are formed by the bone marrow. They live about 9 days.

Platelets (thrombocytes) are needed for blood clotting. They are formed by the bone marrow. There are about 200,000 to 400,000 platelets in a cubic millimeter of blood. A platelet lives about 4 days.

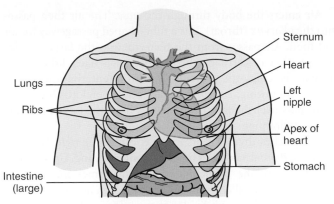

Fig. 5-14 Location of the heart in the chest cavity.

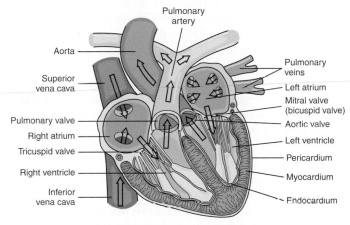

Fig. 5-15 Structures of the heart.

The Heart

The heart is a muscle. It pumps blood through the blood vessels to the tissues and cells. The heart lies in the middle to lower part of the chest cavity toward the left side (Fig. 5-14). The heart is hollow and has three layers (Fig. 5-15):

- The *pericardium* is the outer layer. It is a thin sac covering the heart.
- The *myocardium* is the second layer. It is the thick, muscular part of the heart.
- The *endocardium* is the inner layer. A membrane, it lines the inner surface of the heart.

The heart has four chambers (Fig. 5-15). Upper chambers receive blood and are called *atria*. The *right atrium* receives blood from body tissues. The *left atrium* receives blood from the lungs. Lower chambers are called *ventricles*. Ventricles pump blood. The *right ventricle* pumps blood to the lungs for oxygen. The *left ventricle* pumps blood to all parts of the body.

Valves are between the atria and ventricles. The valves allow blood flow in one direction. They prevent blood from flowing back into the atria from the ventricles. The *tricuspid valve* is between the right atrium and the right ventricle. The *mitral valve (bicuspid valve)* is between the left atrium and left ventricle.

Heart action has two phases:

- *Diastole.* It is the resting phase. Heart chambers fill with blood.
- *Systole.* It is the working phase. The heart contracts. Blood is pumped through the blood vessels when the heart contracts.

The Blood Vessels

Blood flows to body tissues and cells through the blood vessels. There are three groups of blood vessels: arteries, capillaries, and veins.

Arteries carry blood away from the heart. Arterial blood is rich in oxygen. The *aorta* is the largest artery. It receives blood directly from the left ventricle. The aorta branches into other arteries that carry blood to all parts of the body (Fig. 5-16). These arteries branch into smaller parts within the tissues. The smallest branch of an artery is an *arteriole*.

Arterioles connect to **capillaries.** Capillaries are very tiny blood vessels. Food, oxygen, and other substances pass from capillaries into the cells. The capillaries pick up waste products (including carbon dioxide) from the cells. Veins carry waste products back to the heart.

Veins return blood back to the heart. They connect to the capillaries by *venules*. Venules are small veins. Venules branch together to form veins. The many veins also branch together as they near the heart to form two main veins (Fig. 5-16). The two main veins are the *inferior vena cava* and the *superior vena cava*. Both empty into the right atrium. The inferior vena cava carries blood from the legs and trunk. The superior vena cava carries blood from the head and arms. Venous blood is dark red. It has little oxygen and a lot of carbon dioxide.

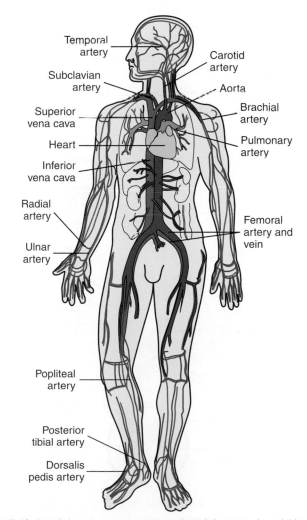

Fig. 5-16 Arterial and venous systems. Arterial system is red. Venous system is blue.

Blood flow through the circulatory system is shown in Fig. 5-15. The path of blood flow is as follows:

- Venous blood, poor in oxygen, empties into the right atrium.
- Blood flows through the tricuspid valve into the right ventricle.
- The right ventricle pumps blood into the lungs to pick up oxygen.
- Oxygen-rich blood from the lungs enters the left atrium.
- Blood from the left atrium passes through the mitral valve into the left ventricle.
- The left ventricle pumps the blood to the aorta. It branches off to form other arteries.
- Arterial blood is carried to the tissues by arterioles and to the cells by capillaries.
- Cells and capillaries exchange oxygen and nutrients for carbon dioxide and waste products.
- Capillaries connect with venules.
- Venules carry blood that has carbon dioxide and waste products.
- Venules form veins.
- Veins return blood to the heart.

THE RESPIRATORY SYSTEM

Oxygen is needed to live. Every cell needs oxygen. Air contains about 21% oxygen. This meets the body's needs under normal conditions. The respiratory system (Fig. 5-17) brings oxygen into the lungs and removes carbon dioxide. **Respiration** is the process of supplying the cells with oxygen and removing carbon dioxide from them. Respiration involves *inhalation* (breathing in) and *exhalation* (breathing out). The terms *inspiration* (breathing in) and *expiration* (breathing out) also are used.

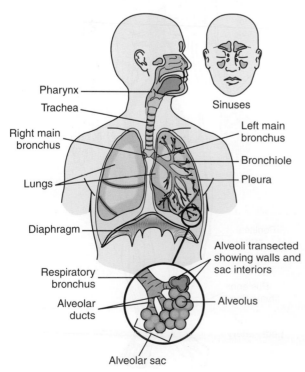

Fig. 5-17 Respiratory system.

Air enters the body through the *nose*. The air then passes into the *pharynx* (throat). It is a tube-shaped passageway for air and food. Air passes from the pharynx into the *larynx* (voice box). A piece of cartilage, the *epiglottis*, acts like a lid over the larynx. The epiglottis prevents food from entering the airway during swallowing. During inhalation, the epiglottis lifts up to let air pass over the larynx. Air passes from the larynx into the *trachea* (windpipe).

The trachea divides at its lower end into the *right bronchus* and the *left bronchus*. Each bronchus enters a lung. Upon entering the lungs, the bronchi divide many times into smaller branches. The smaller branches are called *bronchioles*. Eventually the bronchioles subdivide. They end up in tiny one-celled air sacs called *alveoli*.

Alveoli look like small clusters of grapes. They are supplied by capillaries. Oxygen and carbon dioxide are exchanged between the alveoli and capillaries. Blood in the capillaries picks up oxygen from the alveoli. Then the blood is returned to the left side of the heart and pumped to the rest of the body. Alveoli pick up carbon dioxide from the capillaries for exhalation.

The lungs are spongy tissues. They are filled with alveoli, blood vessels, and nerves. Each lung is divided into lobes. The right lung has three lobes; the left lung has two. The lungs are separated from the abdominal cavity by a muscle called the *diaphragm*.

Each lung is covered by a two-layered sac called the *pleura*. One layer is attached to the lung and the other to the chest wall. The pleura secretes a very thin fluid that fills the space between the layers. The fluid prevents the layers from rubbing together during inhalation and exhalation. A bony framework made up of the ribs, sternum, and vertebrae protects the lungs.

THE DIGESTIVE SYSTEM

The digestive system breaks down food physically and chemically so it can be absorbed for use by the cells. This process is called **digestion.** The digestive system is also called the *gastrointestinal (GI) system.* The system also removes solid wastes from the body.

The digestive system involves the *alimentary canal (GI tract)* and the accessory organs of digestion (Fig. 5-18). The alimentary canal is a long tube. It extends from the mouth to the anus. Its major parts are the mouth, pharynx, esophagus, stomach, small intestine, and large intestine. Accessory organs are the teeth, tongue, salivary glands, liver, gallbladder, and pancreas.

Digestion begins in the *mouth.* The mouth also is called the *oral cavity.* It receives food and prepares it for digestion. Using chewing motions, the *teeth* cut, chop, and grind food into small particles for digestion and swallowing. The *tongue* aids in chewing and swallowing. Taste buds on the tongue's surface contain nerve endings. Taste buds allow sweet, sour, bitter, and salty tastes to be sensed. *Salivary glands* in the mouth secrete *saliva.* Saliva moistens food particles to ease swallowing and begin digestion. During swallowing, the tongue pushes food into the *pharynx.*

The pharynx (throat) is a muscular tube. Swallowing continues as the pharynx contracts. Contraction of the pharynx

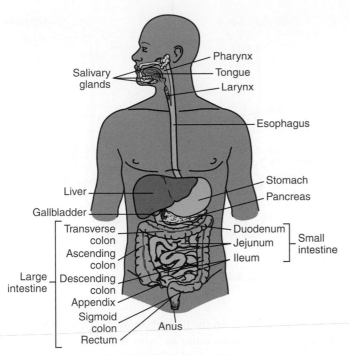

Fig. 5-18 Digestive system.

pushes food into the *esophagus*. The esophagus is a muscular tube about 10 inches long. It extends from the pharynx to the *stomach*. Involuntary muscle contractions called peristalsis move food down the esophagus through the alimentary canal.

The stomach is a muscular, pouch-like sac. It is in the upper left part of the abdominal cavity. Strong stomach muscles stir and churn food to break it up into even smaller particles. A mucous membrane lines the stomach. It contains glands that secrete *gastric juices*. Food is mixed and churned with the gastric juices to form a semi-liquid substance called *chyme*. Through peristalsis, the chyme is pushed from the stomach into the small intestine.

The *small intestine* is about 20 feet long. It has three parts. The first part is the *duodenum*. There more digestive juices are added to the chyme. One is called *bile*. Bile is a greenish liquid made in the *liver*. Bile is stored in the *gallbladder*. Juices from the *pancreas* and small intestine are added to the chyme. Digestive juices chemically break down food so it can be absorbed.

Peristalsis moves the chyme through the two other parts of the small intestine: the *jejunum* and the *ileum*. Tiny projections called *villi* line the small intestine. Villi absorb the digested food into the capillaries. Most food absorption takes place in the jejunum and the ileum.

Some chyme is not digested. Undigested chyme passes from the small intestine into the *large intestine (large bowel* or *colon)*. The colon absorbs most of the water from the chyme. The remaining semi-solid material is called *feces*. Feces contain a small amount of water, solid wastes, and some mucus and germs. These are the waste products of digestion. Feces pass through the colon into the *rectum* by peristalsis. Feces pass out of the body through the *anus*.

THE URINARY SYSTEM

The digestive system rids the body of solid wastes. The lungs rid the body of carbon dioxide. Water and other substances leave the body through sweat. There are other waste products in the blood from cells burning food for energy. The urinary system (Fig. 5-19):
- Removes waste products from the blood
- Maintains water balance within the body

The *kidneys* are two bean-shaped organs in the upper abdomen. They lie against the back muscles on each side of the spine. They are protected by the lower edge of the rib cage.

Each kidney has over a million tiny *nephrons* (Fig. 5-20). Each nephron is the basic working unit of the kidney. Each nephron has a *convoluted tubule*, which is a tiny coiled tubule. Each convoluted tubule has a *Bowman's capsule* at one end. The capsule partly surrounds a cluster of capillaries called a *glomerulus*. Blood passes through the glomerulus and is filtered by the capillaries. The fluid part of the blood is squeezed into the Bowman's capsule. The fluid then passes into the tubule. Most of the water and other needed substances are reabsorbed by the blood. The rest of the fluid and the waste products form *urine* in the tubule. Urine flows through the tubule to a *collecting tubule*. All collecting tubules drain into the *renal pelvis* in the kidney.

A tube, called the *ureter*, is attached to the renal pelvis of the kidney. Each ureter is about 10 to 12 inches long. The ureters carry urine from the kidneys to the *bladder*. The bladder is a hollow, muscular sac. It lies toward the front in the lower part of the abdominal cavity.

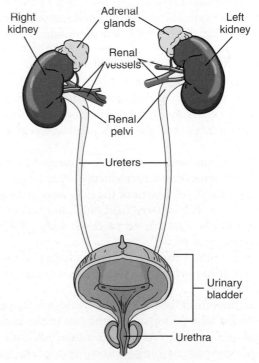

Fig. 5-19 Urinary system.

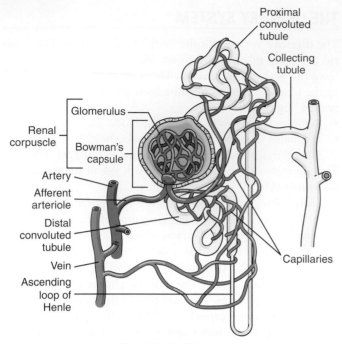

Fig. 5-20 A nephron.

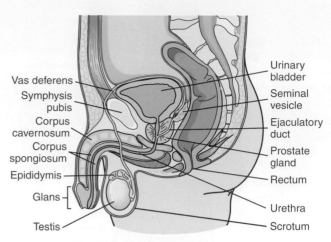

Fig. 5-21 Male reproductive system.

Urine is stored in the bladder until the need to urinate is felt. This usually occurs when there is about a half pint (250 mL) of urine in the bladder. Urine passes from the bladder through the *urethra.* The opening at the end of the urethra is the *meatus.* Urine passes from the body through the meatus. Urine is a clear, yellowish fluid.

THE REPRODUCTIVE SYSTEM

Human reproduction results from the union of a male sex cell and a female sex cell. The male and female reproductive systems are different. This allows for the process of reproduction.

The Male Reproductive System

The male reproductive system is shown in Fig. 5-21. The *testes (testicles)* are the male sex glands. Sex glands also are called *gonads.* The two testes are oval or almond-shaped glands. Male sex cells are produced in the testes. Male sex cells are called *sperm* cells.

Testosterone, the male hormone, is produced in the testes. This hormone is needed for reproductive organ function. It also is needed for the development of the male secondary sex characteristics. These include facial hair; pubic and axillary (underarm) hair; and hair on the arms, chest, and legs. Neck and shoulder sizes increase.

The testes are suspended between the thighs in a sac called the *scrotum.* It lies behind the penis. The scrotum is made of skin and muscle.

Sperm travel from the testis to the *epididymis.* The epididymis is a coiled tube on top and to the side of the testis. From the epididymis, sperm travel through a tube called the *vas deferens.* Each vas deferens joins a seminal vesicle. The two seminal vesicles store sperm and produce *semen.* Semen is a fluid

that carries sperm from the male reproductive tract. The ducts of the seminal vesicles unite to form the *ejaculatory duct.* It passes through the *prostate gland.*

The prostate gland lies just below the bladder. It is shaped like a donut. The gland secretes fluid into the semen. As the ejaculatory ducts leave the prostate, they join the *urethra.* The urethra runs through the prostate gland. The urethra is the outlet for urine and semen. The urethra is contained within the *penis.*

The penis lies in front of the scrotum and has *erectile* tissue. When a man is sexually excited, blood fills the erectile tissue. The penis enlarges and becomes hard and erect. The erect penis can enter a female's vagina. The semen, which contains sperm, is released into the vagina.

The Female Reproductive System

Fig. 5-22 shows the female reproductive system. The female gonads are two almond-shaped glands called *ovaries.* An ovary is on each side of the uterus in the abdominal cavity.

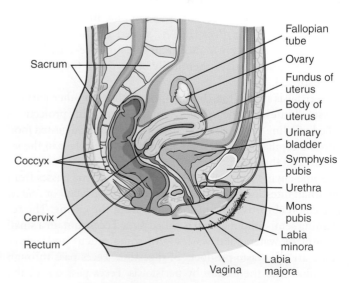

Fig. 5-22 Female reproductive system.

The ovaries contain *ova* or eggs. Ova are the female sex cells. One ovum (egg) is released monthly during the woman's reproductive years. Release of an ovum is called *ovulation.*

The ovaries secrete the female hormones *estrogen* and *progesterone.* These hormones are needed for reproductive system function. They also are needed for the development of secondary sex characteristics in the female. These include increased breast size, pubic and axillary (underarm) hair, slight deepening of the voice, and widening and rounding of the hips.

When an ovum is released from an ovary, it travels through a *fallopian tube.* There are two fallopian tubes, one on each side. The tubes are attached at one end to the uterus. The ovum travels through the fallopian tube to the *uterus.*

The *uterus* is a hollow, muscular organ shaped like a pear. It is in the center of the pelvic cavity behind the bladder and in front of the rectum. The main part of the uterus is the *fundus.* The neck or narrow section of the uterus is the *cervix.* Tissue lining the uterus is called the *endometrium.* The endometrium has many blood vessels. If sex cells from the male and female unite into one cell, that cell implants into the endometrium. There the cell grows into a baby. The uterus serves as a place for the *fetus* (unborn baby) to grow and receive nourishment.

The cervix of the uterus projects into a muscular canal called the *vagina.* The vagina opens to the outside of the body. It is just behind the urethra. The vagina receives the penis during intercourse. It also is part of the birth canal. Glands in the vaginal wall keep it moistened with secretions. In young girls, the external vaginal opening is partially closed by a membrane called the *hymen.* The hymen ruptures when the female has intercourse for the first time.

The external female genitalia are called the *vulva* (Fig. 5-23):

- The *mons pubis* is a rounded, fatty pad over a bone called the *symphysis pubis.* The mons pubis is covered with hair in the adult female.
- The *labia majora* and *labia minora* are two folds of tissue on each side of the vaginal opening.
- The *clitoris* is a small organ composed of erectile tissue. It becomes hard when sexually stimulated.

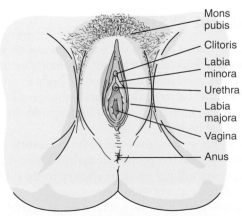

Mons pubis
Clitoris
Labia minora
Urethra
Labia majora
Vagina
Anus

Fig. 5-23 External female genitalia.

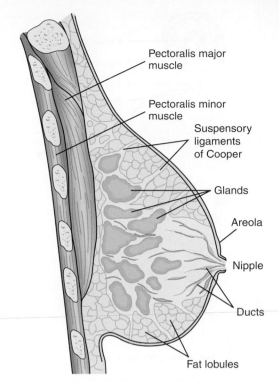

Pectoralis major muscle
Pectoralis minor muscle
Suspensory ligaments of Cooper
Glands
Areola
Nipple
Ducts
Fat lobules

Fig. 5-24 The female breast.

The *mammary glands (breasts)* secrete milk after childbirth. The glands are on the outside of the chest. They are made up of glandular tissue and fat (Fig. 5-24). The milk drains into ducts that open onto the *nipple.*

Menstruation. The endometrium is rich in blood to nourish the cell that grows into a fetus. If pregnancy does not occur, the endometrium breaks up. It is discharged from the body through the vagina. This process is called **menstruation.** Menstruation occurs about every 28 days. Therefore, it is called the *menstrual cycle.*

The first day of the menstrual cycle begins with menstruation. Blood flows from the uterus through the vaginal opening. Menstrual flow usually lasts 3 to 7 days. Ovulation occurs during the next phase. An ovum matures in an ovary and is released. Ovulation usually occurs on or about day 14 of the cycle.

Meanwhile, estrogen and progesterone (the female hormones) are secreted by the ovaries. These hormones cause the endometrium to thicken for pregnancy. If pregnancy does not occur, the hormones decrease in amount. This causes the blood supply to the endometrium to decrease. The endometrium breaks up. It is discharged through the vagina. Another menstrual cycle begins.

Fertilization

To reproduce, a male sex cell (sperm) must unite with a female sex cell (ovum). The uniting of the sperm and ovum into one cell is called *fertilization.* A sperm has 23 chromosomes. An ovum has 23 chromosomes. When the two cells unite, the fertilized cell has 46 chromosomes.

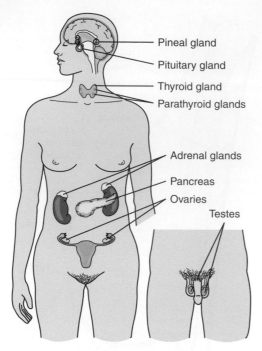

Fig. 5-25 Endocrine system.

During intercourse, millions of sperm are deposited into the vagina. Sperm travel up the cervix, through the uterus, and into the fallopian tubes. If a sperm and an ovum unite in a fallopian tube, fertilization results. Pregnancy occurs. The fertilized cell travels down the fallopian tube to the uterus. After a short time, the fertilized cell implants in the thick endometrium and grows during pregnancy.

THE ENDOCRINE SYSTEM

The endocrine system is made up of glands called the *endocrine glands* (Fig. 5-25). The endocrine glands secrete chemical substances called **hormones** into the bloodstream. Hormones regulate the activities of other organs and glands in the body.

The *pituitary gland* is called the *master gland*. About the size of a cherry, it is at the base of the brain behind the eyes. The pituitary gland is divided into the *anterior pituitary lobe* and the *posterior pituitary lobe*. The anterior pituitary lobe secretes:

- *Growth hormone (GH)*—needed for growth of muscles, bones, and other organs. It is needed throughout life to maintain normal-size bones and muscles. Growth is stunted if a baby is born with deficient amounts of growth hormone. Too much of the hormone causes excessive growth.
- *Thyroid-stimulating hormone (TSH)*—needed for thyroid gland function.
- *Adrenocorticotropic hormone (ACTH)*—stimulates the adrenal gland.

The anterior lobe also secretes hormones that regulate growth, development, and function of the male and female reproductive systems.

The posterior pituitary lobe secretes *antidiuretic hormone (ADH)* and *oxytocin.* ADH prevents the kidneys from excreting excessive amounts of water. Oxytocin causes uterine muscles to contract during childbirth.

The *thyroid gland,* shaped like a butterfly, is in the neck in front of the larynx. *Thyroid hormone (T4, thyroxine)* is secreted by the thyroid gland. It regulates **metabolism.** Metabolism is the burning of food for heat and energy by the cells. Too little T4 results in slowed body processes, slowed movements, and weight gain. Too much T4 causes increased metabolism, excess energy, and weight loss. Some babies are born with deficient amounts of T4. Their physical growth and mental growth are stunted.

The four *parathyroid glands* secrete *parathormone.* Two lie on each side of the thyroid gland. Parathormone regulates calcium use. Calcium is needed for nerve and muscle function. Insufficient amounts of calcium cause *tetany.* Tetany is a state of severe muscle contraction and spasm. If untreated, tetany can cause death.

There are two *adrenal glands.* An adrenal gland is on the top of each kidney. The adrenal gland has two parts: the *adrenal medulla* and the *adrenal cortex.* The adrenal medulla secretes *epinephrine* and *norepinephrine.* These hormones stimulate the body to quickly produce energy during emergencies. Heart rate, blood pressure, muscle power, and energy all increase.

The adrenal cortex secretes three groups of hormones needed for life:

- *Gluco corticoids*—regulate the metabolism of carbohydrates. They also control the body's response to stress and inflammation.
- *Mineralo corticoids*—regulate the amount of salt and water that is absorbed and lost by the kidneys.
- Small amounts of male and female sex hormones—p. 54 & 55.

The *pancreas* secretes *insulin.* Insulin regulates the amount of sugar in the blood available for use by the cells. Insulin is needed for sugar to enter the cells. If there is too little insulin, sugar cannot enter the cells. If sugar cannot enter the cells, excess amounts of sugar build up in the blood. This condition is called *diabetes.*

The *gonads* are the glands of human reproduction. Male sex glands (testes) secrete *testosterone.* Female sex glands (ovaries) secrete *estrogen* and *progesterone.*

THE IMMUNE SYSTEM

The immune system protects the body from disease and infection. Abnormal body cells can grow into tumors. Sometimes the body produces substances that cause the body to attack itself. Microorganisms (bacteria, viruses, and other germs) can cause an infection. The immune system defends against threats inside and outside the body.

The immune system gives the body **immunity**. Immunity means that a person has protection against a disease or condition. The person will not get or be affected by the disease.

There are two types of immunity:

- *Specific immunity* is the body's reaction to a certain threat.

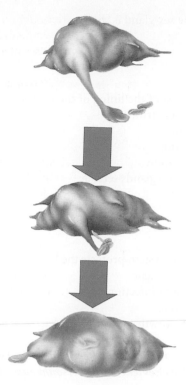

Fig. 5-26 A phagocyte digests and destroys a microorganism. (From Thibodeau, G. A., Patton, K. T., *Structure and Function of the Body,* 11th ed., St Louis, Mosby, 2000.)

- *Non-specific immunity* is the body's reaction to anything it does not recognize as a normal body substance. Special cells and substances function to produce immunity:
- *Antibodies*—normal body substances that recognize abnormal or unwanted substances. They attack and destroy these substances.
- *Antigens*—abnormal or unwanted substances. An antigen causes the body to produce antibodies. The antibodies attack and destroy the antigens.
- *Phagocytes*—white blood cells that digest and destroy microorganisms and other unwanted substances (Fig. 5-26).
- *Lymphocytes*—white blood cells that produce antibodies. Lymphocyte production increases as the body responds to an infection.
- *B lymphocytes (B cells)*—cause the production of antibodies that circulate in the plasma. The antibodies react to specific antigens.
- *T lymphocytes (T cells)*—cells that destroy invading cells. *Killer T cells* produce poisons near the invading cells. Some T cells attract other cells. The other cells destroy the invaders.

When the body senses an antigen (an unwanted substance), the immune system acts. Phagocyte and lymphocyte production increases. Phagocytes destroy the invaders through digestion. The lymphocytes produce antibodies that attack and destroy the unwanted substances.

REVIEW QUESTIONS

Circle the BEST answer.

1. The basic unit of body structure is the:
   a. cell
   b. neuron
   c. nephron
   d. ovum
2. The outer layer of the skin is called the:
   a. dermis
   b. epidermis
   c. integument
   d. myelin
3. Which is *not* a function of the skin?
   a. providing the protective covering for the body
   b. regulating body temperature
   c. sensing cold, pain, touch, and pressure
   d. providing the shape and framework for the body
4. Skeletal muscles:
   a. are under involuntary control
   b. appear smooth
   c. are under voluntary control
   d. appear striped and smooth
5. The highest functions in the brain take place in the:
   a. cerebral cortex
   b. medulla
   c. brainstem
   d. spinal nerves
6. The ear is involved with:
   a. regulating body movements
   b. balance
   c. smoothness of body movements
   d. controlling involuntary muscles
7. The liquid part of the blood is the:
   a. hemoglobin
   b. red blood cell
   c. plasma
   d. white blood cell
8. Which part of the heart pumps blood to the body?
   a. right atrium
   b. left atrium
   c. right ventricle
   d. left ventricle
9. Which carry blood away from the heart?
   a. capillaries
   b. veins
   c. venules
   d. arteries
10. Oxygen and carbon dioxide are exchanged:
    a. in the bronchi
    b. between the alveoli and capillaries
    c. between the lungs and pleura
    d. in the trachea

11. Digestion begins in the:
    a. mouth
    b. stomach
    c. small intestine
    d. colon
12. Most food absorption takes place in the:
    a. stomach
    b. small intestine
    c. colon
    d. large intestine
13. Urine is formed by the:
    a. jejunum
    b. kidneys
    c. bladder
    d. liver
14. Urine passes from the body through the:
    a. ureters
    b. urethra
    c. anus
    d. nephrons
15. The male sex gland is called the:
    a. penis
    b. semen
    c. testis
    d. scrotum
16. The male sex cell is the:
    a. semen
    b. ovum
    c. gonad
    d. sperm
17. The female sex gland is the:
    a. ovary
    b. cervix
    c. uterus
    d. vagina
18. The discharge of the lining of the uterus is called:
    a. the endometrium
    b. ovulation
    c. fertilization
    d. menstruation
19. The endocrine glands secrete:
    a. hormones
    b. mucus
    c. semen
    d. insulin
20. The immune system protects the body from:
    a. low blood sugar
    b. disease and infection
    c. loss of fluid
    d. stunted growth

Answers to these questions can be found on the Evolve Resources site: http://evolve.elsevier.com/Anderson/medasst/

6

Infection Prevention

OBJECTIVES

- Define the key terms and key abbreviations in this chapter.
- Identify what microbes need in order to live and grow.
- List the signs and symptoms of infection.
- Describe healthcare–associated infections and the persons at risk.
- Describe the principles of medical asepsis.
- Describe Standard Precautions and Transmission-Based Precautions.
- Describe the differnt types of Personal Protective Equipment.
- Explain the Bloodborne Pathogen Standard.
- Describe ways to prevent the spread of COVID-19.
- Perform the procedures described in this chapter.

PROCEDURES

- Handwashing
- Hand hygiene using an alcohol-based hand rub
- Removing gloves
- Donning and removing a gown
- Donning and removing a mask

KEY TERMS

antibiotics Drugs that kill microbes that cause infections.

asepsis Being free of disease-producing microbes.

contamination The process of becoming unclean.

cross-contamination Passing microbes from one person to another by contaminated hands, equipment, or supplies.

epidemic A disease that affects a large number of people within a community, population, or region.

healthcare-associated infection An infection a person gets when cared for in any setting where health care is given. The infection is related to receiving health care.

immunity Protection against a disease or condition; the person will not get or be affected by the disease.

infection A disease state resulting from the invasion and growth of microbes in the body.

medical asepsis Practices used to remove or destroy pathogens and to prevent their spread from one person or place to another person or place; clean technique.

normal flora Microbes that live and grow in a certain area.

pandemic An epidemic that has spread to multiple countries or continents.

social distancing Putting space (at least 6 feet) between yourself and others.

spores Bacterium protected by a hard shell.

sterile The absence of all microbes.

sterilization The process of destroying all microbes.

surgical asepsis The practice that keeps items free of *all* microbes; sterile technique.

vaccination Giving a vaccine to produce immunity against an infectious disease.

vaccine A preparation containing dead or weakened microbes.

KEY ABBREVIATIONS

AIDS Acquired immunodeficiency syndrome

AIIR Airborne infection isolation room

ALR Assisted living residence

CDC Centers for Disease Control and Prevention

C. diff *Clostridium difficile*

COVID-19 Novel Coronavirus (2019)

HAI Healthcare-associated infections

HBV Hepatitis B virus

HIV Human immunodeficiency virus

ID Identification

MDRO Multidrug-resistant organisms

MRSA Methicillin-resistant Staphylococcus aureus

OPIM Other potentially infectious materials

OSHA Occupational Safety and Health Administration

PPE Personal protective equipment

TB Tuberculosis

UTI Urinary tract infection

VRE Vancomycin-resistant Enterococcus

WHO World Health Organization

INFECTION

An **infection** is a disease state resulting from the invasion and growth of microbes in the body.

A local infection is in a body part. A systemic infection involves the whole body. (Systemic means entire.) The person has some or all of the signs and symptoms listed in Box 6-1.

Preventing Infection

When administering drugs, you will have contact with many people. You will have contact with their bodies and care equipment. As you go from one person to another, you must protect them and yourself from infection. Some microbes found in the body are harmful and can cause infections. They are called *pathogens*. Some infections are serious and can cause death. *Non-pathogens* are microbes that do not usually cause an infection.

There are five types of microbes.

• Bacteria—single-celled organisms that multiply rapidly. Often called germs. Can cause an infection in any body system.
• Fungi—plants that live on other plants or animals. Mushrooms, yeasts, and molds are common fungi. Fungi can infect the mouth, vagina, skin, feet, and other areas of the body.
• Protozoa—one-celled animals. They can infect the blood, brain, intestines, and other areas of the body.
• Rickettsiae—found in fleas, lice, ticks, and other insects. They are spread to humans through insect bites. Rocky Mountain spotted fever is an example. The person has fever, chills, headache, rash, and other signs and symptoms.
• Viruses—grow in living cells and cause many diseases. The common cold, flu, acquired immunodeficiency syndrome (AIDS), hepatitis, and coronavirus (COVID-19) are examples.

Requirements of Microbes

Microbes need a reservoir to live and grow. The reservoir (host) is the environment in which a microbe lives and grows. People, plants, animals, soil, food, and water are common reservoirs. Microbes need water and nourishment from the reservoir. Most need oxygen to live. A warm and dark environment is needed. Most grow best at body temperature. They are destroyed by heat and light.

Healthcare-Associated Infection

A **healthcare-associated infection** (HAI) is an infection a person gets when cared for in any setting where healthcare is administered. The infection is related to receiving healthcare. Hospitals, nursing centers, clinics, and home care settings are examples. HAIs also are called nosocomial infections. (Nosocomial comes from the Greek word for hospital.) HAIs are caused by microbes passed to the person from other sources. They can also be caused by **normal flora**. Normal flora are non-pathogens that normally live and grow in certain parts of the body. They can stop some pathogens

from causing infections. Normal flora become pathogens if they enter other parts of the body.

For example, E. coli normally infects the colon. Feces contain E. coli. Poor wiping after bowel movements can cause E. coli to enter the urinary system. E. coli in the urinary system can cause a urinary tract infection (UTI). If hand washing is poor, E. coli spreads to any body part or anything the hands touch. It also can be transmitted to other people.

Common sites for HAIs are:
• The urinary system.
• The respiratory system.
• Wounds.
• The bloodstream.

The health team must prevent the spread of infection. HAIs are prevented by:
• Medical asepsis, including hand hygiene.
• Surgical asepsis.
• Standard Precautions.
• Transmission-Based Precautions.
• The Bloodborne Pathogen Standard.
See *Focus on Older Persons: Infection.*

FOCUS ON OLDER PERSONS
Infection

The immune system protects the body from disease and infection. Like other body systems, changes occur in the immune system with aging. Older persons are at risk for infection. When an older person has an infection, they may have only a slight fever or no fever at all. Redness and swelling may be very slight. The person may not complain of pain. Confusion and delirium may occur.

An infection can become life-threatening before the person has obvious signs and symptoms. You must be alert to the most minor changes in the person's behavior or condition. Report any concerns to the nurse at once.

Multidrug-Resistant Organisms

Multidrug-resistant organisms (MDROs) are microbes that can resist the effects of antibiotics. **Antibiotics** are drugs that kill microbes that cause infections. You may be giving people antibiotics to treat their infection (Chapter 35). Some microbes can change their structures, which makes them harder to kill. They can survive in the presence of antibiotics. Therefore, the infections they cause are hard to treat.

MDROs are caused by doctors prescribing antibiotics when they are not needed (overprescribing). Not taking antibiotics for the length of time prescribed is another cause. Three common MDROs are resistant to many antibiotics.

- *Methicillin-resistant Staphylococcus aureus (MRSA). Staphylococcus aureus* ("staph") is a bacterium normally found in the nose and on the skin. MRSA is resistant to antibiotics often used for "staph" infections. It can cause serious wound and bloodstream infections and pneumonia.
- *Vancomycin-resistant Enterococcus (VRE). Enterococcus* is a bacterium normally found in the intestines and in feces. It can be transmitted to others by contaminated hands, toilet seats, care equipment, and other items that the hands touch. When not in their natural site (the intestines), enterococci can cause infection in the urinary tract, wounds, and pelvis. Vancomycin is an antibiotic often used to treat such infections. Enterococci resistant to vancomycin are called vancomycin-resistant enterococci (VRE).

MEDICAL ASEPSIS

Asepsis is being free of disease-producing microbes. Microbes are everywhere. Measures are needed to achieve asepsis. **Medical asepsis (clean technique)** is the practice used to:

- Remove or destroy microbes. The number of pathogens is reduced.
- Prevent microbes from spreading from one person or place to another person or place.

Surgical asepsis (sterile technique) is the practice that keeps items free of *all* microbes. **Sterile** means the absence of *all* microbes—pathogens and non-pathogens. **Sterilization** is the process of destroying *all* microbes (pathogens and non-pathogens) using very high temperatures.

Most healthcare equipment is disposable. Single-use items are used once then discarded. Multi-use items are used by only one person and then discarded. Multi-use items include bedpans, urinals, water pitchers, and some blood pressure cuffs. Do not "borrow" multi-use items for another person. Disposable items help prevent the spread of infections. Non-disposable items are cleaned, disinfected, and sterilized.

Cleaning reduces the number of microbes present. It also removes organic matter such as blood, body fluids, secretions, and excretions. Disinfecting destroys pathogens but does not destroy spores. **Spores** are bacteria protected by a hard shell. Sterilization is the only way to kill spores.

Clostridium difficile (C. diff or *C. difficile)* is a bacteria that produces spores. It commonly affects older adults in long-term care facilities and individuals on antibiotics. In recent years, it has become more frequent and more difficult to treat.

The most common symptoms are watery diarrhea and abdominal cramping. C. diff bacteria are passed in feces and spread to food, surfaces, and objects when people do not wash their hands properly. *Alcohol-based hand sanitizers are not effective in destroying these spores.* When caring for these individuals, it is important to wash your hands vigorously with soap and warm water (See Hand Washing, p. 62).

Contamination is the process of becoming unclean. In medical asepsis, an item or area is clean when it is free of pathogens. The item or area is contaminated if pathogens are present. A sterile item or area is contaminated when pathogens or non-pathogens are present. **Cross-contamination** is passing microbes from one person to another by contaminated hands, equipment, or supplies. When giving drugs to people, it is important to prevent cross-contamination.

Common Aseptic Practices

Aseptic practices prevent the spread of microbes. Remember to wash your hands:

- After urinating or having a bowel movement.
- After changing tampons or sanitary pads.
- After contact with your own or another person's blood, body fluids, secretions, or excretions. This includes saliva, vomitus, urine, feces, vaginal discharge, mucus, semen, wound drainage, pus, and respiratory secretions.
- After coughing, sneezing, or blowing your nose.
- Before and after handling, preparing, or eating food.
- After smoking or vaping.

Hand Hygiene

Hand hygiene is the easiest and most important way to prevent the spread of infection. You use your hands for almost everything. They are easily contaminated. They can spread microbes to other persons or items. *Practice hand hygiene before and after giving drugs or other care measures.* The CDC and WHO report that alcohol-based hand rubs can be more effective than handwashing in ridding the hands of microorganisms. Many hospitals and health care agencies provide alcohol-based hand rubs for personnel to use when hands are not visibly contaminated. See Box 6-2 for the rules of hand hygiene.

See *Promoting Safety and Comfort: Hand Hygiene.*

PROMOTING SAFETY AND COMFORT
Hand Hygiene

Safety

You use your hands for almost every task. They can pick up microbes from any person, place, or thing. Your hands transfer them to other people, places, and things. That is why hand hygiene is so important.

Comfort

You should practice hand hygiene often during your shift. Hand lotions and hand creams help prevent chapping and dry skin. Apply hand lotion or cream as often as needed.

HAND WASHING

Procedure

1. See *Promoting Safety and Comfort: Hand Hygiene p. 61.*
2. Make sure you have soap, paper towels, an orange stick or nail file, and a wastebasket. Collect missing items.
3. Push your watch up your arm 4 to 5 inches. If your uniform sleeves are long, push them up too.
4. Stand away from the sink so your clothes do not touch the sink. Stand so the soap and faucet are easy to reach (see Fig. 6-1). Do not touch the inside of the sink at any time.
5. Turn on and adjust the water until it feels warm.
6. Wet your wrists and hands. Keep your hands lower than your elbows. Be sure to wet the area 3 to 4 inches above your wrists.
7. Apply about 1 teaspoon of soap to your hands.
8. Rub your palms together and interlace your fingers to work up a good lather (see Fig. 6-2). This step should last at least 20 seconds.
9. Wash each hand and wrist thoroughly. Clean well between the fingers.
10. Clean under the fingernails. Rub your fingertips against your palms (see Fig. 6-3).
11. Clean under the fingernails with a nail file or orange stick (see Fig. 6-4). This step is necessary for the first hand washing of the day and when your hands are highly soiled.
12. Rinse your wrists and hands well. Water flows down from the wrists to the fingertips.
13. Repeat steps 7–12, if needed.
14. Dry from your hands to your wrists with a clean, dry paper towel. Pat dry starting at your fingertips.
15. Discard the paper towel into the wastebasket.

16. Turn off the faucets with clean, dry paper towels (see Fig. 6-5). Use a clean paper towel for each faucet. This prevents you from contaminating your hands.
17. Discard the paper towels into the wastebasket.

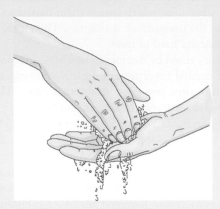

Fig. 6-3 The fingertips are rubbed against the palms to clean under the fingernails.

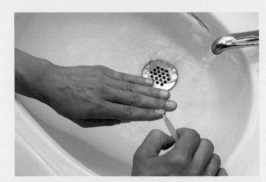

Fig. 6-4 A nail file is used to clean under the fingernails.

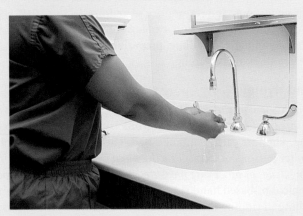

Fig. 6-1 The uniform does not touch the sink. Soap and water are within reach. Hands are lower than the elbows. Hands do not touch the inside of the sink.

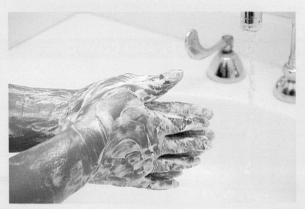

Fig. 6-2 The palms are rubbed together to work up a thick lather.

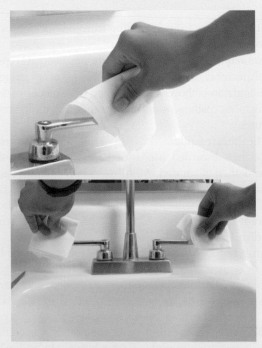

Fig. 6-5 A dry paper towel is used to turn off each faucet.

BOX 6-2 Rules of Hand Hygiene

- Wash your hands with soap and water when they are visibly dirty or soiled with blood, body fluids, secretions, or excretions.
- Wash your hands with soap and water before eating and after using a restroom.
- Wash your hands with soap and water if exposure to the anthrax spore is suspected or proven.
- Use an alcohol-based hand rub to decontaminate your hands if they are not visibly soiled. (If an alcohol-based hand rub is not available, wash your hands with soap and water.) Follow this rule in the following clinical situations:
  - Before having direct contact with a person.
  - After contact with a person's intact skin. For example, after taking a pulse or blood pressure or after moving a person.
  - After contact with body fluids or excretions, mucous membranes, non-intact skin, and wound dressings, if hands are not visibly soiled.
  - When moving from a contaminated body site to a clean body site during care activities.
  - After contact with objects (including equipment) in a person's care setting.
  - After removing gloves.
- Follow these rules for washing your hands with soap and water. See procedure: *Hand Washing,* p. 62.
  - Wash your hands under warm running water. Do not use hot water.
  - Stand away from the sink. Do not let your hands, body, or uniform touch the sink; the sink is contaminated (Fig. 6-1).
  - Do not touch the inside of the sink at any time.
  - Keep your hands and forearms lower than your elbows. Your hands are dirtier than your elbows and forearms. If you hold your hands and forearms up, dirty water runs from your hands to your elbows. Those areas then become contaminated.
- Rub your palms together to work up a thick lather (Fig. 6-2). The rubbing action helps remove microbes and dirt.
- Pay attention to areas often missed during hand washing (thumbs, knuckles, sides of the hands, little fingers, and under the nails).
- Clean fingernails by rubbing the fingertips against your palms (Fig. 6-3).
- Use a nail file or orange stick to clean under fingernails (Fig. 6-4). Microbes easily grow under the fingernails.
- Wash your hands for at least 20 seconds. Wash your hands longer if they are dirty or soiled with blood, body fluids, secretions, or excretions. Use your best judgment.
- Use a clean, dry paper towel to dry your hands.
- Dry your hands starting at the fingertips, working up to your forearms. This way, you will dry the cleanest area first.
- Use a clean, dry paper towel for each faucet to turn the water off (Fig. 6-5). Faucets are contaminated. The paper towels prevent clean hands from becoming contaminated again.
- Follow these rules when decontaminating your hands with an alcohol-based hand rub: See procedure: Hand Hygiene Using an Alcohol-Based Hand Rub, p. 64.
  - Apply the product to the palm of one hand. Follow the manufacturer's instructions for the amount to use.
  - Rub your hands together.
  - Make sure you cover all surfaces of your hands and fingers.
  - Continue rubbing your hands together until your hands are dry.
- Apply hand lotion or cream after hand hygiene. This prevents the skin from chapping and drying. Skin breaks can occur in chapped and dry skin. Skin breaks are portals of entry for microbes.

Modified from Centers for Disease Control and Prevention: Guideline for hand hygiene in health-care settings. *Morbidity and Mortality Weekly Report,* Vol 51, No. RR-16, October 25, 2002.

ISOLATION PRECAUTIONS

Blood, body fluids, secretions, and excretions can transmit pathogens. Sometimes barriers are needed to prevent their escape. The pathogens are kept within a certain area. Usually, the area is the person's designated room or area. This requires isolation procedures.

The *Guideline for Isolation Precautions: Preventing Transmission of Infectious Agents in Healthcare Settings 2007, issued by the CDC,* is followed. Isolation precautions prevent the spread of *communicable diseases (contagious diseases).* They are diseases caused by easily-spread pathogens.

Isolation precautions are based on *clean* and *dirty areas. Clean* areas or objects are free of pathogens. They are not contaminated. *Dirty* areas or objects are contaminated with pathogens. If a *clean* area or object has contact with something *dirty,* the clean area or object is now dirty. *Clean* and *dirty* also depend on how the pathogen is spread.

The CDC's isolation precautions guideline has two tiers of precautions:
- Standard Precautions
- Transmission-Based Precautions

Standard Precautions

Standard Precautions are part of the CDC's *Guideline for Isolation Precautions: Preventing Transmission of Infectious Agents in Health-care Settings 2007* (Box 6-3). They reduce the risk of spreading pathogens. They also reduce the risk of spreading known and unknown infections. *Standard Precautions are used for all persons whenever care is given. This includes when giving drugs.* Standard Precautions prevent the spread of infection from:
- Blood
- All body fluids, secretions, and excretions (except sweat) even if blood is not visible
- Non-intact skin (skin with open breaks)
- Mucous membranes

Follow agency procedures when removing linens, trash, and equipment from the room as they may require special handling.

See *Promoting Safety and Comfort: Standard Precautions.*

PROMOTING SAFETY AND COMFORT

Standard Precautions

Safety

Safe injection practices are part of the CDC's Standard Precautions. If your state and agency allow you to give injections, you need to learn how to safely handle needles and sterile injection equipment. Ask for the necessary education and training.

Transmission-Based Precautions

Some infections require Transmission-Based Precautions (Box 6-4), which are commonly called "isolation precautions."

HAND HYGIENE USING AN ALCOHOL-BASED HAND RUB

Procedure

1. See Promoting Safety and Comfort: Hand Hygiene.
2. Apply the product to the palm of one hand. Follow the manufacturer instructions for the amount to use (Fig. 6-6A).
3. Rub palms together in a circular motion (see Fig. 6-6B).
4. Interlace fingers to spread hand rub on all surfaces of fingers (see Fig. 6-6C and Fig. 6-6D).
5. Rub tips of fingers up and down palm of opposite hand (see Fig. 6-6E).
6. Coat surfaces of each thumb with hand rub (see Fig. 6-6F).
7. Rub fingertips in palm of opposite hand using circular motions (see Fig. 6-6G).
8. Continue rubbing in product until hands are dry (at least 15 seconds or according to manufacturer recommendation). There is no need to use water or paper towels when using alcohol-based hand rubs.
9. Apply hand lotion or cream after hand hygiene. This prevents the skin from chapping and drying.

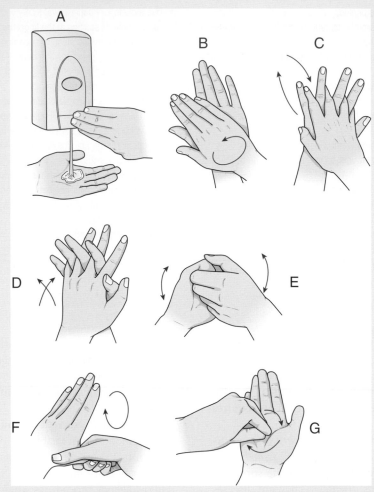

Fig. 6-6 Using an Alcohol-Based Hand Rub: **A,** A palmful of an alcohol-based hand rub is applied into a cupped hand; **B,** The palms are rubbed together; **C,** The palm of 1 hand is rubbed over the back of the other; **D,** The palms are rubbed together with the fingers interlaced; **E,** The fingers are interlocked and rubbed back and forth; **F,** The thumb of 1 hand is rubbed in the palm of the other; and **G,** The fingers of 1 hand are rubbed into the palm of the other hand with circular motions.

Transmission-Based Precautions require wearing personal protective equipment (PPE)—gloves, gown, mask, and goggles or face shield. There are three basic categories of Transmission-Based Precautions:

- Contact precautions
- Droplet precautions
- Airborne precautions

You must understand how certain infections are spread. This helps you understand the different types of transmission-based precautions and why the precautions are needed. Agency policies may differ from those in this text. The rules in Box 6-5 are a guide for administering safe care and drugs when using isolation precautions.

See *Focus on Communication: Isolation Precautions.*
See *Delegation Guidelines: Isolation Precautions.*

BOX 6-3 Standard Precautions

Hand Hygiene
- Follow the rules for hand hygiene.
- Avoid unnecessary touching of surfaces close to the person. This prevents contamination of clean hands from environmental surfaces. It also prevents the transmission of pathogens from contaminated hands to other surfaces.
- Do not wear fake nails or nail extenders if you will have contact with persons at risk for infection or other adverse outcomes.

Personal Protective Equipment (PPE)
- Wear PPE when contact with blood or body fluids is likely.
- Do not contaminate your clothing or skin when removing PPE.
- Remove and discard PPE before leaving the person's room or care setting.

Gloves
- Wear gloves when contact with the following is likely:
  - Blood
  - Potentially infectious materials (e.g., body fluids, secretions, and excretions)
  - Mucous membranes
  - Non-intact skin
  - Skin that may be contaminated (e.g., a person incontinent of stool or urine)
- Wear gloves that fit and are appropriate for the task at hand:
  - Wear disposable gloves to provide direct care to the person
  - Wear disposable gloves or utility gloves for cleaning equipment or care settings
- Remove gloves after contact with the person or the person's care setting. The care setting includes equipment used in the person's care.
- Remove gloves after contact with care equipment.
- Do not wear the same pair of gloves to care for more than one person. Remove gloves after contact with a person and before moving to another person.
- Do not wash gloves for re-use.
- Change gloves during care if your hands will move from a contaminated body site to a clean body site.

Gowns
- Wear a gown that is appropriate to the task.
- Wear a gown to protect your skin and clothing when contact with blood, body fluids, secretions, or excretions is likely to occur.
- Wear a gown during direct contact with a person if he or she has uncontained secretions or excretions.
- Remove the gown and perform hand hygiene before leaving the person's room or care setting.
- Do not re-use gowns, even for repeated contact with the same person.

Mouth, Nose, and Eye Protection
- Wear PPE—masks, goggles, face shields—for procedures and tasks that are likely to cause splashes and sprays of blood, body fluids, secretions, or excretions.
- Wear PPE—mask, goggles, face shield—appropriate for the procedure or task.
- Wear gloves, a gown, and one of the following for procedures that are likely to cause sprays of respiratory secretions:
  - A face shield that fully covers the front and sides of the face
  - A mask with attached shield
  - A mask and goggles

Respiratory Hygiene/Cough Etiquette
- Instruct persons with respiratory symptoms to:
  - Cover the nose and mouth when coughing or sneezing (Fig. 6-13).
  - Use tissues to contain respiratory secretions
  - Dispose of tissues in the nearest waste container after use
  - Perform hand hygiene after contact with respiratory secretions
- Provide visitors with masks according to agency policy.

Care Equipment
- Wear appropriate PPE when handling care equipment that is visibly soiled with blood, body fluids, secretions, or excretions.
- Wear appropriate PPE when handling care equipment that may have been in contact with blood, body fluids, secretions, or excretions.
- Remove organic material before disinfection and sterilization procedures. Use cleaning agents according to agency policy.

Care of the Environment
- Follow agency policies and procedures for cleaning and maintaining surfaces (e.g., environmental surfaces and care equipment). Surfaces near the person may need more frequent cleaning and maintenance (e.g., door knobs, bed rails, overbed tables, and toilet surfaces and surrounding areas).
- Clean and disinfect multi-use electronic equipment according to agency policy. This includes:
  - Items used by residents
  - Items used to give care
  - Mobile devices that are moved in and out of resident rooms
- Follow these rules for toys used by pediatric patients or child play toys in waiting areas:
  - Select play toys that can be easily cleaned and disinfected
  - Do not allow use of stuffed furry toys if they will be share
  - Clean and disinfect large stationary toys (e.g., climbing equipment) at least once weekly and whenever visibly soiled
  - Rinse toys with water after disinfection (or run through a dishwasher) if they are likely to be mouthed by children
  - Clean and disinfect a toy immediately when it requires cleaning; alternatively, store the toy in a labeled container away from toys that are clean and ready for use

Textiles and Laundry
- Handle used textiles and fabrics (linens) with minimum agitation. This is done to avoid contamination of air, surfaces, and other persons.

Worker Safety
- Protect yourself and others from exposure to bloodborne pathogens. This includes how to handle needles and other sharps. Follow federal and state standards and guidelines. See the Bloodborne Pathogen Standard (p. 72).
- Use a mouthpiece, resuscitation bag, or other ventilation device during resuscitation to prevent contact with the person's mouth and oral secretions.

Resident Placement
- A private room is preferred if the person is at risk for transmitting the infection to others.
- Follow the nurse's instructions if a private room is not available.

Modified from Siegel JD, Rhinehart E, Jackson M, Chiarello L, and the Healthcare Infection Control Practices Advisory Committee: *Guideline for Isolation Precautions: Preventing Transmission of Infectious Agents in Healthcare Settings 2007*, June 2007.

BOX 6-4   Transmission-Based Precautions

Contact Precautions

- Used for persons with known or suspected infections or conditions that increase the risk of contact transmission.
- Resident placement:
  - A single room is preferred
  - If a single room is not available, place the resident with another resident who is infected with the same microorganism
  - If a room is shared with another person who is not infected with the same agent:
    - Keep the privacy curtain between the beds closed
    - Change personal protective equipment (PPE) and perform hand hygiene between contact with persons in the same room; do so regardless of whether one or both persons are on Contact Precautions
- Gloves:
  - Don gloves upon entering the person's room or care setting
  - Wear gloves at all times while in the person's room or care setting
  - Wear gloves whenever touching the patient's skin or equipment, surfaces, or items near the person
- Gowns:
  - Don the gown upon entering the person's room or care setting
  - Wear a gown whenever clothing may have direct contact with the person
  - Wear a gown whenever contact is likely with surfaces or equipment near the person
  - Remove the gown and perform hand hygiene before leaving the person's room or care setting
  - After removing the gown, make sure your clothing and skin do not touch potentially contaminated surfaces
- Resident transport:
  - Limit transport and movement of the person outside of the room to medically necessary purposes
  - Cover the area of the person's body that is infected
  - Remove and discard contaminated PPE and perform hand hygiene before transporting the person
  - Don clean PPE to handle the person at the transport destination
- Care equipment:
  - Follow Standard Precautions
  - Use disposable equipment when possible
  - Leave non-disposable equipment in the person's room if possible
  - Clean and disinfect non-disposable and multiple-use equipment before use on another person
  - For home care settings:
    - Limit amount of non-disposable care items brought into the home and leave those required in the home as long as they are needed
    - Clean and disinfect items that cannot be left in the home (e.g., stethoscopes and blood pressure cuffs)
    - Clean and disinfect care items before removing them from the home (or place them in a plastic bag for transport for later cleaning and disinfection)

Droplet Precautions

- Used for persons known or suspected to be infected with pathogens transmitted by respiratory droplets. Such droplets are generated by a person who is coughing, sneezing, or talking.
- Resident placement:
  - A single room is preferred
  - If a single room is not available, place the resident with another resident who is infected with the same microorganism
  - If a room is shared with another person who is not infected with the same agent:
    - Keep the privacy curtain between the beds closed
    - Change personal protective equipment (PPE) and perform hand hygiene between contact with persons in the same room. Do so regardless of whether one or both persons are on Droplet Precautions.
- Personal protective equipment:
  - Don a mask upon entering the person's room or care settin
- Resident transport:
  - Limit transport and movement of the person outside of the room to medically necessary purposes
  - Have the person wear a mask
  - Instruct the person to follow Respiratory Hygiene/Cough Etiquette (Fig. 6-13)
  - No mask is required for health team members transporting the person

Airborne Precautions

- Used for persons known or suspected to be infected with pathogens transmitted by person-to-person by the airborne route. Examples include tuberculosis, coronavirus (COVID-19), measles, chickenpox, smallpox, and severe acute respiratory syndrome (SARS).
- The resident is placed in an airborne infection isolation room (AIIR). If one is not available, the person is transferred to an agency with an available AIIR.
- Health team members susceptible to the infection are restricted from entering the room if immune staff members are available.
- Personal protective equipment:
  - An approved respirator (N95 mask) is worn upon entering the room or home of a person with tuberculosis
  - Respiratory protection is recommended for all health team members when caring for persons with smallpox
- Resident transport:
  - Limit transport and movement of the person outside of the room to medically necessary purposes
  - Have the person wear a surgical mask
  - Instruct the person to follow Respiratory Hygiene/Cough Etiquette (Fig. 6-13)
  - Cover skin lesions infected with the microbe
  - No mask or respirator is required for health team members transporting the person if:
    - The person is wearing a mask or respirator
- Skin lesions are covered

Modified from Siegel JD, Rhinehart E, Jackson M, Chiarello L, and the Healthcare Infection Control Practices Advisory Committee: *Guideline for Isolation Precautions: Preventing Transmission of Infectious Agents in Healthcare Settings 2007,* Centers for Disease Control and Prevention, June 2007.

BOX 6-5 Rules for Isolation Precautions

- Collect all needed items before entering the room.
- Do not contaminate equipment and supplies. Floors are contaminated; therefore, so is any object that touches the floor for any reason.
- Clean floors with mops wetted with a disinfectant solution. Floor dust is contaminated.
- Prevent drafts. Drafts can carry some microbes in the air.
- Use paper towels to handle contaminated items.
- Remove items from the room in leak-proof plastic bags.
- Double-bag items if the outside of the bag is or can be contaminated.
- Follow agency policy to remove and transport disposable and re-usable items.
- Return reusable dishes, drinking vessels, eating utensils, and trays to the food service (dietary) department. Discard disposable dishes, drinking vessels, eating utensils, and trays in the waste container in the person's room.
- Do not touch your hair, nose, mouth, eyes, or other body parts.
- Do not touch any clean area or object if your hands are contaminated.
- Wash your hands if they are visibly dirty or contaminated with blood, body fluids, secretions, or excretions.
- Place clean items on paper towels.
- Do not shake linens.
- Use paper towels to turn faucets on and off.
- Use a paper towel to open the door to the person's room. Immediately discard after use.
- Tell the nurse if you have any cuts, open skin areas, vomiting, diarrhea, or a sore throat.

FOCUS ON COMMUNICATION

Isolation Precautions

Some centers require visitors to wear PPE when visiting a person in need of isolation precautions. Some visitors may question the need for PPE. They may not wear PPE around the person in his or her home or outside the center. They may not understand why it is needed. Some visitors may ignore signs or requests to wear PPE; however, it is important to effectively communicate with patients and visitors about the importance of PPE in this particular setting. You can politely say:

- "Your visitors will need to wear a gown and gloves while in your room."
- "Please wear this mask. It is our policy to protect you, your family member, and others."

Tell the nurse if the patient or visitors have more questions. Also tell the nurse if someone refuses to follow isolation precautions.

DELEGATION GUIDELINES

Isolation Precautions

You may be giving medications to people who require isolation precautions. If so, review the type of precautions needed with the nurse. You also need this information from the nurse:

- What PPE to use.
- What special safety measures are necessary.

PERSONAL PROTECTIVE EQUIPMENT (PPE)

The PPE needed for Standard Precautions depends on the person's drug order. Some routes require the use of gloves. PPE needed also depends on the type of Transmission-Based Precautions ordered for the person. The nurse tells you when other PPE are needed.

According to the CDC's isolation guideline, gloves are always worn when gowns are worn. Sometimes, other PPE is needed when gowns are worn. The isolation guideline shows PPE donned and removed in the following order:

Donning PPE (Fig. 6-7A):

- Gown
- Mask or respirator
- Eyewear (goggles or face shield)
- Gloves

Removing PPE (removed at the doorway before leaving the person's room) (Fig. 6-7B):

- Gloves
- Eyewear (goggles or face shield)
- Gown
- Mask or respirator

Gloves

The skin is a natural barrier. It prevents microbes from entering the body. Small skin breaks on the hands and fingers are common. Some are very small and hard to see. Disposable gloves act as a barrier. They protect you from pathogens in the person's blood, body fluids, secretions, and excretions. They also protect the person from microbes on your hands. Wear gloves whenever contact with blood, body fluids, secretions, excretions, mucous membranes, or nonintact skin is likely. Contact may be direct, or contact may be indirect through items or surfaces contaminated with blood, body fluids, secretions, or excretions.

Wearing gloves is the most common protective measure used with Standard Precautions and Transmission-Based Precautions. Remember the following when using gloves:

- The outside of gloves is contaminated.
- Gloves are easier to put on when your hands are dry.
- Do not tear gloves when putting them on. Carelessness, long fingernails, and rings can tear gloves. Blood, body fluids, secretions, and excretions can enter the glove through the tear. This contaminates your hand.
- You need a new pair for every person.
- Remove and discard torn, cut, or punctured gloves at once. Practice hand hygiene. Then put on a new pair.
- Wear gloves once. Discard them after use.
- Put on clean gloves just before touching mucous membranes or nonintact skin.
- Put on new gloves whenever gloves become contaminated with blood, body fluids, secretions, or excretions. A task may require more than one pair of gloves.
- Change gloves whenever moving from a contaminated body site to a clean body site.
- Change gloves if interacting with a person involves touching portable computer keyboards or other mobile equipment that is transported from room to room.
- Put on gloves last when they are worn with other PPE.
- Make sure gloves cover your wrists. If you wear a gown, make sure gloves cover the cuffs (Fig. 6-8).
- Remove gloves so the inside part is on the outside. The inside is clean.
- Wash your hands after removing gloves.

SEQUENCE FOR PUTTING ON PERSONAL PROTECTIVE EQUIPMENT (PPE)

The type of PPE used will vary based on the level of precautions required, such as standard and contact, droplet or airborne infection isolation precautions. The procedure for putting on and removing PPE should be tailored to the specific type of PPE.

1. GOWN

- Fully cover torso from neck to knees, arms to end of wrists, and wrap around the back
- Fasten in back of neck and waist

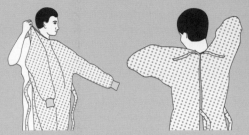

2. MASK OR RESPIRATOR

- Secure ties or elastic bands at middle of head and neck
- Fit flexible band to nose bridge
- Fit snug to face and below chin
- Fit-check respirator

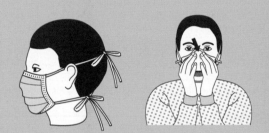

3. GOGGLES OR FACE SHIELD

- Place over face and eyes and adjust to fit

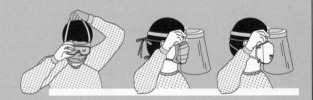

4. GLOVES

- Extend to cover wrist of isolation gown

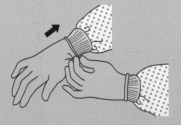

USE SAFE WORK PRACTICES TO PROTECT YOURSELF AND LIMIT THE SPREAD OF CONTAMINATION

- Keep hands away from face
- Limit surfaces touched
- Change gloves when torn or heavily contaminated
- Perform hand hygiene

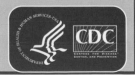

Fig. 6-7A Donning PPE.

HOW TO SAFELY REMOVE PERSONAL PROTECTIVE EQUIPMENT (PPE) EXAMPLE 1

There are a variety of ways to safely remove PPE without contaminating your clothing, skin, or mucous membranes with potentially infectious materials. Here is one example. **Remove all PPE before exiting the patient room** except a respirator, if worn. Remove the respirator **after** leaving the patient room and closing the door. Remove PPE in the following sequence:

1. GLOVES

- Outside of gloves are contaminated!
- If your hands get contaminated during glove removal, immediately wash your hands or use an alcohol-based hand sanitizer
- Using a gloved hand, grasp the palm area of the other gloved hand and peel off first glove
- Hold removed glove in gloved hand
- Slide fingers of ungloved hand under remaining glove at wrist and peel off second glove over first glove
- Discard gloves in a waste container

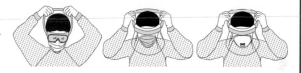

2. GOGGLES OR FACE SHIELD

- Outside of goggles or face shield are contaminated!
- If your hands get contaminated during goggle or face shield removal, immediately wash your hands or use an alcohol-based hand sanitizer
- Remove goggles or face shield from the back by lifting head band or ear pieces
- If the item is reusable, place in designated receptacle for reprocessing. Otherwise, discard in a waste container

3. GOWN

- Gown front and sleeves are contaminated!
- If your hands get contaminated during gown removal, immediately wash your hands or use an alcohol-based hand sanitizer
- Unfasten gown ties, taking care that sleeves don't contact your body when reaching for ties
- Pull gown away from neck and shoulders, touching inside of gown only
- Turn gown inside out
- Fold or roll into a bundle and discard in a waste container

4. MASK OR RESPIRATOR

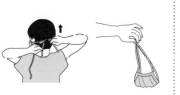

- Front of mask/respirator is contaminated — DO NOT TOUCH!
- If your hands get contaminated during mask/respirator removal, immediately wash your hands or use an alcohol-based hand sanitizer
- Grasp bottom ties or elastics of the mask/respirator, then the ones at the top, and remove without touching the front
- Discard in a waste container

5. WASH HANDS OR USE AN ALCOHOL-BASED HAND SANITIZER IMMEDIATELY AFTER REMOVING ALL PPE

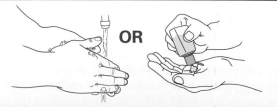

OR

PERFORM HAND HYGIENE BETWEEN STEPS IF HANDS BECOME CONTAMINATED AND IMMEDIATELY AFTER REMOVING ALL PPE

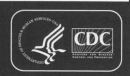

Fig. 6-7B Removing PPE. (From CDC: Sequence for Donning and Removing Personal Protective Equipment, 2014).

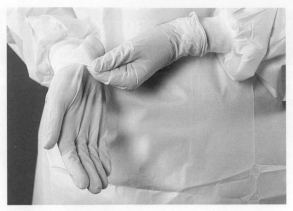

Fig. 6-8 The gloves cover the cuffs of the gown.

REMOVING GLOVES

Procedure

1. See Promoting Safety and Comfort: Gloves.
2. Make sure that glove touches only glove.
3. Grasp a glove on the outside just below the cuff (Fig. 6.9A).
4. Pull the glove down over your hand so it is inside out (see Fig. 6-9B).

5. Hold the removed glove with your other gloved hand.
6. Reach inside the other glove using the first two fingers of the ungloved hand (see Fig. 6-9C).
7. Pull the glove down (inside out) over your hand and the other glove (see Fig. 6-9D).
8. Discard both gloves. Follow agency policy.
9. Perform hand hygiene with soap and water or an alcohol-based hand rub.

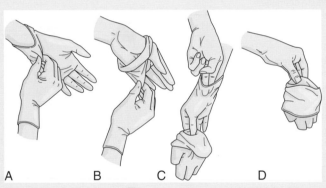

A   B   C   D

Fig. 6-9 Removing Gloves: A, Grasp the glove below the cuff; **B,** Pull the glove down and over the hand so that the glove is inside out; **C,** Insert the fingers of the ungloved hand inside the other glove; and **D,** Pull the glove down and over the other hand and glove so that the glove is inside out.

Gowns

Gowns prevent the spread of microbes. They protect your clothes and body from contact with blood, body fluids, secretions, and excretions. They also protect against splashes and sprays.

Gowns must completely cover you from your neck to your knees. The long sleeves have tight cuffs. The gown opens at the back. It is tied at the neck and waist. The gown front and sleeves are considered to be contaminated. Gowns are used once. A wet gown is contaminated. It is removed and a dry one put on. Disposable gowns are discarded after use.

DONNING AND REMOVING A GOWN

Procedure

1. Remove your watch and all jewelry.
2. Roll up uniform sleeves.
3. Practice hand hygiene.
4. Hold a clean gown out in front of you while letting it unfold. Do not shake the gown.
5. Put your hands and arms through the sleeves (see Fig. 6-7A).

6. Make sure the gown covers you completely from your neck to your knees. It must cover your arms to the end of your wrists.
7. Tie the strings at the back of the neck (see Fig. 6-7A).
8. Overlap the back of the gown to make sure it covers your uniform. The gown should be snug, not loose. (If the gown does not cover your back, you may need to take a second gown and put it on with the opening in the front.)

DONNING AND REMOVING A GOWN—cont'd

9. Tie the waist strings at the back or the side. Do not tie them in front.
10. Put on other PPE: a. Mask or respirator (if needed); b. Goggles or face shield (if needed); c. Gloves (ensure gloves cover gown cuffs).
11. Provide care.
12. Remove and discard the gloves (Fig. 6-9A-D).
13. Remove and discard goggles or face shield if worn.
14. Remove gown. Do not touch the outside of the gown.
    a. Untie the neck and waist strings (see Fig. 6-7B).
    b. Pull the gown down from each shoulder toward the same hand (see Fig. 6-7B).
    c. Turn the gown inside out as it is removed. Hold it at the inside shoulder seams and bring your hands together (Fig. 6-7B).
15. Hold and roll up the gown away from you (see Fig. 6-7B). Keep it inside out.
16. Discard the gown. Follow agency policy.
17. Perform hand hygiene with soap and water or an alcohol-based hand rub.

Masks and Respiratory Protection

You should wear masks for these reasons:
- For protection from contact with infectious materials from a person. Examples include respiratory secretions and sprays of blood or body fluid.
- During sterile procedures to protect the person from infectious agents carried in your mouth or nose.

Masks are disposable. A wet or moist mask is contaminated. Over a period of time, breathing can cause masks to become wet or moist. Apply a new mask when contamination occurs.

A mask fits snugly over your nose and mouth. Practice hand hygiene before putting on a mask. When removing a mask, touch only the ties or elastic bands; the front of the mask is contaminated. Tuberculosis respirators (N95 masks) (Fig. 6-10) are worn when caring for persons with TB and Covid-19.

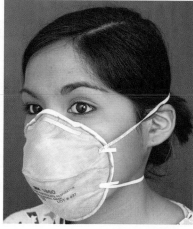

Fig. 6-10 Tuberculosis Respirator (N95 Mask).

DONNING AND REMOVING A MASK

Procedure

1. Practice hand hygiene.
2. Put on a gown if required.
3. Pick up a mask by its upper ties. Do not touch the part that will cover your face.
4. Place the mask over your nose and mouth (see Fig. 6-11A).
5. Place the upper strings above your ears. Tie them at the back at the middle of your head (see Fig. 6-11B).
6. Tie the lower strings at the back of your neck (see Fig. 6-11C). The lower part of the mask is under your chin.
7. Pinch the metal band around your nose. The top of the mask must be snug over your nose. If you wear eyeglasses, the mask must be snug under the bottom of the eyeglasses.
8. Make sure the mask is snug over your face and under your chin.
9. Put on goggles or a face shield (if needed and if not part of the mask).
10. Put on gloves.
11. Provide care. Avoid coughing, sneezing, and unnecessary talking.
12. Change the mask if it becomes wet or contaminated.
13. Remove the mask (see Fig. 6-7B).
    a. Remove the gloves.
    b. Remove the goggles or face shield and gown if worn.
    c. Untie the lower strings of the mask.
    d. Untie the top strings.
    e. Hold the top strings and remove the mask.
14. Discard the mask. Follow agency policy.
15. Perform hand hygiene with soap and water or an alcohol-based hand rub.

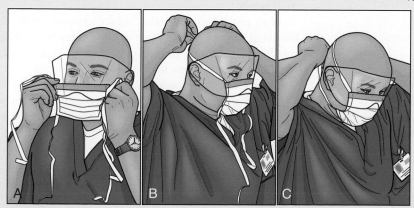

Fig. 6-11 Donning and Removing a Mask (Note: The mask has a face shield.): A, The mask covers the nose and mouth; B, Upper strings are tied at the back of the head; and C, Lower strings are tied at the back of the neck.

Goggles and Face Shields

Goggles and face shields protect your eyes, mouth, and nose from splashing or spraying of blood, body fluids, secretions, and excretions (Fig. 6-11). Splashes and sprays can occur when giving care, cleaning items, or disposing of fluids.

The front of goggles or a face shield is contaminated. The ties, earpieces, or headband used to secure the device are considered "clean." Use them to remove the device after hand hygiene. They are safe to touch with bare hands.

Discard disposable goggles or face shields after use. Reusable eyewear is cleaned before reuse. It is washed with soap and water. Then a disinfectant is used.

See *Promoting Safety and Comfort: Goggles and Face Shields.*

PROMOTING SAFETY AND COMFORT

Goggles and Face Shields

Safety
Eyeglasses and contact lenses do not provide adequate eye protection. If you wear eyeglasses, use a face shield that fits over your glasses with minimal gaps. Goggles do not provide splash or spray protection to other parts of your face.

THE BLOODBORNE PATHOGEN STANDARD

The human immunodeficiency virus (HIV) and the hepatitis B virus (HBV) are major health concerns. The health team is at risk for exposure to these viruses. The Bloodborne Pathogen Standard is intended to protect them from exposure. It is a regulation of the Occupational Safety and Health Administration (OSHA).

HIV and HBV are found in the blood; they are bloodborne pathogens. They exit the body through blood. They are spread to others by blood. Other potentially infectious materials (OPIM) also spread the viruses:

- Human body fluids—semen, vaginal secretions, cerebrospinal fluid, synovial fluid, pleural fluid, pericardial fluid, peritoneal fluid, amniotic fluid, saliva in dental procedures, any body fluid that is visibly contaminated with blood, and all body fluids when it is difficult or impossible to differentiate between them.
- Any tissue or organ (other than intact skin) from a human (living or dead).
- HIV-containing cell or tissue cultures, organ cultures, and HIV- or HBV-containing culture medium or other solutions; blood, organs, or other tissues from animals experimentally infected with HIV or HBV.

EXPOSURE CONTROL PLAN

The agency must have an exposure control plan. It identifies staff at risk for exposure to blood or OPIM. All caregivers and the laundry, central supply, and housekeeping staffs are at risk. The exposure control plan includes actions to take for an exposure incident.

Staff at risk receive free training. Training first occurs upon employment and then yearly. Training is also required for new or changed tasks involving exposure to bloodborne pathogens. Training must include:

- An explanation of the standard and where to get a copy
- The causes, signs, and symptoms of bloodborne diseases
- How bloodborne pathogens are spread
- The tasks that might cause exposure
- An explanation of the exposure control plan and where to get a copy
- How to know which tasks might cause exposure
- The use and limits of safe work practices, engineering controls, and personal protective equipment
- Information about the hepatitis B vaccination
- Who to contact and what to do in an emergency
- Information on reporting an exposure incident, post-exposure evaluation, and follow-up
- Information on warning labels and color-coding

PREVENTIVE MEASURES

Preventive measures reduce the risk of exposure. Such measures follow.

Hepatitis B Vaccination

Hepatitis B is a liver disease. It is caused by the hepatitis B virus (HBV). HBV is spread by blood and sexual contact.

The hepatitis B vaccine produces immunity against hepatitis B. **Immunity** means protection against a certain disease. He or she will not get the disease.

A **vaccination** involves administering a vaccine to produce immunity against an infectious disease. A **vaccine** is a preparation containing dead or weakened microbes. The hepatitis B vaccination involves 3 injections. The second injection is given 1 month after the first. The third injection is given 6 months after the second. The vaccination can be given before or after exposure to HBV.

You can receive the hepatitis B vaccination within 10 working days of being hired (it is paid for by the agency). You have the right to refuse the vaccination. If you do so, you must sign a statement refusing the vaccine. You can have the vaccination at a later date.

Engineering and Work Practice Controls

Engineering controls reduce employee exposure in the workplace. Special containers for contaminated sharps (needles, broken glass) and specimens remove and isolate the hazard from staff. Containers are puncture-resistant, leak-proof, and color-coded in red. They are clearly marked with the *BIOHAZARD* symbol.

Work practice controls also reduce exposure risks. All tasks involving blood or OPIM are done in ways to limit splatters, splashes, and sprays. Producing droplets also is avoided. OSHA requires these work practice controls:

- Do not eat, drink, smoke, apply cosmetics or lip balm, or handle contact lenses in areas of occupational exposure.
- Do not store food or drinks where blood or OPIM are kept.
- Practice hand hygiene after removing gloves.
- Wash hands as soon as possible after skin contact with blood or OPIM.
- Never recap, bend, or remove needles by hand. When recapping, bending, or removing contaminated needles is required, use mechanical means (forceps) or a one-handed method.

- Never shear or break contaminated needles.
- Discard contaminated needles and sharp instruments (such as razors) in containers that are closable, puncture-resistant, and leak-proof. Containers are color-coded in red and are marked with the *BIOHAZARD* symbol. Containers must be upright and must not be over-filled.

Personal Protective Equipment (PPE)

This includes gloves, goggles, face shields, masks, laboratory coats, gowns, shoe covers, and surgical caps. Blood or OPIM must not pass through them. PPE protect your clothes, undergarments, skin, eyes, mouth, and hair.

PPE is free to employees. Correct sizes are available. The agency makes sure that PPE is cleaned, laundered, repaired, replaced, or discarded. OSHA requires these measures for the safe handling and use of PPE:

- Remove PPE before leaving the work area.
- Remove PPE when a garment becomes contaminated.
- Place used PPE in marked areas or containers when being stored, washed, decontaminated, or discarded.
- Wear gloves when you expect contact with blood or OPIM.
- Wear gloves when handling or touching contaminated items or surfaces.
- Immediately replace worn, punctured, or contaminated gloves.
- Never wash or decontaminate disposable gloves for re-use.
- Discard utility gloves that show signs of cracking, peeling, tearing, or puncturing. Utility gloves are decontaminated for re-use if the process will not ruin them.

Equipment

Contaminated equipment is cleaned and decontaminated. Decontaminate work surfaces with a proper disinfectant:

- Upon completing tasks
- Immediately following obvious contamination
- After any spill of blood or OPIM
- At the end of the work shift when surfaces have become contaminated since their last cleaning

Use a brush and dustpan or tongs to clean up broken glass. Never pick up broken glass with your hands – not even with gloves. Discard broken glass into a puncture-resistant container.

Waste

Special measures are required when discarding regulated waste:

- Liquid or semi-liquid blood or OPIM
- Items contaminated with blood or OPIM
- Items caked with blood or OPIM
- Contaminated sharps

Closable, puncture-resistant, and leak-proof containers are used. Containers are color-coded in red. They display the *BIOHAZARD* symbol.

Housekeeping

The agency must be kept clean and sanitary. A cleaning schedule is required. It includes decontamination methods and the tasks and procedures to be done.

Laundry

OSHA requires these measures for contaminated laundry:

- Handle it as little as possible.
- Wear gloves or other needed PPE.
- Bag contaminated laundry where it is used.
- Mark laundry bags or containers with the *BIOHAZARD* symbol for laundry sent off-site.
- Place wet, contaminated laundry in leak-proof containers before transport. The containers are color-coded in red or display the *BIOHAZARD* symbol.

EXPOSURE INCIDENTS

An *exposure incident* is any eye, mouth, other mucous membrane, non-intact skin, or parenteral contact with blood or OPIM. *Parenteral* means piercing the mucous membranes or the skin barrier. Piercing occurs through needle sticks, human bites, cuts, and abrasions.

Report exposure incidents at once. Medical evaluation, follow-up, and required tests are free. Your blood is tested for HIV and HBV. If you refuse testing, the blood sample is kept for at least 90 days. Testing may be done later if you change your mind.

Confidentiality is important. You are told of the evaluation results. You also are told of any medical conditions that may need treatment. You receive a written opinion of the medical evaluation within 15 days after its completion.

The *source individual* is the person whose blood or body fluids are the source of an exposure incident. His or her blood is tested for HIV or HBV. State laws vary about releasing the results. The agency informs you about laws affecting the source's identity and test results.

STOPPING THE SPREAD OF INFECTION

In January 2020, an outbreak of the deadly coronavirus (COVID-19), or novel coronavirus, was first reported in the United States at a nursing center. The virus infected many of the residents and the staff. Several people from the nursing center died from the infection. There may be times when you are working where certain infections spread through a nursing center. Other examples of these types of illnesses are influenza (flu) and gastroenteritis. The strict use of PPE and hand hygiene are needed to prevent the spread of the illness to other residents, visitors, staff, and yourself.

When this happens, it may be necessary to take the following actions to stop the spread of the infection:

- Restrict visitors
- Serve meals in the person's room instead of in a common dining room
- Isolate the infected residents from those not infected
- Require workers and volunteers to get vaccinated
- Require residents to get vaccinated
- Stay home if you have signs and symptoms of illness; you could expose residents and other employees to the illness

Most nursing centers and agencies already require workers, volunteers, and residents to receive vaccines.

EPIDEMIC AND PANDEMIC

An **epidemic** is a disease that affects a large number of people within a community, population, or region. For example, in December 2019, COVID-19 began spreading throughout China and was considered an epidemic. By January 2020, the disease spread to many other countries, infecting millions all over the world and killing hundreds of thousands of people. COVID-19 was then declared a **pandemic**. A pandemic is an epidemic that has spread to multiple countries or continents.

During the COVID-19 pandemic, the Centers for Disease Control and Prevention (CDC) issued the following recommendations to slow the spread of infection (Fig. 6-12):

- Get vaccinated
- Avoid close contact with people who are sick
- Cover your cough or sneeze with a tissue, then throw the tissue in the trash (Fig. 6-13)
- Avoid touching your eyes, nose, and mouth
- When in public, wear a cloth face covering over your nose and mouth
- Clean and disinfect frequently touched objects and surfaces
- Stay home when you are sick (except to get medical care)
- Wash your hands often with soap and water for at least 20 seconds
- **Social Distancing**—putting space (at least 6 feet) between yourself and others. (Fig. 6-14)

While this list was created to slow the spread of COVID-19, most of these recommendations can also prevent the spread of other infections.

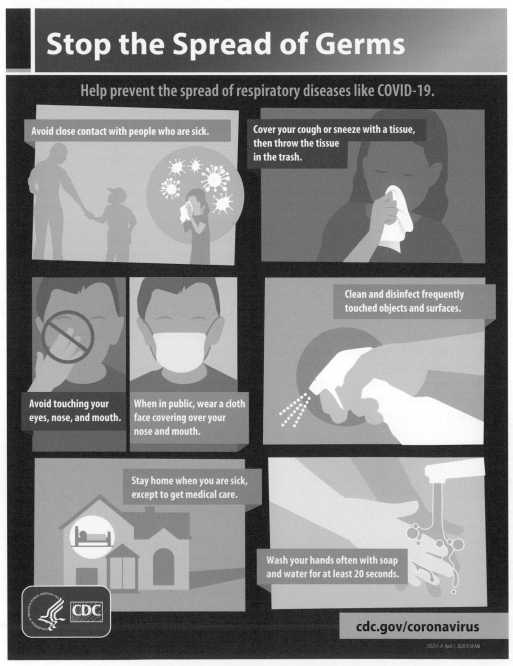

Fig. 6-12 Stop the Spread of Germs. (From CDC.gov/coronavirus, 2020)

Stop the spread of germs that make you and others sick!

Cover your Cough

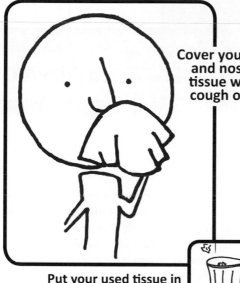

Cover your mouth and nose with a tissue when you cough or sneeze

or

cough or sneeze into your upper sleeve, not your hands

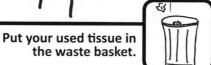

Put your used tissue in the waste basket.

You may be asked to put on a surgical mask to protect others.

Clean your Hands
after coughing or sneezing.

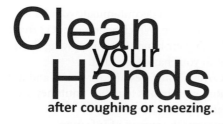

Wash with soap and water

or
clean with alcohol-based hand sanitizer.

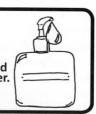

DEPARTMENT OF HEALTH

Infectious Disease Epidemiology, Prevention and Control
PO Box 64975, St. Paul, MN 55164
651-201-5414 or 1-877-676-5414
www.health.state.mn.us

APIC
ASSOCIATION FOR PROFESSIONALS IN
INFECTION CONTROL AND EPIDEMIOLOGY, INC.

3/2020

Fig. 6-13 Respiratory Hygiene/Cough Etiquette. (From CDC Posters for Schools about Flu Prevention, 2019)

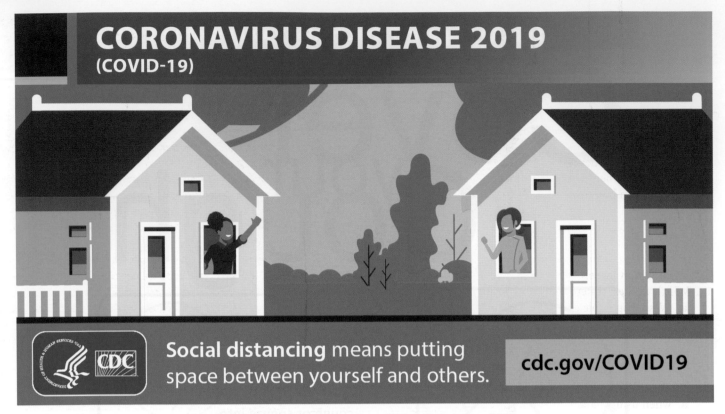

CORONAVIRUS DISEASE 2019
(COVID-19)

Social distancing means putting space between yourself and others.

cdc.gov/COVID19

Fig 6-14 Social Distancing. (From CDC.gov/coronavirus, 2020)

REVIEW QUESTIONS

Circle the BEST answer.

1. Which is not considered a microbe?
   a. bacteria
   b. fungi
   c. viruses
   d. ants
2. What does a microbe need to live and grow?
   a. a cold environment
   b. Reservoir
   c. light
   d. water
3. Which does not prevent healthcare-associated infections?
   a. hand hygiene before and after giving care
   b. sterilizing all care items
   c. surgical asepsis
   d. standard Precautions
4. Which will not prevent the spread of HAIs?
   a. taking prescribed antibiotics
   b. Standard Precautions
   c. hand hygiene
   d. Transmission-Based Precautions
5. These statements are about older persons with an infection. Which is false?
   a. They may have a slight fever or no fever at all.
   b. They may become confused.
   c. Their immune system becomes stronger with age.
   d. Their infection can become life-threatening before they have signs and symptoms.

6. Your hands are soiled with blood. What should you do?
   a. Wash your hands with soap and water.
   b. Decontaminate your hands.
   c. Rinse your hands.
   d. Use hand sanitizer.
7. During care, you move from a contaminated body site to a clean body site. Your hands are not visibly soiled. What should you do?
   a. Wash your hands.
   b. Decontaminate your hands.
   c. Rinse your hands.
   d. Put on sterile gloves.
8. You are going to decontaminate your hands with an alcohol-based hand rub. Which action is not correct?
   a. Wash your hands before applying the hand rub.
   b. Rub your hands together.
   c. Cover all surfaces of your hands and fingers.
   d. Rub your hands together until they are dry.
9. Isolation precautions:
   a. prevent the spread of infection
   b. destroy pathogens
   c. keep pathogens within a certain area
   d. destroy all microbes
10. Standard Precautions:
    a. are used for all persons
    b. prevent the spread of pathogens through the air
    c. require gowns, masks, gloves, and goggles
    d. require a doctor's order

11. When administering drugs, you must practice all of the following, *except*:
    a. hand hygiene
    b. Standard Precautions
    c. surgical asepsis
    d. the Bloodborne Pathogen Standard
12. Gloves are:
    a. easier to put on when your hands are wet
    b. worn by several people until they are visibly soiled
    c. put on first when wearing other PPE
    d. changed when moving from a contaminated body site to a clean body site
13. A mask:
    a. can be reused
    b. is clean on the inside
    c. is contaminated when moist
    d. should fit loosely for breathing
14. Which of these statements about PPE is false?
    a. Wash disposable gloves for reuse.
    b. Remove PPE before leaving the work area.
    c. Discard cracked or torn utility gloves.
    d. Wear gloves when touching contaminated items or surfaces.
15. Goggles or a face shield is worn:
    a. when using Standard Precautions
    b. when splashing body fluids is likely
    c. if you have an eye infection
    d. when assisting with sterile procedures
16. According to the Bloodborne Pathogen Standard, you should not:
    a. wear gloves
    b. discard sharp items into a biohazard container
    c. store food and blood in different places
    d. eat and drink in care settings
17. You were exposed to a bloodborne pathogen. Which is true?
    a. You do not have to report the exposure.
    b. You pay for required tests.
    c. You can refuse HIV and HBV testing.
    d. The source individual can refuse testing.
18. If an outbreak of COVID-19 happens at the nursing center where you are working, you should:
    a. Serve all meals in the common dining room.
    b. Come to work even if you are sick.
    c. Ask visitors to visit their family members more frequently.
    d. Isolate the infected residents from those not infected.

Circle T if the statement is true. Circle F if the statement is false.

19. T F   Microbes are pathogens in their natural sites
20. T F   E. coli are normal flora when found in the colon
21. T F   A pathogen can cause an infection
22. T F   An infection results when microbes invade and grow in the body
23. T F   An item is sterile if non-pathogens are present
24. T F   A healthcare-associated infection (HAI) is also called a nosocomial infection
25. T F   You cannot prevent cross-contamination when administering drugs
26. T F   You hold your hands and forearms up while washing hands
27. T F   You should wipe your hands with a paper towel after using an alcohol-based hand rub
28. T F   A clean towel lands on the floor; the towel is now dirty
29. T F   You do not need to wear personal protective equipment when administering drugs to people who require isolation precautions
30. T F   A pandemic is an epidemic that has spread to multiple countries or continents
31. T F   You only need to cover your cough if you have a fever
32. T F   Social distancing was recommended by the CDC to slow the spread of COVID-19 infections

Answers to these questions can be found on the Evolve Resources site: http://evolve.elsevier.com/Anderson/medasst/

7

Basic Pharmacology

Pharmacology is the study of drugs and their actions on living organisms. There are thousands of drugs; new ones are developed every year.

DRUG NAMES

All drugs have different names, but many have similar spellings. The exact name and spelling of a drug are of the utmost importance so as to give the right drug to the right person.

Drugs have the following names (Fig. 7-1):
- *Chemical name*—the exact chemical structure of a drug.
- *Generic name*—the drug's common name. A generic drug is a copy of a brand name drug. The generic drug is the same in dosage, safety, strength, how it is taken, quality, performance, and intended use. All manufacturers of the drug use the generic name. The first letter is not capitalized.
- *Official name*—the name under which the drug is listed by the Food and Drug Administration (FDA). It is almost always the generic name.
- *Brand name*—the *trademark* or *trade name* of the drug. This name is often followed by the symbol ®. Only the manufacturer who owns the drug can use the brand or trade name. Brand or trade names are easier to spell, pronounce, and remember. The first letter is capitalized.

EXAMPLE OF GENERIC AND BRAND NAMES FOR DRUGS

Generic name: cetirizine
Brand name: Zyrtec Allergy

Fig. 7-1 Different names of the same drug. From Willihnganz, Gurevits, & Clayton: Clayton's Basic Pharmacology for Nurses, ed 18, St. Louis, Elsevier 2020.

DRUG CLASSIFICATIONS

Classification means a group or category. Things in a group or category are similar and have common attributes and qualities. Drugs are classified by:
- *Body system.* Drugs are classified according to the body system they affect. Examples include drugs affecting the central nervous system (CNS) and drugs affecting the cardiovascular system.
- *Therapeutic use or clinical indications.* The word "therapeutic" relates to treating or curing a disease or disorder. Clinical indications relate to the signs or reasons for using a drug. For example, when a person has an infection, the doctor may order an antibiotic. An antibiotic is a drug that kills microbes and cures infections. (*Anti* means *against. Biotic* means *life.*)
- *Physiologic or chemical action.* The action relates to what the drug does in the body. Calcium channel blockers reduce calcium flow across the cell membranes in smooth muscles.

They are used to prevent coronary artery spasm. This promotes blood flow through the coronary arteries to the heart muscle.
- *Prescription or non-prescription.* Prescription drugs require an order from a health professional licensed to prescribe—doctors, dentists, nurse practitioners, physician assistants, and pharmacists. The manufacturer's label contains the phrase "Rx only" or "Caution: Federal Law Prohibits Dispensing Without a Prescription." Non-prescription drugs also are called *over-the-counter (OTC) drugs.* These drugs do not require a prescription. They are sold in drug stores, grocery stores, and other stores.
- *Illegal drugs.* These are drugs or chemical substances used for non-therapeutic reasons. They are obtained illegally and are not approved for use by the FDA. They also are called *recreational drugs.*

BASIC PRINCIPLES

Drugs act in the human body in the following ways:
- Drugs change a physiologic activity within the body. They do not create new responses. Drug response is stated in relation to the physiologic activity before drug therapy. For example, when a drug is given to lower blood pressure, the therapy is considered successful if blood pressure is lower during therapy than before therapy. The person's blood pressure is measured before and during drug therapy. The doctor and nurse use the measurements to evaluate whether or not drug therapy was effective in lowering the person's blood pressure.
- Usually, a drug forms chemical bonds within specific sites *(receptors)* within the body. The relationship between a drug and a receptor is similar to that of a key and a lock (Fig. 7-2, *A*).
- Drugs that interact with a receptor to cause a response are *agonists* (Fig. 7-2, *B*). Drugs that attach to a receptor but do not cause a response are *antagonists* (Fig. 7-2, *C*). Drugs that interact with a receptor to cause a response but prevent other responses are *partial agonists* (Fig. 7-2, *D*).
- Once given, all drugs go through four stages: *a*bsorption, *d*istribution, *m*etabolism, and *e*xcretion (ADME).

Routes of Drug Administration

The three most common routes of drug administration are the enteral, parenteral, and percutaneous routes.
- **Enteral route**—drugs are administered directly into the gastrointestinal (GI) tract. *Enteral* means *bowel.* Enteral drugs are given through the oral, rectal, and nasogastric routes.

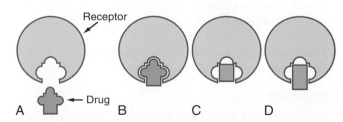

Fig. 7-2 A, Drugs act by forming a chemical bond with a specific receptor site. This process works like a key and a lock. B, The better the fit of the key into the lock, the better the response. Those drugs with complete attachment are called *agonists.* C, *Antagonists* are drugs that attach but do not cause a response. D, *Partial agonists* attach and cause a small response. They also block other responses.

- **Parenteral route**—drugs bypass the GI tract. (*Para* means *beyond*. *Enteral* means *bowel*.) Parenteral routes include:
  - **Subcutaneous (subcut)**—beneath (*sub*) the skin (*cutaneous*).
  - **Intramuscular (IM)**—within (*intra*) a muscle (*muscular*).
  - **Intravenous (IV)**—within (*intra*) a vein (*venous*).
- **Percutaneous route**—drugs are administered through (*per*) the skin (*cutaneous*) or a mucous membrane. Prime examples include sublingual drugs (under the tongue) and topical drugs (on the skin). Inhalation is also a common route, along with vaginal and rectal drug administration.

Absorption

Absorption is the process by which a drug is transferred from its site of body entry to circulating body fluids (blood, lymph) for distribution. The rate of absorption depends on:

- The route of administration
- Blood flow through the tissue where the drug was given
- How well the drug can dissolve (solubility)

In order to promote absorption, it is important to give oral drugs with enough fluid. Eight ounces of water is usually sufficient. It is also important to reconstitute and dilute drugs as recommended by the manufacturer. **Reconstitute** means adding water or other liquid to a powder or solid form of a drug. **Dilute** means adding the correct amount of water or other liquid. If the drug is given as an injection, it needs to be given into the correct tissue.

A drug must dissolve in body fluids before it can be absorbed into body tissues. For example, a solid drug taken orally must be absorbed into the bloodstream for transport to the site of action. First it must dissolve in the GI fluids. Then, it must be transported across the stomach or intestinal lining into the blood. A liquid is absorbed faster than a tablet or capsule because it does not need to dissolve first.

The rate of absorption for parenteral drugs depends on the blood flow through the tissues. Circulatory problems and respiratory distress may lead to vasoconstriction. (*Vaso* means *blood vessel*. *Constriction* means *to narrow*.) Therefore, the nurse does not give an injection at a site where circulation is impaired. Subcutaneous injections have the slowest absorption rate. IM injections are more rapidly absorbed. Blood flow to muscle is greater than to subcutaneous tissue. Drugs are dispersed throughout the body most rapidly when given by IV injection.

Absorption of drugs applied to the skin (topical route) is influenced by:

- The amount given and strength of the drug
- Length of contact time
- Size of the affected area
- Thickness of the skin surface
- Tissue hydration (amount of water in the tissues)
- Skin condition (intact or non-intact)

Distribution

Distribution refers to the ways drugs are transported by circulating body fluids to the sites of action (receptors) and to the sites of metabolism and excretion. Organs with the greatest blood supply (heart, liver, kidneys, and brain) receive the drug most rapidly. Areas with lesser blood supplies (muscle, skin, and fat) receive the drug more slowly.

After a drug has dissolved, it is absorbed into the blood. Its distribution is determined by the chemical properties of the drug and how it is affected by the blood and tissues with which it comes into contact.

A blood sample may be studied to determine the amount of a drug present in the blood. This amount is known as a **drug blood level.** If the drug blood level is too low, the dosage is increased, or the drug is given more often. If the drug blood level is too high, the person may show signs of toxicity. (*Toxin* means *poison*. **Toxicity** means exposure to large amounts of a substance that should not cause problems in smaller amounts.) The dosage is reduced, or the drug is given less often.

The amount of drug that actually gets to the receptor sites determines the extent of the response. If a small amount of the drug actually reaches and binds to the receptor sites, the response is minimal.

Metabolism

Metabolism is the process by which the body inactivates drugs. The liver is the primary site for drug metabolism. Other tissues and organs, such as white blood cells, GI tract, and lungs, metabolize drugs to a minor extent. Genetic, environmental, and physiologic factors help regulate drug metabolism. Illness, age, and use of other drugs are a few other factors affecting metabolism.

Excretion

Excretion is the elimination of a drug from the body. Urine and feces are the primary routes of excretion. Others routes include evaporation from the skin, exhalation from the lungs, and secretion into saliva and breast milk.

DRUG ACTION

No drug has a single action. When a drug is absorbed and distributed, the **desired action** (expected response) usually occurs. All drugs can affect more than one body system; therefore, side effects and adverse drug reactions can occur.

- **Side effects**—unintended reactions to a drug given in a normal dosage. The effect is usually not desired. Nausea, dry mouth, dizziness, blurred vision, and ringing in the ears (*tinnitus*) are common side effects. When side effects are severe, the reaction is sometimes called **toxicity.**
- **Adverse drug reaction** (ADR), or adverse effect—an unintended effect on the body from using a legal drug, an illegal drug, or two or more drugs. Rash, itching, high blood sugar (*hyperglycemia*), and a reduced number of platelets (*thrombocytopenia*) are common ADRs. Sadly, ADRs are a leading cause of death in the United States; however, most can be prevented.

Each drug has parameters (measures)—therapeutic actions to expect, side effects to expect, ADRs to report, and probable drug interactions. The health team monitors the parameters. Dosages are adjusted for the best therapeutic effect and to reduce side effects and ADRs. Always follow agency policy for reporting ADRs.

Idiosyncratic reactions and allergic reactions can occur. An **idiosyncratic reaction** is something unusual or abnormal that happens when a drug is first given. (*Idio* means *own*. *Syncratic* means *mixing together*.) The person has an over-response to the drug's action. This uncommon response usually occurs because the person cannot metabolize the drug.

An **allergic reaction** is an unfavorable response to a substance that causes a hypersensitivity reaction. *Hypersensitivity* means an exaggerated (*hyper*) response (*sensitivity*). Allergic reactions can occur in persons previously exposed to a drug. This happens because the person has developed antibodies to the drug; on re-exposure, the antibodies cause a reaction.

The most common allergic reaction is **urticaria (hives)**—raised, irregularly shaped patches on the skin and severe itching (Fig. 7-3). Some people experience **anaphylaxis (anaphylactic reaction)**—a severe, life-threatening sensitivity to an antigen (an unwanted substance). (*Ana* means *without*. *Phylaxis* means *protection*.). This is a medical emergency, as the following signs and symptoms can occur within seconds:

- Sweating
- Shortness of breath
- Low blood pressure
- Irregular pulse
- Respiratory congestion
- Swelling of the larynx (laryngeal edema)
- Hoarseness
- Dyspnea

A mild allergic reaction is a warning not to take the drug again. The reactive person is at risk for anaphylaxis from their next exposure to the drug. It is important for the person to receive information about the drug so that they may report the reaction to any other necessary health professionals. The person must never use the drug again. In addition, a medic alert bracelet or necklace may be worn to explain the allergy.

See *Focus on Older Persons: Drug Action.*

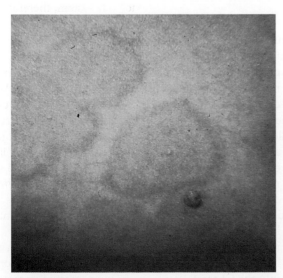

Fig. 7-3 Urticaria (Hives).(Courtesy Dr. Donald W. Kress, Children's Hospital of Pittsburgh. From Zitelli BJ, Davis HW: *Atlas of pediatric physical diagnosis*, ed 4, St Louis, 2002, Mosby.)

Factors Influencing Drug Action

Exact responses to drug therapy are hard to predict. Drugs have strong effects in some people while others show little response to the same dosage. Some people react differently to the same dosage given at different times. The following factors may affect a person's response to drugs:

- *Age.* Infants and older persons are the most sensitive to drugs. The ADME of drugs differs in premature infants, full-term newborns, and children. Bodily changes due to aging may affect the older person's response to drug therapy.
- *Body weight.* Very heavy persons may need higher dosages to attain the desired response while persons who are underweight may need lower dosages for the desired response. Weight and height measurements are needed; the doctor uses them to determine drug dosages (Chapter 4).

FOCUS ON OLDER PERSONS
Drug Action

Older persons may not tolerate drug side effects well. For example, dizziness may cause an older person to decrease activity because he or she has fears of falling. Additionally, a dry mouth can cause problems with dentures, taste, and chewing. Nutrition can suffer as a result.

Many drugs cause depression, confusion, and delirium in older persons. Confusion is often the first and only sign of a drug-induced problem.

Always report signs, symptoms, and behavior changes to the nurse. The doctor may need to adjust the person's drug therapy.

- *Metabolic rate.* *Metabolism* is the burning of food for heat and energy by the cells. *Metabolic rate* is the amount of energy used in a given amount of time. People with a high metabolic rate tend to metabolize drugs faster and therefore need larger doses more often. The opposite is true for those with a low metabolic rate.
- *Illness.* Illness may affect ADME. For example, persons in shock have reduced circulation and absorb IM or subcutaneous drugs slowly. With vomiting present, drugs may not stay in the stomach long enough for absorption. Some persons do not have enough proteins in the blood to adequately distribute drugs. Many drugs are excreted by the kidneys; persons with kidney failure need lower dosages.
- *Willingness to take drugs.* Some diseases have rapid effects if therapy is ignored. Diabetes is one example. Persons with diabetes usually take drugs as prescribed. Persons with high blood pressure may not have signs and symptoms and therefore may not take drugs as prescribed.
- *Placebo effect.* A **placebo,** commonly called a "sugar pill," is a drug dosage form that has no active ingredients. Positive expectations about treatment and care can affect good therapy outcomes. Therefore, when taken, the person may report the desired response. This is called the *placebo effect.* In Latin, *placebo* means *shall please*. The American Pain Society recommends avoiding the deceitful (not honest) use of placebos to manage pain because it violates the person's right to the highest quality of care possible.
- *Tolerance.* Tolerance occurs when a person begins to need higher dosages to produce the same effects that lower dosages

once gave. For example, over time, a heroin-addicted person may require increasingly larger dosages to achieve the same "high." Tolerance can be caused by psychologic dependence, or the body may metabolize a drug faster than before. Tolerance also causes the effects of drugs to diminish faster.

- *Dependence.* Drug dependence (addiction or habituation) occurs when a person cannot control their ingestion of drugs. Dependence may be physiologic. The person develops withdrawal symptoms if the drug is not taken for a certain period of time. Psychological dependence is when the person is emotionally attached to the drug. Drug dependence is most common with scheduled or controlled drugs (Chapter 3). Many people worry about becoming addicted to pain-relief drugs. They may not take them even when needed as a result of this concern. However, the risk of addiction is low. For the person's well-being, they should be as pain-free as possible.
- *Cumulative effect.* A drug may accumulate in the body if the next dose is given before the previous one has been metabolized or excreted, and may result in toxicity. For example, a person drinking alcohol becomes "drunk" when he or she drinks faster than the rate of alcohol metabolism and excretion.

DRUG INTERACTIONS

A **drug interaction** occurs when the action of one drug is altered by the action of another drug. This happens in two ways:
- Drugs, when combined, *increase* the actions of one or both drugs.
- Drugs, when combined, *decrease* the effectiveness of one or both drugs.

Some drug interactions are beneficial. For example, caffeine is a CNS stimulant. An antihistamine is a CNS depressant. When combined, the caffeine counteracts the drowsiness from the antihistamine. The desired antihistamine effects are allowed.

DRUG INFORMATION

There are thousands of drugs in existence; you simply cannot memorize information about all of them. Many drug resources are available in print and online. Be sure the resources you use are accurate and current by checking for a current date on the resource. Also check other current resources to make sure the information is correct.

Know where to find other resources on your nursing unit. The following online resources are helpful:
- *United States Pharmacopeia (USP)/National Formulary (NF).* This online resource provides standards for the identity, quality, strength, and purity of substances used in healthcare practice. It is published annually and contains over 10,000 drug names. The standards described in the USP/NF are enforced by the FDA.
- *Drug Facts and Comparisons.* This resource is available online or in print. It is arranged in a table by body systems. It allows for comparison of similar products, brand names, manufacturers, and available dosages.
- *Handbook of Nonprescription Drugs: An Interactive Approach to Self-Care.* This resource is available online or in print. It is the most comprehensive text about over-the-counter medications that can be purchased in the United States.
- *Natural Medicines Comprehensive Database.* This resource is only available online. It is considered the scientific gold standard for evidence-based information about herbal medicines and combination products involving herbal medicines.
- *Physicians' Desk Reference (PDR).* More than 3000 drugs are presented. Divided into six sections, each section has a different page color. The Product Identification Guide contains actual-size color photos of tablets and capsules provided by the manufacturers. The Product Information Section contains reprints of package inserts. The inserts describe the drug's action, uses, administration, dosages, contraindications, and other information.

■ REVIEW QUESTIONS

Circle the BEST answer.

1. The brand name of a drug is:
   a. its trade name
   b. its chemical structure
   c. its common name
   d. the name listed by the FDA
2. A prescription drug:
   a. affects one body system
   b. has one use
   c. needs a doctor's order
   d. is not approved for use by the FDA
3. Over-the-counter drugs:
   a. are called recreational drugs
   b. are sold without a prescription
   c. have no therapeutic use
   d. require the phrase "Rx only" on the label
4. Drugs act in the human body by:
   a. forming a chemical bond within specific sites
   b. creating new body responses
   c. reconstituting a body fluid
   d. diluting a body fluid
5. The process by which the body inactivates a drug is called:
   a. absorption
   b. distribution
   c. metabolism
   d. excretion
6. A drug administered through the enteral route is given:
   a. into a vein
   b. into a muscle
   c. beneath the skin
   d. into the GI tract

7. The nurse tells you that the blood level of a drug is too high. You know that the:
   a. person is taking illegal drugs
   b. person is at risk for toxicity
   c. the rate of absorption is low
   d. the rate of excretion is high
8. Most drugs are metabolized:
   a. in the kidneys
   b. by white blood cells
   c. by the GI tract
   d. in the liver
9. Most drugs leave the body through:
   a. the skin
   b. the lungs
   c. saliva
   d. urine and feces
10. Which is life-threatening?
    a. an allergic reaction
    b. an adverse drug reaction
    c. an idiosyncratic drug reaction
    d. an anaphylactic reaction
11. A person complains of severe itching. You observe raised, irregular patches on the person's skin. This is called:
    a. a side effect
    b. an adverse drug reaction
    c. anaphylaxis
    d. hives

12. A hypersensitivity to a drug is called:
    a. an allergic reaction
    b. an adverse effect
    c. a side effect
    d. an anaphylactic reaction
13. Which has no active ingredients?
    a. IM
    b. IV
    c. subcutaneous
    d. placebo
14. A person needs higher dosages of a drug to produce the same effects that lower dosages once gave. This is called:
    a. tolerance
    b. dependence
    c. cumulative effect
    d. a drug interaction
15. When checking drug information, you must use:
    a. the *PDR*
    b. package inserts
    c. the most current resource
    d. online resources

Answers to these questions can be found on the Evolve Resources site: http://evolve.elsevier.com/Anderson/medasst/

8

Life Span Considerations

OBJECTIVES

- Define the key terms and abbreviations used in this chapter.
- Know the age ranges for each age group.
- Identify the factors that affect drug absorption in children and older adults.
- Identify the factors that affect drug distribution in children and older adults.
- Identify the factors that affect drug metabolism in children and older adults.
- Identify the factors that affect drug excretion in children and older adults.

- Explain the purpose of therapeutic drug monitoring.
- Explain how to assist the nurse with therapeutic drug monitoring.
- Explain the factors and guidelines related to giving drugs to children.
- Identify the causes of drug toxicity in older adults.
- Explain how to help older adults with drug therapy.
- Explain how to help pregnant women and breastfeeding mothers with drug therapy.

KEY TERMS

enzymes Substances produced by body cells; using oxygen, enzymes break down glucose and other nutrients to release energy for cellular work

metabolite A product of drug metabolism
therapeutic drug monitoring The measurement of a drug's concentration in body fluids

KEY ABBREVIATIONS

FDA Food and Drug Administration

GI Gastrointestinal

Gender (male; female) affects drug therapy. Men and women respond to drugs differently. They also react to and experience disease differently.

The person's age can greatly affect drug therapy. See the different age groups in Box 8-1. Children and older adults require special considerations when administering drugs.

BOX 8-1	Age Groups
Less than 38 weeks gestation	Premature
0 to 1 month	Newborn; neonate
1 to 24 months	Infant; toddler
3 to 5 years	Young child
6 to 12 years	Older child
13 to 18 years	Adolescent
19 to 54 years	Adult
55 to 64 years	Older adult
65 to 74 years	Elderly
75 to 84 years	The aged
85 years and older	The very old

DRUG ABSORPTION

Absorption is the process by which a drug is transferred from its site of body entry to circulating body fluids (blood, lymph) for distribution (Chapter 7).

Drugs Applied to the Skin

Absorption of drugs applied to the skin (topical drugs) is usually effective in infants. The outer skin layer is not fully developed. The skin is more fully hydrated (has more water) at this age. Skin absorption is enhanced when infants wear plastic-coated diapers. The plastic increases hydration of the skin. Inflammation of the skin also increases the amount of drug absorbed. Diaper rash is one example of skin inflammation.

On the other hand, skin absorption in older adults is often hard to predict. Skin thickness decreases with aging and may enhance absorption. However, numerous factors may lessen absorption, including:

- Dry skin
- Wrinkled skin
- Decreased number of hair follicles
- Decreased cardiac output; decreased amount of blood flow to tissues

Drugs Given Orally

Most drugs are given orally. However, some tablet and capsule forms are too large for children and older adults to swallow safely. With the nurse's permission, some tablets can be crushed to mix with food or a liquid form is ordered. Taste is a factor when administering oral liquids because the liquid comes into contact with the taste buds.

Certain oral drug forms must not be crushed; doing so affects the absorption rate. Toxicity also is a risk. Examples of noncrushable oral drug forms are discussed in Chapter 11 and include:

- Timed-release tablets
- Enteric-coated tablets
- Sublingual tablets

Loose teeth are common in children and older adults; infants and some older adults may not have enough teeth for chewable drugs. Always inquire about loose teeth and do not give chewable tablets to anyone with loose teeth.

Saliva flow is often decreased in older adults, making chewing and swallowing harder for them.

Gastrointestinal (GI) absorption of drugs is influenced by disease processes and many factors, including:

- *Gastric pH*—how much acid is in the stomach. Older adults have fewer acid-secreting cells, which in turn gives them a higher gastric pH (the lower the pH, the more acid in the stomach). Some drugs are destroyed by gastric acid. Older adults have less gastric acid to destroy such drugs. Therefore, drugs destroyed by gastric acid are absorbed faster in older adults. Blood levels also are higher in older adults. Penicillin is one example of this. Other drugs, such as Aspirin, depend on gastric acid for absorption. They are poorly absorbed and have lower blood levels in older adults.
- *Gastric emptying*—how fast the stomach empties. The stomach empties more slowly in older adults than it does in younger people. As a result, drugs may have a longer time period of tissue contact. This allows increased absorption, which leads to a higher blood level. Toxicity is a risk from extended contact time in the stomach. The risk of ulcers increases with some drugs.
- *Motility of the GI tract*—how fast digested food and fluids move through the GI tract. GI motility is decreased in older adults. Decreased motility can alter the absorption of drugs. Constipation or diarrhea can occur.
- *Blood flow*—the amount of blood that reaches the stomach and intestines. Blood flow decreases in older adults. Lower blood flow can alter the absorption of drugs; constipation or diarrhea can occur.

DRUG DISTRIBUTION

Distribution refers to the ways drugs are transported by circulating body fluids to the sites of action (receptors) and to the sites of metabolism and excretion (Chapter 7). Most drugs are transported using the following methods:

- The drug is dissolved in the circulating body water (in blood). The amount of body water changes with age. About 74% of an infant's body is composed of water. About 60% of an adult man's body is composed of body water. This figure drops to 50% in older adults.

- The drug is bound to plasma proteins within the blood. Albumin and globulins are plasma proteins. After age 40, protein composition begins to change. Albumin concentrations gradually decrease, and globulins increase. As albumin levels decrease, the amount of unbound, active drug increases. Some liver and kidney diseases may lower albumin levels. If the albumin level is low, the person needs lower doses of certain drugs. The doctor may then slowly increase the dosage. The drug effect may be greater at first because there is more active drug available. However, the duration of action may be reduced. When the drug is not bound to protein, there is more drug available for metabolism and excretion.

DRUG METABOLISM

Metabolism is the process by which the body inactivates drugs. Enzymes are a major factor in drug metabolism. **Enzymes** are substances produced by body cells. Using oxygen, enzymes break down glucose and other nutrients to release energy for cellular work. Enzyme systems in the liver provide the major pathway for drug metabolism. All enzyme systems are present at birth. However, they mature at different rates. Some enzyme systems may take only weeks to fully develop while others may take one year to fully develop.

Drug metabolism is slower in older adults due to the fact that liver weight, liver blood flow, and the number of functioning liver cells decrease with age. Therefore, reduced metabolism is made more serious by the presence of liver disease and heart failure. Drugs metabolized by the liver can have longer action if liver blood flow is reduced. Dosages are usually reduced or the time between doses is extended to address this issue. An appropriately adjusted dosage prevents the accumulation of active drugs and the risk of toxicity.

Regardless of age, drug metabolism is also affected by genetics, smoking, diet, gender, liver disease, and use of other drugs. The doctor orders liver function tests, and dosages are adjusted as needed.

DRUG EXCRETION

Excretion is the elimination of a drug from the body. Metabolites of drugs, and sometimes the drug itself, are eventually excreted from the body (a **metabolite** is a product of drug metabolism). Metabolites are excreted mainly through the urine and feces. Other possible routes of excretion include through the skin, lungs, saliva, and breast milk.

At birth, a full-term newborn has about 35% of the kidney capacity of an adult; full adult function is achieved at 9 to 12 months of age. Some drugs are excreted mainly by the kidneys. As the child grows, dosages of such drugs are increased or given more often to maintain therapeutic blood levels.

Changes in the kidneys occur naturally with aging. Kidney blood flow, kidney function, and cardiac output all decrease with age. The doctor orders kidney function tests as needed. Drug dosages are decreased or given less often to maintain therapeutic blood levels.

THERAPEUTIC DRUG MONITORING

Therapeutic drug monitoring is the measurement of a drug's concentration in body fluids. It is done to determine the drug dosage and the blood level of the drug in relation to the body's response. Blood testing is a commonly used method; saliva tests are also used for some drugs.

Therapeutic drug monitoring is essential in newborns, infants, children, and adults with certain health problems. Heart failure and abnormal heart rhythms are examples. The doctor adjusts the dosage and how often the drug is given to maintain desired drug levels.

Blood levels are measured if drug toxicity is suspected. The doctor uses the blood level to decide how to treat the toxicity.

Blood and urine samples can be obtained for legal purposes if drug abuse is suspected.

Assisting with the Nursing Process

Vital signs and urinary output are used to plan dosages and monitor the effects of drug therapy in all persons. Accurate measurements are essential. You must know the normal ranges for the person and report abnormal measurements at once.

Health teaching is important for all drugs. The nurse involves family members and caregivers in the health teaching plan as needed. Patients need to understand the purpose of the drugs they are taking. They also need to know the complications that may occur if they stop taking the drug.

Children. Infants and children are at great risk for complications from drug therapy because their bodies and organ functions are still developing. Remember the following when administering drugs to children:

- They are at risk for dehydration from fever, vomiting, and diarrhea.
- They grow rapidly and have growth spurts. The doctor may need to adjust dosages according to the child's weight; accurate height and weight measurements are important.
- Report your observations to the nurse (e.g., vital signs, appetite, appearance, responsiveness, and intake and output measurements).
- Use appropriate devices when administering liquid drugs (e.g., medicine cup, oral dropper, or oral syringe) (Fig. 8-1).
- Around age 5, children can usually begin swallowing tablets and capsules. Many tablets that are not timed-release or enteric-coated can be crushed instead of directly swallowed. Most capsules can be opened and their contents sprinkled on small amounts of food (e.g., applesauce, jelly, or pudding).
- Dilute oral drugs in powder form according to the manufacturer's instructions.
- Many drugs are not approved by the Food and Drug Administration (FDA) for use in children. Doctors may legally prescribe some drugs for what is called *off-label use.* The nurse must question a specific dose if it is not readily available for cross-checking in drug information resources. Before administering the drug for off-label use, the nurse documents in the child's medical record that the drug order was verified. The nurse may need to give the drug; be sure to follow agency policy.

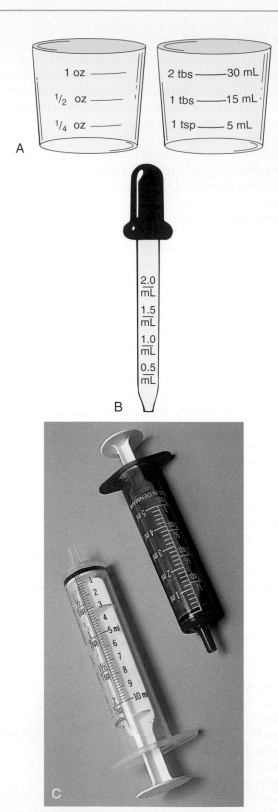

Fig. 8-1 Devices for giving oral drugs to children. **A,** Medicine cup. **B,** Oral dropper. **C,** Oral syringe.

- In general, salicylates (aspirin) should not be given to children until after the teenage years. Taking aspirin puts children at risk for Reye's syndrome (a life-threatening illness). Reye's syndrome is a risk when a child takes aspirin at the time of or shortly after chickenpox or influenza is present.

Ibuprofen (Advil) and acetaminophen (Tylenol) are routinely used to relieve pain or reduce fever in children.

- Allergic reactions can occur rapidly in children. Reactions most often occur with use of antibiotics, especially penicillins. Closely observe the child's response to the drug. Report any adverse signs and symptoms to the nurse at once. Intense anxiety, weakness, sweating, and shortness of breath are common at first. Other symptoms that may occur include hypotension, shock, abnormal heart rhythms, respiratory congestion, laryngeal edema, nausea, and defecation. Call for the nurse at once if any of the aforementioned symptoms occurs. Start cardiopulmonary resuscitation if necessary.

See Box 8-2 for guidelines when giving oral drugs to children.

Older Adults. Older adults are at great risk for drug interactions or drug toxicity. Causes include:

- Reduced liver function
- Reduced kidney function
- Chronic illnesses that require many drugs
- Poor nutrition
- Also reduced muscle mass that may affect drug distribution or cause inaccurate lab levels (example: serum creatinine).
- Reduced muscle mass

Remember the following when assisting older adults with drug therapy:

- Drug organizers (Fig. 8-3) and calendars are reminders for when to take drugs. Smartphone apps are also available to help remind people when to take their drugs. Apps are useful for persons who can take their own drugs.
- Help the person get rid of old prescriptions. This helps prevent confusion with current drug therapy.
- Older adults may have problems swallowing large tablets or capsules. You can crush them with the nurse's approval, or you can break them in half if there is a "score" mark on the tablet (Fig. 8-4). A *score* is a groove or indentation used to divide the tablet. A scored tablet can be easily broken in half. Remember, timed-release tablets, enteric-coated tablets, and sublingual tablets are never crushed. Crushing these types of drugs affects the absorption rate and increases the risk of toxicity. When crushed drugs are appropriate, give with applesauce, ice cream, or jelly, as the person's diet allows.

Pregnant Women. Drug therapy during pregnancy is avoided whenever possible because many drugs can injure the developing fetus. However, many women take at least one drug while pregnant, most of which are non-prescription, self-care remedies. Pain-relief drugs, antacids, and cold and allergy products are commonly taken by pregnant women. Some drugs may cause birth defects and are therefore contraindicated during pregnancy.

When assisting a pregnant woman with drug therapy, remind her to:

- Only take drugs ordered by the doctor.
- Avoid drinking alcohol. Excessive use may cause the child to be born with fetal alcohol syndrome (a lifelong condition with psychological, behavioral, and physical effects). Women planning to become pregnant should stop drinking alcohol 2 to 3 months before conception.
- Avoid the use of tobacco, including vaping. Mothers who smoke have a higher frequency of miscarriages, stillbirths,

---

BOX 8-2 Guidelines for Giving Oral Drugs to Children

Infants
- Use a calibrated dropper or oral syringe (see Fig. 8-1).
- Support the infant's head while holding him or her in your lap (Fig. 8-2).
- Give small amounts of the drug at a time to prevent choking.
- Give oral medications before feeding, unless instructed otherwise.
- Rock the baby before and after drug administration.

Toddlers
- Ask other parents what techniques have worked for them.
- Let the toddler choose a position in which to take the drug.
- Disguise the drug's taste with a small amount of food or flavored drink. Let the child drink water or a flavored drink to help remove an unpleasant aftertaste.
- Use age-appropriate language to explain what you are doing. For example, "This will make you feel better. Open up. Yummy, yummy."
- Never refer to the drugs as "candy."
- If more than one drug is being taken, let the toddler choose which drug to take first.
- Use verbal and physical responses to promote the child's cooperation.
- Let the child become familiar with and inspect the oral dosing device.
- Praise the child for cooperating.

Older Children
- Place a tablet or capsule near the back of the tongue. Then provide water or a flavored drink to help the child swallow the drug.
- Chewable tablets are avoided if the child has loose teeth; tell the nurse if this is the case.
- Explain to the child how the drug will help them.
- Let the child rinse with water or a drink a flavored beverage to remove an unpleasant aftertaste.
- Involve the child in the process by letting them decide which drug to take first, what to drink with it, and where they feel comfortable taking the drug(s).
- Praise the child for cooperating.

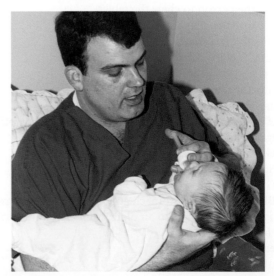

Fig. 8-2 The infant's head is supported while being given an oral drug.

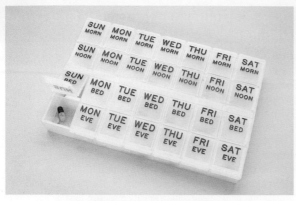

Fig. 8-3 Drug organizer.

 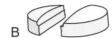

Fig. 8-4 A, A scored tablet. **B,** The scored tablet is broken in half.

premature births, and low-birth-weight infants.
- When treating morning sickness, try the following non-drug treatments first:
  - Lay down when feeling nauseated
  - Eat crackers or sip small amounts of liquids before arising
  - Eat small, frequent meals high in carbohydrates and low in fat
  - Avoiding spicy foods, dairy products, and smells or situations that may cause vomiting
  - Avoid herbal medicines that have not been scientifically tested on humans during pregnancy

Breastfeeding Women. Many drugs will enter the breast milk of nursing mothers and may harm the infant. If the breastfeeding mother is taking any drugs, the best times to take them are:
- Right after the infant finishes breastfeeding
- Just before the infant's longer sleep period

Remind the mother about adverse effects that may occur in the infant.

REVIEW QUESTIONS

Circle the BEST answer.

1. Skin absorption of drugs is enhanced in infants. This is because their skin:
   a. is thinner
   b. has more water
   c. is dry
   d. has few hair follicles

2. You are giving drugs to an older adult. Which of the following may enhance skin absorption?
   a. thin skin
   b. dry skin
   c. wrinkled skin
   d. decreased blood flow to the skin

3. A tablet is too large for a person to swallow. With the nurse's permission, you can:
   a. crush the tablet and mix it with food
   b. give a liquid form of the same drug
   c. ask the person to chew the tablet
   d. dissolve the drug in water

4. Before giving a chewable tablet, you should:
   a. taste the drug
   b. ask about the person's saliva flow
   c. mix the drug with food
   d. ask about loose teeth

5. These statements are about gastrointestinal absorption of drugs in older adults. Which is *false?*
   a. Gastric acid secretion increases.
   b. Stomach emptying is slower.
   c. GI motility is slower.
   d. Blood flow to the stomach and intestines is decreased.

6. Drugs are given orally to an older adult. They are at risk for the following, *except:*
   a. enzymes
   b. ulcers
   c. constipation
   d. diarrhea

7. Drug distribution is likely to be greater in:
   a. infants
   b. persons with liver disease
   c. persons with kidney disease
   d. older adults

8. In persons with liver or kidney disease, you should expect drug dosages to be:
   a. increased
   b. decreased
   c. within the normal range
   d. half the normal range

9. Therapeutic drug monitoring is done to measure:
   a. metabolites
   b. enzymes
   c. a drug's concentration in body fluids
   d. drug toxicity

10. You may assist the nurse with therapeutic drug monitoring by measuring:
    a. vital signs and urinary output
    b. gastric pH
    c. blood pH
    d. drug blood levels

11. The following are used to give oral drugs to children, *except:*
    a. medicine cups
    b. oral droppers
    c. oral syringes
    d. pacifiers

12. A child cannot swallow a capsule. With the nurse's permission, you can:
    a. sprinkle the contents onto small amounts of applesauce, jelly, or pudding
    b. sprinkle the contents into a flavored drink
    c. dilute the capsule following the manufacturer's instructions
    d. have the child chew the drug

13. From birth until after the teenage years, children should *not* be given:
    a. Tylenol
    b. Advil
    c. penicillin
    d. aspirin
14. When giving drugs to an infant, you should:
    a. support the child's head
    b. let the child choose which drug to take first
    c. place a tablet near the back of the child's tongue
    d. use a straw if the drug can stain teeth
15. To remove an unpleasant aftertaste, you should let the child:
    a. have candy
    b. rinse with water or have a flavored drink
    c. choose which drug form to take
    d. choose where to take the drug
16. Which is a useful reminder for when to take drugs?
    a. medicine cup
    b. oral dropper
    c. oral syringe
    d. drug organizer

17. A tablet may be scored. What does "scored" mean?
    a. You keep track of the number of tablets given to the person.
    b. The tablet can be broken in half.
    c. A "score" means 20. There are 20 doses in the tablet.
    d. The tablet is timed-release.
18. A pregnant woman should do the following, *except:*
    a. try non-drug treatments before trying drugs
    b. take only drugs ordered by the doctor
    c. have one alcoholic drink a day
    d. take prescribed drugs after the infant is done breastfeeding

Answers to these questions can be found on the Evolve Resources site: http://evolve.elsevier.com/Anderson/medasst/

9

Drug Orders and Prescriptions

OBJECTIVES

- Define the key terms and key abbreviations used in this chapter.
- Identify the members of the health team who can give drug orders.
- List the components of a drug order.
- Explain four different types of drug orders.
- Identify abbreviations commonly used in drug orders and prescriptions.
- Know the weights and measurements used in drug orders and prescriptions.
- Identify common drug administration times.

- Describe the information on a prescription label.
- Describe the information contained in a person's medical record.
- Describe each part of a medication administration record.
- Describe each part of a PRN or unscheduled medication record.
- Identify which information to record when giving a PRN drug.
- Explain the purpose of a Kardex.
- Explain how the nurse verifies and transcribes a drug order.
- Explain how to accurately transcribe a drug order.

KEY TERMS

chart   See "medical record"

clinical record   See "medical record"

drug order   An order for a drug written on the agency's (e.g., hospital, nursing center) physician's order form or entered electronically into the agency's computer system for a patient; medication order

electronic health record (EHR)   An electronic version of a person's medical record; electronic medical record

electronic medical record (EMR)   See "electronic health record"

Health Insurance Portability and Accountability Act (HIPAA)   An act created in 1996 that protects people's privacy and health information. A HIPAA violation may result in severe fines.

medical record   The written or electronic account of a person's condition and response to treatment and care; chart or clinical record

medication order   See "drug order"

prescription   A drug or drugs ordered for a person leaving the hospital or nursing center or for a person seen in a clinic or doctor's office; it can be written on a prescription pad or it can be called in, faxed, or emailed to the pharmacy by the prescriber

PRN order   The nurse decides when to give the drug based on the person's needs

routine order   A drug given as prescribed until cancelled by the prescriber, or the prescribed number of doses has been given; scheduled medication

single order   A drug is to be given at a certain time and only one time

STAT order   The drug is to be given at once and only one time

KEY ABBREVIATIONS

CPOE   computerized physician (or provider) order entry
EHR   electronic health record
EMR   electronic medical record
HIPAA   Health Insurance Portability and Accountability Act
ISMP   Institute for Safe Medication Practices
IV   Intravenous; intravenously

MAR   Medication administration record
mEq   milliequivalent
PRN   When necessary; as needed
STAT   Immediately; at once
TO   Telephone order
VO   Verbal order

Healthcare providers such as licensed doctors, dentists, nurse practitioners, and physician's assistants order necessary drugs for patients. Providers who write drug orders or prescriptions are called *prescribers*.

- A drug order (medication order) is an order for a drug written on the agency's (e.g., hospital, nursing center) physician's order form for a patient (Fig. 9-1). The order form is part of the person's medical record. An electronic version of a person's medical record is known as an electronic health record (EHR) or electronic medical record (EMR). In agencies with EHRs, the order is entered into the system by the prescriber. The order is filled in the agency's pharmacy and then is sent to the nursing unit.

PHYSICIAN'S ORDER FORM

Addressograph here:

016-28-3978
Joseph Lorenzo
18 Bush Ave.
Hometown, USA

Martindale Hometown Hospital
Hometown, USA

Dr. M. Martin
Unit-6W, Rm. 621

Please Indicate Allergies

None	Codeine	Penicillin	Sulfa	Aspirin	Others

Date	Time	Prob. No.	Physician's Orders	Physician	Progress Record
1/6	1500	6	Erythromycin 250 mg, PO		
			q6h × 8 days	M. Martin	

Fig. 9-1 Physician's Order Form.

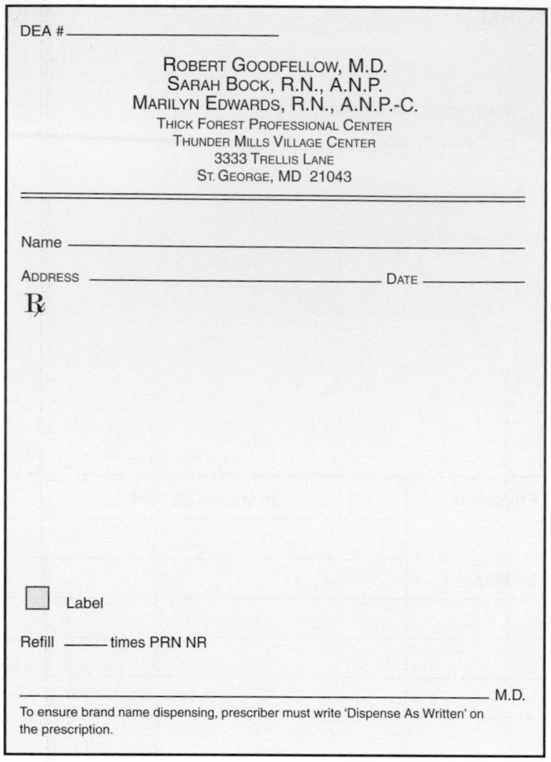

DEA # _____

ROBERT GOODFELLOW, M.D.
SARAH BOCK, R.N., A.N.P.
MARILYN EDWARDS, R.N., A.N.P.-C.
THICK FOREST PROFESSIONAL CENTER
THUNDER MILLS VILLAGE CENTER
3333 TRELLIS LANE
ST. GEORGE, MD 21043

Name _____

ADDRESS _____ DATE _____

℞

☐ Label

Refill _____ times PRN NR

_____ M.D.
To ensure brand name dispensing, prescriber must write 'Dispense As Written' on
the prescription.

Fig. 9-2 Prescription pad. (From Edmunds MW: Introduction to clinical pharmacology, ed 5, St Louis, 2006, Mosby.)

A **prescription** is a drug or drugs ordered for a person leaving the hospital or nursing center. A prescription may also be written for a person seen in a clinic or doctor's office. The prescription can be written on a prescription pad, called in, faxed, or e-mailed to the pharmacy by the prescriber (Fig. 9-2). A written prescription must be taken to a local pharmacy (drug store) to be filled.

Drug orders and prescriptions are essentially the same. They differ for:

- Where they are used (e.g., hospital, nursing center, home setting)
- Where they are filled (i.e., within or outside the agency)

PARTS OF A DRUG ORDER

All drug orders and prescriptions must contain the:

- Person's full name
- Current date
- Drug name
- Dose
- Route of administration (Chapters 11, 12, 13, and 14)
- Frequency of use
- Duration of the order (or number of refills)
- Prescriber's signature

TYPES OF DRUG ORDERS

There are four types of drug orders.

- **STAT order.** *STAT* comes from the Latin word *statim*, meaning *immediately* or *at once*. The drug is to be given at once and only one time. For example, if a person has a seizure, the ordered drug is given at once to stop the seizure. STAT orders are usually given for emergency or urgent situations.
- **Single order.** A drug is to be given at a certain time and only once. For example, a drug to reduce fluid retention is ordered to be given at 0700.
- **PRN order.** *PRN* comes from the Latin term *pro re nata*, meaning *when necessary* or *as needed*. The nurse decides when to give the drug based on the person's needs.
- **Routine order.** Also known as a scheduled medication. A drug is to be given as prescribed until it is cancelled by the prescriber, or after the total prescribed number of doses has been given. For example, an antibiotic is ordered to be given daily for 10 days; the doctor must renew the order if they want the drug to be given over a longer period of time.

ORDERING METHODS

Prescribers can give drug orders in several ways.

- *Written order.* The prescriber writes the order on the doctor's order form or prescription pad. The prescriber then signs the order with their name. A copy of the order form is sent to the pharmacy. Some written orders may be hard to read; if unsure of what is written, the nurse checks with the doctor before transcribing the order (see Box 9-2). The pharmacist contacts the prescriber if they have any questions.
- *Verbal order (VO).* The prescriber verbally gives the drug order to a nurse, who then writes the order on the physician's order form or enters it into the electronic health record (EHR). 'VO' is written on the order to communicate that it was verbally given, and the prescriber signs the order later. Verbal orders are reserved for emergencies. Most agencies strongly discourage them, while others may not accept verbal orders at all.
- *Telephone order (TO).* The prescriber gives the order to a nurse over the phone. The nurse writes the order on the physician's order form or enters it into the EHR. 'TO' is written on the order to show that it was given orally over the phone, and the prescriber signs the order later.
- *Faxed orders.* An order is faxed from a doctor's office to the nursing unit in which the person is a patient. The prescriber signs the orders at the agency within 24 hours of sending the fax.
- *Computerized Physician (or Provider) Order Entry* (CPOE). The healthcare provider enters patient drug orders, as well as other treatments, into the EHR. The computerized system then communicates the drug order to the pharmacy.

See *Focus on Older Persons: Ordering Methods.*
See *Promoting Safety and Comfort: Ordering Methods.*

FOCUS ON OLDER PERSONS
Ordering Methods

Some hospital patients may be transferred to nursing centers. When this occurs, faxed orders are often sent to the nursing center before the person arrives there. This allows the center to prepare for the person's arrival. The person brings the original signed order to the nursing center as well.

PROMOTING SAFETY AND COMFORT

Ordering Methods

Safety

As an MA-C, you do not accept verbal or telephone orders from doctors. This is the nurse's responsibility. Politely give your name and title and ask the doctor to wait for a nurse. Promptly find a nurse to speak with the doctor.

ABBREVIATIONS

Abbreviations are commonly used in writing drug orders and prescriptions (Table 9-1). The Joint Commission and the Institute for Safe Medication Practices (ISMP) recommend using only agency-approved abbreviations. If other abbreviations are used, they can lead to confusion and drug errors. Each agency is required to have a "Do Not Use" list to avoid such confusion (Table 9-2).

WEIGHTS AND MEASUREMENTS

The household and metric systems of measurement are used to calculate, prepare, and administer drugs (Box 9-1). See Appendix A for how to calculate dosages using these systems.

A person's weight is measured in pounds (lb) or kilograms (kg). Follow your agency's protocol for recording weight.

The *unit* and *milliequivalent (mEq)* are other measures used in drug orders. These quantities are stated with a number followed by "units" or "mEq." Examples include the following:

- 300,000 units of penicillin
- 40 mEq of potassium chloride

ADMINISTRATION TIMES

Agencies have standard drug administration times. A standard administration time helps prevent drug errors and ensures that drugs are given safely and on time. Standard times may vary among agencies; always use the standard times outlined by your agency.

Examples of administration times are listed in Table 9-3. The times are listed in military time and the conventional time is in parentheses.

PRESCRIPTION LABELS

All healthcare agencies have drug distribution systems (Chapter 10). Prescriptions filled in local pharmacies are labeled with the following information (Fig. 9-3):

- The person's name, address, and phone number
- The pharmacy's name, address, and phone number
- Prescription number
- Date the prescription was filled
- Original date of the prescription
- Doctor's name
- Brand name of the drug
- Generic name of the drug
- Manufacturer's name
- Drug dosage
- Amount in the container
- How often to take the drug
- Directions for use
- Warnings
- Number of refills allowed
- Expiration date or when to discard

Always read the label carefully and make sure it is complete before administering the drug. If it is not complete, tell the nurse at once. Read and follow warnings and directions on the label. Check the expiration date; if the date has passed, do not give the drug.

THE MEDICAL RECORD

The **medical record (chart; clinical record)** is the written or electronic account of a person's condition and response to treatment and care. Medical records are written on paper forms or patient

TABLE 9-1 Common Abbreviations Used in Writing Prescriptions	
Abbreviation	**Meaning**
ac	Before meals
ad lib	Freely
BID or bid	Twice a day
g or gm	Gram
gtt	Drops
H or hr	Hour
I.D.	Intradermal
IM	Intramuscular
IV	Intravenous
IVPB	Intravenous piggyback
Kg	Kilogram
KVO	Keep vein open
L	Liter
Mcg	Microgram
mEq	Milliequivalent
mL	Milliliter
MDI	Metered-dose inhaler
NGT	Nasogastric tube
PCA	Patient-controlled analgesia
pc	After meals
PR	Per rectum
PRN or prn	As needed
Q	Every
q2h; q4h; q6h; q8h; q12h	Every 2 hours; every 4 hours; every 6 hours; every 8 hours; every 12 hours
QID or qid	Four times a day
Rx	Take
STAT or stat	Immediately
Subling or SL	Sublingual
Sub-Q or subcut	Subcutaneous
SR	Sustained release
TID or tid	Three times a day

Modified from deWit's Fundamental Concepts and Skills for Nursing, ed 6, St. Louis, deWit, 2022.

TABLE 9-2   The Joint Commission "Do Not Use" List of Abbreviations

OFFICIAL "DO NOT USE" LIST[1]

Do Not Use	Potential Problem	Use Instead
U, u (unit)	Mistaken for "0" (zero), the number "4" (four) or "cc"	Write "unit"
IU (International Unit)	Mistaken for IV (intravenous) or the number 10 (ten)	Write "International Unit"
Q.D., QD, q.d., qd (daily)	Mistaken for each other	Write "daily"
Q.O.D., QOD, q.o.d, qod (every other day)	Period after the Q mistaken for "I" and the "O" mistaken for "I"	Write "every other day"
Trailing zero (X.o mg)*	Decimal point is missed	Write X mg
Lack of leading zero (.X mg)		Write o.X mg
MS	Can mean morphine sulfate or magnesium sulfate	Write "morphine sulfate"
MSO$_4$ and MgSO$_4$	Confused for one another	Write "magnesium sulfate"

[1]Applies to all orders and all medication-related documentation that is handwritten (including free-text computer entry) or on pre-printed forms.
*Exception: A "trailing zero" may be used only where required to demonstrate the level of precision of the value being reported, such as for laboratory results, imaging studies that report size of lesions, or catheter/tube sizes. It may not be used in medication orders or other medication-related documentation.
(From The Joint Commission, 2020. Reprinted with permission.)

BOX 9-1   Weights and Measurements

Household Measurements
1 quart = 4 cups
1 pint = 2 cups
1 cup = 8 ounces
1 teacup = 6 ounces
1 tablespoon = 3 teaspoons
1 teaspoon = approximately 5 mL

Metric System
Units of Length (Meter)
1 millimeter = 0.001 (meaning 1/1000)
1 centimeter = 0.01 (meaning 1/100)
1 decimeter = 0.1 (meaning 1/10)
1 meter = 1 (meter)

Units of Volume (Liter)
1 milliliter = 0.001 (meaning 1/1000)
1 centiliter = 0.01 (meaning 1/100)
1 deciliter = 0.1 (meaning 1/10)
1 liter = 1 (liter)

Units of Weight (Gram)
1 microgram = 0.000001 (meaning 1/1,000,000)
1 milligram = 0.001 (meaning 1/1000)
1 centigram = 0.01 (meaning 1/100)
1 gram = 1 (gram)
1 kilogram (kg) = 1000 grams
1 kilogram = 2.2 pounds (lb)

TABLE 9-3   Examples of Standard Drug Administration Times

Order	Times	Order	Times
Daily; once daily	0900 (9:00 AM)	Every 6 hours	0600 (6:00 AM), 1200 (12:00 PM, noon), 1800 (6:00 PM), and 2400 (12:00 AM; midnight)
Bedtime; nightly, at bedtime	2100 (9:00 PM)	Every 8 hours	0800 (8:00 AM), 1600 (4:00 PM), and 2400 (12:00 AM; midnight)
Twice a day	0900 (9:00 AM) and 1700 (5:00 PM)	Every 12 hours	0900 (9:00 AM) and 2100 (9:00 PM)
Three times a day	0900 (9:00 AM), 1300 (1:00 pm), and 1700 (5:00 PM)	Before meals	0700 (7:00 AM), 1100 (11:00 AM), and 1600 (4:00 PM)
Four times a day	0900 (9:00 AM), 1300 (1:00 PM), 1700 (5:00 PM), and 2100 (9:00 PM)	After meals	0800 (8:00 AM), 1200 (12:00 PM, noon), and 1800 (6:00 PM)

information is entered electronically into the EHR through the use of computers. In time, all medical records will be electronic.

The medical record allows the health team to share necessary information about the person. The record is a permanent legal document. It can be used years later if the person's health history is needed. It can be used as evidence in a court of law of the person's problems, treatment, and care.

The paper record has many forms and the EHR has many sections. The forms and sections are organized for easy use.

Each form includes the person's name, date of birth, room and bed number, along with any other identifying information. This helps prevent errors and improper placement of records. The paper record includes the person's:

- Admission form
- Health history
- Physical examination results
- Doctor's orders
- Doctor's progress notes

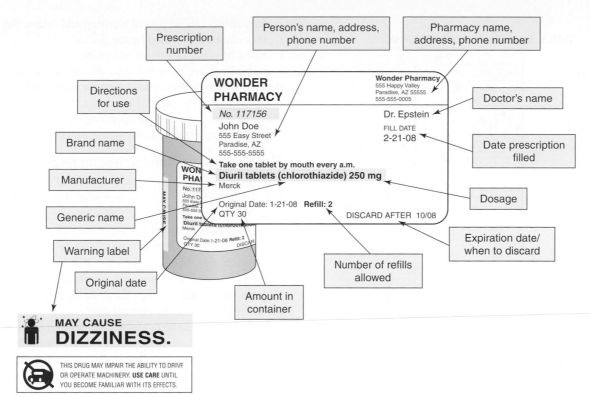

Fig. 9-3 Drug Label.

- Nursing team's and health team's progress notes
- Graphic sheets and flowsheets
- Laboratory and x-ray reports
- Therapy records: IV (intravenous), respiratory, and others
- Consultation reports: specialty doctors, surgery, anesthesia, and others
- Assessments from social services, dietary services, and physical, occupational, speech, and recreational therapies
- Consent forms
- Medication administration record (MAR): Routine, PRN, STAT, and single order drugs

The health team records information on the forms for their departments. Other health team members read the information. It describes the care provided and the person's response.

Agencies have policies about medical records and who can see them. Such policies address:
- Who records
- When to record
- Abbreviations
- How to correct errors
- Ink color
- How to make and sign entries

You have an ethical and legal duty to keep the person's information confidential. You have no right to review the person's chart unless you give medical care to that person (even if they are a friend or family member). To do so is an invasion of privacy. In 1996, the Health Insurance Portability and Accountability Act (HIPAA) was created to protect people's privacy and health information. The rules under HIPAA protect the way patient information is shared with other health care providers and how it is stored. You can only share a person's health information with family members, friends, or other individuals if the person gives their consent. Severe fines may be imposed if patient confidentiality is breached.

Patients have the right to information in their medical records. The person or the person's legal representative may ask to see the chart at any time. Report the request to the nurse; he or she deals with the request.

The following parts of the medical record relate to your work as an MA-C.

The Graphic Sheet

The *graphic sheet* is used to record measurements and observations made every day, every shift, or three to four times a day. Depending on your agency's medical record system, your graphic sheet may be handwritten (Fig. 9-4) or electronic (Fig. 9-5). Information includes vital signs (temperature, pulse, respirations, blood pressure) and may also include the person's weight, intake and output, bowel movements (feces), and doctor's visits.

You may need to check the graphic sheet before giving a drug. For example, it may be necessary for you to check the person's pulse, blood pressure, intake and output, daily weight, or when the person last had a bowel movement.

Progress Notes

Progress notes describe the care given as well as the person's response and progress (Fig. 9-6). Sometimes called *nurses' notes*, the nursing team uses this form to record:
- The person's signs and symptoms
- Information about treatments and drugs
- Information about PRN drugs that have been given

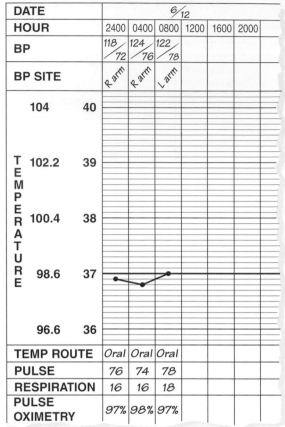

DAILY SUMMARY AND GRAPHIC

DATE			6/12			
HOUR	2400	0400	0800	1200	1600	2000
BP	118/72	124/76	122/78			
BP SITE	R arm	R arm	L arm			

TEMPERATURE							
104	40						
102.2	39						
100.4	38						
98.6	37						
96.6	36						

TEMP ROUTE	Oral	Oral	Oral			
PULSE	76	74	78			
RESPIRATION	16	16	18			
PULSE OXIMETRY	97%	98%	97%			

Fig. 9-4 Graphic sheet. (Courtesy OSF St. Joseph Medical Center, Bloomington, Ill.)

- Information about patient teaching and counseling
- Procedures performed by the doctor
- Visits by other health team members

PRN drugs are recorded right *after* they are given. The date, time, medication, dose, and reason for administering the drug is recorded in the Progress Notes. Later, the patient's response to the drug is also recorded. Depending on the drug, the person's vital signs may be taken and documented before giving the drug.

The Medication Administration Record

The *medication administration record* is called a *MAR*. It can be handwritten (Fig. 9-7A) or electronic (Fig. 9-7B). It is sometimes referred to as an *eMAR*. Some agencies refer to this record as the *medication profile*. The MAR lists all drugs to be given to a person. MARs are kept in a notebook or clipboard file on the medication cart. MARs may be for a shift (8, 10, or 12 hours), for 24 hours, or for as long as 1 month. The eMAR is accessed through the agency's computer or EHR. It usually displays the medications due for the current shift.

The MAR should be organized and written clearly to minimize errors. The drugs are sometimes organized in the following groups:

- *Scheduled medications.* These drugs are scheduled on a regular basis. Daily, every 6 hours, twice a day, and at bedtime are examples of common drug schedules.
- *Parenteral medications. Parenteral* involves piercing the skin or mucous membranes through a needle stick. Injections ("shots") and drugs given intravenously (IV) are in this group.
- *STAT medications.* These drugs are given at once after receiving the order.
- *Preoperative medications.* These drugs are given before surgery.
- *PRN medications.* These drugs are given as needed. They are usually listed at the bottom of the MAR or on a separate page.

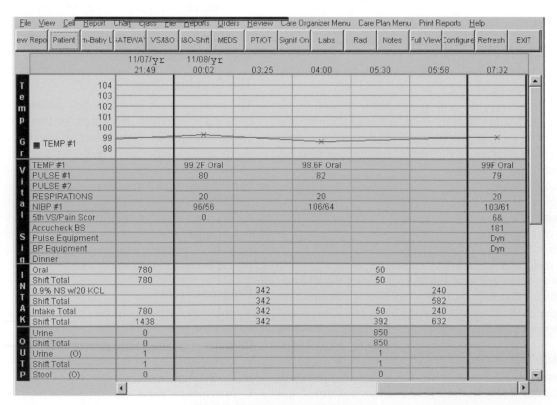

Fig. 9-5 Electronic graphic sheet.

Date	Time	Nursing Margin / Other Depts Margin
3-19	1700	Out with family for dinner. Jane Doe, LPN
3-19	1930	Returned from outing accompanied by her son. States she had a pleasant time. Mary Smith, CNA
3-20	0900	In bed. Complains of headache. T 98.4 orally, radial pulse 72 and regular, respirations 18 and unlabored. BP 134/84 left arm lying down. Alice Jones, RN Notified of resident complaint and vital signs. Ann Adams, CNA
3-20	0910	In bed resting. States she has had a headache for about 1/2 hour. Denies nausea and dizziness. No other complaints. PRN Tylenol given. Instructed resident to use call light if headache worsens or other symptoms occur. Alice Jones, RN
3-20	0945	Resting quietly. Denies headache at this time. T 98.4 orally, radial pulse 70 and regular, respirations 18 and unlabored. BP 132/84 left arm lying down. Alice Jones, RN

Fig. 9-6 Progress notes. Note that other members of the health team also can record on this form.

Write your initials, your signature, and job title in the space provided (Fig. 9-7A). Some agencies use a PRN or unscheduled MAR (Fig. 9-8). The following information is recorded on the PRN MAR after giving the drug:

- Date and time
- Drug given
- Dose given
- Drug administration route
- Your initials and signature

Agencies with an EHR may use a bar code medication administration system. The patient is issued a bracelet with a bar code on it. Each drug is packaged individually, and each package contains a bar code. The patient's bar code as well as each individual drug are scanned before the drug is given. In some systems, you may also need to scan the bar code on your identification badge. The system then documents that you have given this drug to the patient.

See Promoting Safety and Comfort: The Medication Administration Record.

MARTINDALE HOMETOWN HOSPITAL

MEDICATION ADMINISTRATION RECORD

NAME: Joseph Lorenzo RM-BD: 621-2
ID NO. 016-28-3978 AGE: 62
DIAGNOSIS Myocardial Infarction SEX: M
PHYSICIAN M. Martin, M.D. Ht: 6' Wt: 200 lbs

Init	Signature	Title

DATES:	MEDICATION—STRENGTH—FORM—ROUTE	0701-1500	1501-2300	2301-0700
	SCHEDULED MEDICATIONS			
1/25	RANITIDINE ZANTAC 150 MG TABLET ORAL TWICE A DAY	0900	1700	
1/25	DILTIAZEM HYDROCHLORIDE CARDIZEM 90 MG TABLET ORAL 4 TIMES DAILY-HOLD FOR HR LESS THAN 60	0900 1300	1700 2100	
1/25	WARFARIN SODIUM COUMADIN 1 MG TABLET ORAL EVERY OTHER DAY	NOT GIVEN	TODAY	
	IV AND PIGGYBACK ORDERS			
1/25	CEFTAZIDIME (FORTAZ) 1 G IVPB SODIUM CHLORIDE 0.9% 50 ML EVERY 8 HOURS RATE: 100 ML/HR	0800	1600	2400
1/25	GENTAMICIN PREMIX 80 MG IVPB SODIUM CHLORIDE 0.9% 100 ML EVERY 12 HOURS RATE: 100 ML/HR	0900	2100	
1/25	BY IV PUMP 1 IV D5 0.9% NACL 1000 ML RATE: 100 ML/HR			
	PRN MEDICATIONS			
1/25	ACETAMINOPHEN TYLENOL 650 MG TABLET ORAL EVERY 4 HOURS AS NEEDED PRN TEMP > 101°F			
1/25	MAGNESIUM HYDROXIDE MILK OF MAGNESIA 60 ML (CONC) ORAL CONC AS NEEDED PRN CONSTIPATION			
1/25	ALBUTEROL PROVENTIL INHALER 90 MCG/INH AEROSOL INH 2 PUFFS AS NEEDED PRN SHORTNESS OF BREATH SEE RESPIRATORY THERAPY NOTES			

Age/Sex	HT	WT	Date	ALLERGIES CODEINE
62/ M	6'0"	200 lbs	1/25	
Room-Bd	Name			
621 2	Joseph Lorenzo			

A

Fig. 9-7 Medication administration records. **A,** A computer-generated MAR. Recordings are handwritten.

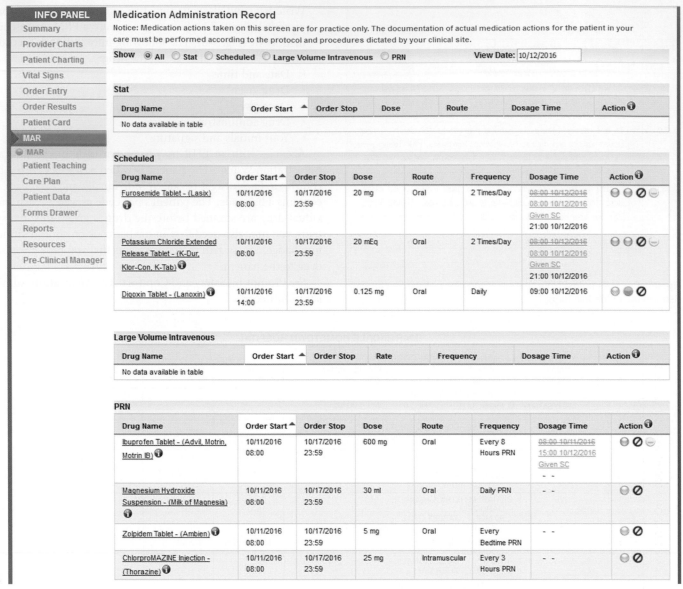

B

Fig. 9-7, cont'd **B,** A computer generated MAR. Recordings are computerized. (Williams: deWit's Fundamental Concepts and Skills for Nursing, ed 6, St. Louis, Elsevier, 2022.).

C

MEDICATION ADMINISTRATION RECORD

Nursing Home Name _____

Mo. _____ Yr. _____

PHARMACY PROVIDER		INIT. = GIVEN R = REFUSED V = VOMITED H = HELD O = HOME	INIT.	SIGNATURE	INIT.	SIGNATURE	INIT.	SIGNATURE	INIT.	SIGNATURE

RX#—DATE ORDERED MEDICATION—DOSE—ROUTE	TIME	1	2	3	4	5	6	7	8	9	10	11	12	13	14	15	16	17	18	19	20	21	22	23	24	25	26	27	28	29	30	31

ALLERGIES

DIAGNOSIS

LAST NAME	FIRST	INIT.	LEVEL OF CARE	ROOM-BED	SEX	BIRTHDATE	DIET	IDENTIFICATION #	PHYSICIAN

DATE OF MED. REVIEW _____

REVIEWED BY _____ (RPh)

_____ (RN)

Fig. 9-7, cont'd C, An MAR used in a nursing center.

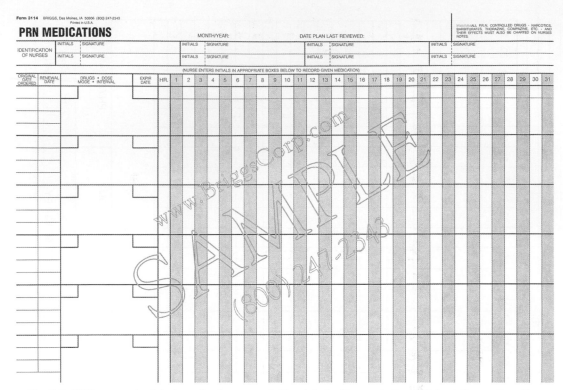

Fig. 9-8 PRN or unscheduled medication record. (Reprinted with permission of Briggs Corporation, Des Moines, Iowa, [800] 247-2343.)

PROMOTING SAFETY AND COMFORT

The Medication Administration Record

Safety

The MAR includes a place to note the person's allergies (see Fig. 9-7. A and C). Before giving a drug, always compare it to the allergies listed. Tell the nurse at once if the person is allergic to a drug ordered. If unsure, check with the nurse before giving the drug.

Medication Records in Assisted Living Residences. People living in assisted living residences manage and take their own drugs if able. Some residents need help. A medication record is kept for each person needing help with drugs. The record includes:

- The person's name
- Drug name, dose, directions, and route of administration
- Designated date and time to take the drug
- Date and time help was given
- Signature or initials of the person assisting

The Kardex

The *Kardex* is a type of card file. It summarizes information found in the medical record—drugs, treatments, diagnoses, routine care measures, equipment, and special needs. The Kardex is a quick, easy source of information about the person (Fig. 9-9).

Often completed in pencil, it is updated regularly. Old information or orders are erased and new ones are added. Keep in mind that the Kardex is not a formal, legal part of the medical record and is destroyed when the person is discharged from the agency.

In an EHR, a Dashboard or Patient Summary tab typically contains the information found on a Kardex. The nurse updates this information within the computer system.

THE NURSE'S ROLE

A nurse verifies and transcribes the drug order. To *transcribe* means *to copy*. To *verify* an order means to make sure the drug order is safe for the person taking it. The nurse makes professional judgments regarding:

- The type of drug
- The drug's therapeutic intent
- The usual dosage of the drug
- The person's ability to tolerate the dosage form ordered
- If the person has any known allergies to the drug

The nurse decides if the drug is safe to give. If the drug order is deemed safe, the nurse sends the drug order to the pharmacy. If it is not deemed safe, the prescriber is contacted and the nurse explains why the nursing team cannot give the drug. In this scenario, the prescriber will usually rewrite the order. If not, the nurse follows agency policy for refusing to administer a drug.

After verifying the order, it is transcribed. Transcribing is necessary to put the order into action. The transcription process involves:

- Copying the order onto the Kardex and medication profile or entering it into the computer. This may be done by the nurse or unit secretary. In some states and agencies, you may be allowed to transcribe orders.
- Signing the order. Some agencies call this *noting the order* or *acknowledging the order*. The nurse reviews the transcription to make sure it is correct. Then the nurse signs, dates, and times the transcription on the original order. This means that the order has been received and verified.
- Sending the order to the pharmacy following agency policy. This involves sending a hard copy or duplicate copy of the physician's order form to the pharmacy. If the agency uses an

DIET	NOURISHMENT/SPECIAL FEEDING	INTAKE/OUTPUT
Regular	Health shake at Bedtime	Encourage/Restrict Fluids 2000 mL/24 Hr.
Hold:		7-3 1000 3-11 800 11-7 200

FUNCTIONAL STATUS

	SELF	ASSIST	TOTAL	OTHER	SPECIFY
Feeding		X			
Bathing		X			
Toileting		X			
Oral Care		X			
Positioning	X				
Transferring	X				
Wheeling					
Walking	X				

ACTIVITIES
Bedrest & BRP ____
Bedside Commode ____
Up ad Lib X
Chair ____
Ambulatory X
Ambulate & Assist ____
Turn ____
Dangle ____
Mode of Travel ____

ELIMINATION
Bladder - Cont. (Incont)
Catheter ____
Date Changed ____
Irrigations ____
Bowel - Cont./Incont.
Ostomy ____
Irrigations ____

VITALS
Temp. qid
Pulse qid
Resp. qid
BP qid
Weight daily
Other: Pulse OX daily

COMMUNICATION DEFICITS ☐ None
Hearing Hard-of-hearing
Vision Impaired
Speech
Language Impaired

PROSTHESIS ☐ None
Glasses X Dentures X
Contacts ____ Limb ____
Hearing Aid L ear

SPECIAL CONDITIONS (Paralysis, Pressure Ulcers, Etc.)

SAFETY/SUPPORTIVE MEASURES
Bed rails: ☐ Nights Only ☐ Constant ☐ No Need
Restraints: ☐ PRN ☐ Constant
Support Devices: ☐ PRN ☐ Constant

RESPIRATORY THERAPY
Aerosol
IPPB
Ultrasonic
Rx Med ____

OXYGEN
2 Liter/Minute
X PRN ☐ Constant
Tent ____ Catheter
Mask X Cannula

SPECIAL EQUIPMENT/PROCEDURES/ANCILLARY SERVICES/ETC.
Speech therapy 3 times/wk.

DATE	TREATMENTS/MISCELLANEOUS

ORDERED	SCHEDULED	COMPLETED	X-RAY AND SPECIAL DIAGNOSTIC EXAMS
10-20	10-20	10-20	Chest x-ray

START DATE	SCHEDULED MEDICATIONS	STOP DATE	RENEW	START DATE	STOP OR RENEW	SITE	IV FLUID & RATE	TUBING	DRESS.	SITE
10-19	Lasix 40 mg PO daily									
10-19	Lanoxin 0.25 mg PO daily									

DATE	ONE TIME ORDERS

DATE	DAILY/REPEATING ORDERS
10-20	Serum potassium daily

DATE	TIME	PRN MEDICATIONS
10-19	2100	Ativan 0.25 mg PO q4h PRN anxiety

MISCELLANEOUS

ALLERGIES: X None Known

NURSING ALERTS:

EMERGENCY CONTACT:
Name: Parker, Marie Telephone No. Home: 555-1212
Relationship: Wife Bus:

ROOM	NAME	PHYSICIAN	ADMITTING DIAGNOSIS/PROBLEM	HOSP. NO.
310	Parker, Edwin	Dr. S Epstein	1. CHF 2. Dementia	1035B

Fig. 9-9 A sample Kardex. (Reprinted with permission of Briggs Corporation, Des Moines, Iowa [800] 247-2343.)

BOX 9-2   Guidelines for Transcribing

General Rules

- Make sure your state and agency allow you to transcribe drug orders.
- Make sure you have received the necessary education and training to transcribe drug orders.
- Make sure that a nurse reviews and completes the transcription process.
- Follow agency policy whenever transcribing. Remember that agency policies may vary from the rules listed in this box.
- Make sure the form includes the person's identifying information.
- Make sure the form includes the person's current diagnoses.
- Make sure the form lists any known allergies.
- Follow the rules for reporting and recording. (See Chapter 4.)
- Use only the abbreviations allowed in your agency. Tell the nurse if an abbreviation on the "Do Not Use" list is used.
- Use only the standard drug administration times approved for use in your agency.
- Immediately tell the nurse of any STAT order.
- Use the ink color required by your agency. Never use pencil on a doctor's order form or MAR.
- Write clearly and neatly. Your writing must be legible.
- Ask a nurse to clarify if you cannot read or are not sure of something on the order.
- Place a check-mark next to each order transcribed. Do this *after* transcribing each order; the checkmark shows that the order was transcribed.
- Write "noted" or "acknowledged," and sign, date, and time the doctor's order form after transcribing all orders. This tells the nurse that:
  - You have transcribed all orders.
  - The orders are ready for the nurse to review and sign. After checking for accuracy, the nurse will write "verified" and sign, date, and time when this was done.
- When using EHRs, the provider enters orders in the computer. Drug orders are automatically sent to the pharmacy and the drugs are put on the electronic MAR. The nurse must still verify and note or acknowledge each order.

Adding a New Drug

- Transfer the following information from the drug order to the MAR:
  - The name of the drug. Some agencies require both the brand and generic names.
  - The strength of the drug. This is the amount of drug in each tablet or capsule.
  - The dose and amount of the drug to give.

- How to give the drug (which route to use).
- What time(s) to give the drug or how many times a day to give the drug.
- When the order was written.
- When to start the drug (if written). This is usually the day the drug was ordered.
- When to stop the drug (if written).
- Special instructions or precautions. For example: "Hold if apical pulse is less than 60 per minute."
- Note the times to give the drug. Use the agency's standard set of times (p. 94). For example, if a drug is ordered four times a day, an agency may give drugs ordered at 0900 (9:00 am), 1300 (1:00 pm), 1700 (5:00 pm), and 2100 (9:00 pm).
- Put an X through every date and time not included in the order.

Discontinuing a Drug

- Draw a diagonal or straight line through the drug order and all dates affected on the MAR.
- Write "discontinued" and the date above or next to the diagonal or straight line.
- Sign your name next to or under "discontinued" and the date.
- Use a highlighter to mark out the line and the dates affected according to agency policy.
- Drugs discontinued in the EHR are marked as discontinued on the MAR. Typically, the dates and times are greyed out on the MAR.

Changing an Order

- Discontinue the current order.
- Transcribe the new order on a new line or in a new box on the MAR.
- Put an X through every date and time not included in the order.
- When a drug order is changed in the EHR, the drug is marked as discontinued and the remaining dates and times are greyed out. A new entry appears on the MAR that includes the prescribed changes.

Stat or "One-Time Only" Orders

- Transfer all information from the drug order to the MAR.
- Put an X through every date and time not included in the order.
- When STAT or "One-Time Only" orders are entered in the EHR, the date and time indicated on the MAR matches the date and time the provider entered the order. Once the drug is given, it is marked as discontinued on the MAR.

EHR, the order is sent by computer. Nursing centers will fax or email the order to a local pharmacy.

Assisting With Transcription

Some states and agencies may allow you to transcribe drug orders from the doctor's order form to the Kardex and MAR or computer. *Accuracy* is a must. When transcribing, follow the guidelines in Box 9-2. Also follow agency policies and procedures. The nurse is still responsible for verifying all aspects of the drug order.

▉ REVIEW QUESTIONS

Circle the BEST answer.

1. Drug orders written on a prescription pad are usually filled:
   a. on the nursing unit
   b. in the hospital pharmacy
   c. at a local pharmacy
   d. at the doctor's office
2. A STAT drug order is to be given:
   a. at once
   b. as needed
   c. at a certain time
   d. at bedtime

3. A PRN order means that a drug is given:
   a. at once
   b. as needed
   c. at a certain time
   d. at bedtime
4. A routine drug order is given:
   a. at once
   b. as needed
   c. as prescribed until it is cancelled
   d. at bedtime

5. The electronic health record is:
   a. an electronic version of a person's medical record
   b. the list of PRN medication
   c. sent home with the person at discharge
   d. only seen by the pharmacist

6. A healthcare provider enters a drug order into the computer. What ordering method is this?
   a. written order
   b. telephone order
   c. faxed order
   d. Computerized Physician (or Provider) Order Entry (CPOE)

7. In the evening, the clock shows 4:25. In military time (or the 24-hour clock), this time is:
   a. 0425
   b. 4:25 PM
   c. 1625
   d. 1425

8. A drug order states to administer the drug if the person has not had a bowel movement for 3 days. Where will you find information about the drug order?
   a. the Kardex
   b. the graphic sheet
   c. the progress notes
   d. the care plan

9. You gave a PRN drug as directed by the nurse. Besides the MAR, where should you record giving the drug?
   a. the Kardex
   b. the graphic sheet
   c. the progress notes
   d. the care plan

10. Where do you record giving a drug?
    a. the Kardex
    b. the MAR
    c. the graphic sheet
    d. a flow sheet

11. When do you record giving a drug?
    a. before giving the drug
    b. after giving the drug
    c. at the end of your shift
    d. when you have time

12. Before giving a drug, you must:
    a. check the person's allergies
    b. take the person's pulse
    c. measure the person's blood pressure
    d. check the care plan

13. When is a copy of the order sent to the pharmacy?
    a. as soon as it is written
    b. after it is transcribed
    c. at the end of the shift
    d. at the time noted by the doctor

14. A drug order contains an abbreviation on the agency's "Do Not Use" list. What should you do?
    a. Transcribe the order as written.
    b. Tell the nurse.
    c. Call the pharmacist.
    d. Call the doctor.

15. You are not sure of something on a drug order. What should you do?
    a. Transcribe the order as written.
    b. Tell the nurse.
    c. Call the pharmacist.
    d. Call the doctor.

16. After transcribing a drug order, you should do all of the following, *except*:
    a. place a check mark by the order
    b. write "noted" or "acknowledged" on the order
    c. sign, date, and time the order
    d. give the drug

17. A drug is to be given daily. What time should you include on the MAR?
    a. 0900
    b. the agency's standard time for a drug given daily
    c. the time the drug was ordered
    d. the time preferred by the person

18. A drug order was changed from daily to twice a day. When transcribing the new order to the MAR, you should do all of the following, *except*:
    a. erase the first order
    b. discontinue the first order
    c. put an X through every date and time not included in the order
    d. transcribe the new order on a new line

Circle T if the statement is true. Circle F if the statement is false.

19. T F   Only doctors can order or prescribe drugs.
20. T F   The doctor's order form is a permanent part of the person's medical record.
21. T F   All drug orders must contain the prescriber's signature.
22. T F   All drug orders must include the route of administration.
23. T F   You can accept telephone orders from doctors.
24. T F   You can accept verbal orders from doctors.
25. T F   Verbal orders are reserved for emergencies and are strongly discouraged.
26. T F   According to HIPAA, you can discuss the person's drug orders with anyone in the agency.
27. T F   The Kardex is a permanent part of the person's medical record.
28. T F   You can verify drug orders.
29. T F   You can use a pencil to transcribe a drug order to the MAR.
30. T F   A healthcare provider orders a drug using CPOE. The computerized system communicates the drug order to the pharmacy.

Answers to these questions can be found on the Evolve Resources site: http://evolve.elsevier.com/Anderson/medasst/

10

Medication Safety

OBJECTIVES

- Define the key terms and key abbreviations used in this chapter.
- Describe four different drug distribution systems.
- Describe the Bar Code Medication Administration system.
- Explain how controlled substances are distributed.
- Explain how to dispose of an unused portion of a controlled substance.
- Describe the narcotics count process.
- Explain how to safely store drugs.
- List the reasons for disposing of drugs.
- Explain how to dispose of drugs.
- Explain the Six Rights of Drug Administration.
- Explain your role in self-directed medication management.
- Identify common drug errors.
- Describe the rules for administering drugs safely.

KEY TERMS

dose The amount of drug to give
drug diversion Taking a person's drugs for your own use
medication reminder Reminding the person to take drugs, observing them being taken as prescribed, and charting that they were taken

route How and where the drug enters the body

KEY ABBREVIATIONS

ADE adverse drug event
ADM automated dispensing machine
ALR assisted living residence
BCMA Bar Code Medication Administration
EHR electronic health record
FDA Food and Drug Administration
ID identification
IM intramuscular

ISMP Institute for Safe Medication Practices
IV intravenous
MAR medication administration record
mg milligram
NDC National Drug Code
PRN when necessary; as needed
STAT at once; immediately
subcut subcutaneous; subcutaneously

Medication safety is freedom from preventable harm from drugs. It also involves the correct dispensing of the drug, correct storage, and correct disposal. Preventing drug errors must be a top priority. To prevent drug errors and give drugs safely, you must follow the *Six Rights of Drug Administration*. The *right* person must receive the *right* drug at the *right* time in the *right* dose using the *right* route. *Right* documentation follows immediately after giving a drug.

DRUG DISTRIBUTION SYSTEMS

The pharmacy processes and fills drug orders. Then they are distributed (dispensed) to the nursing unit. Each agency has its own drug distribution system. The following systems are common.

See *Promoting Safety and Comfort: Drug Distribution Systems.*

Floor or Ward Stock System

With the *floor* or *ward stock system*, frequently used drugs are kept on the nursing unit in stock containers (Fig. 10-1). Dangerous and rarely used drugs are kept in the pharmacy. Small hospitals and some nursing centers may use this system. Some government hospitals may use this system if drugs are not charged directly to the patient.

Ordered drugs are readily available using this system. There is no waiting or lag time for the pharmacy to process, fill, and send the drug order to the nursing unit. There are several safety issues to keep in mind:

- Many drugs are stocked on the nursing unit, which increases the risk for drug errors. You must be careful to select the right drug and the right dose from all the drugs stocked.
- Monitoring drug expiration dates can be difficult. Over time, the chemical nature of a drug can change. In other words, the drug deteriorates. A once helpful drug can turn harmful.

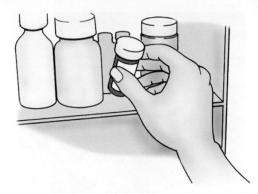

Fig. 10-1 Floor or ward stock system. (From Edmunds MW: *Introduction to clinical pharmacology,* ed 5, St Louis, 2006, Mosby.)

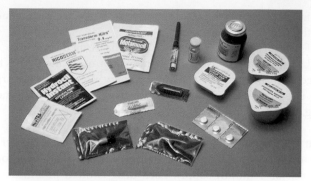

Fig. 10-2 Unit dose packages.

- The nursing unit may not have enough space to store all drugs safely.
- Agency personnel have access to many drugs; drug diversion is a risk.

Individual Prescription Order System

The *individual prescription order system* also involves storing drugs in the nursing unit. For a patient or resident, the pharmacy sends a 3- to 5-day supply of an ordered drug to the nursing unit. The drugs are stored in small bins in a cabinet in the nursing unit. Each person has a bin. Bins are arranged alphabetically by the person's last name. Some agencies may arrange the bins by room and bed numbers.

This system is safer than the floor or ward stock system because:

- A pharmacist and a nurse review the order before the drug is given.
- The pharmacy monitors drug expiration dates. This lessens the danger of drug deterioration.
- Fewer drugs are available for possible drug diversion.

Like the floor or ward stock system, drugs are available for STAT or PRN use. While fewer drugs are available, drug diversion remains a risk.

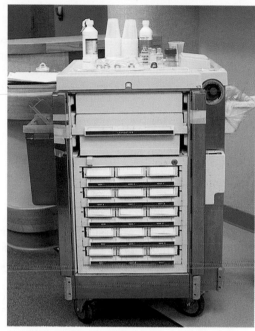

Fig. 10-3 Unit dose cart. Each drawer is labeled with a person's name and room and bed number.

PROMOTING SAFETY AND COMFORT

Drug Distribution Systems

Safety

Always check drugs received from the pharmacy. Compare the pharmacy label against the drug order on the medication administration record (MAR) and check that the number of doses is correct. If the number of doses is not correct, tell the nurse before continuing. It is possible that:

- The drug was discontinued.
- Another staff member gave the drug.
- The pharmacy omitted a dose.
- The drug was given to the wrong person.
- The drug was diverted by a staff member. **Drug diversion** is taking a person's drugs for your own use. This is illegal.

Follow agency policy for reporting a drug error (p. 113).

Unit Dose System

With the *unit dose system,* a single-unit dose package of a drug is dispensed for each dose ordered (Fig. 10-2). Placed in a packet, each packet is labeled according to agency policy. A 24-hour supply is provided in hospitals. For example, a person receives a drug four times a day. Four doses are included in the packet. The pharmacist refills the drawers every 24 hours.

A drawer in a drug cart is labeled with the person's name and room and bed number (Fig. 10-3). The cart is kept at the nurses' station and is wheeled to each person's room to give the drugs. In some institutions, individualized drawers or envelopes containing drugs are locked in a cabinet in the patient's room.

The unit dose system is very common. It is safe and cost and time efficient:

- The nursing team spends less time preparing to administer drugs.
- The pharmacy has a list of all drugs ordered for a person. The pharmacist can check for drug interactions and/or contraindications.
- The pharmacist determines the correct dosage. For example, 100 mg (milligrams) of a drug is ordered and the drug is supplied in 50 mg tablets. Therefore, the pharmacist determines that two tablets are needed.

• Every dose must be accounted for on the MAR. This reduces the risk of drug diversion.
• Fewer drugs are available for potential drug diversion.

Unit dose carts have compartments for medicine bottles too large to fit in the person's drawer. There also are storage areas for supplies (e.g., medicine cups, drinking cups, and straws [Fig. 10-4].

The Unit Dose System in Nursing Centers. Each drawer in the drug cart is large enough to hold drug containers for a 1-week or 1-month supply. Each drug is often provided in a bubble pack. In long-term care facilities, these drawers are usually exchanged on a 3- or 7-day schedule. Each drawer is labeled with the person's name, room and bed number, pharmacy name and phone number, and the facility's name.

The pharmacist fills a container with the prescribed drug. Each container has sections for each day of the week, and each section contains the number of doses for that day.

Some systems have color codes for different times of day. For example:

• Purple—0600 (6:00 AM)
• Pink—0800 (8:00 AM)
• Yellow—1200 (12:00 PM; noon)
• Green—1400 (2:00 PM) or 1600 (4:00 PM)
• Orange—early evening
• Red—PRN

With a color coding system, you can remove the drug containers for a certain time of day. For example, if a person receives four drugs at 0800, you can remove the four pink containers for 0800.

Computer-Controlled Dispensing System

A common system for ordering and administering medication is a *computer-controlled dispensing system* (Fig. 10-5). Also

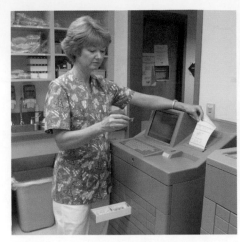

Fig. 10-5 MA-C obtaining medication from an automated dispensing unit.

known as an automated dispensing machine (ADM), these systems are typically kept in a locked medication room. ADMs commonly seen are the Pyxis, Omnicell, and Cerner systems. They use the unit-dose system. Unit-dose packets are supplied and stocked daily in the ADM by the pharmacy. Use your security code and password to access the system. In some agencies, you may use a thumbprint or fingerprint. When you select your patient's name, their medication profile is displayed and the drugs ordered for that person are listed. You select the drugs scheduled at that time from the machine. The drugs are then dispensed; they are opened and administered at the person's bedside. This method decreases the chances of medication errors and increases patient safety.

Bar Code Medication Administration (BCMA)

In 2004, the Food and Drug Administration (FDA) issued a rule titled *Bar Code Label Requirements for Human Drug Products and Biological Products.* The rule is intended to improve safety by reducing drug errors. This FDA rule requires bar codes to be present on most prescription drugs and on over-the-counter drugs commonly used in hospitals. The bar codes must contain the drug's National Drug Code (NDC). Bar Code Medication Administration (BCMA) systems are electronic scanning systems that can catch a drug error before the drug is given. BCMA is usually linked with the eMAR, which makes documentation quick and easy. It automatically documents a drug is given in the electronic health record (EHR).

Bar Code Medication Administration (BCMA) works as follows:

• You receive a bar-coded identification (ID) bracelet when admitted to the agency. The bar code on the ID bracelet is linked to your EHR.
• The agency has bar code scanners (bar code readers) linked to the computer system.
• Log onto the system and bring up the person's computerized medical record.
• Drug orders appear on the screen; you select the drugs to be given at that time. A section of the cart opens for you to remove the person's drugs from the cart.

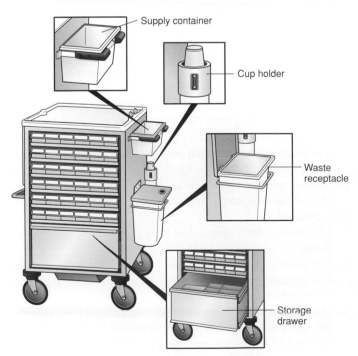

Supply container

Cup holder

Waste receptacle

Storage drawer

Fig. 10-4 Storage areas on a unit dose drug cart.

At the bedside, use a handheld bar code scanner to read the bar code on your ID badge, the person's ID bracelet, and the unit-dose packet. All information is linked to the person's database.

- *If there is an error*—An alarm sounds, or an error message appears. Error examples include the wrong drug, wrong dose, wrong time, or wrong person. If none of these errors apply, the person's drug orders may have changed.
- *If the process is correct*—There is automatic documentation in the person's MAR once you "file" or "save" your entry.

Computer-controlled systems are safe and time efficient. However, the systems can be costly.

Narcotic Control Systems

As explained in Chapter 3, federal laws regulate the use of controlled substances. These laws are strictly enforced.

In hospitals and nursing centers, controlled substances are dispensed in single-unit packages. The packages are stored in a locked cabinet in the medicine room or in a locked drawer in the drug cart. If a computer-controlled dispensing system is not used, the nurse manager or charge nurse is responsible for the key to the medicine cabinet or drawer. The key is commonly called the "narcotics key." The cabinet or drawer is then locked, and the key returned to the nurse once the dose has been obtained and the paperwork is complete. Never leave the key in the lock.

An inventory control sheet lists each type of controlled substance and the number of doses issued (Fig. 10-6). The nurse receiving the drug supply will:

- Count and verify the number and types of drugs received
- Sign a form indicating that the count is accurate
- Lock the controlled substances in a designated cabinet or drug cart drawer

The inventory control sheet is used to account for each drug and dose given. When a drug is removed from the locked storage area to give to a patient or resident, the following are documented on the inventory control sheet:

- The time
- The person's name
- The drug
- The dose
- The signature of the nurse or MA-C removing the drug

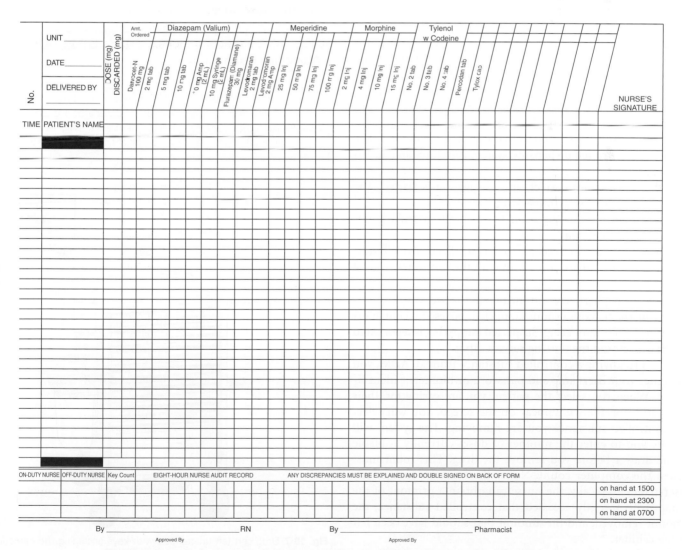

Fig. 10-6 Controlled substances inventory control sheet. (Courtesy The Nebraska Medical Center.)

Sometimes the prescribed dose is smaller than that supplied. Disposal procedures are followed for the unused portion. When a nurse gives the drug, another nurse must check:

- The dose
- How the drug is prepared
- Disposal of the unused portion

Both nurses then sign the inventory control sheet. If you are giving the drug, a nurse checks the drug. You and the nurse then sign the inventory control sheet.

With computer-controlled dispensing systems, all controlled drugs are kept in the automated dispensing machine. The system provides a detailed record of:

- The drug dispensed
- The date and time the drug was dispensed
- Who accessed the drug

If the entire dose was not used, a nurse must witness one of the following:

- The disposal of the portion not used
- The return of the portion not used to the automated dispensing machine

The inventory control sheet is a legal document. Follow the rules for recording (Chapter 4).

Narcotics Count. Controlled substances are inventoried at the end of each shift. A nurse from the incoming shift counts the drugs with a nurse going off-duty. Each container and remaining doses are counted. For each drug, the number remaining is added to the number used. The total should equal the number issued by the pharmacy. For example, if the pharmacy issues 10 doses of a drug and 4 were used during the shift, 6 should remain in the container. The computer-controlled dispensing system generates an end-of-shift report.

If the count is not correct, an investigation is started. The nurse manager or charge nurse will:

- Check with the nursing team to see if all controlled substances were charted
- Check all medical records to see if all controlled substances recorded are consistent with the inventory control sheet
- Contact the pharmacy and the nursing service office

During the narcotics count, unopened boxes and containers are inspected for tampering. Suspected tampering is reported to the pharmacy and the nursing service office.

When removing a controlled substance from an ADM, you will enter your username and password or biometric identification. When you select the patient you are caring for, their medication profile will appear on the screen. You will select the controlled substance you are removing. The system will require you to enter the number of doses currently available in the drawer before you remove the drug. This count must match the computer count. Notify the nurse at once of any discrepancy. Typically, the nurse can obtain a printout of the nurses who recently accessed that controlled substance, the amount removed, and the amount that should have been left in the cabinet.

See *Promoting Safety and Comfort: Narcotics Count.*

STORING DRUGS

All drugs must be safely stored. If the nursing unit has a medicine room, only authorized staff may enter the room. The room is locked when not in use.

Drug carts are locked when not in use. If you need to leave the drug cart to go into a person's room, lock the cart first. Always keep the keys with you; do not leave keys in the lock or on the cart (Fig. 10-7).

Follow these rules to properly store drugs:

- Open only one bin or drawer at a time. This prevents you from mistakenly taking the wrong drugs or putting drugs back in the wrong bin or drawer.
- When removing drugs from an ADM, prepare drugs for only one person at a time.
- Once you have administered those drugs, return to the ADM and remove drugs for the next person.
- Store drugs in their original containers or unit dose packets.
- Store drugs as noted on the label or unit dose packet. Some drugs are stored in a refrigerator, which is to be used for drugs only; not food or fluids.
- Keep drug containers closed tightly. Moisture and heat may destroy some drugs.

Narcotics Count

Safety

Before removing a controlled substance to prepare for a person, count the remaining doses, then add that number to the number used. The total should equal the number issued by the pharmacy. If a dose is missing, tell the nurse at once. Finding the problem early saves a lot of time at the end of the shift when the narcotics count is done.

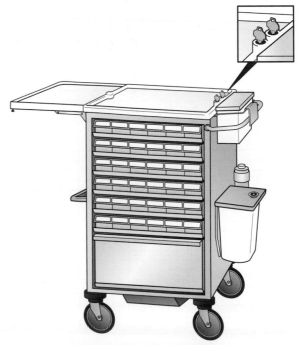

Fig. 10-7 Drug cart left unattended with keys (including the narcotics key) in the lock. This is a very unsafe practice.

Assisted Living Residences

Many residents use drug organizers in assisted living residences (ALRs) (Chapter 8). These organizers include sections for days and times. Some may be for a week, while others may be for a month. This helps to ensure that the person takes the right drugs on the right day at the right time.

Drugs are always kept in a secure location. This prevents unauthorized persons from taking them. If the ALR stores the drugs, they are kept in a locked container, cabinet, or area.

Some persons may manage and store their own drugs. If a resident's room is shared, each person's ability to safely have drugs is assessed. If safety is a factor, drugs are kept in a locked container.

Drug containers must include the original pharmacy label and be stored as directed on the label. For example, some drugs are refrigerated, and others are kept away from light. The label also displays an expiration date. To dispose of expired or discontinued drugs, follow the ALR's procedures.

DISPOSING OF DRUGS

Drugs are disposed of for many reasons. They include:
- A person refuses to take a drug after it is ready to be given.
- A drug is dropped on the floor or bed.
- You are to give only part of a drug dispensed.
- The drug's expiration date has passed.
- A drug became contaminated.
- The person was discharged.
- The person died.
- The doctor discontinued the drug.

To dispose of a drug, follow agency policy. Do not return an unused dose or an unused portion to a stock supply bottle. Do not flush prescription drugs down the toilet unless specifically instructed to do so by the manufacturer. Always follow agency policy recording drug disposal.

See *Promoting Safety and Comfort: Disposing of Drugs.*

PROMOTING SAFETY AND COMFORT
Disposing of Drugs

Safety
Drug diversion is a crime. To protect yourself from being suspected or accused of drug diversion, have someone observe you dispose of a drug every time you do so. When recording, include the full name and title of the person who witnessed the disposal. A computer-controlled dispensing system requires the witness to enter their username and password into the system. This process proves that another nurse witnessed you properly disposing of the drug.

THE SIX RIGHTS

When giving drugs, always protect the person's safety. This involves the *Six Rights of Drug Administration:*
- Right person
- Right drug
- Right dose
- Right time
- Right route
- Right documentation

Right Person

To make sure you have the right person, compare the information on the MAR against the person's ID bracelet. Do not only check the person's name; some people may have the same name or similar names. For example, John Smith is a very common name. A similar name is Jon Smith. When identifying the person, also check for drug allergies. The person wears another bracelet to signify drug allergies.

The Joint Commission requires using at least two identifiers. An identifier cannot be the person's room or bed number. Some agencies require that the person state his or her name and birth date. Others require using the person's ID number. Always follow agency policy.

See *Focus on Older Persons: Right Person.*
See *Promoting Safety and Comfort: Right Person.*

FOCUS ON OLDER PERSONS
Right Person

Alert and oriented nursing center residents may choose not to wear ID bracelets. This is noted on the person's care plan. Follow center policy and the care plan to identify the person.

Some nursing centers have photo ID systems (Fig. 10-8). The person's photo is taken on admission, then placed in the person's medical record. If your center uses such a system, learn to use it safely.

PROMOTING SAFETY AND COMFORT
Right Person

Safety
ID bracelets may become damaged from water, spilled food and fluids, and everyday wear and tear. Make sure you can read the information on the ID bracelet. If you cannot, tell the nurse; they can have a new bracelet made for the person.

Identify the person every time you give a drug. Always do so right before administering the drug. Do not identify the person and then leave the room to get the drug or to collect supplies; this could lead to you mistakenly entering the wrong room and giving the drug to the wrong person. The person for whom the drug was intended would not receive it, which may cause harm.

Use at least two identifiers when identifying a person. Have the person state their name and date of birth and compare what is said with their ID bracelet. More than one identifier is necessary because confused, disoriented, drowsy, hard-of-hearing, or distracted persons may answer to any name. You may also compare the name and the person's ID number on the MAR to the person's ID bracelet.

Comfort
Make sure the person's ID bracelet is not too tight. For an ideal fit, you should be able to slide one or two fingers under the bracelet. If it is too tight, tell the nurse.

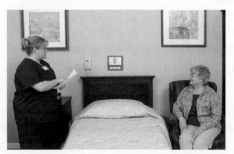

Fig. 10-8 The person's photo is at the headboard. Her name is under the photo. The MA-C is using the photo to identify the person.

Right Drug

Many drugs have similar names and spellings and some drugs have similar-looking packaging. Serious harm or even death may occur if the wrong drug is given.

Do not assume that the pharmacist provided the right drug. Before giving any drug, compare the exact spelling of the prescribed drug and dosage against the MAR. Always read the drug label:

- Before removing the drug from the unit dose cart, ADM, or from the shelf
- Before preparing or measuring the prescribed dose
- Before returning the drug to the shelf or before opening a unit dose packet (open the unit dose right before giving the drug)

Right Dose

You must give the right dose. The **dose** is the amount of drug to give. The person may suffer harm if too much or too little of a drug is given. To give the right dose:

- Compare the dose on the pharmacy label against the MAR
- Use the correct measuring device for drugs in liquid form (e.g., medicine cup or medicine dropper)
- Report nausea and vomiting to the nurse; the nurse will likely instruct you to hold oral drugs

PROMOTING SAFETY AND COMFORT

Calculating Drug Dosages

Safety

If you calculate a drug dosage, always have a nurse check the dose, even for very simple drug calculations. Nurses also have their drug calculations checked by another nurse; safety is the goal.

Also check drug calculations done by a pharmacist or nurse. If you find a mistake, tell the nurse before you give the drug. The nurse will recheck the calculation.

Calculating Drug Dosages. Sometimes the nursing team must calculate a drug dosage. For example, if a drug is supplied in 25 mg tablets and the doctor ordered 50 mg of the drug, a calculation is necessary to determine how many tablets to give.

Some states and agencies do not allow MA-Cs to complete drug calculations. Other states and agencies allow MA-Cs to perform or check simple drug calculations. See Appendix A for a review of arithmetic.

See *Promoting Safety and Comfort: Calculating Drug Dosages.*

Right Time

Many factors are involved in giving a drug at the right time. These factors include the drug order, standard administration times (Chapter 8), blood levels, drug absorption, and diagnostic tests.

- The drug order states how often to give the drug. Standard abbreviations are often used (Chapter 8).
- Each agency has standard drug administration times. Standard times help prevent drug errors and help the nursing and health teams plan care activities. For example, all drugs ordered four times a day are given at 0900, 1300, 1700, and 2100 (9:00 AM, 1:00 PM, 5:00 PM, and 9:00 PM).

- Some drugs are given at specific times. This allows laboratory and diagnostic tests to be completed and the results reported before the drug is given. For example, if a drug affects the time it takes for blood to clot and another dose is given when the blood level is too high, the person is at risk for severe bleeding or hemorrhage. Therefore, the drug is given only if the person's clotting time is within a certain range. Laboratory staff obtain a blood specimen and report the results before the nurse lets you give the drug. Sometimes laboratory or diagnostic tests are done before starting a drug or before continuing drug therapy.
- Some drugs require a consistent blood level to be effective. Such drugs are given on a regular basis (e.g., every 6 hours). If the drug is not given on time, the blood level lowers, and the drug is less effective.
- Drugs must be properly absorbed by the body. Some drugs are absorbed better when the stomach is empty and are therefore given 1 to 2 hours after meals. Drugs that irritate the stomach are given with food. Other drugs may not be given with dairy products or antacids.

See *Promoting Safety and Comfort: Right Time.*

PROMOTING SAFETY AND COMFORT

Right Time

Safety

It is often impossible to give every person drugs at precisely the right time. For example, if 10 people have drugs ordered for 0900, you cannot be with 10 people at exactly 0900. Agency policies usually allow drugs to be given within a certain time range. This range is usually 30 minutes before the scheduled time and 30 minutes after the scheduled time (e.g., if a drug is ordered for 0900, you can give it anytime between 0830 and 0930).

Whenever possible, give drugs on time or as close as possible to the scheduled time. Remember that some drugs must be given at certain times for proper absorption or to maintain a certain blood level. Follow the agency's policy for acceptable drug administration times.

PRN, One-Time-Only, and STAT Orders. Before giving a drug ordered PRN (when necessary; as needed), one-time-only, or STAT (at once; immediately), make sure no one else has administered the drug. These measures are in place to prevent a drug overdose. Check the person's chart and the MAR.

For a PRN order, also make sure that the time between doses has passed. For example, if a drug for pain relief is ordered every 4 hours and only 2 hours have passed since the last dosage, you cannot give the drug. Remember to record PRN drugs at once on both the MAR and the progress notes.

Right Route

The drug order states the route for administration. The **route** is how and where the drug enters the body. Table 10-1 lists the various routes of drug administration.

Not every drug can be given by every route. Never change the route of administration or the dosage form. Only the doctor can make such changes by changing the drug order.

The absorption rate varies with the route used:

- Intravenous (IV)—the drug is given directly into the bloodstream. This route has the most rapid onset of action. It presents the greatest risk for adverse effects.

TABLE 10-1 Routes for Giving Drugs

Route	Name
Mouth	Oral
Skin	Topical
Under the tongue	Sublingual
Between the cheek and molar teeth	Buccal
Eye	Ophthalmic
Ear	Otic
Nose	Nasal
Respiratory tract	Inhalation
Vagina	Vaginal
Stomach	Gastric
Rectum	Rectal
Dermal skin layer	Intradermal
Between the dermis and muscle layer	Subcutaneous
Muscle	Intramuscular
Vein	Intravenous

- Intramuscular (IM)—after the IV route, the IM route provides the next fastest onset of action.
- Subcutaneous (subcut; subcutaneously)—after the IV and IM routes, it provides the next fastest onset of action.
- Intradermal—a small volume of drug is injected into the dermal skin layer. Absorption is slow.

As an MA-C, you can only give drugs by certain routes. You must know what your state and agency allow you to do. A nurse gives the drugs that you are not allowed to give. Remember the following:

- Always give the drug by the route stated on the order, the MAR, and the pharmacy label. Make sure the information from the three sources is the same. If not, check with the nurse.
- Never change the route of administration.
- Never give a drug using a route not allowed by your state and agency. For example, if your state and agency do not allow MA-Cs to give IV drugs, you should never give a drug IV. Likewise, if your state or agency do not allow you to give injections, you should never give drugs through the intramuscular, subcutaneous, and intradermal routes.

See *Promoting Safety and Comfort: Right Route.*

PROMOTING SAFETY AND COMFORT

Right Route

Safety
The oral route is usually safe if the person is conscious and can swallow. It is not safe if the person is unconscious or has *dysphagia* (difficulty swallowing). To safely swallow oral drugs, the person must be awake, alert, sitting upright, able to understand direction, and able to swallow. Tell the nurse at once if the person shows signs of an altered level of consciousness, confusion, disorientation, or swallowing problems. The nurse will give the drug or ask the doctor to change the route ordered.

Right Documentation

You must record the administration of a drug as soon as possible; otherwise, it may be assumed that the drug was not given.

A nurse or another MA-C may give another dose thinking that the drug was not given. An overdose can cause the person serious harm or even death.

When using unit dose and computer charting systems, document on the MAR right after giving the drug. For the "right documentation," follow the rules in Box 10-1.

THE SELF-ADMINISTRATION OF DRUGS

In some agencies and settings, patients and residents take their own drugs. This is called *self-directed medication management.* The person knows his or her drugs by name, color, or shape. The person knows what drugs to take, the correct doses, and when and how to take them. The person is able to question changes in the usual drug routine. For example, if the person comments that a pill is not broken in half or that a pill looks different, report these comments or questions to the nurse.

Your role may involve one or more of the following:
- Reminding the person that it is time to take a drug
- Reading the drug label to the person
- Opening containers for persons who cannot do so themselves
- Checking the dosage against the drug label
- Providing water, juice, milk, crackers, applesauce, or other food and fluids as needed
- Making sure the person takes the right drug, the right dose, at the right time, by the right route
- Charting that the person took or refused to take the drug (right documentation)
- Storing drugs

Many people find that drug organizers are helpful. Some people need medication reminders. A **medication reminder** means reminding the person to take drugs, observing them being taken as prescribed, and then charting that they were taken. Many smartphone apps are available to help people remember to take their medications. You may assist with downloading an app and setting the reminders on the person's smartphone.

BOX 10-1 Rules for "Right Documentation"

- Follow the rules for recording. See Chapter 4.
- Follow agency policy for recording drugs.
- Record as soon as possible after giving the drug.
- Record the following for every drug you give:
  - Date and time you gave the drug
  - The name of the drug
  - The dose
  - The route
  - The site of administration
- Record PRN drugs on the MAR or on the PRN or unscheduled medication record. Also record PRN drugs in the progress notes. See Chapter 8 for instructions on recording PRN drugs.
- Record when and why a drug was not given.
- Record a person's refusal to take a drug and include the reason for the refusal.
- Do not record a drug until after it is taken by the person.
- Follow agency policy for reporting drug errors.

See *Focus on Communication: The Self-Administration of Drugs.*

FOCUS ON COMMUNICATION

The Self-Administration of Drugs

To remind a person to take his or her drugs, you can say:
- "Ms. Epstein, it's time to take your 8 o'clock pills."
- "Mr. Ladd, you'll need to take your pills in about 10 minutes."
- "Mrs. Young, are you ready to take your pills?"

To read a drug label to a person, read the following:
- The name of the person on the drug label
- The name of the drug
- How to take the drug (e.g., by mouth, with food, with a full glass of water, apply to the skin, or rectally)
- The dosage
- When to take the drug (e.g., before meals, with meals, or after meals)
- How often to take the drug
- Warnings and other information on the drug label

PREVENTING DRUG ERRORS

Drug errors can cause the person serious harm or even death. These errors are known as adverse drug events (ADEs). Box 10-2 lists examples of drug errors. You can prevent drug errors by following the:
- Six Rights of Drug Administration
- Rules listed in Box 10-3

BOX 10-2 Examples of Drug Errors

Prescribing Errors
- Prescribing the wrong drug for the person's diagnosis
- Prescribing a drug to which the person is allergic
- Prescribing the wrong dose for the person's diagnosis

Transcription Errors
- Misinterpreting or misunderstanding the drug ordered or the directions
- Interpreting handwriting that is not legible
- Using unapproved abbreviations
- Omitting a drug order
- Misspelling
- Recording the wrong dates or times

Dispensing
- Sending the wrong drug or dose to the nursing unit
- Using the wrong formulation
- Using the wrong dosage form

Giving Drugs
- Giving the wrong drug
- Giving the wrong dose
- Giving an extra dose
- Giving a drug not ordered for the person
- Missing or skipping a dose
- Giving a drug at the wrong time
- Giving the drug through the wrong route
- Not recording that a drug was given

BOX 10-3 Safety Rules for Giving Drugs

- Follow the Six Rights of Drug Administration pp. 109–111.
- Store all drugs properly (p. 108).
- Make sure you have good lighting; you must be able to read the MA and drug labels correctly.
- Stay focused. Do not allow yourself to become distracted. Ask other staff not to interrupt you unless the situation is critical.
- Keep your working area clean and orderly.
- Check the container label for the drug name, dose, and route.
- Check the person's chart, Kardex, MAR, and ID bracelet for allergies. Before giving a drug, ask the person if he or she has any allergies.
- Check the person's chart, Kardex, and MAR for rotation schedules for drugs applied to the skin (Chapter 12).
- Know why the drug was ordered. Also know its side effects and possible adverse reactions.
- Calculate drug dosages accurately (if allowed by your state and agency). Ask a nurse to check your calculation.
- Identify the person before giving any drug.
- Position the person for the route of administration. For example, to receive an oral drug, the person should be sitting or in a Fowler's position to promote swallowing. Check the care plan and with the nurse for any position limits.
- Have correct fluids ready for the person to swallow oral drugs.
- Stay with the person to make sure that all drugs have been swallowed. If necessary, check the person's mouth—under the tongue and between teeth and the cheeks.
- Follow agency policy for self-administered drugs.
- Never leave a drug in the person's room for the person to take later (unless there is a doctor's order to do so). Always make sure the person takes the drug in your presence.
- Never leave a drug unattended.
- Refer any questions about the person's drug or treatment plan to the nurse.
- Do not prepare or give a drug if:
  - The container is not properly labeled
  - You cannot fully or clearly read the label
- Give only those drugs that your state and agency allow you to give.
- Only give drugs prepared by a pharmacist. Do not give drugs prepared by a nurse or another MA-C. Do not assume that the nurse or MA-C followed the six rights.
- Check the drug name, dose, how often to give the drug, and the route against the order.
- Do not return an unused portion or drug dose to a stock supply container.
- Do not give any oral drug to a person who is comatose or is having difficulty swallowing.
- Do not mix a drug in liquid form with water or other fluid unless directed to do so.
- Ask the nurse if you have questions or if you are not sure about any aspect of giving a drug to any person.
- Perform hand hygiene:
  - Before preparing a person's drugs
  - After contact with the person or items in his or her care setting
- Never touch the actual drug with your hands.
- Do not let the drug container touch any part of a medicine cup or other device (Fig. 10-9).
- Check the drug carefully; many drugs and drug forms look alike.
- Listen to the person; they may know drugs by name, color, or shape. The person may also know what drugs to take, the correct doses, and when and how to take them. The person may question changes in the usual drug routine. For example, if the person comments that a tablet is not broken in half or that a tablet looks different, report these comments or questions to the nurse.
- Observe the person for possible side effects or adverse reactions.
- Leave the medicine room or drug cart neat and orderly. Clean and straighten the area as needed. Restock medicine cups, straws, and other supplies.
- Make sure the drug cabinet or drug cart is locked. Do not leave the key in the lock.

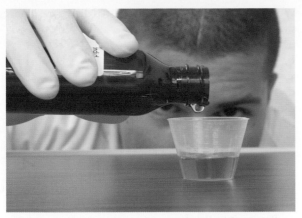

Fig. 10-9 The drug container does not touch the medicine cup. (From Perry AG, Potter PA: *Clinical nursing skills & techniques*, ed 6, St. Louis, 2006, Mosby.)

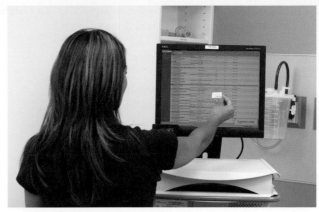

Fig. 10-10 The pharmacy label on the unit-dose packet is compared against the MAR.

GIVING DRUGS

As listed in Box 10-1, drugs can be given by different routes. No matter the route used, safe administration is always the priority. Box 10-4 lists the rules for giving drugs safely. Always use the 6 Rights of Drug Administration (pp. 109–111) and complete 3 safety checks before giving drugs to a person. See *Promoting Safety and Comfort: 3 Safety Checks Before Giving Drugs*

PROMOTING SAFETY AND COMFORT

3 Safety Checks Before Giving Drugs

Safety

The medication administration procedures in this book include three safety checks:
- Before you start, check the drug order.
- *First safety check:* When removing the drug from the shelf or unit dose cart, compare the unit-dose packet against the MAR (Fig. 10-10).
- *Second safety check:* Before preparing or measuring the prescribed dose, compare the unit-dose packet against the MAR (Fig. 10-10).
- *Third safety check:* Before replacing the drug on the shelf or before opening a unit dose container. compare the unit-dose packet against the MAR (Fig. 10-10). In other words, just before giving the drug to the person.

The Institute for Safe Medication Practices (ISMP) recommends opening and giving unit doses one drug at a time. The ISMP gives the following reasons for this practice:
- A drug is harder to identify when removed from its packaging.
- A drug that is not labeled is at greater risk of being mistaken for another drug.
- A drug removed from its packaging cannot be returned to the drawer, floor stock, or pharmacy.

Reporting Drug Errors

If you do make a drug error, notify the nurse immediately. You will need to complete an incident report; agency policy will require that you describe exactly what happened. Do not include your opinions regarding why the error occurred. To help prevent future errors, report the events of the error accurately. In the incident report, include:
- The date and time
- The time the drug was ordered
- The drug name, dosage, and route of administration
- How you found out about the error
- The person's response
- Signs and symptoms of adverse reactions
- The date and time that you reported the error to the nurse

Do not record the error in the progress notes. The nurse will contact the doctor about the error.

▮ REVIEW QUESTIONS

Circle the BEST answer.

1. Medication safety includes all of the following *except*:
   a. freedom from preventable harm from drugs
   b. writing drug orders
   c. the correct dispensing of drugs
   d. the correct storage and disposal of drugs

2. A drug is dispensed in a packet for each drug ordered. This is done using the:
   a. floor stock system
   b. individual prescription order system
   c. unit dose system
   d. narcotic control system

3. The pharmacy sends a 3- to 5-day supply of an ordered drug to the nursing unit. This is done using the:
   a. floor stock system
   b. individual prescription order system
   c. unit dose system
   d. computer-controlled dispensing system

4. Ordered drugs are readily available with the:
   a. floor stock system
   b. individual prescription order system
   c. unit dose system
   d. narcotic control system

5. A staff member is accused of diverting a person's drugs. Drug diversion is:
   a. returning a person's drugs to the medication cart
   b. giving the wrong dose of a drug
   c. giving a drug through the incorrect route
   d. taking a person's drugs for your own use

6. When using a Bar Code Medication Administration (BCMA) system, you must do all of the following, *except*:
   a. complete an inventory control sheet
   b. use the agency's bar code scanner to scan the person's ID bracelet
   c. use the agency's bar code scanner to scan the unit dose package
   d. log onto the system and bring up the person's computerized medical record

7. Only a portion of a controlled substance dose is ordered. What should you do with the unused portion?
   a. Return it to the pharmacy.
   b. Return it to the medicine room.
   c. Ask a nurse to watch you dispose of the unused portion.
   d. Save the unused portion for the next dose.

8. A narcotics count is required:
   a. at the end of each shift
   b. every week
   c. every month
   d. whenever a dose is removed

9. The pharmacy issued 12 doses of a controlled substance. Eight were used. How many should remain?
   a. 2
   b. 4
   c. 6
   d. 8

10. You need to leave a drug cart to go into a person's room. What should you do?
    a. Lock the cart and take the keys with you.
    b. Lock the cart and leave the keys in the lock.
    c. Leave the cart open if you can see it from the bedside.
    d. Ask a coworker to guard the cart.

11. The following statements are about storing drugs. Which is *false*?
    a. Drugs are stored in their original containers.
    b. Refrigerated drugs are stored with food and fluids.
    c. Drug containers are kept tightly closed.
    d. One drug bin or drawer is open at a time.

12. Which is commonly used in assisted living residences to store drugs?
    a. medicine room
    b. drug cart
    c. drug organizer
    d. bedside drawer

13. Controlled substances are:
    a. stored in a locked cabinet
    b. kept with the nurse
    c. stored in the person's drawer or bin
    d. kept in the pharmacy

14. You have a drug ready to give but the person refuses to take the drug. What should you do with the drug?
    a. Return it to the drug cart.
    b. Send it to the pharmacy.
    c. Leave it at the person's bedside.
    d. Dispose of it following agency policy.

15. You dropped a drug on the floor. What should you do?
    a. Dispose of the drug.
    b. Decontaminate the drug.
    c. Sterilize the drug.
    d. Keep the drug for yourself.

16. To give the right drug, always compare the exact spelling of the drug on the label against the:
    a. MAR
    b. Kardex
    c. progress notes
    d. doctor's order form

17. To give the right drug, you always read the drug label before all of the following, *except*:
    a. removing the drug from the drug cart or from the shelf
    b. preparing the prescribed dose
    c. returning the drug to the shelf
    d. charting that you gave the drug

18. A drug was ordered to be given one-time-only. You should:
    a. check to see if it was given
    b. give the drug as soon as it arrives from the pharmacy
    c. ask the person when he or she would like to take the drug
    d. give the drug with those ordered for 0800

19. A drug is supplied in 25 mg tablets. The doctor ordered 50 mg of the drug. How much should you give?
    a. ½ of a tablet
    b. 2 tablets
    c. 2 teaspoons
    d. 2 tablespoons

20. To make sure you give the right drug to the right person, you must use:
    a. two identifiers
    b. the person's name and room number
    c. the person's name
    d. the person's name and bed number

21. Before giving a drug, when should you identify the person?
    a. right before giving the drug
    b. when you arrive at the person's bedside
    c. before you open the person's drug bin
    d. after deciding how to give the drug

22. The drug route is:
    a. where the drug is absorbed in the body
    b. how and where the drug enters the body
    c. how the drug is supplied
    d. the supplies used to give the drug
23. Which route provides the fastest absorption rate?
    a. IV
    b. IM
    c. subcutaneous
    d. oral
24. You are using a unit dose system. When should you record giving a drug?
    a. when the drug is ready to give
    b. after giving the drug
    c. after returning to the nurses' station
    d. at the end of your shift
25. Self-directed medication management means that patients and residents:
    a. order their own drugs
    b. take their own drugs
    c. buy their own drugs
    d. record their own drugs
26. Your role in self-directed medication management may involve the following, *except*:
    a. ordering drugs
    b. assisting with downloading an app and setting the reminders on the person's smartphone
    c. checking the dosage against the drug label
    d. charting that the person took or refused to take a drug
27. You made a drug error. You must complete:
    a. an inventory control sheet
    b. the MAR
    c. an incident report
    d. the required part of the progress notes
28. Which action is *not* safe?
    a. having good lighting to read the MAR and drug labels
    b. leaving drugs in a room for the person to take later
    c. giving drugs prepared only by a pharmacist
    d. making sure the drug cart is locked

29. Examples of drug errors include the following, *except*:
    a. prescribing errors
    b. transcription errors
    c. completing an incident report
    d. giving the wrong drug
30. How many safety checks are done when giving drugs?
    a. 1
    b. 2
    c. 3
    d. 4

Circle T if the statement is true. Circle F if the statement is false.

31. **T   F**   A drug is ordered for 0900 and 2100. You must give the doses exactly at 0900 and 2100.
32. **T   F**   A PRN drug is ordered to be given every 4 hours as needed. Three hours have passed since the last dose. You may now give another dose.
33. **T   F**   Your state does not allow you to give IV drugs. However, you are allowed to give an IV drug in an emergency.
34. **T   F**   Giving the wrong drug is a drug error.
35. **T   F**   In order to access drugs in an automated dispensing machine (ADM), you must enter your username and password into the system.
36. **T   F**   Giving the drug at the wrong time is a drug error.
37. **T   F**   Giving a drug to the wrong person is a drug error.
38. **T   F**   Not record administration of a drug is a drug error.
39. **T   F**   When giving drugs, you should help your co-workers give care.
40. **T   F**   Before giving any drug, you should check if the person has allergies.
41. **T   F**   You calculated a drug dosage. You should ask another MA-C to check your calculation.
42. **T   F**   Oral drugs are ordered for a person who is comatose; you can administer the oral drugs.

Answers to these questions can be found on the Evolve Resources site: http://evolve.elsevier.com/Anderson/medasst/

Oral, Sublingual, and Buccal Drugs

OBJECTIVES

- Define the key terms and key abbreviations used in this chapter.
- Identify solid and liquid oral dose forms.
- Explain how to use the equipment for giving oral dose forms.
- Know the equivalents for household, apothecary, and metric measurements.
- Explain how to give oral, sublingual, and buccal drugs.
- Perform the procedures described in this chapter.

PROCEDURES

- Giving an Oral Drug—Solid Form
- Giving an Oral Drug—Liquid Form

KEY TERMS

buccal Inside the cheek *(bucco)*

capsule A gelatin container that holds a drug in a dry powder or liquid form

elixir A clear liquid made up of a drug dissolved in alcohol and water

emulsion An oral dose form containing small droplets of water-in-oil or oil-in-water

lavage Washing out the stomach

lozenge A flat disk containing a medicinal agent with a flavored base; troche

medicine cup A plastic container with measurement scales

medicine dropper A small glass or plastic tube with a hollow rubber ball at one end

meniscus The lowest point of liquid in a medicine cup.

soufflé cup A small paper or plastic cup used for solid drug forms

sublingual Under *(sub)* the tongue *(lingual)*

suspension A liquid containing solid drug particles

syringe A plastic measuring device with three parts—tip, barrel, and plunger

syrup An oral dose form containing a drug dissolved in sugar

tablet A dried, powdered drug compressed into a small disk

troche See "lozenge"

KEY ABBREVIATIONS

GI Gastrointestinal

ISMP Institute for Safe Medication Practices

ODT Orally disintegrating tablets

PO By mouth (per os)

Oral drugs are given by mouth—the *oral route*. Drugs are given directly into the gastrointestinal (GI) tract. The oral route is commonly used for giving drugs and offers the following advantages:

- Most drugs have oral dose forms.
- Oral drugs are easy to administer.
- Most people can swallow oral drugs easily.
- The procedure is noninvasive, meaning:
  - The skin is not pierced as for an injection.
  - Nothing is inserted into a body opening (e.g., vagina, rectum).
- The drug can be retrieved from the stomach to lessen adverse drug events. If necessary, an orogastric or nasogastric tube is inserted to wash out (lavage) the stomach.

However, oral drugs do have their share of problems and limitations:

- They have the slowest rate of absorption and onset of action.
- Some may harm or discolor the teeth.

- Some may have an unpleasant taste or smell.
- Some may cause nausea.
- They cannot be given if the person:
  - Is vomiting
  - Has gastric or intestinal suction
  - Is at risk for aspiration
  - Is unconscious or comatose
  - Cannot swallow

An order for an oral drug is written as one of the following:

- PO—per os (*per* means *by*; *os* means *mouth*)
- By mouth
- Orally

See p. 122 for sublingual and buccal drugs.

See *Promoting Safety and Comfort: Oral Drugs.*

ORAL DOSE FORMS

Oral drugs come in the following dose forms:

- *Capsule.* A **capsule** is a small, cylindrical gelatin container that holds a drug in a dry powder or liquid form. This form is used for drugs that have an unpleasant odor or taste. You can identify a drug by the size, color, and shape, as well as the manufacturer's symbol on the capsule (Fig. 11-1). *Timed-release or sustained-release capsules* contain granules (Fig. 11-2). The granules dissolve at different rates and, over a period of time, there is a continuous release of the drug. Fewer doses are needed per day; usually every 12 or 24 hours.
- *Tablets.* A **tablet** is a dried, powdered drug compressed into a small disk.
  - *Scored* tablets are grooved for use in dividing the dose (Fig. 11-3, *A*).
  - *Layered* tablets have layers (Fig. 11-3, *B*). More than one drug is given at the same time.
  - *Enteric-coated* tablets have a special coating (Fig. 11-3, *C*) that prevents the tablet from dissolving in the stomach. The tablet dissolves in the small intestine. It should not be crushed or chewed.
  - *Caplets* are tablets shaped in the form of a capsule.
  - *Orally disintegrating tablets* (ODT) are placed under the tongue and dissolve rapidly (usually within seconds). They are used for rapid onset of action, meaning the drug starts working very quickly.
- *Sublingual Film or Strips.* A film or strip placed under the tongue that dissolves quickly. No additional liquid is needed to take a drug in this form. The drug dissolves quickly upon

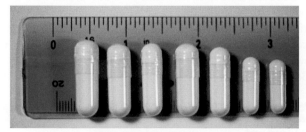

Fig. 11-1 Capsules.

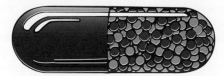

Fig. 11-2 Timed-release capsule.

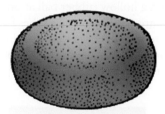

Fig. 11-3 A, Scored tablet. **B**, Layered tablet. **C**, Enteric-coated tablet.

Color coat
Acid-resistant coat
Active ingredient

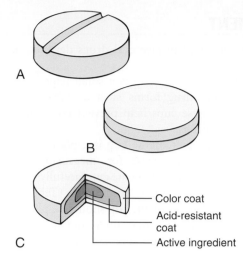

Fig. 11-4 Lozenge. (From Edmunds MW: *Introduction to clinical pharmacology*, ed 5, St Louis, 2006, Mosby.)

contact with a wet surface (e.g., the tongue). This is especially useful for people who have trouble swallowing.

- *Lozenges.* A **lozenge** (**troche**) is a flat disk containing a medicinal agent with a flavored base (Fig. 11-4). The base is a hard or soft sugar candy. Lozenges are held or sucked in the mouth to slowly dissolve; the ingredients of the lozenge are released slowly.
- *Elixirs.* An **elixir** is a clear liquid made up of a drug dissolved in alcohol and water. A flavor is added to improve the taste.
- *Emulsions.* An **emulsion** contains small droplets of water-in-oil or oil-in-water. This form is used to mask bitter tastes or to increase the ability to dissolve.
- *Suspensions.* A **suspension** is a liquid containing solid drug particles. Before giving a suspension, shake the bottle well to thoroughly mix the particles. Many oral liquid antacids and liquid antibiotics are suspensions.
- *Syrups.* A **syrup** contains drugs dissolved in a sugar solution. The sugar helps mask the drug's bitter taste. Syrups are most commonly used for children.

See *Focus on Communication: Oral Dose Forms.*

EQUIPMENT

The equipment used to give oral drugs depends on the dose form ordered.

- *Soufflé cups.* A **soufflé cup** is a small paper or plastic cup used for solid drug forms such as tablets and capsules (Fig. 11-5). These cups help prevent contamination while handling the drugs.
- *Medicine cups.* A **medicine cup** is a plastic container with measurement scales used for measuring liquid drugs (Fig. 11-6). Check the medicine cup carefully before pouring any drug. You must use the proper scale (Table 11-1) for the dose ordered. The medicine cup should be placed on a hard, flat surface. The medicine cup is not accurate for doses smaller than 1 teaspoon. For smaller doses, use an oral syringe.
- *Medicine droppers.* A **medicine dropper** is a small glass or plastic tube with a hollow rubber ball at one end (Fig. 11-7). Measurements are marked on the tube. Drops vary in size from dropper to dropper. *Only use the dropper supplied by the manufacturer of the drug ordered.* Once you draw the drug into the tube, do not turn the dropper upside down;

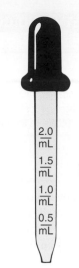

Fig. 11-7 Medicine dropper.

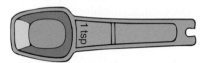

Fig. 11-8 Measuring teaspoon.

when the dropper is turned upside down, some of the drug flows into the bulb and the person receives less than the amount ordered. Also, do not transfer the drug from the medicine dropper to another container. This results in part of the drug remaining in the container and the person receives less than the amount ordered.

- *Teaspoon.* Many liquid drugs are ordered using a teaspoon as the unit of measure. In hospitals and nursing centers, a teaspoon measure is converted into a metric measure (Table 11-1). For example, 1 teaspoon is equal to 5 mL. If 2 teaspoons are ordered, you give 10 mL of the drug. For home use, use an oral syringe, medicine cup, or a measuring teaspoon normally used for baking (Fig. 11-8). Never use a teaspoon (kitchen spoon) that is used for eating.
- *Oral syringes.* A **syringe** is a plastic measuring device with three parts—tip, barrel, and plunger (Fig. 11-9). Measurements are marked on the barrel. To withdraw a liquid, pull back on the plunger; to give a liquid, push the plunger forward. Oral syringes measure volumes from 0.1 mL to 15 mL. Choose the correct size syringe for the amount ordered. Note that a needle will not fit on the tip of an oral syringe.

See *Promoting Safety and Comfort: Equipment.*

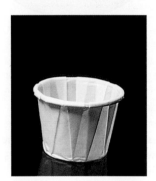

Fig. 11-5 Soufflé cup.

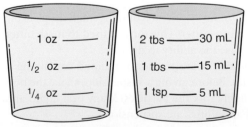

Fig. 11-6 Medicine cup.

TABLE 11-1	Measurement Equivalents	
Household Measurement	**Apothecary Measurement**	**Metric Measurement**
2 tbsp (tbsp = tablespoon)	1 oz (oz = ounce)	30 mL (mL = milliliters)
1 tbsp (tbsp = tablespoon)	½ oz (oz = ounce)	15 mL (mL = milliliters)
2 tsp (tsp = teaspoon)	⅓ oz (oz = ounce)	10 mL (mL = milliliters)
1 tsp (tsp = teaspoon)	⅙ oz (oz = ounce)	5 mL (mL = milliliters)

PROMOTING SAFETY AND COMFORT

Equipment

Safety

Always use *oral syringes* to give an oral drug by syringe. Oral syringes cannot be connected to an IV port or catheter. The ISMP has reported drug errors in which parenteral syringes were used for oral drugs. In these instances, nurses gave the oral drugs by the IV route when an oral syringe was left on the drug cart or when more than one drug was prepared. These were serious drug errors that must be avoided.

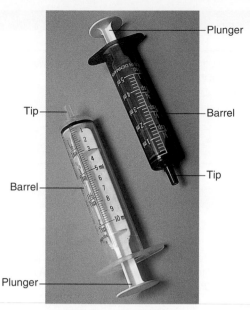

Fig. 11-9 Oral syringe.

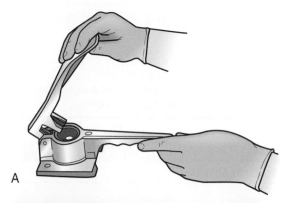

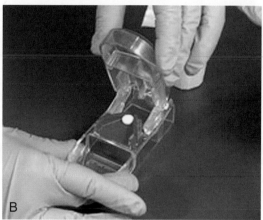

Fig. 11-10 A, Pill crusher. **B,** Pill cutter.

GIVING ORAL DRUGS

When giving oral drugs, always practice medication safety (Chapter 10). Remember to:

- Follow the Six Rights of Drug Administration.
- Prevent drug errors.
- Prevent infection.
- Follow the rules for giving oral drugs listed in Box 11-1. See *Delegation Guidelines: Giving Oral Drugs*. See *Promoting Safety and Comfort: Giving Oral Drugs*.

BOX 11-1 Rules for Giving Oral Drugs

General Rules

- Give the most important drug first (e.g., antibiotics or drugs affecting the heart).
- Give solid drugs first, then liquid drugs.
- Do not mix solid drugs with liquid drugs.
- Stay with the person while he or she takes the drug. Do not leave the drug at the bedside unless there is a doctor's order to do so.
- Do not let the container touch any part of a soufflé cup, medicine cup, or measuring teaspoon.
- Place a container (or bottle cap or lid) upside down on a clean surface. Do not touch the inside of the cap or lid.

Solid Form

- Use the same soufflé or medicine cup for all of the person's tablets and capsules with the nurse's approval.
- Use a separate cup for a drug affecting the heart.
- Use a separate cup for a drug affecting blood pressure.
  - Check with the nurse before crushing tablets or opening capsules. To crush a tablet:
  - Wear gloves.
  - Place the tablet in the pill crusher and crush the drug as per manufacturer instructions (Fig. 11-10, A).
- Wash the pill crusher after each use. This removes powder or particles left in or on the device.
- Check with the nurse before cutting a scored tablet. To cut a scored tablet:
- Wear gloves.

- Use a disposable pill cutter (Fig. 11-10, B). It should be labeled with the person's name. Do not use the person's pill cutter for another patient or resident.
- Wash (with water) and dry the pill cutter if it is not disposable. This removes powder or particles left on the device.
- Do not mix a drug with food or fluids unless ordered to do so.
- Do not give a drug with food unless ordered to do so.
- Let the person drink a small amount of water before taking a drug; this moistens the mouth to make swallowing the drug easier.
- Have the person place the drug far back on the tongue. Assist as needed. (Wear gloves if assisting the person.)
- Give the person fluids to swallow the drug.
- Have the person keep his or her head forward (as while eating) when swallowing. Tilting the head back usually does not help the person swallow the drug.
- Encourage the person to drink a full glass of fluid; this helps the drug reach the stomach and helps dilute the drug to decrease the risk of stomach irritation.
- Remind the person to suck on a lozenge. Lozenges should not be swallowed whole.

Liquid Form

- Do not dilute (add water or other fluid) a liquid drug unless ordered to do so.
- Do not mix liquid drugs together. Pour each liquid into a separate medicine cup or measuring teaspoon. If using oral syringes, use a different syringe for each liquid.
- Give cough syrup last if administering more than one liquid drug. Cough syrup is given to coat and soothe the throat.
- Do not return extra liquid poured into a medicine cup or measuring teaspoon back to the bottle. Dispose of the drug according to agency policy.

DELEGATION GUIDELINES

Giving Oral Drugs

When giving oral drugs is delegated to you, you need the following information from the nurse, the care plan, and the MAR:

- Which drugs to give first.
- Which tablets are crushed for a person.
- Which capsules are opened for a person.
- What to use to give crushed tablets or opened capsules (e.g., applesauce, pudding, custard, jelly, strained fruit, or ice cream).

- Whether or not the sitting or Fowler's position is allowed. If not, how to properly position the person.
- When to report observations.
- What specific patient or resident concerns to report immediately.

PROMOTING SAFETY AND COMFORT

Giving Oral Drugs

Safety

When crushed tablets or opened capsules are mixed with food, use a teaspoon to give the drug. Unless otherwise ordered, the teaspoon should only be one-third full. This portion is usually swallowed easily; however, some people may need a smaller portion. Follow the care plan. The person must ingest all of the food in which the drug is mixed. Otherwise, the person receives less than the amount of drug ordered. You may need to fill the teaspoon two or three times to complete the process.

Comfort

A crushed tablet or opened capsule does not have a pleasant taste. Mix the drug with food as directed by the nurse, care plan, and MAR. (See *Delegation Guidelines: Giving Oral Drugs.*)

GIVING AN ORAL DRUG—SOLID FORM

Quality of Life

Remember to:

- Knock before entering the person's room.
- Address the person by name.
- Introduce yourself by name and title.
- Explain the procedure to the person before and during the procedure.
- Protect the person's rights during the procedure.
- Handle the person gently during the procedure.

Pre-procedure

1. Follow *Delegation Guidelines: Giving Oral Drugs.* See *Promoting Safety and Comfort: Giving Oral Drugs.*
2. Check the most recent drug order and compare the drug order to the medication profile. Focus on the 6 Rights of Drug Administration (Chapter 10).
3. Check with the nurse if you have any questions.
4. Perform hand hygiene.
5. Collect the following:
   - MAR
   - Water glass and water or other ordered liquid
   - Drinking straw
   - Soufflé cups

Procedure

6. Read the order on the MAR.
7. Select the right drug from the drug cart/system.
8. Compare the drug order on the MAR against the pharmacy label on the drug container or unit-dose packet. **(First safety check.)** Review the 6 Rights of Drug Administration (Chapter 10).
9. Check the drug container or unit-dose packet for an expiration date.
10. Compare the drug order on the MAR against the pharmacy label on the drug container or unit-dose packet. **(Second safety check.)** Review the 6 Rights of Drug Administration (Chapter 10).

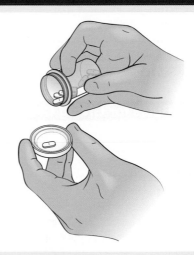

Fig. 11-11 A drug is poured from a container into the container lid. The lid does not touch the container.

11. Prepare the drug. (Note: unit dose packets are placed in a soufflé cup [or a small plastic bag]. Do not open the unit-dose packets until you are at the person's bedside.)
    a. Open the container.
    b. Gently tap on the container to pour the ordered dosage into the container cap or lid. Do not let the container touch the cap or lid. See Figure 11-11.
    c. Return extra tablets or capsules back into the container. Do not let the cap or lid touch the container. For example, if 1 tablet is ordered but 3 tablets are poured from the container into the cap, return 2 tablets to the container.
    d. Pour the drug from the lid into the soufflé cup.
    e. Close the container.
    f. Return the container to the drug system or drug cart.

GIVING AN ORAL DRUG—SOLID FORM—cont'd

12. Compare the drug order on the MAR against the pharmacy label on the drug container. **(Third safety check.)** Review the 6 Rights of Drug Administration (Chapter 10).
13. Repeat steps 6–12 for each drug ordered for the person. You can use the same soufflé cup for all tablets and capsules if the nurse approves. However, you should always:
    - Use a separate cup for a drug affecting the heart
    - Use a separate cup for a drug affecting blood pressure
14. Bring all drugs and supplies to the person's bedside.
15. Provide for privacy.
16. Identify the person and call them by their name. Check the ID bracelet against the MAR. Make sure you use at least two identifiers according to agency policy. If using a barcode scanner, sign into the computer system and scan the person's ID band.
17. Obtain required measurements as noted on the MAR. For example, measure the person's blood pressure or pulse and note the measurement on the MAR.
18. Position the person in a sitting position, Fowler's position, or in the position directed by the nurse, care plan, and MAR.
19. Let the person drink a small amount of water. Provide a straw if preferred.
20. Give the person the drugs. If using a unit dose system:
    a. Hand the drug package to the person and ask him or her to read the label out loud.
    b. Ask the person to hand the package back to you.
    c. Open the package.
    d. Place the contents into the soufflé cup or directly into the person's hand.
21. Give the person a full glass of water or other ordered fluid. Provide a straw if preferred. Encourage the person to drink all of the water or other provided fluid.
22. Stay with the person to make sure he or she swallows all of the drugs. If necessary, check the person's mouth—under the tongue and between the teeth and the cheeks. (Wear gloves if checking the person's mouth.)

Post-procedure

23. Discard the soufflé cup or unit-dose packages.
24. Provide for comfort and complete a safety check before leaving the room. (See the inside back cover of this book.)
25. Unscreen the person.
26. Perform hand hygiene.
27. Record the *right documentation* on the MAR:
    - The date, time, drug name, dosage, and route of administration
    - Your name or initials
28. Report and record any specific patient or resident observations or concerns to the nurse.

GIVING AN ORAL DRUG—LIQUID FORM

Quality Of Life

Remember to:
- Knock before entering the person's room.
- Address the person by name.
- Introduce yourself by name and title.
- Explain the procedure to the person before and during the procedure.
- Protect the person's rights during the procedure.
- Handle the person gently during the procedure.

Pre-procedure

1. Follow *Delegation Guidelines: Giving Oral Drugs*. See *Promoting Safety and Comfort: Giving Oral Drugs*.
2. Check the most recent drug order. Compare the drug order to the medication profile. Focus on the 6 Rights of Drug Administration (Chapter 10).
3. Check with the nurse if you have any questions.
4. Perform hand hygiene.
5. Collect the following:
   - MAR
   - Medicine cup
   - Oral syringe in the correct size (if needed)
   - Tray (if needed)
   - Paper towels

Procedure

6. Read the order on the MAR.
7. Select the right drug from the drug cart/system.
8. Compare the drug order on the MAR against the pharmacy label on the drug container or unit-dose container. **(First safety check.)** Review the 6 Rights of Drug Administration (Chapter 10).
9. Check the drug container or unit-dose container for an expiration date.
10. Compare the drug order on the MAR against the pharmacy label on the drug container or unit-dose container. **(Second safety check.)** Review the 6 Rights of Drug Administration (Chapter 10).
11. Prepare the drug. (Note: do not open a unit-dose container until you are at the person's bedside. Place the unit-dose container in a small plastic bag if preparing other drugs for the same person.)
    a. Shake the bottle or container only if directed to do so on the label. Make sure the lid is secure before shaking a bottle.
    b. Open the container.
    c. Place the lid on a clean surface on the drug cart so that the outside of the lid is facing down and the inside of the lid is facing up.
    d. Hold the bottle so that the label is in the palm of your hand; this prevents the contents from running down and smearing the label during pouring.
12. *For a medicine cup:*
    a. Locate the scale to be used on the medicine cup.
    b. Locate the exact place where the liquid drug should be measured.
    c. Place the medicine cup on a hard surface.
    d. Pour the prescribed dose into the medicine cup at eye level (Fig 11-12).
    e. Measure the dose at the **meniscus**. The meniscus is the lowest point of the liquid in the medicine cup (Fig. 11-13).
    f. Set the medicine cup on the drug cart.

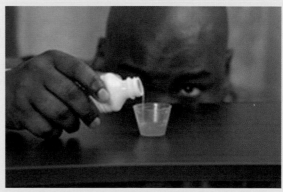

Fig. 11-12 Medicine cup on hard surface. Pour liquid at eye level.

Continued

GIVING AN ORAL DRUG—LIQUID FORM—cont'd

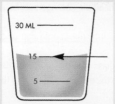

Fig. 11-13 The dose is measured at the meniscus, which is the lowest level of liquid in the medicine cup.

13. *For a syringe:*
    a. Follow steps 12 a–e.
    b. Pull back on the plunger to withdraw the drug from the medicine cup into the barrel (Fig. 11-14).
    c. Set the syringe on the tray or a paper towel.
14. Wipe off any liquid from the bottle top and close the bottle.
15. Return the bottle to the drug cart or system.
16. Compare the drug order on the MAR against the pharmacy label on the drug container. **(Third safety check.)** Review the 6 Rights of Drug Administration (Chapter 10).
17. Repeat steps 6–16 for each liquid drug ordered for the person.
18. Bring all drugs and supplies to the person's bedside.
19. Provide for privacy.
20. Identify the person and call them by name. Check the ID bracelet against the MAR. Make sure you use at least two identifiers according to agency policy. If using a barcode scanner, sign into the computer system and scan the person's ID band.
21. Obtain required measurements as noted on the MAR. For example, measure the person's blood pressure or pulse and note the measurement on the MAR.
22. Position the person in a sitting position, Fowler's position, or position the person as directed by the nurse, care plan, and MAR.
23. Give the person the medicine cup.
24. Observe while the person ingests the drug.
    If using a unit dose system:
    a. Hand the drug container to the person. Ask him or her to read the label out loud.
    b. Ask the person to hand the container back to you.
    c. Shake the container, then open it carefully.
    d. Give the container to the person.
    e. Have the person drink the drug.

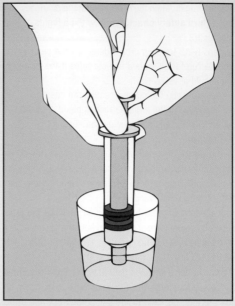

Fig. 11-14 The plunger is pulled back to withdraw a liquid drug from a medicine cup into the syringe barrel.

25. If using a medicine dropper or an oral syringe:
    a. Place the dropper or syringe inside the mouth by the tongue.
    b. Dispense the liquid in small amounts. Allow time for the person to swallow.
    c. Return the dropper to the bottle.

Post-procedure

26. Discard the medicine cup, unit-dose container, or oral syringe.
27. Provide for comfort and complete a safety check before leaving the room. (See the inside back cover of this book.)
28. Unscreen the person.
29. Perform hand hygiene.
30. Record the *right documentation* on the MAR:
    • The date, time, drug name, dosage, and route of administration
    • Your name or initials
31. Report and record any specific patient or resident observations or concerns to the nurse.

SUBLINGUAL AND BUCCAL DRUGS

Sublingual means under *(sub)* the tongue *(lingual)*. Sublingual tablets are placed under the tongue and are then dissolved and absorbed through the many blood vessels in that area.

Buccal means inside the cheek *(bucco)*. Buccal tablets are placed between the cheek and the molar teeth. A buccal tablet is absorbed by the blood vessels in the cheek.

The onset of action is rapid because drugs are quickly absorbed through the sublingual and buccal routes.

To give a sublingual or buccal tablet, follow these steps:

1. Perform hand hygiene.
2. Put on a glove.
3. For a sublingual drug, place the tablet under the tongue (Fig. 11-15, *A*).
4. For a buccal drug, place the tablet between the upper molar and the cheek (Fig. 11-15, *B*).
5. Do not give the person water to drink.
6. Encourage the person to:
   a. Allow the drug to dissolve where placed and remind the person not to move the drug to another part of the mouth.
   b. Hold saliva in the mouth until the tablet is dissolved.
7. Remove and properly discard the glove.
8. Perform hand hygiene.

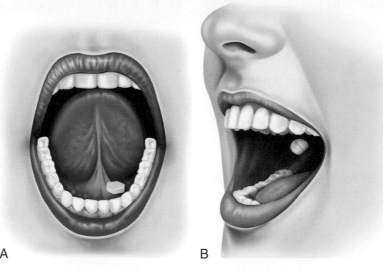

A   B

Fig. 11-15 A, A sublingual tablet is placed under the tongue. **B,** A buccal tablet is placed between the cheek and upper molar.

REVIEW QUESTIONS

Circle the BEST answer.

1. The wrong oral drug was given to a person. If necessary, how is the drug retrieved?
   a. by giving an enema
   b. by giving water to dilute the drug
   c. by lavage
   d. through surgery

2. Which person can receive oral drugs?
   a. the person who is alert, oriented
   b. the person who is vomiting
   c. the person who is at risk for aspiration
   d. the person who is comatose

3. To receive oral drugs, the person must be able to:
   a. state his or her name
   b. identify the drug
   c. sit in a Fowler's position
   d. swallow

4. Oral drug orders may be written as follows. Which should you question?
   a. 10 mL PO
   b. 10 mL per os
   c. 10 mL orally
   d. 10 mL by mouth

5. Which dose form is a tablet that is shaped in the form of a capsule?
   a. tablet
   b. capsule
   c. caplet
   d. lozenge

6. Which dose form is placed under the tongue and dissolves quickly?
   a. tablet
   b. capsule
   c. timed-release capsule
   d. sublingual film

7. Another name for a lozenge is:
   a. elixir
   b. emulsion
   c. troche
   d. suspension

8. Which is not a liquid dose form?
   a. elixir
   b. emulsion
   c. lozenge
   d. syrup

9. Which of the following prevents a tablet from dissolving in the stomach?
   a. scoring
   b. layering
   c. granules
   d. enteric coating

10. Which dose form should you shake before pouring the drug?
   a. suspension
   b. timed-release capsule
   c. elixir
   d. syrup

11. Which has a hollow rubber ball at one end?
   a. soufflé cup
   b. medicine cup
   c. medicine dropper
   d. oral syringe

12. Which is *not* a part of an oral syringe?
   a. tip
   b. barrel
   c. plunger
   d. bulb

13. How many milliliters (mL) are in 1 teaspoon?
   a. 5
   b. 10
   c. 15
   d. 30

14. How many milliliters (mL) are in half an ounce?
    a. 5
    b. 10
    c. 15
    d. 30
15. A person has four drugs ordered for 0900. Which should you give first?
    a. the liquid drug
    b. a drug in a unit dose package
    c. a solid drug
    d. the most important drug
16. Before giving a person a solid dose form, you should have the person:
    a. eat some food
    b. drink a small amount of water
    c. drink a full glass of water
    d. tilt his or her head back

Circle T if the statement is true. Circle F if the statement is false.

17. T F   You can mix solid dose forms with liquid dose forms.
18. T F   You can mix liquid drugs together.
19. T F   You can leave a drug at the bedside if there is a doctor's order to do so.
20. T F   A medicine cup can touch the drug container or bottle.
21. T F   A bottle cap is placed upside down on a clean surface.
22. T F   A person has four drugs ordered for 1300. The drugs are in tablet and capsule form. You can use the same soufflé cup for all the drugs if the nurse approves.
23. T F   You can give all ordered drugs with food.
24. T F   You are giving two liquid drugs; one is cough syrup. The cough syrup is given last.
25. T F   You pour extra liquid into a medicine cup. You can return the extra liquid to the bottle.

Answers to these questions can be found on the Evolve Resources site: http://evolve.elsevier.com/Anderson/medasst/

Topical Drugs

OBJECTIVES

- Define the key terms and key abbreviations used in this chapter.
- Identify the factors that affect topical drug absorption.
- List the reasons for topical drug applications.
- Describe the topical dose forms.
- Explain the rules for applying topical dose forms.
- Explain how to safely apply nitroglycerin ointment.
- Explain how to safely apply a transdermal patch.
- Perform the procedures described in this chapter.

PROCEDURES

- Applying a Cream, Lotion, Ointment, and Powder
- Applying Nitroglycerin Ointment

KEY TERMS

cream A semi-solid emulsion containing a drug
debride To remove
lotion A watery preparation containing suspended particles
ointment A semi-solid preparation containing a drug in an oily base
powder A finely ground drug in a talc base

topical Refers to a surface of a part of the body
transdermal Through *(trans)* the skin *(dermal)*
transdermal patch A patch applied to the skin that provides continuous, gradual absorption of a drug through the skin and into the bloodstream; transdermal disk

KEY ABBREVIATIONS

ID identification

MAR medication administration record

Topical refers to a surface of a part of the body. Drugs given by the topical route are applied directly to the area of the skin requiring treatment. The action of the drug is usually short and requires frequent application. Sometimes, the drugs may be messy and difficult to apply.

The absorption of a topical drug is affected by:
- The strength of the drug
- How long the drug is in contact with the skin
- The size of the area of application
- Skin thickness
- Amount of water in the tissues
- Amount of skin breakdown or irritation

Drugs are topically applied to:
- Clean and debride a wound. **Debride** means to remove. Wounds are debrided to remove dirt, damaged tissue, foreign objects, and drainage. This process helps prevent infection and promotes healing.
- Hydrate (add water to) the skin.
- Reduce inflammation.
- Relieve itching or a rash.
- Provide a protective barrier to the skin.
- Reduce thickening of the skin (e.g., callous formation).

TOPICAL DOSE FORMS

Creams, lotions, ointments, and powders are common topical dose forms.
- *Creams.* A **cream** is a semi-solid emulsion containing a drug. An *emulsion* contains small droplets of water-in-oil or oil-in-water. The cream base is usually non-greasy. Creams are removed with water.
- *Lotions.* A **lotion** is a watery preparation containing suspended particles. All lotions need to be well-shaken prior to application. Gently but firmly pat the lotion onto the skin. Do not rub the lotion into the skin; rubbing increases circulation and itching while also causing friction, thus irritating the skin. Lotions are used to:
  - Soothe and protect the skin.
  - Relieve rashes and itching.
  - Cleanse the skin.
- *Ointments.* An **ointment** is a semi-solid preparation containing a drug in an oily base. Because ointments are not easily removed with water, the drug has longer contact with the skin.
- *Powders.* A **powder** is a finely ground drug in a talc base. Powders are used to absorb moisture. They also dry, cool, and protect the skin. Powder is applied to dry skin in a thin, even layer.

BOX 12-1 Rules for Applying Creams, Lotions, Ointments, and Powders

- Perform hand hygiene before and after application.
- Follow the 6 Rights of Medication Administration (Chapter 10).
- Follow Standard Precautions.
- Follow isolation precautions as ordered (Chapter 6).
- Wear gloves.
- Do not let the dose form touch your skin.
- Provide for privacy.
- Position the person to expose the application site. Avoid unnecessary exposure.
- Clean and dry the skin as directed by the nurse before applying a dose form. Soap and water are typically used if the person's skin condition allows. Make sure previous applications are thoroughly removed.
- Observe the skin. Report and record your observations. See *Delegation Guidelines: Applying Creams, Lotions, Ointments, and Powders*.

- See *Promoting Safety and Comfort: Applying Creams, Lotions, Ointments, and Powders*.
- Shake lotions thoroughly. The lotion should have a uniform color throughout.
- Apply the dose form to clean, dry skin.
- Apply the correct amount. Use a sterile tongue blade or sterile cotton-tipped applicator to remove the dose from a jar. If applying the drug by gloved hand or finger, use the tongue blade or cotton-tipped applicator to transfer the dose to your hand or finger.
- Do not let the drug container touch the person's skin.
- Cover the site with gauze or other covering as directed by the nurse, care plan, and MAR. Ointments and creams may stain or soil garments and linens.
- See procedure: *Applying Nitroglycerin Ointment*, p. 128-129.

Applying Creams, Lotions, Ointments, and Powders

Each topical dose form is applied differently. Lotions are dabbed on the skin with gauze or a cotton ball. Use a tongue blade, cotton-tipped applicator, or a gloved hand or finger to apply ointments and creams. Powders are applied in a thin, even layer. To safely apply a topical dose form, follow the rules in Box 12-1. Also practice medication safety (Chapter 10). To apply a nitroglycerin ointment, see p. 128-129.

See *Focus on Older Persons: Applying Creams, Lotions, Ointments, and Powders.*

See *Delegation Guidelines: Applying Creams, Lotions, Ointments, and Powders.*

See *Promoting Safety and Comfort: Applying Creams, Lotions, Ointments, and Powders.*

FOCUS ON OLDER PERSONS

Applying Creams, Lotions, Ointments, and Powders

Increasingly dry skin occurs with aging. Long-term use of soap also dries the skin. Dry skin is easily damaged. Thorough rinsing is needed when using soap. If necessary, the nurse and care plan may direct you to use a different cleansing agent.

DELEGATION GUIDELINES

Applying Creams, Lotions, Ointments, and Powders

Before applying a topical dose form, you need the following information from the nurse, care plan, and MAR:
- Whether or not isolation precautions are required. If yes:
  - What type of precaution.
  - What personal protective equipment is needed.
  - Special measures for cleaning and drying the skin.
  - What cleansing agent to use.
  - The exact site of application.
- What to use to apply the drug (e.g., tongue blade, cotton-tipped applicator, or gloved hand or finger).
- Whether or not you need to cover the application. If yes, how to cover the application site (e.g., gauze, see-through dressing and tape, and so on).

- What observations to report and record:
  - Color of the skin
  - Locations and descriptions of rashes
  - Dry skin
  - Bruises or open skin areas
- Pale or reddened areas, particularly over bony parts
- Blisters
- Drainage or bleeding from wounds or body openings
- Skin temperature
- Complaints of pain or discomfort
- When observations should be reported
- Which specific patient or resident concerns to immediately report

PROMOTING SAFETY AND COMFORT

Applying Creams, Lotions, Ointments, and Powders

Safety

Use caution when applying powder; accidentally inhaling powder can irritate the airway and lungs. Do not shake or sprinkle powder onto the person's skin. To safely apply powder:
- Turn away from the person.
- Sprinkle a small amount of powder onto your hands or a cloth.
- Apply the powder in a thin layer.
- Make sure powder does not get on the floor; powder is slippery and may cause falls.

Comfort

A skin area is exposed to apply topical dose forms. Provide for privacy. Screen the person and close all doors and window coverings (e.g., drapes, shades, blinds, and shutters). Avoid unnecessary exposure; expose only the needed area.

The person may have a rash or skin lesion. Skin disorders may be contagious; the person knows the disease can be spread to others. As a result, self-esteem may suffer. Be sure to treat the person with dignity and respect.

APPLYING A CREAM, LOTION, OINTMENT, AND POWDER

Quality of Life
Remember to:
- Knock before entering the person's room.
- Address the person by name.
- Introduce yourself by name and title.
- Explain the procedure to the person before and during the procedure.
- Protect the person's rights during the procedure.
- Handle the person gently during the procedure.

Pre-procedure
1. Follow *Delegation Guidelines: Applying Creams, Lotions, Ointments, and Powders.* See *Promoting Safety and Comfort: Applying Creams, Lotions, Ointments, and Powders.*
2. Check the most recent drug order and compare to the medication profile. Focus on the 6 Rights of Drug Administration (Chapter 10).
3. Check with the nurse if you have any questions.
4. Perform hand hygiene.
5. Collect necessary items:
   - Soap or other cleansing agent
   - Washcloth and towel
   - Wash basin with warm water
   - Gauze squares or cotton balls
   - Sterile tongue blade
   - Sterile cotton-tipped applicator
   - Gloves
   - MAR

Procedure
6. Read the order on the MAR.
7. Select the right drug from the drug cart/system.
8. Compare the drug order on the MAR against the pharmacy label on the drug container. **(First safety check.)** Review the 6 Rights of Drug Administration (Chapter 10).
9. Check the drug container for an expiration date and bring the drug to the person's bedside.
10. Provide for privacy.
11. Identify the person by checking the ID bracelet against the MAR. Make sure you use at least two identifiers according to agency policy. Call the person by name. Follow agency policy if using a barcode scanner.
12. Put on gloves.
13. Position the person to expose the application site; then, expose the site.
14. Clean and dry the application site.
15. Observe the application site.
16. Remove and discard gloves. Perform hand hygiene. Put on new, clean gloves.
17. Compare the drug order on the MAR against the pharmacy label on the drug container. **(Second safety check.)** Review the 6 Rights of Drug Administration (Chapter 10).
18. Shake the lotion thoroughly.
19. Open the container and place the lid or cap upside down on a clean surface. For an ointment or cream:
    a. *From a jar:* use a tongue blade to remove the ordered amount.
    b. *From a tube:* squeeze the ordered amount onto a tongue blade or cotton-tipped applicator.
20. Close the container. Compare the drug order on the MAR against the pharmacy label on the drug container. **(Third safety check.)** Review the 6 Rights of Drug Administration (Chapter 10).

21. Apply the topical dose form:
    a. Lotion:
       (1) Hold the bottle in your non-dominant hand with the label in the palm of your hand. This prevents the contents from smearing the label during pouring.
       (2) Pour some lotion onto a cotton ball or gauze square. Do not let any part of the container touch the cotton ball.
       (3) Gently but firmly dab the lotion onto the skin. Do not rub.
       (4) Repeat steps 21 a (1)–(3) with a new cotton ball or gauze square until the area is covered.
    b. Cream or ointment:
       (1) Transfer the cream or ointment from the tongue blade or cotton-tipped applicator to your gloved hand or index finger (if necessary).
       (2) Apply the agent to the skin with the tongue blade, cotton-tipped applicator, or your gloved hand or finger (Fig. 12-1).
       (3) Apply the agent in a thin layer in the direction of hair growth. Use firm, gentle strokes.
    c. Powder:
       (1) Apply in a thin, even layer with your gloved hand.
       (2) Smooth over the area for even coverage.
23. Return the container to the drug cart/system.

Post-procedure
24. Discard the used supplies or unit-dose packages.
25. Follow agency policy for soiled linen.
26. While wearing gloves, empty and clean the wash basin. Return it and other supplies to their proper location.
27. Remove the gloves and perform hand hygiene.
28. Provide for comfort and complete a safety check before leaving the room. (See the inside back cover of this book.)
29. Unscreen the person.
30. Record the *right documentation* on the MAR:
    - The date, time, drug name, dosage, and route of administration
    - The application site
    - Your name or initials
31. Report and record any specific patient or resident observations or concerns to the nurse.

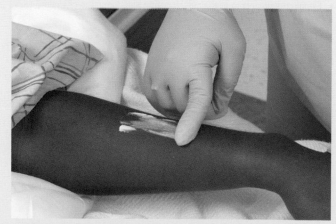

Fig. 12-1 A cream is applied with a gloved index finger. (Courtesy Rick Brady, from Lilley LL and others: *Pharmacology and the nursing process,* ed 5, St Louis, 2007, Mosby.)

Applying Nitroglycerin Ointment

Nitroglycerin ointment is used to prevent angina (chest pain). It relaxes the heart's blood vessels and increases the blood and oxygen supply to the heart. See Chapter 21.

The dosage applied must be accurate. To properly apply nitroglycerin ointment, follow these rules:

- Wear gloves. Do not let any ointment touch any part of your skin.
- Check for an old application:
  - Check the MAR
  - Ask the person for the location of an existing application
- Do not assume that there are no applications or that one has fallen off. Carefully check the person's skin. This is especially important if the person is confused, sedated, or nonresponsive.
- Remove the old application before applying a new one. Check the person carefully to make sure there is only one old application. If you find more than one, tell the nurse at once. Remove all applications before applying a new one.
- Rotate the application site. Different sites are used to prevent skin irritation. Check the MAR or care plan for the rotation schedule.
- Apply the drug to clean, dry skin that has little or no hair (Fig. 12-2).
- Do not shave an area to apply the ointment, as shaving can cause skin irritation.
- Do not apply the ointment to irritated, scarred, open, broken, or calloused skin areas. Such areas can negatively affect drug absorption.

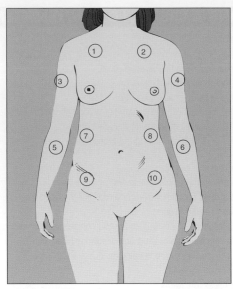

Fig. 12-2 Sites for applying nitroglycerin ointment. The sites also are used for a transdermal patch.

- Do not rub or massage the ointment into the skin.
- Date, time, and sign your name and title to the tape securing the new application. Also include the drug name and dosage. Do not use a ball-point pen, as they can easily puncture the application.
- Document the application site on the MAR.

See *Promoting Safety and Comfort: Applying Nitroglycerin Ointment.*

APPLYING NITROGLYCERIN OINTMENT

Quality Of Life

Remember to:

- Knock before entering the person's room.
- Address the person by name.
- Introduce yourself by name and title.
- Explain the procedure to the person before and during the procedure.
- Protect the person's rights during the procedure.
- Handle the person gently during the procedure.

Pre-procedure

1. Follow *Delegation Guidelines: Applying Creams, Lotions, Ointments, and Powders.* See *Promoting Safety and Comfort:*
   - *Applying Creams, Lotions, Ointments, and Powders*
   - *Applying Nitroglycerin Ointment.*
2. Check the most recent drug order and compare to the medication profile. Focus on the 6 Rights of Drug Administration (Chapter 10).
3. Check with the nurse if you have any questions.
4. Perform hand hygiene.
5. Collect necessary items:
   - Soap or other approved cleansing agent
   - Washcloth and towel
   - Wash basin with warm water
   - Applicator paper
   - See-through dressing
   - Non-allergic tape
   - Gloves
   - MAR

Procedure

6. Read the order on the MAR.
7. Select the nitroglycerin ointment from the drug cart/system.
8. Compare the drug order on the MAR against the pharmacy label on the nitroglycerin tube or unit-dose packet. **(First safety check.)** Review the 6 Rights of Drug Administration (Chapter 10).
9. Check the drug container for an expiration date. Bring the drug to the person's bedside.
10. Provide for privacy.
11. Identify the person. Check the ID bracelet against the MAR. Make sure you use at least two identifiers according to agency policy and call the person by name. Follow agency policy if using a barcode scanner.
12. Put on gloves.
13. Position the person to expose the old application site. Expose the site.
14. Remove the old application. Fold the old application in half with the sticky sides together. Discard the application according to agency policy. Make sure that no one can access the old application.
15. Clean and dry the old application site.
16. Observe the old application site.
17. Position the person to expose the new application site. Expose and observe the site.
18. Clean and dry the new application site. Follow agency policy.
19. Remove and discard the gloves. Perform hand hygiene.
20. Put on clean gloves.
21. Compare the drug order on the MAR against the pharmacy label on the drug container or unit-dose packet. **(Second safety check.)** Review the 6 Rights of Drug Administration (Chapter 10).

APPLYING NITROGLYCERIN OINTMENT—cont'd

22. Use the dose-measuring paper (which includes a ruler along the side or in the middle) to measure the ordered dose (Fig. 12-3, *A*). The print side should be *down*.
23. Squeeze a ribbon of ointment on the paper for the amount ordered (Fig. 12-3, *B*). For example, if the order is for 2 inches, squeeze a ribbon length of 2 inches using the ruler on the dose-measuring paper.
24. Close the container. Compare the drug order on the MAR against the pharmacy label on the drug container. **(Third safety check.)** Review the 6 Rights of Drug Administration (Chapter 10).
25. Apply the paper, ointment side down, to the application site (Fig. 12-3, *C*).
26. Use the paper to spread a thin, uniform layer of ointment under the paper. *Do not rub the ointment into the skin.*
27. Leave the paper in place.
28. Cover the paper and application site with a see-through dressing. Tape the dressing in place.
29. Date, time, and sign your name and title to the tape. Include the drug name and dosage.

30. Return the container to the drug cart/system.

Post-procedure
31. Discard the used supplies.
32. Follow agency policy for soiled linen.
33. While wearing gloves, empty and clean the wash basin. Return it and other supplies to their proper location.
34. Remove the gloves. Perform hand hygiene.
35. Provide for comfort and complete a safety check before leaving the room. (See the inside back cover of this book.)
36. Unscreen the person.
37. Record the *right documentation* on the MAR:
    - The removal of an old application and from what site
    - The date, time, drug name, dosage, and route of administration
    - The application site
    - Your name or initials
38. Report and record any specific patient or resident observations or concerns to the nurse.

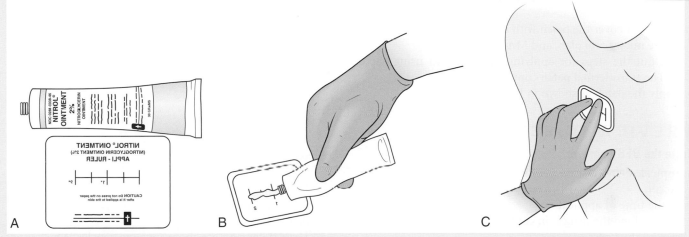

Fig. 12-3 A, Nitroglycerin ointment and application paper. **B,** The ordered amount is squeezed onto the paper. **C,** The ointment is applied to the skin. (Redrawn and modified from Edmunds MW: *Introduction to clinical pharmacology,* ed 5, St Louis, 2006, Mosby.)

PROMOTING SAFETY AND COMFORT

Applying Nitroglycerin Ointment

Safety
Some people may have more body hair than others. Check with the nurse about the application sites; the nurse may have you clip hair at an application site. Remember, do not let the drug touch any part of your skin. If contact occurs, the drug will absorb into your skin and blood and you will feel its effect.

TRANSDERMAL PATCH

Transdermal means through *(trans)* the skin *(dermal)*. A **transdermal patch** (also called a transdermal disk) provides continuous, gradual absorption of a drug through the skin and into the bloodstream; the effect is systemic. *Systemic* relates to the whole body.

A transdermal disk or patch provides controlled release of a drug (Fig. 12-4). The drug is slowly absorbed over several hours or days. The dose released depends on the drug and the size of the skin area covered.

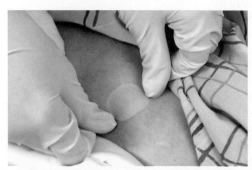

Fig. 12-4 Transdermal patch. (Courtesy Rick Brady, from Lilley LL and others: *Pharmacology and the nursing process,* ed 5, St Louis, 2007, Mosby.)

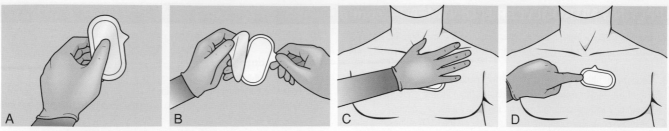

Fig. 12-5 Applying a transdermal patch. **A,** Pick up the patch with the clear plastic backing facing you. Some patches include tabs to assist with removal. **B,** Remove the clear plastic backing. Do not touch the inside of the exposed patch. **C,** Place the exposed adhesive side of the patch onto the skin. Press firmly with the palm of your hand. **D,** Circle the outside edge of the patch with one or two fingers; this helps secure the patch to the skin.

To apply a transdermal patch:
- Follow the rules in Box 12-1.
- Follow the rules listed for "Applying Nitroglycerin Ointment." p. 128.
- Follow the procedure: *Applying Nitroglycerin Ointment.* p. 128-129.
  - Do not cover the patch with a dressing unless directed by the nurse, care plan, and MAR.
  - Omit the steps for applying the ointment using paper. The transdermal patch contains the drug.
- Apply the patch as shown in Fig. 12-5.

See *Promoting Safety and Comfort: Transdermal Patch.*

PROMOTING SAFETY AND COMFORT
Transdermal Patch

Safety

Always carefully look for the old transdermal patch before applying a new one. Patches may be hard to see on the skin because:
- Many patches are clear
- The drug name printed on the patch may have rubbed off

REVIEW QUESTIONS

Circle the BEST answer.

1. Topical drug absorption is affected by the following, *except:*
   a. the time of application
   b. how long the drug is in contact with the skin
   c. skin thickness
   d. amount of water in the skin tissue
2. A topical drug is applied to debride a wound. Debriding is done to:
   a. relieve itching
   b. provide a protective barrier to the skin
   c. reduce inflammation
   d. promote healing
3. Which of the following is a watery preparation?
   a. cream
   b. lotion
   c. ointment
   d. powder
4. Which of the following do you shake before use?
   a. cream
   b. lotion
   c. ointment
   d. powder
5. Lotions are used for the following reasons, *except:*
   a. absorb moisture
   b. soothe and protect the skin
   c. relieve itching
   d. cleanse the skin

6. Which topical dose form is dabbed onto the skin?
   a. cream
   b. lotion
   c. ointment
   d. powder
7. These statements are about applying powder. Which is *false?*
   a. You may shake or sprinkle powder onto the person.
   b. Powder is applied in a thin layer.
   c. Powder is slippery and can cause falls.
   d. Smooth over the area after applying powder for even coverage.
8. Before applying a topical dose form, always:
   a. provide for the person's privacy
   b. follow isolation precautions
   c. shave the application site
   d. clip hair at the application site
9. An ointment is in a jar. What should you use to remove the amount ordered?
   a. your hand
   b. a sterile tongue blade
   c. a syringe
   d. a measuring spoon
10. These statements are about nitroglycerin ointment and transdermal patches. Which is *false?*
   a. An old application is removed before applying a new one.
   b. Ointment is rubbed or massaged into the skin.
   c. The application site is rotated.
   d. The drug is applied to a skin site with little or no hair.

11. Which is used to measure the ordered dose of nitroglycerin ointment?
    a. a measuring spoon
    b. a medicine cup
    c. dose-measuring paper
    d. a transdermal patch

Circle T if the statement is true. Circle F if the statement is false.

12. T F A person gets a drug through the topical route. The drug action is usually short and requires frequent application.

13. T F You must wear gloves to apply a topical dose form.
14. T F It's okay if a topical dose form touches your skin.
15. T F Topical drugs are applied to clean, dry skin.
16. T F You can use your gloved hand to apply creams and ointments as directed by the nurse.
17. T F Creams and ointments are applied in the direction of hair growth.
18. T F It's okay if nitroglycerin ointment touches your skin.
19. T F A transdermal patch requires a dressing.

Answers to these questions can be found on the Evolve Resources site: http://evolve.elsevier.com/Anderson/medasst/

13

Eye, Ear, Nose, and Inhaled Drugs

OBJECTIVES

- Define the key terms and key abbreviations used in this chapter.
- Explain the safety rules for giving eye, ear, nose, and inhaled drugs.
- Perform the procedures described in this chapter.

PROCEDURES

- Applying Medications to the Eye
- Instilling Ear Drops
- Giving Nose Medications
- Giving Inhaled Medications

KEY TERMS

cerumen Ear wax
instill To enter drop by drop
nasal Pertains to the nose

ocular Pertains to the eye
ophthalmic Pertains to the eye
otic Pertains to the ear

KEY ABBREVIATIONS

ID Identification
ISMP Institute for Safe Medication Practices

MAR Medication administration record
MDI Metered-dose inhaler

The eyes, ears, and nose contain mucous membranes. Drugs are well absorbed across such surfaces. Inhaled drugs are also well-absorbed through the mucous membranes. To safely give eye, ear, nose, and inhaled medications, follow the rules in Box 13-1.

EYE MEDICATIONS

Ophthalmic and **ocular** are terms that pertain to the eye (*Opthalmo* means *eye; ocular* also means *eye.*) Ocular drugs are usually in the form of drops or ointments.

See *Delegation Guidelines: Eye Medications.*
See *Promoting Safety and Comfort: Eye Medications.*

DELEGATION GUIDELINES

Eye Medications

Before applying drugs to the eye, you need the following information from the nurse, care plan, and MAR:

- How many eye medications are ordered
- If more than one drug is ordered for the eyes, which should be given first, second, third, etc.
- If the drug is to be given in the left eye, right eye, or both eyes.
- How long to wait before applying more than one eye medication (if ordered); usually 1 to 5 minutes between applications

- Observations to report and record:
  - Color of the sclera
  - Redness
  - Irritation
  - Drainage
  - Complaints of pain or discomfort
- When to report observations
- What specific patient or resident concerns to report immediately

PROMOTING SAFETY AND COMFORT

Eye Medications

Safety
If a drug ordered for the eye is not labeled "ophthalmic," do not administer the drug to the eye. Check with the nurse.

The drug order should read "right eye," "left eye," or "each eye." According to the Institute for Safe Medication Practices (ISMP), the following error-prone abbreviations should be avoided: OD (right eye), OS (left eye), and OU (each eye). If a drug order contains such abbreviations, check with the nurse before giving the drug.

BOX 13-1 Administering Eye, Ear, Nose, and Inhaled Drugs

General Rules

- Perform hand hygiene.
- Follow Standard Precautions and the Bloodborne Pathogen Standard (Chapter 6).
- Wear gloves.
- Use only the dropper supplied by the drug manufacturer.
- Do not let the dropper touch the eye, ear, nose, face, or other body part.
- Use a separate bottle or tube for each person.

Eye Medications

- Position the person properly:
- Supine, sitting, or Fowler's position.
- The head is tilted back slightly. The face is directed toward the ceiling.
- Remove eye secretions with saline and gauze squares, cotton balls, or a washcloth. Clean from the inner aspect of the eye to the outer aspect.
- Give eye drops at room temperature.
- Do not allow the container tip to touch the eye, face, or other body part.
- Apply the drops or ointment to the conjunctival sac (Fig. 13-1). Do not apply the drug directly onto the eyeball.
- Have the person gently close the eye after the application.
- Use a tissue to blot medication that runs out of the eye. Do not rub or wipe the eye.

Ear Medications

- Give ear drops at room temperature. If refrigerated, allow the container to warm to room temperature. This may take about 30 minutes.
- Position the person in a side-lying position. The affected ear is up.
- Remove excessive amounts of cerumen (ear wax). Use a wet washcloth.

Nasal Medications

- Explain that the medication may cause a burning or stinging feeling.
- Position the person properly:
- For nose drops: supine with the head over the edge of the mattress
- For nasal spray: sitting or Fowler's position
- Remind the person not to blow his or her nose after receiving a nasal medication.

Inhaled Medications

- Follow the manufacturer's instructions for the inhaler used.
- Give a bronchodilator (Chapter 25) before giving a corticosteroid (Chapter 29).
- Check inside the inhaler after removing the cap. Look for and remove foreign matter.
- Have the person rinse his or her mouth after inhaling a corticosteroid. This helps prevent a fungal infection in the mouth.
- Clean the inhaler and spacer after use. Follow the manufacturer's instruction.

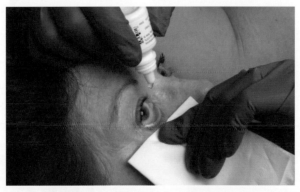

Fig. 13-1 The lower conjunctival sac is exposed. (From Elkin MK, Perry AG, Potter PA: *Nursing interventions & clinical skills,* ed 4, St Louis, 2007, Mosby.)

APPLYING MEDICATIONS TO THE EYE

Quality of Life

Remember to:

- Knock before entering the person's room.
- Address the person by name.
- Introduce yourself by name and title.
- Explain the procedure to the person before beginning and during the procedure.
- Protect the person's rights during the procedure.
- Handle the person gently during the procedure.

Pre-procedure

1. Follow *Delegation Guidelines: Eye Medications.* See *Promoting Safety and Comfort: Eye Medications.*
2. Check the most recent drug order. Compare the drug order to the medication profile. Focus on the 6 Rights of Drug Administration (Chapter 10).
3. Check with the nurse if you have any questions.
4. Perform hand hygiene.
5. Collect the following:
   - Gauze squares, cotton balls, or a washcloth
   - Saline solution
   - Tissues
   - Gloves
   - MAR

Procedure

6. Read the order on the MAR.
7. Select the right drug from the drug cart/system.
8. Compare the drug order on the MAR against the pharmacy label on the drug container or unit-dose packet. **(First safety check.)** Review the 6 Rights of Drug Administration (Chapter 10).
9. Check the drug container for an expiration date. Bring the drug to the person's bedside.
10. Provide for privacy.
11. Identify the person. Check the ID bracelet against the MAR. Make sure you use at least two identifiers according to agency policy. Also call the person by name. Follow agency policy if using a bar code scanner.
12. Put on gloves.
13. Position the person supine or in a sitting position. The head is tilted back slightly.
14. Remove eye drainage as needed. Clean from the inner aspect to the outer aspect. Use a new gauze square or cotton ball with saline for each wipe. If using a washcloth, use a clean part of the washcloth for each wipe.

Continued

APPLYING MEDICATIONS TO THE EYE—cont'd

15. Observe the eye.
16. Remove and discard the gloves. Perform hand hygiene. Put on clean gloves.
17. Compare the drug order on the MAR against the pharmacy label on the drug container. **(Second safety check.)** Review the 6 Rights of Drug Administration (Chapter 10).
18. Open the container. For ointment, place the lid or cap upside down on a clean surface.
19. Compare the drug order on the MAR against the pharmacy label on the drug container. **(Third safety check.)** Review the 6 Rights of Drug Administration (Chapter 10).
20. Ask the person to look up toward the ceiling.
21. Expose the lower conjunctival sac with your non-dominant hand. Gently pull down on the lower lid (see Fig. 13-1). Use a gauze square, cotton ball, or tissue if desired.
22. Apply eye drops:
    a. Hold the container in your dominant hand.
    b. Hold the dropper ½ to ¾ inch above the conjunctival sac. Avoid touching the dropper to any part of the eye.
    c. Drop the ordered number of drops into the conjunctival sac (Fig. 13-2, *A*).
    d. Release the lower lid.
    e. Apply gentle pressure to the inner corner of the eyelid on the bone for 1 to 2 minutes (Fig. 13-2, *B*). Use a clean cotton ball or tissue. This promotes proper absorption.
23. Apply eye ointment:
    a. Squeeze the ointment in a strip fashion into the conjunctival sac (Fig. 13-3). Start at the inner aspect and move toward the outer aspect. Avoid touching the container to any part of the eye.
    b. Release the lower lid.
    c. Ask the person to:
       (1) Gently close the eyes.
       (2) Move the eyes with the lids shut as if looking around the room. This spreads the medication over the eye.
24. Cap and return the container to the drug cart/system.

Post-procedure

25. Discard the supplies.
26. Follow agency policy for soiled linen.
27. Remove the gloves. Perform hand hygiene.
28. Provide for comfort and complete a safety check before leaving the room. (See the inside back cover of this book.)
29. Unscreen the person.
30. Record the *right documentation* on the MAR:
    - The date, time, drug name, dosage, and route of administration
    - The application site
    - Your name or initials
31. Report and record any specific patient or resident observations or concerns to the nurse.

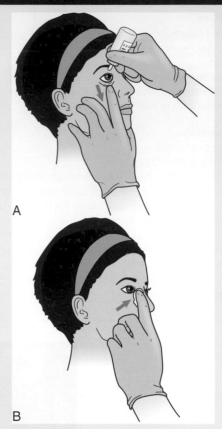

Fig. 13-2 Eye drops. **A,** Drops are given into the conjunctival sac. **B,** Pressure is applied to the inner corner of the eyelid on the bone.

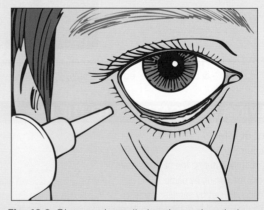

Fig. 13-3 Ointment is applied to the conjunctival sac.

EAR MEDICATIONS

Otic pertains to the ear *(oto)*. Otic (ear) drops are used to treat ear inflammations and infections. They also are used to soften ear wax (cerumen).

Ear drops are instilled into the ear. To instill means to enter drop by drop.

See *Delegation Guidelines: Ear Medications.*
See *Promoting Safety and Comfort: Ear Medications.*

DELEGATION GUIDELINES
Ear Medications

Before applying drugs to the ear, you need this information from the nurse, care plan, and MAR:
- How long to wait before instilling ear drops in the other ear (if ordered)—usually 5 to 10 minutes.
- How long the person needs to remain in the side-lying position after receiving the ear drops—usually 5 to 10 minutes.
- If you need to insert a cotton plug into the ear. If yes, how long should it remain in place—usually about 15 minutes.
- What observations to report and record:
  - Redness
  - Irritation
  - Drainage
  - Complaints of pain or discomfort
- When to report observations.
- What specific patient or resident concerns to report at once.

PROMOTING SAFETY AND COMFORT
Ear Medications

Safety

If a drug ordered for the ear is not labeled "otic," *do not administer the drug to the ear. Check with the nurse.*

The drug order should read "right ear," "left ear," or "each ear." According to the ISMP, the following error-prone abbreviations should be avoided: AD (right ear), AS (left ear), and AU (each ear). If a drug order contains such abbreviations, check with the nurse before giving the drug.

If you can see excess ear wax, remove it with a wet washcloth. Do not insert cotton swabs or cotton-tipped applicators into the ear. If you cannot remove the wax, call for the nurse.

Comfort

Ear drops are given at room temperature. Cold ear drops can cause nausea, pain, and dizziness.

INSTILLING EAR DROPS

Quality of Life
Remember to:
- Knock before entering the person's room.
- Address the person by name.
- Introduce yourself by name and title.
- Explain the procedure to the person before beginning and during the procedure.
- Protect the person's rights during the procedure.
- Handle the person gently during the procedure.

Pre-procedure
1. Follow *Delegation Guidelines: Ear Medications.* See *Promoting Safety and Comfort: Ear Medications.*
2. Check the most recent drug order. Compare the drug order to the medication profile. Focus on the 6 Rights of Drug Administration (Chapter 10).
3. Check with the nurse if you have any questions.
4. Perform hand hygiene.
5. Collect needed items:
   - Wet washcloth
   - Cotton plug
   - Gloves
   - MAR

Procedure
6. Read the order on the MAR.
7. Select the right drug from the drug cart/system.
8. Compare the drug order on the MAR against the pharmacy label on the drug container. **(First safety check.)** Review the 6 Rights of Drug Administration (Chapter 10).
9. Check the drug container for an expiration date. Bring the drug to the person's bedside.
10. Provide for privacy.
11. Identify the person. Check the ID bracelet against the MAR. Make sure you use at least two identifiers according to agency policy. Also call the person by name. Follow agency policy if using a bar code scanner.
12. Put on gloves.
13. Position the person in a side-lying position. The affected ear is up.
14. Remove excess ear wax with a wet washcloth.
15. Observe the ear.

16. Compare the drug order on the MAR against the pharmacy label on the drug container. **(Second safety check.)** Review the 6 Rights of Drug Administration (Chapter 10).
17. Shake the container.
18. Draw medication into the dropper.
19. Compare the drug order on the MAR against the pharmacy label on the drug container. **(Third safety check.)** Review the 6 Rights of Drug Administration (Chapter 10).
20. Apply ear drops (for persons 3 years of age and older):
    a. Pull the ear upward and back (Fig. 13-4). This straightens the external auditory canal.
    b. Instill the ordered number of drops along the side of the ear canal.
    c. Return the dropper to the container.
21. Insert a cotton plug loosely into the ear if ordered. This prevents the medication from flowing out of the ear.
22. Have the person remain in the side-lying position for 5 to 10 minutes or as directed by the nurse and the care plan.
23. Return the container to the drug cart/system.

Post-procedure
24. Discard the supplies or unit dose packages.
25. Follow agency policy for soiled linen.

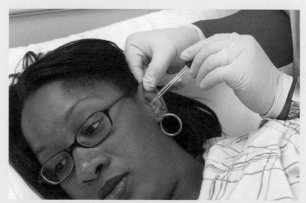

Fig. 13-4 The adult's ear is pulled upward and back. Ear drops are instilled. (Courtesy Rick Brady, from Lilley LL and others: *Pharmacology and the nursing process,* ed 5, St Louis, 2007, Mosby.)

Continued

INSTILLING EAR DROPS—cont'd

26. Remove the gloves. Perform hand hygiene.
27. Provide for comfort and complete a safety check before leaving the room. (See the inside back cover of this book.)
28. Unscreen the person.
29. Record the *right documentation* on the MAR:
    - The date, time, drug name, dosage, and route of administration

- The application site
- Your name or initials

30. Report and record any specific patient or resident observations or concerns to the nurse.
31. Remember to wear gloves when you return to the person's room to remove the cotton plug.

NOSE MEDICATIONS

Nasal means nose *(naso)*. Nose drops and nasal sprays are used to administer drugs to the mucous membranes of the nose.

See *Delegation Guidelines: Nose Medications.*
See *Promoting Safety and Comfort: Nose Medications.*

DELEGATION GUIDELINES

Nose Medications

Before applying drugs to the nose, you need this information from the nurse, care plan, and MAR:
- If the person needs to blow his or her nose before receiving the drug.
- If the person can be positioned with his or her head over the edge of the mattress for nose drops. If not, how to position the person.
- How long the person needs to remain in the supine position after receiving nose drops—usually 5 minutes.
- How long the person must wait to blow his or her nose after receiving the drug.

- What observations to report and record:
  - Redness
  - Irritation
  - Drainage
  - Bleeding
  - Nasal congestion
  - Complaints of pain or discomfort
- When to report observations.
- What specific patient or resident concerns to report at once.

PROMOTING SAFETY AND COMFORT

Nose Medications

Safety
Certain conditions make blowing the nose unsafe. Nasal surgery and head injuries or surgeries are examples. Blowing the nose can increase pressure inside the person's head. Always check with the nurse and the care plan before asking a person to blow his or her nose.

GIVING NOSE MEDICATIONS

Quality of Life

Remember to:
- Knock before entering the person's room.
- Address the person by name.
- Introduce yourself by name and title.
- Explain the procedure to the person before beginning and during the procedure.
- Protect the person's rights during the procedure.
- Handle the person gently during the procedure.

Pre-procedure

1. Follow *Delegation Guidelines: Nose Medications.* See *Promoting Safety and Comfort: Nose Medications.*
2. Check the most recent drug order. Compare the drug order to the medication profile. Focus on the 6 Rights of Drug Administration (Chapter 10).
3. Check with the nurse if you have any questions.
4. Perform hand hygiene.
5. Collect needed items:
   - Tissues
   - Gloves
   - MAR

Procedure

7. Read the order on the MAR.
8. Select the right drug from the drug cart/system.
9. Compare the drug order on the MAR against the pharmacy label on the drug container. **(First safety check.)** Review the 6 Rights of Drug Administration (Chapter 10).
10. Check the drug container for an expiration date. Bring the drug to the person's bedside.
11. Provide for privacy.
12. Identify the person. Check the ID bracelet against the MAR. Make sure you use at least two identifiers according to agency policy. Also call the person by name. Follow agency policy if using a bar code scanner.
13. Put on gloves.
14. Observe the nose.
15. Compare the drug order on the MAR against the pharmacy label on the drug container. **(Second safety check.)** Review the 6 Rights of Drug Administration (Chapter 10).
16. Open the container. For nasal spray, place the lid or cap upside down on a clean surface.

GIVING NOSE MEDICATIONS—cont'd

17. Compare the drug order on the MAR against the pharmacy label on the drug container. **(Third safety check.)** Review the 6 Rights of Drug Administration (Chapter 10).
18. Give the drug:
    a. Nose drops (for adults and older children):
       (1) Ask the person to gently blow the nose (Fig. 13-5, *A*). Provide tissues.
       (2) Position the person supine with the head over the edge of the mattress. Or position the person as directed by the nurse and the care plan.
       (3) Draw medication into the dropper (Fig. 13-5, *B*).
       (4) Hold the dropper about ½ inch above the nostril.
       (5) Instill the number of drops ordered (Fig. 13-5, *C*).
       (6) Repeat steps 18 a (3)–(5) for the other nostril.
       (7) Have the person remain as positioned for 5 minutes. Or for as long as directed by the nurse and the care plan.
    b. Nasal spray:
       (1) Provide tissues. Ask the person to gently blow the nose.
       (2) Position the person in a sitting or Fowler's position.
       (3) Block one nostril (Fig. 13-6, *A*).
       (4) Hold the spray bottle upright. Shake the bottle.
       (5) Insert the bottle tip into the nostril.

       (6) Ask the person to take a deep breath through the nose.
       (7) Squeeze a puff of spray into the nostril as the person is taking a deep breath (Fig. 13-6, *B*).
       (8) Wipe the bottle tip if you need to spray the other nostril. Then repeat steps 18 b (3)–(7).
19. Provide the person with tissues for blotting drainage. Remind the person not to blow his or her nose for several minutes.
20. Return the container to the drug cart/system.

Post-procedure

21. Discard the supplies or unit dose packages.
22. Follow agency policy for soiled linen.
23. Remove the gloves. Perform hand hygiene.
24. Provide for comfort and complete a safety check before leaving the room. (See the inside back cover of this book.)
25. Unscreen the person.
26. Record the *right documentation* on the MAR:
    • The date, time, drug name, dosage, and route of administration
    • The application site
    • Your name or initials
27. Report and record any specific observations or concerns to the nurse.

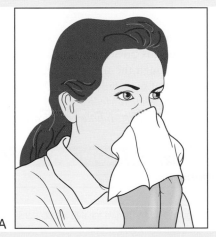
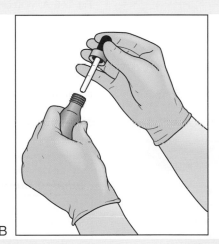
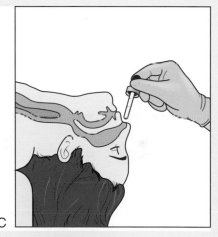

Fig. 13-5 Nose drops. **A,** The person blows her nose. **B,** Drops are drawn into the dropper. **C,** Drops are instilled into the nose.

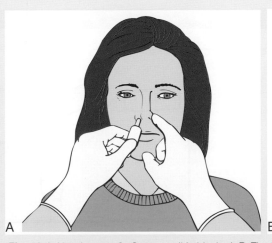
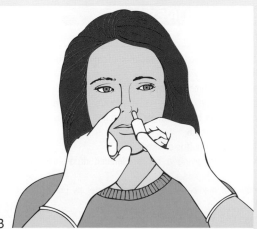

Fig. 13-6 Nasal spray. **A,** One nostril is blocked. **B,** The bottle tip is inserted into the person's nose. A puff of spray is squeezed into the nose as the person takes a deep breath.

INHALED MEDICATIONS

Some corticosteroids (Chapter 28) and bronchodilators (Chapter 24) are inhaled into the respiratory tract through the mouth. Inhaled drugs affect the bronchial smooth muscle. Therefore, absorption and onset of action are rapid.

Metered-dose inhalers (MDIs) are commonly used (Fig. 13-7). (*Meter* means *measure*.) An MDI is a small pressurized canister that contains a spray, mist, or fine powder. A measured (metered) amount of the drug is released for inhalation each time the dispensing valve is pushed or squeezed. MDIs can be used with or without a *spacer* (Fig. 13-8 A & B). A spacer is a tube that attaches to the inhaler. It traps or holds the dose sprayed by the MDI. Part of the dose is not sprayed into the air. The spacer lets the person inhale more slowly and more completely. More of the drug gets into the person's airway. For some people, MDIs are easier to use with spacers.

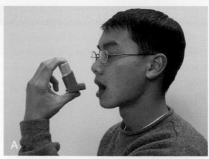

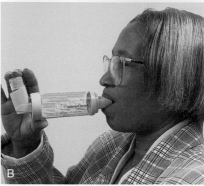

Fig. 13-8 **A,** MDI being used without a spacer. **B,** MDI being used with a spacer.

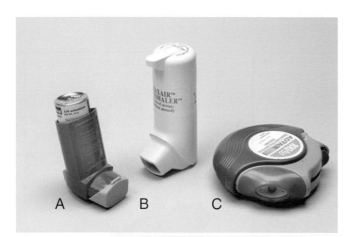

Fig. 13-7 **A,** Metered-dose inhaler (MDI). **B,** Automated, or breath-activated, MDI. **C,** Dry powder inhaler. It delivers powdered medication. (Courtesy Rick Brady, from Lilley LL and others: *Pharmacology and the nursing process,* ed 5, St Louis, 2007, Mosby.)

The automated, or breath-activated, MDI is a pressurized canister with a mouthpiece. It is breath activated. That means when the person inhales through the mouthpiece, the inhaler automatically releases a mist of medication.

See *Delegation Guidelines: Inhaled Medications.*
See *Promoting Safety and Comfort: Inhaled Medications.*

PROMOTING SAFETY AND COMFORT
Inhaled Medications

Safety
Some states and agencies do not let MA-Cs give inhaled medications. Make sure you know what your state and agency allow.

DELEGATION GUIDELINES
Inhaled Medications

Before giving an inhaled medication, you need this information from the nurse, care plan, and MAR:
- If the person uses the MDI himself or herself.
- How many times to shake the canister—usually four or five times.
- If the person can hold his or her breath for 10 seconds. If not, how long can the person hold his or her breath.
- How long to wait if a repeat puff is ordered.
- How long to wait before giving a second inhaled drug—usually 1 to 3 minutes.
- Measure the amount of medication left in the canister by immersing it in water (Fig. 13-9).
- What observations to report and record.
- When to report observations.
- What specific patient or resident concerns to report at once.

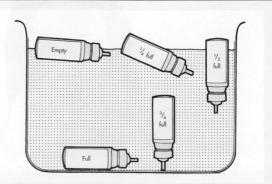

Fig. 13-9 The canister is immersed in water to measure the amount of medication remaining. (From Elkin MK, Perry AG, Potter PA: *Nursing interventions & clinical skills,* ed 4, St Louis, 2007, Mosby.)

GIVING INHALED MEDICATIONS

Quality of Life

Remember to:

- Knock before entering the person's room.
- Address the person by name.
- Introduce yourself by name and title.
- Explain the procedure to the person before beginning and during the procedure.
- Protect the person's rights during the procedure.
- Handle the person gently during the procedure.

Pre-procedure

1. Follow *Delegation Guidelines: Inhaled Medications.* See *Promoting Safety and Comfort: Inhaled Medications.*
2. Check the most recent drug order. Compare the drug order to the medication profile. Focus on the 6 Rights of Drug Administration (Chapter 10).
3. Check with the nurse if you have any questions.
4. Perform hand hygiene.
5. Collect needed items:
   - Tissues
   - Gloves
   - MAR

Procedure

6. Read the order on the MAR.
7. Select the right inhaler from drug cart/system.
8. Compare the drug order on the MAR against the pharmacy label on the drug container. **(First safety check.)** Review the 6 Rights of Drug Administration (Chapter 10).
9. Check the inhaler for an expiration date. Bring the drug to the person's bedside.
10. Provide for privacy.
11. Identify the person. Check the ID bracelet against the MAR. Make sure you use at least two identifiers according to agency policy. Also call the person by name. Follow agency policy if using a bar code scanner.
12. Put on gloves.
13. Compare the drug order on the MAR against the pharmacy label on the drug container. **(Second safety check.)** Review the 6 Rights of Drug Administration (Chapter 10).
14. Position the person so that they are upright—standing, sitting, or Fowler's position.
15. Remove the cap from the inhaler. Place the lid or cap upside down on a clean surface.
16. Compare the drug order on the MAR against the pharmacy label on the drug container. **(Third safety check.)** Review the 6 Rights of Drug Administration (Chapter 10).
17. Hold the inhaler upright.. Use your thumb and first 1 or 2 fingers.
18. Give the drug:
    a. *MDI without a spacer* (Fig. 13-8A):
       (1) Shake the inhaler the number of times as directed by the nurse.
       (2) Ask the person to open his or her mouth. Also ask the person to tilt his or her head back slightly.
       (3) Ask the person to exhale.
       (4) Place the inhaler 1 to 2 inches in front of the person's mouth.
       (5) Push down on or squeeze the dispensing valve. This releases the dose. Ask the person to inhale deeply and slowly for 3 to 5 seconds.
       (6) Ask the person to hold his or her breath for about 10 seconds.
       (7) Ask the person to exhale slowly through his or her mouth.
       (8) Repeat the puffs as ordered:
          (a) Shake the inhaler again.
          (b) Repeat steps 18 a (2)–(7).
    b. *MDI with a spacer* (Fig. 13-8B):
       (1) Insert the inhaler into the spacer.
       (2) Shake the inhaler and spacer the number of times as directed by the nurse.
       (3) Ask the person to open his or her mouth. Also ask the person to tilt his or her head back slightly.
       (4) Ask the person to exhale.
       (5) Ask the person to place the spacer mouthpiece in his or her mouth. Then ask the person to close their lips around the mouthpiece.
       (6) Push down on or squeeze the dispensing valve. This releases the dose. Ask the person to inhale deeply and slowly for 3 to 5 seconds.
       (7) Ask the person to hold his or her breath for about 10 seconds.
       (8) Ask the person to exhale slowly through his or her mouth.
       (9) Repeat the puffs as ordered:
          (a) Shake the inhaler again.
          (b) Repeat steps 18 b (3)–(8).
    c. Automated or breath-activated *MDI*:
       (1) Remove the cap over the mouthpiece.
       (2) Ask the person to exhale.
       (3) Ask the person to place the mouthpiece in their mouth. Then ask the person to close their lips around the mouthpiece.
       (4) Ask the person to inhale deeply through the mouth with a steady, moderate force. You will hear a click and they will feel a mist when their breath activates the medication .
       (5) Ask the person to hold their breath for about 10 seconds.
       (6) Ask the person to exhale slowly through the mouth.
       (7) Repeat the puffs as ordered:
          (a) Repeat steps 18 c (2)–(6).
19. Remove the spacer (if used). Replace the cap on the inhaler.
20. Have the person rinse their mouth with water if they inhaled a corticosteroid.
21. Clean the inhaler and spacer. Follow the manufacturer's instructions. (Wear gloves for this step.)
22. Return the inhaler and spacer to the drug cart/system.

Post-procedure

23. Remove the gloves. Perform hand hygiene.
24. Provide for comfort and complete a safety check before leaving the room. (See the inside back cover of this book.)
25. Unscreen the person.
26. Record the *right documentation* on the MAR:
    - The date, time, drug name, dosage, and route of administration
    - Your name or initials
27. Report and record any specific patient or resident observations or concerns to the nurse.

REVIEW QUESTIONS

Circle the BEST answer.

1. Otic medications are administered to the:
   a. eye
   b. ear
   c. nose
   d. throat

2. To give eye, ear, or nose medications, you should wear:
   a. gloves
   b. a gown
   c. a face mask
   d. a surgical cap

3. Eye drops are ordered. You should use:
   a. a syringe
   b. a dropper from the supply cart
   c. the dropper supplied by the drug manufacturer
   d. a squeeze bottle

4. A person has two eye medications ordered for the same eye. You can usually give the second medication:
   a. immediately
   b. after 1 to 5 minutes
   c. after 5 to 10 minutes
   d. after 10 to 15 minutes

5. Which is *not* a position for giving eye medications?
   a. supine
   b. sitting
   c. Fowler's
   d. with the head over the edge of the mattress

6. A drug order states that a medication is to be given "OS." What should you do?
   a. Give the drug in the left eye.
   b. Give the drug in the right eye.
   c. Give the drug in both eyes.
   d. Check with the nurse.

7. An eye dropper is held:
   a. ½ inch above the eye
   b. 1 inch above the eye
   c. 1½ inches above the eye
   d. 2 inches above the eye

8. After eye ointment is applied, the person should:
   a. wipe the eye
   b. rub the eye
   c. close the eyes gently
   d. stare straight ahead

9. Ear medications are given:
   a. cold
   b. at room temperature
   c. after being heated
   d. directly from the refrigerator

10. To give ear drops, the person is positioned:
    a. in a side-lying position with the affected ear up
    b. in a side-lying position with the affected ear down
    c. supine with the head over the edge of the mattress
    d. sitting with the head turned to one side

11. What should you use to remove excess cerumen?
    a. tongue blade
    b. cotton-tipped applicator
    c. gauze and saline
    d. wet washcloth

12. To instill a drug means to give:
    a. a puff by squeezing a tube
    b. a spray by squeezing a container
    c. it drop by drop
    d. it in a strip fashion

13. Ear drops are ordered for both ears. How long should you wait before giving ear drops in the second ear?
    a. No waiting required.
    b. Wait 1 to 5 minutes.
    c. Wait 5 to 10 minutes.
    d. Wait 10 to 15 minutes.

14. You inserted a cotton plug after giving ear drops. How long should the plug remain in place?
    a. 1 minute
    b. 5 minutes
    c. 10 minutes
    d. 15 minutes

15. After receiving nose drops, how long should the person remain in the supine position?
    a. 1 minute
    b. 5 minutes
    c. 10 minutes
    d. 15 minutes

16. Which is the position for giving nasal spray?
    a. supine
    b. side-lying
    c. Fowler's
    d. with the head over the edge of the mattress

17. To give a nasal spray, you give a puff of spray as the person:
    a. blows his or her nose
    b. takes a deep breath
    c. exhales deeply
    d. holds his or her breath

18. Nasal spray is ordered for both nostrils. What should you do to give the drug in the second nostril?
    a. Get a new spray bottle.
    b. Wipe the bottle tip.
    c. Get a new dropper.
    d. Ask the nurse.

19. Before a person uses an MDI with a spacer, you should:
    a. squeeze the dispensing valve to remove foreign objects
    b. shake the MDI and spacer
    c. ask the person to inhale
    d. have the person rinse out his or her mouth with water

20. The mouthpiece of an MDI spacer is:
    a. placed 1 to 2 inches in front of the person's mouth
    b. placed 3 to 4 inches in front of the person's mouth
    c. positioned near the person's lips
    d. placed in the person's mouth

21. After using an MDI, the person does the following, *except:*
    a. holds his or her breath for about 10 seconds
    b. exhales slowly through the mouth
    c. inhales more puffs immediately
    d. rinses the mouth with water if a corticosteroid was inhaled

Circle T if the statement is true. Circle F if the statement is false.

22. T   F   Eye drops are applied to the eyeball.
23. T   F   Eye ointment is applied from the inner aspect of the conjunctiva to the outer aspect.

24. T   F   To give ear drops to an adult, the ear is pulled upward and back.
25. T   F   A person should blow the nose after receiving a nasal medication.
26. T   F   When using an MDI, you measure the dose released.
27. T   F   When using an automated or breath-activated MDI, when you exhale into the mouthpiece, a dose of the drug is delivered.

Answers to these questions can be found on the Evolve Resources site: http://evolve.elsevier.com/Anderson/medasst/.

14

Vaginal and Rectal Drugs

OBJECTIVES

- Define the key terms listed in this chapter.
- Explain the safety rules for giving vaginal and rectal drugs.
- Perform the procedures described in this chapter.

PROCEDURES

- Giving Vaginal Drugs
- Giving a Rectal Suppository

KEY TERMS

gynecologic Pertains to diseases of the female reproductive organs and breasts

suppository A cone-shaped, solid drug that is inserted into a body opening; melts at body temperature

---

The vagina and rectum are lined with mucous membranes. Vaginal drugs are usually given for a local effect (meaning that the site of action is in the vagina). Rectal drugs may be given for either local or systemic effects. They are given to treat or prevent:

- Constipation
- Anal itching
- Hemorrhoids
- Vomiting
- Fever
- Bladder spasms

Vaginal drugs are usually packaged in the form of creams, gels, tablets, foams, suppositories, or irrigations. A *douche* is used for vaginal irrigation. A douche helps wash the vagina using a topical solution. It is not done for normal female hygiene. It may be required if a vaginal infection and discharge are present. Rectal drugs are usually in the form of suppositories. A **suppository** is a cone-shaped, solid drug that is inserted into a body opening and melts at body temperature. As shown in Fig. 14-1, vaginal suppositories are larger than rectal suppositories. Vaginal suppositories also have a more oval shape than rectal ones.

Suppositories are stored in a cool place to prevent softening. If one becomes soft and the package is sealed, do one of the following until it hardens:

- Hold the foil-wrapped suppository under cold running water
- Place the foil-wrapped suppository in ice water

To properly administer vaginal and rectal drugs, follow the rules listed in Box 14-1.

VAGINAL DRUGS

Vaginal drugs are ordered for some gynecologic disorders. **Gynecologic** pertains to diseases of the female reproductive organs and breasts. (*Gyneco* means *woman*.)

Vaginal creams, gels, tablets, foams, and some suppositories are inserted with applicators provided by the manufacturers (Fig. 14-4). A gloved index finger is often used to insert a suppository.

See *Delegation Guidelines: Vaginal Drugs*.
See *Promoting Safety and Comfort: Vaginal Drugs*.

DELEGATION GUIDELINES
Vaginal Drugs

Before giving a vaginal drug, you will need the following information from the nurse, care plan, and MAR:

- Whether or not the woman can self-administer the drug
- If a perineal pad or panty shield should be applied after administration
- How to position the woman after administering the drug and for how long; usually, the supine position with the hips elevated for 5 to 10 minutes
- If the applicator is to be discarded or washed with soap and water
- How and where to store a reusable applicator
- Observations to report and record:
- Redness, swelling, discharge, bleeding, or irritation
- Color and amount of discharge or bleeding
- Odor
- Complaints of pain, burning, or other discomfort
- Amount and length of symptom relief
- When to report observations
- What specific patient or resident concerns to report immediately

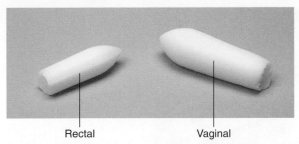

Fig. 14-1 Rectal and vaginal suppositories. (Courtesy Rick Brady, from Lilley LL and others: *Pharmacology and the nursing process*, ed 5, St Louis, 2007, Mosby.)

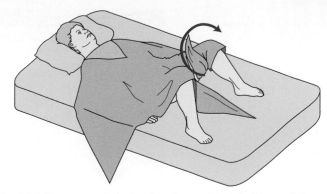

Fig. 14-2 The woman is in the dorsal recumbent position and draped.

BOX 14-1 Administering Vaginal and Rectal Drugs

General Rules
- Practice hand hygiene before and after the application.
- Follow Standard Precautions and the Bloodborne Pathogen Standard (Chapter 6).
- Follow Transmission-Based Precautions as ordered (Chapter 6).
- Wear gloves.
- Provide for privacy.
- Insert the rounded end of the suppository first.
- Remind the person of the nurse's instructions if self-administration is allowed.

Vaginal Drugs
- Administer vaginal suppositories at room temperature.
- Have the woman void before the procedure; a full bladder may cause discomfort.
- Position the woman in the dorsal recumbent position using a pillow to elevate her hips. Drape her as for perineal care. See Fig. 14-2.
- Apply a perineal pad or panty shield after administering the drug. This protects clothing and linens from soiling or staining.
- Have the woman remain supine with her hips elevated for 5 to 10 minutes to allow the suppository to melt and spread within the vagina.

Rectal Drugs
- Ask the person to have a bowel movement (if possible) before the procedure.
- Position the person in the modified left lateral recumbent position. Use the left side-lying position if the person cannot tolerate the modified left prone recumbent position.
- Do not insert the suppository into feces (Fig. 14-3, *A*). The suppository must have contact with the rectal wall (Fig. 14-3, *B*).
- Have the person remain in the modified left prone recumbent position or a left side-lying position for 15 to 20 minutes. The suppository melts and is absorbed during this time.

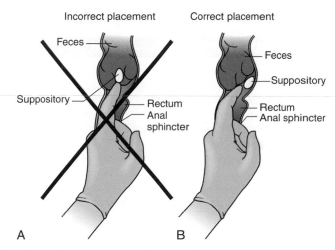

Incorrect placement   Correct placement

A   **B**

Fig. 14-3 A, Do not insert a rectal suppository into feces. **B,** Insert a rectal suppository along the rectal wall. (Modified from deWit SC: *Fundamental concepts and skills for nursing*, ed 2, Philadelphia, 2005, Saunders.)

PROMOTING SAFETY AND COMFORT

Vaginal Drugs

Comfort

Vaginal drugs are often ordered to be administered at bedtime. Doing so allows the drug to remain in place longer and avoids partial loss of the dosage by accidental leakage (which may occur while sitting or standing). Bedtime administration also helps avoid any potential discomfort or embarrassment due to vaginal leakage.

Many women may prefer to self-administer vaginal drugs. The nurse, care plan, and MAR can provide information about self-administration.

GIVING VAGINAL DRUGS

Quality of Life
Remember to:
- Knock before entering the person's room.
- Address the person by name.
- Introduce yourself by name and title.
- Explain the procedure to the person before and during the procedure.
- Protect the person's rights during the procedure.
- Handle the person gently during the procedure.

Pre-procedure
1. Follow *Delegation Guidelines: Vaginal Drugs*. See *Promoting Safety and Comfort: Vaginal Drugs*.

2. Check the most recent drug order and compare it to the medication profile. Focus on the 6 Rights of Drug Administration (Chapter 10).
3. Check with the nurse if you have any questions.
4. Perform hand hygiene.
5. Collect needed items:
   - Vaginal applicator
   - Water-soluble lubricant
   - Pillow
   - Perineal pad or panty shield
   - Gloves
   - Paper towels
   - MAR

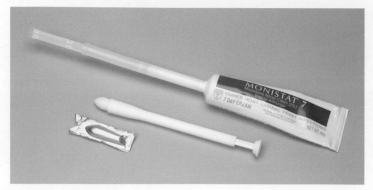

Fig. 14-4 Vaginal cream and suppository with applicators provided by the manufacturers. (Courtesy Rick Brady, from Lilley LL and others: *Pharmacology and the nursing process*, ed 5, St Louis, 2007, Mosby.)

GIVING VAGINAL DRUGS—cont'd

Procedure

6. Read the order on the MAR.
7. Select the right drug from the drug cart/system.
8. Compare the drug order on the MAR against the pharmacy label on the drug container. **(First safety check.)** Review the 6 Rights of Drug Administration (Chapter 10).
9. Check the drug container for an expiration date. Bring the drug to the person's bedside.
10. Provide for privacy.
11. Identify the person. Check the ID bracelet against the MAR. Make sure you use at least two identifiers according to agency policy. Always call the person by name. Follow agency policy if using a barcode scanner.
12. Compare the drug order on the MAR against the pharmacy label on the drug container. **(Second safety check.)** Review the 6 Rights of Drug Administration (Chapter 10).
13. Put on gloves.
14. Position and drape the woman in the dorsal recumbent position with her hips on a pillow.
15. Prepare the drug:
    a. *Cream, foam, or gel with an applicator:*
       (1) Open the container. Place the lid or cap upside down on a clean surface.
       (2) Attach the applicator to the container.
       (3) Squeeze the container to fill the applicator.
       (4) Lubricate the applicator tip using the water-soluble lubricant.
       (5) Set the applicator on a paper towel.
    b. *Suppository:*
       (1) Open and remove the wrapper containing the suppository.
       (2) Insert the suppository into an applicator (if using one).
       (3) Lubricate the suppository using the water-soluble lubricant.
       (4) Set the suppository on a paper towel.
16. Close the container. Compare the drug order on the MAR against the pharmacy label on the drug container. **(Third safety check.)** Review the 6 Rights of Drug Administration (Chapter 10).
17. Expose the perineum.
18. Observe the perineum and vaginal opening.
19. Administer the dose form:
    a. *Cream, foam, gel, or suppository with an applicator:*
       (1) Spread the labia to expose the vagina using your non-dominant hand.
       (2) Insert the applicator as far as possible into the vagina.
       (3) Push the plunger to deposit the drug (Fig. 14-5).
       (4) Remove the applicator.
       (5) Wrap the applicator in the paper towel.

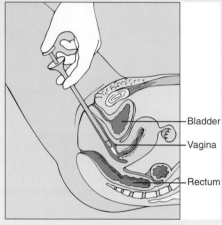

Fig. 14-5 Administering a vaginal cream.

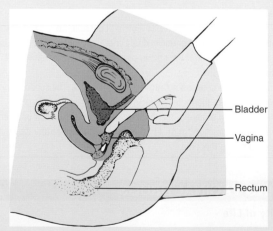

Fig. 14-6 Administering a vaginal suppository. (Modified from Lilley LL and others: *Pharmacology and the nursing process*, ed 5, St Louis, 2007, Mosby.)

    b. *Suppository without an applicator:*
       (1) Lubricate your gloved index finger (if not using an applicator) using the water-soluble lubricant.
       (2) Spread the labia to expose the vagina using your non-dominant hand.
       (3) Use your gloved finger to insert the suppository as far as possible into the vagina (Fig. 14-6).

GIVING VAGINAL DRUGS—cont'd

20. Apply a perineal pad or panty shield.
21. Remove and discard the gloves.
22. Perform hand hygiene.
23. Assist the woman into the supine position with her hips elevated. Ask her to remain in this position for 5 to 10 minutes or position her as directed by the nurse, care plan, or MAR.
24. Put on gloves.
25. Wearing the gloves, empty and clean the applicator. Store it according to agency policy and discard the paper towel.
26. Return the container to the drug cart/system.

Post-procedure

27. Discard the supplies or unit dose packages.
28. Follow agency policy for soiled linen.

29. Remove the gloves. Perform hand hygiene.
30. Provide for comfort and complete a safety check before leaving the room. (See the inside back cover of this book.)
31. Unscreen the person.
32. Record the *right documentation* on the MAR:
    - The date, time, drug name, dosage, and route of administration
    - Your name or initials
33. Report and record any specific patient or resident observations or concerns to the nurse.

RECTAL DRUGS

Suppositories are the most common rectal drugs. They generally are not used:
- After recent prostate surgery
- After recent rectal surgery
- After recent rectal trauma
- If the person has rectal bleeding
- If the person has diarrhea
  See *Delegation Guidelines: Rectal Drugs.*
  See *Promoting Safety and Comfort: Rectal Drugs.*

DELEGATION GUIDELINES

Rectal Drugs

Before administering a rectal drug, you will need the following information from the nurse, care plan, and MAR:
- Whether or not the person can self-administer the drug
- How to position the person after administering the drug and for how long; usually the modified left prone recumbent position or left side-lying position for 15 to 20 minutes
- What observations to report and record for the drug ordered:
  - Redness, swelling, discharge, bleeding, or irritation
  - Color and amount of discharge or bleeding
  - Odor

- Complaints of pain, burning, or other discomfort
- Nausea
- Vomiting
- Respiratory rate
- Temperature
- Color, amount, consistency, shape, and odor of stools
- Amount and length of relief from pain, nausea, or vomiting
- When to report observations
- What specific patient or resident concerns to report immediately

PROMOTING SAFETY AND COMFORT

Rectal Drugs

Comfort

Some people prefer to self-administer rectal drugs; doing so is less embarrassing. The nurse, care plan, and MAR can provide information about self-administration.

GIVING A RECTAL SUPPOSITORY

Quality of Life

Remember to:
- Knock before entering the person's room.
- Address the person by name.
- Introduce yourself by name and title.
- Explain the procedure to the person before and during the procedure.
- Protect the person's rights during the procedure.
- Handle the person gently during the procedure.

Pre-procedure

1. Follow *Delegation Guidelines: Rectal Drugs.* See *Promoting Safety and Comfort: Rectal Drugs.*

2. Check the most recent drug order. Compare the drug order to the medication profile. Focus on the 6 Rights of Drug Administration (Chapter 10).
3. Check with the nurse if you have any questions.
4. Perform hand hygiene.
5. Collect needed items:
   - Water-soluble lubricant
   - Gloves
   - Paper towels
   - Toilet tissue
   - MAR

GIVING A RECTAL SUPPOSITORY—cont'd

Procedure

6. Read the order on the MAR.
7. Select the right drug from the drug cart/system.
8. Compare the drug order on the MAR against the pharmacy label on the drug container. **(First safety check.)** Review the 6 Rights of Drug Administration (Chapter 10).
9. Check the drug container for an expiration date. Bring the drug to the person's bedside.
10. Provide for privacy.
11. Identify the person. Check the ID bracelet against the MAR. Make sure you use at least two identifiers according to agency policy and call the person by name. Follow agency policy if using a bar code scanner.
12. Compare the drug order on the MAR against the pharmacy label on the drug container. **(Second safety check.)** Review the 6 Rights of Drug Administration (Chapter 10).
13. Put on gloves.
14. Position and drape the person in a modified left prone recumbent position or a left side-lying position. Bend the uppermost leg toward the waist.
15. Open and remove the wrapper containing the suppository (Fig. 14-7, *A*).
16. Lubricate the suppository (Fig. 14-7, *B*).
17. Set the suppository on a paper towel.

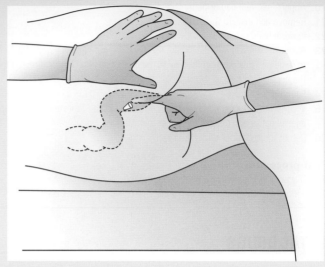

Fig. 14-8 Inserting a rectal suppository. (Modified from Perry AG, Potter PA: *Clinical nursing skills and techniques,* ed 6, St Louis, Mosby.)

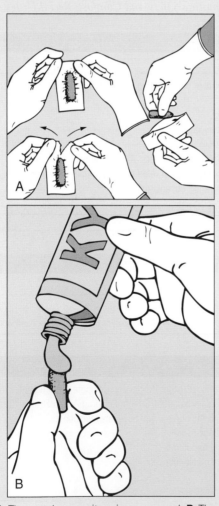

Fig. 14-7 A, The rectal suppository is unwrapped. **B,** The suppository is lubricated with water-soluble lubricant.

18. Compare the drug order on the MAR against the pharmacy label on the drug container. **(Third safety check.)** Review the 6 Rights of Drug Administration (Chapter 10).
19. Expose the rectal area.
20. Observe the rectal area.
21. Insert the suppository:
    a. Raise the upper buttock to expose the anus (Fig. 14-8).
    b. Ask the person to take a deep breath.
    c. Place the rounded tip of the suppository into the anus and rectum. Insert it about 1 inch into the rectum along the rectal wall (see Fig. 14-3, *B*).
22. Wipe the anus with toilet tissue to remove excess lubricant.
23. Ask the person to remain in a left side-lying position for 15 to 20 minutes or position them as directed by the nurse, care plan, or MAR.

Post-procedure

24. Discard the supplies or unit dose packages.
25. Follow agency policy for soiled linen.
26. Remove the gloves. Perform hand hygiene.
27. Provide for comfort and complete a safety check before leaving the room. (See the inside back cover of this book.)
28. Unscreen the person.
29. Record the *right documentation* on the MAR:
    • The date, time, drug name, dosage, and route of administration
    • Your name or initials
30. Report and record any specific patient or resident observations or concerns to the nurse.

REVIEW QUESTIONS

Circle the BEST answer.

1. A cone-shaped solid drug inserted into a body opening is called a:
   a. tablet
   b. foam
   c. gel
   d. suppository

2. Vaginal drugs are given for:
   a. constipation
   b. bladder spasms
   c. vomiting
   d. gynecologic disorders

3. When giving vaginal or rectal drugs, you should always:
   a. wear gloves
   b. wear a gown
   c. wear a mask
   d. wear gloves, a gown, and a mask

4. When giving a vaginal drug, the woman is positioned in:
   a. the dorsal recumbent position
   b. modified left prone recumbent position
   c. a left side-lying position
   d. the supine position

5. A vaginal irrigation (douche) may be given:
   a. to treat constipation
   b. using a suppository
   c. as normal feminine hygiene
   d. if a vaginal infection and discharge are present

6. Before administering a vaginal drug, you should have the woman:
   a. void after the procedure
   b. fill the bladder by drinking extra water
   c. void before the procedure
   d. lay on her right side

7. After receiving a vaginal drug, the woman is positioned in:
   a. the dorsal recumbent position
   b. modified left prone recumbent position
   c. a left side-lying position
   d. the supine position

8. Which is used to give a vaginal cream, gel, or foam?
   a. a gloved finger
   b. an applicator provided by the manufacturer
   c. a cotton-tipped swab
   d. a suppository

9. To protect garments and bed linens after giving a vaginal drug, you can:
   a. apply a perineal pad or panty shield
   b. place a waterproof pad under the buttocks
   c. elevate the woman's hips on pillows
   d. ask the woman to use the bedpan or toilet

10. To give a rectal drug, the person is positioned in:
    a. the dorsal recumbent position
    b. modified left prone recumbent position
    c. a right side-lying position
    d. the supine position

11. A rectal suppository usually melts within:
    a. 5 to 10 minutes
    b. 15 to 20 minutes
    c. 20 to 25 minutes
    d. 25 to 30 minutes

12. A rectal suppository can be given:
    a. for a fever
    b. after rectal surgery
    c. after prostate surgery
    d. if the person has diarrhea

13. Which is used to give a rectal suppository?
    a. a gloved finger
    b. an applicator provided by the manufacturer
    c. a cotton-tipped applicator
    d. an enema tube

Circle T if the statement is true. Circle F if the statement is false.

14. T F Suppositories are stored in a cool place.
15. T F The rounded end of a suppository is inserted first.
16. T F Vaginal suppositories are given at room temperature.
17. T F Vaginal drugs are often ordered to be administered at bedtime.
18. T F A rectal suppository can be inserted into feces.

Answers to these questions can be found on the Evolve Resources site: http://evolve.elsevier.com/Anderson/medasst/

15

Drugs Affecting the Nervous System

OBJECTIVES

- Define the key terms and key abbreviations used in this chapter.
- Review the structures and functions of the nervous system.
- Describe adrenergic agents and their uses.
- Explain how to assist with the nursing process when adrenergic agents are used.
- Describe alpha- and beta-adrenergic blocking agents and their uses.
- Explain how to assist with the nursing process when beta-adrenergic blocking agents are used.
- Describe cholinergic agents and their uses.
- Explain how to assist with the nursing process when cholinergic agents are used.
- Describe anticholinergic agents and their uses.
- Explain how to assist with the nursing process when anticholinergic agents are used.
- Describe sedative-hypnotic drugs and their uses.

- Describe barbiturates and their uses.
- Explain how to assist with the nursing process when barbiturates are used.
- Describe the benzodiazepines.
- Explain how to assist with the nursing process when benzodiazepines are used.
- Describe nonbarbiturate, nonbenzodiazepine sedative-hypnotic agents.
- Explain how to assist with the nursing process when nonbarbiturate, nonbenzodiazepine sedative-hypnotic agents are used.
- Describe the drugs used for Parkinson's disease.
- Explain how to assist with the nursing process when drugs for Parkinson's disease are used.
- Describe the drugs used to treat Alzheimer's disease.
- Explain how to assist with the nursing process when drugs to treat Alzheimer's disease are used.

KEY TERMS

adrenergic fibers   Nerve endings that release the neurotransmitter norepinephrine

adrenergic blocking agent   A drug that inhibits adrenergic effects

agonist   A drug that acts on a certain type of cell to produce a predictable response

anticholinergic agent   A drug that blocks or inhibits cholinergic activity

barbiturate   A drug that depresses the central nervous system, respirations, blood pressure, and temperature

cholinergic fibers   Nerve endings that release the neurotransmitter acetylcholine

homeostasis   A constant internal environment

hypnotic   A drug that produces sleep

inhibitor   A drug that prevents or restricts a certain action

insomnia   A chronic condition in which the person cannot sleep or stay asleep all night

neuron   The basic nerve cell of the nervous system

neurotransmitter   A chemical substance that transmits nerve impulses

sedative   A drug that quiets the person by giving a feeling of relaxation and rest

synapse   The junction between one neuron and the next

KEY ABBREVIATIONS

AD   Alzheimer's disease
CNS   Central nervous system
COMT   Catechol O-methyltransferase
g   Gram
GI   Gastrointestinal
IM   Intramuscular
IV   Intravenous

mcg   Microgram
mg   Milligram
MI   Myocardial infarction
mL   Milliliter
mm Hg   Millimeters of mercury
ODT   Orally disintegrating tablet

The nervous system regulates the body's ongoing activities. See Chapter 5 for a review of the structures and functions of the nervous system.

See *Delegation Guidelines: Drugs Affecting the Nervous System.*

DRUGS AFFECTING THE AUTONOMIC NERVOUS SYSTEM

A **neuron** is the basic nerve cell of the nervous system. Each nerve is composed of a series of segments called neurons. The junction between one neuron and the next is called a **synapse.** Chemical substances called **neurotransmitters** (transmitters of nerve impulses) cause nerve signals or impulses:
- A neurotransmitter is released into the synapse at the end of a neuron.
- Receptors on the next neuron in the chain or at the end of the nerve chain are activated.
- The target organ (e.g., the heart) is stimulated.

Neurotransmitters are excitatory (excite) or inhibitory (inhibit). *Excite* means to stimulate. If the neurotransmitter is excitatory, the neuron is stimulated. *Inhibit* means to slow down, interfere with, or reduce chemical activity. If the neurotransmitter is inhibitory, the neuron's action is slowed. A single neuron releases only one type of neurotransmitter. Therefore, different types of neurons secrete separate neurotransmitters. Regulating neurotransmitters with medication is a way to control diseases caused by an excess or deficiency of neurotransmitters.

Except for skeletal muscle, the autonomic nervous system controls most tissue functions (e.g., blood pressure, gastrointestinal [GI] secretion and motility, urinary bladder function, sweating, and body temperature). The autonomic nervous system maintains a constant internal environment (**homeostasis**) and responds to emergencies. There are two major neurotransmitters released by the autonomic nervous system:
- *Norepinephrine* (nohr ep' in ef' rin). Nerve endings that release norepinephrine are called **adrenergic** (ad' rin er' gek) **fibers.** Drugs that cause effects like those produced by adrenergic neurotransmitters are called *adrenergic, sympathomimetic,* or *catecholamine drugs.* They mimic the action produced by stimulation of the sympathetic nervous system. Those that inhibit adrenergic effects are called **adrenergic blocking agents.**
- *Acetylcholine* (ah se' til koh' leen). Nerve endings that release acetylcholine are called **cholinergic** (koh' lin er' gek) **fibers.** Drugs that cause effects like those produced by acetylcholine are called *cholinergic* or *parasympathomimetic drugs.* They cause the same action produced by stimulation of the parasympathetic nervous system. Drugs that block or inhibit cholinergic activity are called **anticholinergic agents.**

Most organs contain both adrenergic and cholinergic fibers, which produce opposite responses. For example, adrenergic agents increase the heart rate, while cholinergic agents slow the heart rate. In the eyes, adrenergic agents cause the pupils to dilate, and cholinergic agents cause the pupils to constrict.

See Box 15-1 for the clinical uses of drugs affecting the autonomic nervous system.

DRUG CLASS: Adrenergic Agents

There are two broad classes of adrenergic agents: *catecholamines* (kat eh col' 'ah meens) and *noncatecholamines.* Naturally occurring catecholamines are:
- Norepinephrine—secreted from the nerve terminals
- Epinephrine—secreted from the medulla
- Dopamine—secreted at selected sites within the brain, kidneys, and GI tract

These three agents are given to produce the same effects as those naturally secreted. Noncatecholamines have actions similar to the catecholamines. Noncatecholamines are more selective for certain types of receptors, do not act as fast, and have a longer duration.

The autonomic nervous system has *alpha, beta,* and *dopaminergic* (doh' pah min er' gek) receptors. When stimulated by chemicals of certain shapes, the receptors will produce a certain action.
- Alpha-1 receptors—stimulation causes the blood vessels to constrict
- Alpha-2 receptors—prevent further release of norepinephrine
- Beta-1 receptors—increase the heart rate
- Beta-2 receptors—relax the smooth muscle in the bronchi (bronchodilation), uterus, and peripheral arterial blood vessels (vasodilation)
- Dopaminergic receptors:
  - In the brain—improve the symptoms of Parkinson's disease (p. 156)
  - In the kidneys—increase urine output due to better renal blood flow

Many drugs act on more than one type of adrenergic receptor. However, each agent can be used for a certain purpose without many adverse effects. If recommended doses are exceeded, certain receptors may be stimulated excessively, causing serious adverse effects. For example, terbutaline is primarily a beta stimulant. It is an effective bronchodilator when taken in normal doses. Aside from bronchodilation, higher doses of terbutaline cause CNS stimulation, resulting in insomnia and wakefulness. See Table 15-1 for clinical uses of adrenergic agents.

BOX 15-1 Clinical Uses of Drugs Affecting the Autonomic Nervous System

Angina. Angina *(pain)* is chest pain that occurs when the heart needs more oxygen. Chest pain may be described as a tightness, pressure, squeezing, or burning in the chest. The person may appear pale, feel faint, and perspire. Nausea, fatigue, weakness, and difficulty breathing may occur. Some persons complain of "gas" or indigestion.

Aortic stenosis. The left ventricle is enlarged. There is constriction or narrowing *(stenosis)* in the aortic valve.

Arrhythmia. An abnormal heart rhythm.

Asthma. The airway becomes inflamed and narrow, making it difficult for the person to breathe. Extra mucus is produced. Wheezing and coughing are common. The chest may feel tight. Symptoms are mild to severe and are usually triggered by allergies.

Biliary colic. Smooth muscle pain associated with the passing of stones through the bile ducts.

Bronchospasm. Smooth muscles of the lungs contract. The airway narrows and becomes blocked. Coughing and wheezing may occur. See "Asthma."

Emphysema. A lung disease. Oxygen and carbon dioxide exchange cannot occur in affected alveoli. The person has shortness of breath and a cough. Sputum may contain pus. Fatigue is common. The person uses extra effort to breathe in and out, and the body does not get enough oxygen. Breathing is easier when the person sits upright and slightly forward.

Enuresis. Urinary incontinence in bed at night.

Heart failure. Heart failure or congestive heart failure occurs when the heart is weakened and cannot pump normally. Blood backs up and tissue congestion occurs.

Hypertension. In a person with hypertension *(high blood pressure)*, the resting blood pressure is too high. The systolic pressure is 130 mm Hg (millimeters of mercury) or higher *(hyper)*, or the diastolic pressure is 80 mm Hg or higher. Such measurements must occur several times for accurate diagnosis. Narrowed blood vessels are a common cause; the heart pumps with more force to move blood through narrowed vessels.

Hypotension. The systolic blood pressure is below *(hypo)* 90 mm Hg and the diastolic pressure is below 60 mm Hg.

Indigestion. A vague feeling of discomfort above the stomach after eating. Fullness, heartburn, bloating, and nausea are common symptoms.

Irritable bowel syndrome. This disorder may come and go. Nerves that control muscles in the GI tract are too active and the GI tract becomes sensitive to food, feces, gas, and stress. The person experiences abdominal pain, bloating, and constipation or diarrhea.

Migraine. A recurring vascular headache resulting in an intense pulsing or throbbing pain in one area of the head. During a migraine, the person may be sensitive to light and sound. They may experience nausea and vomiting.

Myasthenia gravis. Means *grave muscle weakness*. It is a neuromuscular disease in which the affected person experiences weakness of the skeletal muscles. Muscle weakness increases during activity and improves with rest. Muscles that control the eye and eyelid movement, facial expression, chewing, talking, and swallowing are commonly involved. Muscles that control breathing and movement in the neck, arms, and legs may be affected.

Myocardial infarction (MI). *Myocardial* refers to the heart muscle. *Infarction* means tissue death. When MI occurs, part of the heart muscle dies. Sudden cardiac death *(sudden cardiac arrest)* can occur. Blood flow to the heart muscle is suddenly blocked, and the person may have severe chest pain, usually on the left side. The pain is often described as crushing, stabbing, or squeezing. Pain or numbness in one or both arms, the back, neck, jaw, or stomach may occur. Other signs and symptoms may include indigestion, dyspnea, nausea, dizziness, perspiration, and cold, clammy skin.

Mydriasis. Dilation of the pupil of the eye.

Parkinson's disease. The area of the brain that controls muscle movement is affected.

Peptic ulcer. A sore in the lining of the esophagus, stomach, or duodenum of the small intestine.

Pylorospasm. A spasm of the pyloric sphincter in the stomach.

Tremors. Quivering movements resulting from involuntary contraction and relaxation of skeletal muscles.

Urethral colic. Sharp pain caused by obstruction or smooth muscle spasm of the urethra.

Ventricular dysrhythmia. An abnormal heart rhythm occurring in the heart's ventricles.

TABLE 15-1 Adrenergic Agents

Generic Name	Brand Name	Dose Forms	Clinical Use	Adult Oral Dose
albuterol	Proventil, Ventolin	Aerosol: 90 mcg per puff Tablets: 2, 4 mg Syrup: 2 mg/5 mL Tablets: extended-release 4, 8 mg	Asthma, emphysema	PO: 2-4 mg three to four times daily Inhale: two inhalations q4-6h
ephedrine		Capsules: 25 mg	Nasal decongestant, hypotension	25-50 mg q3-4h
metaproterenol	Alupent	Aerosol: 0.65 mg/puff	Bronchospasm	See manufacturer's recommendations
phenylephrine	Neo-Synephrine	Ophthalmic drops: 2.5%, 10% Nasal solutions: 0.25%, 0.5%, 1% Tablets: 10 mg Syrup: 2.5 mg/5 mL	Shock, hypotension, nasal decongestant, ophthalmic vasoconstrictor, mydriatic	PO: 10-20 mg q4-6h PRN Nasal: 2-3 drops or sprays in each nostril q4h; use for less than 3 days Eyes: 1-2 drops two to three times daily
terbutaline	Brethine, Bricanyl	Tablets: 2.5, 5 mg	Emphysema, asthma, premature labor	5 mg q6h

Modified from Willihnganz M: Clayton's Basic Pharmacology for Nurses, ed 18, St Louis, 2020, Elsevier.

Assisting With the Nursing Process. When giving adrenergic drugs, you will assist the nurse with the nursing process.

Assessment
- Measure heart rate and blood pressure.
- See "Assisting With the Nursing Process" for respiratory tract diseases, bronchodilators, and decongestants (Chapter 25).

Planning. See Table 15-1 for "Dose Forms."

Implementation. See Table 15-1 for "Action" and "Clinical Use."

Evaluation. Side effects are usually dose related and are resolved when the dosage is reduced or the drug is discontinued. Persons with liver disease, thyroid disease, hypertension, and heart disease are at risk for side effects. Persons with diabetes may have more frequent episodes of hyperglycemia. Report and record the following:
- *Palpitations, tachycardia, skin flushing, dizziness, and tremors.* These are usually mild and tend to resolve with continued therapy.
- *Orthostatic hypotension.* This is generally mild when it occurs. Dizziness and weakness may occur when the drug is started. Blood pressure is measured daily in the supine and standing positions. Provide for safety. Remind the person to rise slowly from a supine or sitting position. Have the person sit or lie down to rest if feeling faint.
- *Dysrhythmias, chest pain, severe hypotension, hypertension, angina, nausea, vomiting.* Report these side effects at once; the nurse needs to alert the doctor.

DRUG CLASS: Alpha- and Beta-Adrenergic Blocking Agents

Alpha- and beta-adrenergic blocking agents plug alpha or beta receptors to prevent other agents (usually naturally occurring catecholamines) from stimulating specific receptors.

There are nonselective and selective beta blockers.
- *Nonselective blocking agents.* Inhibit beta-1 and beta-2 receptors.
- *Selective beta-1 blocking agents.* Act against the heart's beta-1 receptors (cardioselective).

The primary action of alpha-receptor stimulants is vasoconstriction (constriction of blood vessels.) Therefore, alpha blocking agents (alpha blockers) are used in persons with diseases associated with vasoconstriction. Alpha blockers cause vasodilation (dilation of blood vessels). Some alpha blockers are used to treat hypertension.

Beta blocking agents (beta blockers) are commonly used after myocardial infarction (MI) and to treat angina, dysrhythmias, and hyperthyroidism. Beta blockers must be used with extreme caution in persons with respiratory disorders (e.g., bronchitis, emphysema, asthma, and allergies). Beta blockers can produce severe bronchoconstriction and may increase wheezing, especially during the pollen season.

Assisting With the Nursing Process. When giving beta blockers, you will assist the nurse with the nursing process.

Assessment
- Measure heart rate and rhythm.
- Measure blood pressure.
- See "Assisting with the Nursing Process" for persons with:

- Hypertension (Chapter 20)
- Antidysrhythmic therapy (Chapter 21)

Planning. See Table 15-2 for "Oral Dose Forms."

Implementation
- See Table 15-2 for "Adult Dosage Range."
- The onset of action is fairly rapid. However, it may take several days or weeks for the desired level of improvement and to stabilize on the lowest dose needed to control the disorder. Angina and MI are risks if the drug is suddenly discontinued. To safely discontinue the drug, the doctor reduces the dosage over 1 to 2 weeks.

Evaluation. Most adverse effects from beta blockers are related to dosage and resolve when the dosage is adjusted. Report and record the following:
- Bradycardia, peripheral vasoconstriction (purple, mottled skin), heart failure (increase in edema, dyspnea, bradycardia, and orthopnea)
- Bronchospasm, wheezing
- Signs and symptoms of hypoglycemia: headache, weakness, decreased coordination, general apprehension, sweating, hunger, or blurred/double vision

DRUG CLASS: Cholinergic Agents

Cholinergic (parasympathomimetic) agents produce effects similar to acetylcholine. Some cholinergic agents directly stimulate the parasympathetic nervous system. Others inhibit acetylcholinesterase—the enzyme that metabolizes acetylcholine when released by a nerve ending. Such agents are *indirect-acting cholinergic agents.*

Cholinergic actions may include:
- Slowed heartbeat
- Increased GI motility and secretions
- Increased urinary bladder contractions with relaxation of muscle sphincter
- Increased secretions and contractility of bronchial smooth muscle
- Sweating
- Miosis of the eye, which reduces intraocular pressure. This causes the pupil to become smaller.
- Increased force of skeletal muscle contractions
- Decreased blood pressure

Cholinergic agents are used to diagnose and treat myasthenia gravis (See Box 15-1).

Assisting With the Nursing Process. When giving cholinergic agents, you will assist the nurse with the nursing process.

Assessment
- Measure heart rate and blood pressure.
- See "Assisting With the Nursing Process" for persons with:
- Respiratory tract disease (Chapter 25)
- Urinary disorders (Chapter 31)
- Eye disorders (Chapter 32)

Planning. See Table 15-3 for "Oral Dose Forms."

Implementation. See Table 15-3 for "Clinical Use."

Evaluation. Cholinergic fibers are present throughout the body, meaning most body systems are affected. Because all receptors do not respond to the same dosage, adverse effects are not

TABLE 15-2   Beta-Adrenergic Blocking Agents

Generic Name	Brand Name	Oral Dose Forms	Clinical Use	Adult Oral Dose
acebutolol	Sectral	Capsules: 200, 400 mg	Hypertension, ventricular dysrhythmias	Initial, 400 mg daily; maintenance, 600-1200 mg daily
atenolol	Tenormin	Tablets: 25, 50, 100 mg	Hypertension, angina, after myocardial infarction	Initial, 50 mg daily; maintenance, up to 200 mg daily
betaxolol		Tablets: 10, 20 mg	Hypertension	Initial, 10 mg daily; maintenance, 20 mg daily
bisoprolol		Tablets: 5, 10 mg	Hypertension	Initial, 5 mg daily; maintenance, 10-20 mg daily
carvedilol	Coreg	Tablets: 3.125, 6.25, 12.5, 25 mg	Hypertension, heart failure, myocardial infarction	Initial, 6.25 mg twice daily; maintenance, up to 50 mg daily
labetalol	Normodyne, Trandate	Tablets: 100, 200, 300 mg	Hypertension	Initial, 100 mg two times daily; maintenance, up to 2400 mg daily
metoprolol	Lopressor, Toprol XL	Tablets: 25, 37.5, 50, 75, 100 mg Tablets, extended release: 25, 50, 100, 200 mg	Hypertension, myocardial infarction, angina, heart failure	Initial, extended release: 100 mg two times daily; maintenance, 100-450 mg daily Initial: regular release: 25-50 mg two times daily; maintenance, 100-400 mg/day given in 2 divided doses.
nadolol	Corgard	Tablets: 20, 40, 80, 120, 160 mg	Angina pectoris, hypertension	Initial, 40 mg once daily; maintenance, 40-320 mg daily; maximum, 320 mg/day
nebivolol	Bystolic	Tablets: 2.5, 5, 10, 20 mg	Hypertension	Initial, 5 mg daily; maintenance, up to 40 mg daily
penbutolol	Levatol	Tablets: 20 mg	Hypertension	Initial, 20 mg daily; maintenance, 20 mg daily
pindolol	Visken	Tablets: 5, 10 mg	Hypertension	Initial, 5 mg twice daily; maximum, 60 mg/day
propranolol	propranolol HCl, Inderal LA, Inderal XL	Tablets: 10, 20, 40, 60, 80 mg Sustained-release capsules: 60, 80, 120, 160 mg	Dysrhythmias, hypertension, angina pectoris, myocardial infarction, migraine, tremors, hypertrophic subaortic stenosis	PO, immediate release: Initial, 40 mg two times daily; maintenance, 120-240 mg daily PO, sustained release: Initial, 80 mg daily; maintenance, 120-160 mg; maximum 640 mg daily
sotalol	Betapace	Tablets: 80, 120, 160, 240 mg	Dysrhythmias	Initial, 80 mg two times daily; maintenance, up to 320 mg daily
timolol	timolol	Tablets: 5, 10, 20 mg	Hypertension, myocardial infarction, migraine, angina pectoris	Initial, 10 mg twice daily; maintenance, up to 30 mg twice daily

Modified from Willihnganz M: Clayton's Basic Pharmacology for Nurses, ed 18, St Louis, 2020, Elsevier.

always apparent. The risk for adverse effects increases with higher dosages. Report and record the following:

- *Nausea, vomiting, diarrhea, abdominal cramping.* These symptoms are dose related.
- *Dizziness, hypotension.* The person's pulse and blood pressure are monitored. The person should rise slowly from a supine or sitting position. They should perform exercises to prevent blood pooling while standing or sitting in one position for prolonged periods. The person should sit or lie down if feeling faint.
- *Bronchospasm, wheezing, bradycardia.* The nurse may tell you to withhold the next dose until the doctor can evaluate the person.

DRUG CLASS: Anticholinergic Agents

Anticholinergic agents are also called *cholinergic blocking agents* or *parasympatholytic agents.* They block the action of acetylcholine

in the parasympathetic nervous system. These drugs occupy receptor sites at parasympathetic nerve endings. By doing so, they prevent the action of acetylcholine, and the parasympathetic response is thereby reduced.

Anticholinergic effects may include:

- Dilation of the pupil with increased intraocular pressure in persons with glaucoma
- Dry, thick secretions of the mouth, nose, throat, and bronchi
- Decreased secretions and motility of the GI tract
- Increased heart rate
- Decreased sweating

Anticholinergic agents are used to treat GI disorders, eye disorders, genitourinary disorders, bradycardia, and Parkinson's disease. They are used preoperatively to:

- Decrease respiratory secretions to prevent aspiration
- Prevent vagal stimulation from skeletal muscle relaxants or placement of an endotracheal tube

TABLE 15-3   Cholinergic Agents

Generic Name	Brand Name	Oral Dose Forms	Clinical Use	Adult Oral Dose
bethanechol	Urecholine	Tablets: 5, 10, 25, 50 mg	Restore bladder tone and urination	10 to 50 mg two to four times daily; Maximum 120 mg daily
neostigmine	Prostigmin	Tablets: 15 mg	Treatment of myasthenia gravis	15 mg three times daily; maintenance, 15 to 375 mg daily
pilocarpine	Isopto Carpine, Pilocar, Salagen tablets	Tablets: 5, 7.5 mg Opthalmic solution: 1, 2, 4%	Treat symptoms of dry mouth to salivary gland hypofunction following radiation therapy Glaucoma	5 mg four times daily; Maximum dosage 30 mg daily. Eyes: 1 drop in affected eye up to four times daily
pyridostigmine	Mestinon, Regonol	Tablets: 60 mg Syrup: 60 mg/5 mL Sustained-release tablets: 180 mg	Treatment of myasthenia gravis	Immediate release: 60 to 1500 mg daily (usually 600 mg/day divided into five or six doses) Sustained-release: 180 to 540 mg once or twice daily at least 6 hours apart

Modified from Willihnganz M: Clayton's Basic Pharmacology for Nurses, ed 18, St Louis, 2020, Elsevier.

TABLE 15-4   Anti-Cholinergic Agents

Generic Name	Brand Name	Oral Dose Forms	Clinical Use	Adult Oral Dose
dicyclomine	Bentyl Bentylol	Tablets: 20 mg Capsules: 10 mg Solution: 10 mg/5 mL	Irritable bowel syndrome	20 mg orally every 6 hours; may increase up to 40 mg every 6 hours; if efficacy not achieved in 2 weeks or adverse effects require dose less than 80 mg/day, therapy should be discontinued; safety data not available for doses greater than 80 mg/day for periods longer than 2 weeks 10-20 mg intramuscularly (IM) every 6 hours; not to exceed 80 mg/day IM
glycopyrrolate	Robinul	Tablets: 1, 2 mg	Reduce salivation. Treatment of peptic or duodenal ulcers. Treatment of irritable bowel syndrome.	PO: 1 mg twice daily to reduce salivation. PO: 1-2 mg two to three times daily for treatment of irritable bowel syndrome and peptic or duodenal ulcers.

Modified from Willihnganz M: Clayton's Basic Pharmacology for Nurses, ed 18, St Louis, 2020, Elsevier.

Assisting With the Nursing Process. When giving anticholinergic agents, you will assist the nurse with the nursing process.

Assessment
- Measure heart rate and blood pressure.
- See "Assisting With the Nursing Process" for:
- Drugs used for Parkinson's disease (p. 156)
- Persons taking antihistamines (Chapter 25)
- Persons with eye disorders (Chapter 32)

   Planning. See Table 15-4 for "Oral Dose Forms."

   Implementation. See Table 15-4 for "Clinical Use."

   Evaluation. Cholinergic fibers are present throughout the body and therefore affect most body systems. Because all receptors do not respond to the same dosage, adverse effects are not always apparent. The risk for adverse effects increases with higher dosages. Report and record the following:
- *Blurred vision; glaucoma; constipation; urinary retention; dryness of the mouth, nose, and throat.* Provide for safety if the person has blurred vision. Follow the care plan for constipation and urinary retention. If dryness of the mouth, nose, or throat occurs, the nurse may allow the person to suck on hard candy or ice chips or chew gum.
- *Confusion, depression, nightmares, hallucinations.* Provide for safety.
- *Orthostatic hypotension.* This is generally mild when it occurs. Dizziness and weakness may occur when the drug is started. Blood pressure is measured daily in the supine and standing positions. Provide for safety. Remind the person to rise slowly from a supine or sitting position. Have the person sit or lie down if feeling faint.
- *Palpitations, dysrhythmias.* Alert the nurse at once.

SEDATIVE-HYPNOTIC DRUGS

Insomnia is a chronic condition in which the person affected cannot sleep or stay asleep all night. Changes in lifestyle or environment are common causes. Insomnia may also be caused by pain, illness, stress, excessive consumption of caffeine and alcohol, or eating a large meal before bedtime.

Sedative-hypnotics are drugs used for altered sleep patterns. A **hypnotic** is a drug that produces sleep. A **sedative** is a drug that quiets the person by providing a feeling of relaxation and rest. Most sedative-hypnotics increase total sleeping time.

Sedatives and hypnotics are not always different drugs. Their effects depend on the dose and the person's condition (e.g., a small dose may act as a sedative whereas a larger dose of the same drug may act as a hypnotic and produce sleep).

Sedative-hypnotics can be used to:
- Treat insomnia and improve sleep
- Decrease anxiety level, increase relaxation, and promote sleep before diagnostic or surgical procedures

   See *Promoting Safety and Comfort: Sedative-Hypnotic Drugs.*

PROMOTING SAFETY AND COMFORT
Sedative-Hypnotic Drugs

Safety
Sedative-hypnotic drugs depress the central nervous system. Assist the nurse with assessment of the person's level of alertness, orientation, and ability to perform motor functions. Practice safety measures and follow the care plan to provide for the person's safety.

A person should not take these drugs while performing any task that requires mental alertness, such as working around machines, driving a car, or administering drugs.

Many of these drugs can cause severe allergic reactions or sleep-related behaviors such as sleep-driving (driving while not fully awake after taking a sedative-hypnotic). The affected person will have no memory of the event. Follow the care plan to provide for safety.

DRUG CLASS: Barbiturates

A **barbiturate** is a drug that depresses the central nervous system, respirations, blood pressure, and temperature. It acts as a sedative or hypnotic. Some barbiturates are used in anesthesia and to treat seizures (Chapter 17).

Depending on the dose of barbiturate, CNS depression can range from mild sedation to deep coma and death. Other factors that may affect CNS depression are the route of administration, tolerance from previous use, CNS excitability, and the person's current condition. The risk of addiction is high.

Barbiturates are rarely used for sleep or sedation. Short-acting barbiturates (e.g., pentobarbital, secobarbital) are used for sedation before diagnostic procedures. The long-acting barbiturate, phenobarbital, is also used as an anticonvulsant (Chapter 17).

Assisting With the Nursing Process. When giving barbiturates, you will assist the nurse with the nursing process.

Assessment
- Measure pulse, respirations, and blood pressure.
- Observe the person's level of alertness.
- Ask the person about pain or discomfort.
  Planning. See Table 15-5 for "Oral Dose Forms."

Implementation
- See Table 15-5 for "Adult Oral Dose."
- Suddenly discontinuing the drug after long-term use of high dosages may cause symptoms similar to alcohol withdrawal, varying from weakness and anxiety to delirium and grand mal seizures. Withdrawal of the drug should be a gradual process over 2 to 4 weeks.

Evaluation. Barbiturates can cause drowsiness, lethargy, headache, muscle or joint pain, and mental depression. Report and record the following:
- *Hangover, sedation, lethargy.* Patients may complain of "morning hangover," blurred vision, or dizziness on arising. *Lethargy* is a state of feeling dull, sleepy, sluggish, or very drowsy. The person may have problems with coordination. If so, have the person rise to a sitting position, gain balance, and then stand. Assist with walking as needed.
- *Excitement, restlessness, confusion.* Older persons and those in severe pain may respond to barbiturates in ways that can prevent sedation or sleep. Provide for safety and help calm and orient them to person, time, and place.
- *Allergic reactions.* Report hives, itching (pruritus), rash, fever, or inflammation of mucous membranes at once. Do not give the drug again until the nurse gives approval.

DRUG CLASS: Benzodiazepines

Benzodiazepines have actions similar to CNS depressants. However, they act more selectively at specific sites, allowing for a variety of uses—sedative-hypnotic, muscle relaxant, antianxiety, and anticonvulsant.

Benzodiazepines are the most commonly used sedative-hypnotics. When therapy is started, the person feels a sense of deep or refreshing sleep. However, the quality of sleep decreases over time. These agents should be used for no more than 4 weeks. When therapy is discontinued, the person may have strange dreams and insomnia.

Drugs in this class are used:
- To produce mild sedation
- For short-term use to produce sleep
- For preoperative sedation (IM and IV dose forms)

TABLE 15-5	Barbiturates			
Generic Name	**Brand Name**	**Oral Dose Forms**	**Clinical Use**	**Adult Oral Dose**
butabarbital	Butisol	Tablets: 15, 30, 50, 100 mg Elixir: 30 mg/5 mL	Primarily a daytime sedative and bedtime hypnotic	Sedation: 15-30 mg three or four times daily Hypnosis: 50-100 mg at bedtime
mephobarbital	Mebaral	Tablets: 32, 50, 100 mg	Primarily an anticonvulsant; may also be used as a daytime sedative	Sedation: 32-100 mg three or four times daily Anti-convulsant: 400-600 mg daily
phenobarbital	Solfoton	Tablets: 15, 16.2, 30, 32.4, 60, 64.8, 97.2, and 100 mg Elixir: 15, 20 mg/5 mL	Most common as an anticonvulsant; may also be used as a daytime sedative, preanesthetic, or hypnotic agent	Sedation: 8-30 mg two or three times daily Hypnosis: 100-320 mg Anti-convulsant: 60-100 mg two or three times daily
secobarbital	Seconal	Capsules: 100 mg	Primarily a daytime sedative or bedtime hypnotic Therapy is not recommended for longer than 15 days	Hypnosis: 100-200 mg at bedtime

Modified from Willihnganz M: Clayton's Basic Pharmacology for Nurses, ed 18, St Louis, 2020, Elsevier.

TABLE 15-6 Benzodiazepines Used for Sedation-Hypnosis

Generic Name	Brand Name	Oral Dose Forms	Clinical Use	Adult Oral Dose
estazolam		Tablets: 1, 2 mg	Hypnosis: 1-2 mg at bedtime	Used to treat insomnia
flurazepam	Flurazepam Apo-Flurazpam	Capsules: 15, 30 mg	Hypnosis: 15-30 mg at bedtime	Used for short-term treatment of insomnia
lorazepam	Ativan Apo-Lorazepam	Tablets: 0.5, 1, 2 mg Oral solution: 2 mg/mL	Hypnosis: 2-4 mg at bedtime	Used primarily to treat insomnia but may also be used for preoperative anxiety, status epilepticus
quazepam	Doral	Tablets: 15 mg	Hypnosis: 7.5-15 mg at bedtime	Used to treat insomnia
temazepam	Restoril	Capsules: 7.5, 15, 22.5, 30 mg	Hypnosis: 15-30 mg at bedtime	Used to treat insomnia
triazolam	Halcion	Tablets: 0.125, 0.25 mg	Hypnosis: 0.125-0.5 mg at bedtime	Used to treat insomnia but tends to lose effectiveness within 2 weeks

Modified from Willihnganz M: Clayton's Basic Pharmacology for Nurses, ed 18, St Louis, 2020, Elsevier.

Assisting With the Nursing Process. When giving benzodiazepines, you will assist the nurse with the nursing process.

Assessment
- Measure vital signs.
- Measure blood pressure in the sitting and supine positions.
- Ask the person to rate their pain using the agency's pain rating scale.
Planning. See Table 15-6 for "Oral Dose Forms."

Implementation
- See Table 15-6 for "Adult Oral Dose."
- The habitual use of these drugs results in physical and psychologic dependence. Rapidly discontinuing the drug after long-term use may cause symptoms similar to alcohol withdrawal (e.g., weakness, anxiety, delirium, and seizures). The symptoms may not appear for several days. Treatment consists of gradual withdrawal of the drug over 2 to 4 weeks.

Evaluation. Benzodiazepines can cause drowsiness, hangover, sedation, and lethargy. Report and record the following:
- *Confusion, agitation, hallucinations, amnesia.* All drugs in this class can cause these symptoms. Older persons who have taken high doses for a prolonged time are at risk.
- *Hypotension.* Remind the person to rise slowly from a supine or sitting position.
- *Liver toxicity.* Symptoms include anorexia, nausea, vomiting, jaundice, and abnormal liver function tests.

DRUG CLASS: Nonbarbiturate, Nonbenzodiazepine Sedative-Hypnotic Agents

These drugs depress the central nervous system and are used to produce sleep. Daytime drowsiness is generally not a problem with these agents.

Drugs in this class are used:
- To produce mild sedation
- For short-term use to produce sleep

Assisting With the Nursing Process. When giving drugs in this class, you will assist the nurse with the nursing process.

Assessment
- Measure vital signs.
- Measure blood pressure in the sitting and supine positions.
- Ask the person to rate their pain using the agency's pain rating scale.
Planning. See Table 15-7 for "Dose Forms."

Implementation
- See Table 15-7 for "Adult Oral Dose."
- Zaleplon, zolpidem, and eszopiclone have a very rapid onset of action. The dose should be taken right before going to bed. The dose may also be taken after the person has gone to bed but is struggling to fall asleep.

Evaluation. General side effects of these drugs include drowsiness, lethargy, headache, muscle or joint pain, and mental depression. Some persons may have short-term restlessness and anxiety before falling asleep. Dullness, moodiness, and coordination problems may also occur. Report and record the following:
- *Hangover, sedation, lethargy.* Patients may complain of "morning hangover," blurred vision, or dizziness on arising. *Lethargy* is a state of feeling dull, sleepy, sluggish, or very drowsy. The person may have problems with coordination. Have the person rise to a sitting position, gain balance, and then stand. Assist with walking as needed.
- *Restlessness, anxiety.* These symptoms are usually mild.
- *Excitement, restlessness, confusion.* Older persons and those in severe pain may respond in ways that directly oppose sedation or sleep. Provide for safety and help calm and orient them to person, time, and place.

DRUGS USED FOR PARKINSON'S DISEASE

Parkinson's disease is a slow, progressive disorder with no cure. The area of the brain that controls muscle movement is affected. Persons over the age of 50 are at risk, with slightly more men than women being affected. All races and ethnic groups are affected. Signs and symptoms of Parkinson's disease become worse over time (Fig. 15-1). They include:
- *Tremors*—often start in one finger and spread to the whole arm. Pill-rolling movements—rubbing the thumb and index finger—may occur. The person may have trembling in the hands, arms, legs, jaw, and face.
- *Rigid, stiff muscles*—in the arms, legs, neck, and trunk.
- *Slow movements*—the person has a slow, shuffling gait.
- *Stooped posture and impaired balance*—it is hard to walk. Falls are a risk.
- *Mask-like expression*—the person cannot blink and smile. A fixed stare is common.

TABLE 15-7   Nonbarbiturate, Nonbenzodiazepine Sedative-Hypnotic Agents

Generic Name	Brand Name	Oral Dose Forms	Clinical Use	Adult Oral Dose
diphenhydramine	Benadryl	Tablets: 25, 50 mg Capsules: 25, 50 mg Strips, orally disintegrating: 12.5 mg ODT: 25 mg Elixir: 12.5 mg/5 mL Syrup: 12.5 mg/5 mL	Used for mild insomnia for up to 1 week. Used to treat seasonal allergies	Sedation: 25-50 mg at bedtime; Seasonal allergies: 25-50 mg at bedtime.
doxepin	Silenor	Tablets: 3, 6 mg	Used to treat insomnia	Hypnosis: 3-6 mg once daily within 30 min of bedtime
doxylamine	Unisom	Tablets: 25 mg	Short-term treatment of insomnia	Sedation: 25 mg at bedtime
eszopiclone	Lunesta	Tablets: 1, 2, 3 mg	Used to treat insomnia	Hypnosis: 2-3 mg
melatonin			See Chapter 36	
ramelteon	Rozerem	Tablets: 8 mg	Used to treat insomnia	Hypnosis: 8 mg within 30 minutes of bedtime
suvorexant	Belsomra	Tablets: 5, 10, 15, 20 mg	Helps people who are having problems falling asleep and staying asleep	Hypnosis: 10 mg once daily within 30 min of bedtime; may increase to a maximum of 20 mg once daily
valerian			See Chapter 36	
tasimelteon	Hetlioz	Capsule: 20 mg	Used to treat non–24-hour sleep-wake disorders in blind persons	Hypnosis: 20 mg once daily at the same time each night before bedtime
zaleplon	Sonata	Capsules: 5, 10 mg	Used to treat insomnia	Hypnosis: 10 mg at bedtime
zolpidem	Ambien Ambien CR	Tablets: 5, 10 mg Controlled-release tablets: 6.25, 12.5 mg	Used to treat insomnia	Hypnosis: 5-10 mg at bedtime Hypnosis: 6.25-12.5 mg at bedtime

Modified from Willihnganz M: Clayton's Basic Pharmacology for Nurses, ed 18, St Louis, 2020, Elsevier.

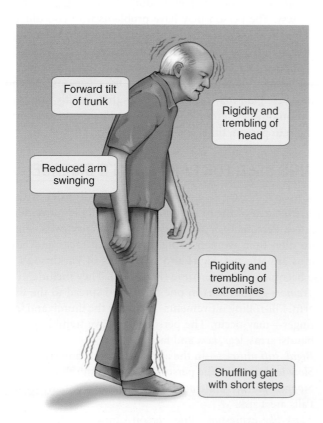

Fig. 15-1 Signs of Parkinson's disease. (From Thibodeau GA, Patton KT: *The human body in health and disease*, ed 4, St Louis, 2005, Mosby.)

Other signs and symptoms develop over time. Symptoms may include excessive salivation due to swallowing and chewing problems, constipation, and bladder problems. Memory loss, slow thinking, sleep problems, depression, and emotional changes (e.g., fear, insecurity) can also occur. The person may have slurred, monotone, and soft speech. Some people may have a tendency to talk too fast or repeat what they say.

Symptoms are caused by a deficiency of dopamine, which is an inhibitory neurotransmitter. A deficiency of dopamine causes an increase in acetylcholine activity.

Parkinson's disease has no cure. All drugs prescribed for Parkinson's disease affect the central nervous system. The goals of treatment are to:
- Relieve signs and symptoms to the extent possible
- Restore dopamine activity to as close to normal as possible

The lowest dosages possible are used. As the disease progresses, dosages are increased. Other drugs are added as needed.

See *Promoting Safety and Comfort: Drugs Used for Parkinson's Disease.*

PROMOTING SAFETY AND COMFORT
Drugs Used for Parkinson's Disease

Safety
Orthostatic hypotension is common with most drugs used to treat Parkinson's disease. Safety measures are needed. Remind the person to rise slowly from a supine or sitting position. Have the person sit or lie down if they feel faint.

DRUG CLASS: Dopamine Agonists

An **agonist** is a drug that acts on a certain type of cell. It produces a predictable response. The following dopamine agonists are used in the treatment of Parkinson's disease:

- Amantadine hydrochloride (ah man' ta deen); Gocovri (go cover ee) and Osmolex ER (oz mo' lex)
- Carbidopa (kar bi doe' pa), levodopa (lee voe doe' 'pa); Sinemet (sin' eh met) and Rytary (ry' tar ee)
- Pramipexole (pra mi pex' ole); Mirapex (mihr' ah pex)
- Ropinirole (roh pin' ihr ol); Requip (re' kwip)
- Rotigotine (ro tig' o teen); Neupro (new pro)

Amantadine Hydrochloride (Gocovri and Osmolex ER)

Amantadine hydrochloride seems to slow the destruction of dopamine, thus making the small amount of dopamine present more effective. It may also help release dopamine from its storage sites. The drug is used to relieve the symptoms of Parkinson's disease.

Assisting With the Nursing Process. When giving amantadine hydrochloride, you will assist the nurse with the nursing process.

Assessment. Measure blood pressure in the supine and standing positions.

Planning. The oral dose forms are:

- 100 mg capsules
- 100 mg tablets
- 50 mg/5 mL syrup
- 68.5 and 137 mg extended-release (24 hr) capsules (Gocovri)
- 129, 193, and 258 mg extended-release (24 hr) tablets (Osmolex ER)

Implementation

- Adults are initially given 100 mg two times a day. The maximum daily adult dose is 400 mg.
- Gocovri (amantadine) ER: Initially 137 mg; after 1 week, increase to the recommended daily dosage of 274 mg
- Osmolex (amantadine) ER: Initially 129 mg orally once daily in the morning; may be increased in weekly intervals to a maximum daily dose of 322 mg once daily in the morning
- Insomnia is a side effect. Therefore, the last dose is usually ordered for late in the afternoon rather than at bedtime.

Evaluation. Most adverse effects are related to dosage and can be reversed. Report and record the following:

- *Confusion, disorientation, hallucinations, mental depression.* Provide for safety.
- *Dizziness, lightheadedness, anorexia, nausea, abdominal discomfort.* These symptoms are usually mild and tend to resolve with continued therapy. Provide for safety when the person is lightheaded or dizzy.
- *Skin mottling.* Mottling means mixed colors. Rose-colored mottling of the skin usually occurs in the extremities. Mottling is worse when the person is standing or exposed to cold. Ankle edema is also often present.
- *Liver disease.* Signs and symptoms include anorexia, nausea, vomiting, jaundice, and abnormal liver function tests.
- *Seizure disorders, psychosis.* Provide for safety.
- *Dyspnea and edema.* The person with heart failure is weighed regularly.

Carbidopa, Levodopa (Sinemet and Rytary)

Sinemet and Rytary are a combination of carbidopa and levodopa. Carbidopa reduces the metabolism of levodopa. This lets more levodopa reach the desired receptor sites. Carbidopa has no effect when used alone and must be used with levodopa. The intent of these drugs is to deliver more dopamine to brain cells.

Assisting With the Nursing Process. When giving carbidopa, levodopa (Sinemet or Rytary), you will assist the nurse with the nursing process.

Assessment

- Ask the nurse about the person's signs and symptoms and response to therapy.
- Measure vital signs.
- Report hallucinations, nightmares, anxiety, or confusion.

Planning. Sinemet and Rytary contain carbidopa and levodopa. For example, Sinemet 10/100 mg tablets have 10 mg of carbidopa and 100 mg of levodopa.

- Sinemet oral dose forms:
  - 10/100 mg tablets
  - 25/100 mg tablets
  - 25/250 mg tablets
- Sinemet CR oral dose forms:
  - 25/100 mg tablets
  - 50/200 mg tablets
- Rytary extended-release oral dose forms:
  - 23.75/95 mg capsules
  - 36.25/145 mg capsules
  - 48.75/195 mg capsules
  - 61.25/245 mg capsules

Implementation

- Sinemet CR tablets and Rytary capsules are sustained-released and must be swallowed whole. Do not crush the tablet or have the person chew the tablet. Do not open the capsule.
- The dosage is adjusted according to the person's response and tolerance.
- Therapy is started in small doses and the dosage is gradually increased.
- Sinement is usually given three to four times a day. Sinemet CR is usually given two to three times a day. Rytary capsules are usually given three times a day.
- Give the drug with food or milk to reduce stomach irritation.

Evaluation. Carbidopa has no effect when used alone and must be used with levodopa. Carbidopa allows more levodopa to reach the brain.

The many possible side effects are related to dosage. Side effects may also depend on the stage of the disease. Report and record the following:

- *Nausea, vomiting, anorexia.* Give the drug with food or milk.
- *Orthostatic hypotension.* This may occur when therapy is started and may resolve after a few weeks of therapy. See *Promoting Safety and Comfort: Drugs Used for Parkinson's Disease.*
- *Chewing motions, bobbing, facial grimacing, rocking movements.* These are involuntary movements.
- *Nightmares, depression, confusion, hallucinations.* Orient the person to person, time, and place. Provide for safety.
- *Tachycardia, palpitations.* Take the person's pulse, taking note of its rhythm and force.

Pramipexole (Mirapex and Mirapex ER)

This drug stimulates dopamine receptors in the brain. The intent of the drug is to increase motor function and the person's ability to perform daily activities. It also helps manage tremors, rigidity, slow body movements, and balance.

Assisting With the Nursing Process. When giving pramipexole (Mirapex), you will assist the nurse with the nursing process.

Assessment
- Measure vital signs.
- Report hallucinations, nightmares, anxiety, or confusion.

Planning
- Mirapex oral dose forms are:
  - 0.125 mg tablets
  - 0.25 mg tablets
  - 0.5 mg tablets
  - 0.75 mg tablets
  - 1 mg tablets
  - 1.5 mg tablets
- Mirapex ER oral dose forms are:
  - 0.375 mg tablets
  - 0.75 mg tablets
  - 1.5 mg tablets
  - 2.25 mg tablets
  - 3 mg tablets
  - 3.75 mg tablets
  - 4.5 mg tablets

Implementation
- The dosage is adjusted according to the person's response and tolerance.
- Therapy is started in small doses and the dosage is gradually increased.
- Immediate-release tablets are usually given three times a day. Extended-release tablets are given once a day.
- Give the drug with food or milk to reduce stomach irritation.
- If pramipexole is to be discontinued, decrease the dose gradually over 1 week.

Evaluation. The many possible side effects are related to dosage and depend on the stage of the disease and other drugs the person takes. Report and record the following:
- *Nausea, vomiting, anorexia.* Give the drug with food or milk.
- *Orthostatic hypotension.* See *Promoting Safety and Comfort: Drugs Used for Parkinson's Disease.*
- *Chewing motions, bobbing, facial grimacing, rocking movements.* These are involuntary movements.
- *Nightmares, depression, confusion, hallucinations.* Orient the person to person, time, and place. Provide for safety.
- *Tachycardia, palpitations.* Take the person's pulse. Note its rhythm and force.
- *Sudden sleep events.* These are described as sleep attacks or sleep episodes, including daytime sleep. Sudden sleep events can cause accidents.
- *Impulsive behaviors.* Notify the nurse immediately.

Ropinirole (Requip and Requip XL)

This drug stimulates dopamine receptors. It is used alone to manage the early signs and symptoms of Parkinson's disease. It is also used with levodopa to manage signs and symptoms

when the disease is advanced. The intent of the drug is to increase motor function and the person's ability to perform daily activities.

Assisting With the Nursing Process. When giving ropinirole (Requip and Requip XL), you will assist the nurse with the nursing process.

Assessment
- Measure vital signs.
- Report hallucinations, nightmares, anxiety or confusion.

Planning
- Requip oral dose forms are:
  - 0.25 mg tablets
  - 0.5 mg tablets
  - 1 mg tablets
  - 2 mg tablets
  - 3 mg tablets
  - 4 mg tablets
  - 5 mg tablets
- Requip XL oral dose forms are:
  - 2 mg tablets
  - 4 mg tablets
  - 6 mg tablets
  - 8 mg tablets
  - 12 mg tablets

Implementation
- The dosage is adjusted according to the person's response and tolerance.
- Therapy is started in small doses and the dosage is gradually increased.
- Requip is usually given three times a day. Requip XL is usually given once a day.
- Give the drug with food or milk to reduce stomach irritation.
- If ropinirole is to be discontinued, decrease the dose gradually over 1 week.

Evaluation. The many possible side effects are related to dosage. Side effects depend on the stage of the disease and other drugs the person takes. Report and record the following:
- *Nausea, vomiting, anorexia.* Give the drug with food or milk.
- *Orthostatic hypotension.* See *Promoting Safety and Comfort: Drugs Used for Parkinson's Disease.*
- *Chewing motions, bobbing, facial grimacing, rocking movements.* These are involuntary movements.
- *Nightmares, depression, confusion, hallucinations.* Orient the person to person, time, and place. Provide for safety.
- *Tachycardia, palpitations.* Take the person's pulse. Note its rhythm and force.
- *Sudden sleep events.* These are described as sleep attacks or sleep episodes, including daytime sleep. Sudden sleep events can cause accidents.
- *Impulsive behaviors.* Alert the nurse immediately.

Rotigotine (Neupro)

This drug stimulates dopamine receptors. It is used to manage early-stage and late-stage Parkinson's disease.

Assisting With the Nursing Process. When giving rotigotine (Neupro), you will assist the nurse with the nursing process.

Assessment
- Measure vital signs.
- Report hallucinations, nightmares, anxiety, or confusion.
Planning. The transdermal dose forms of rotigotine (Neupro) are:
- 1 mg/24 hr patch
- 2 mg/24 hr patch
- 3 mg/24 hr patch
- 4 mg/24 hr patch
- 6 mg/24 hr patch
- 8 mg/24 hr patch
Implementation
- The dosage is adjusted according to the person's response and tolerance.
- Therapy is started in small doses and the dosage is gradually increased.
- Change the patch at the same time every day.
- The patch contains aluminum and must be removed before magnetic resonance imaging (MRI) or cardioversion to avoid skin burns.
- Do not apply heat (such as heating pads or electric blankets) to the application site.

Evaluation. Rotigotine causes many adverse effects, but most are related to dosage and are reversible. Adverse effects vary greatly depending on the stage of the disease and the use of other medicines. Report and record the following:
- *Nausea, vomiting, anorexia.* Effects can be reduced by slowly increasing the dosage.
- *Orthostatic hypotension.* See *Promoting Safety and Comfort: Drugs Used for Parkinson's Disease.*
- *Redness, swelling, and itching where the patch is placed.* Be sure to rotate application sites.

DRUG CLASS: COMT Inhibitor

COMT stands for catechol O-methyltransferase, the enzyme that breaks down levodopa. An **inhibitor** is a drug that prevents or restricts a certain action. By preventing or restricting the breakdown of levodopa, the duration of the drug is longer. Remember, levodopa replaces the dopamine deficiency in the brain. Therefore, a COMT inhibitor allows more dopamine to reach the brain.

These COMT inhibitors are used to treat Parkinson's disease:
- entacapone (en ta' ka pone); Comtan (com' tan) and Stalevo (stah lee' voh)

Entacapone (Comtan and Stalevo)

These drugs reduce the destruction of dopamine in peripheral tissues. More dopamine can reach the brain. Comtan is given with carbidopa-levodopa, as it does not affect Parkinson's disease when given alone. Stalevo contains carbidopa, levodopa, and entacapone.

Assisting With the Nursing Process. When giving entacapone (Comtan and Stalevo), you will assist the nurse with the nursing process.
Assessment
- Measure blood pressure in the supine and sitting positions.
- Observe the person's level of alertness and orientation to person, time, and place.
- Report bowel or GI symptoms.

Planning. Oral dose forms are:
- Comtan: 200 mg tablets
- Stalevo oral dose forms are:
  - 12.5/50/200 mg tablets
  - 18.75/75/200 mg tablets
  - 25/100/200 mg tablets
  - 31.25/125/200 mg tablets
  - 37.5/150/200 mg tablets
  - 50/200/200 mg tablets

Implementation. The dosage is adjusted according to the person's response and tolerance.

Evaluation. Side effects can be reduced by controlling the dosage of levodopa. Report and record the following:
- *Diarrhea.* May develop 1 to 2 weeks after therapy is started.
- *Drowsiness and lethargy.* Observe the person's level of alertness, orientation, and ability to perform basic motor functions. Provide for safety. People working around machines, driving a car, pouring and giving drugs, or performing other duties that require mental alertness should not take these drugs while working.
- *Brownish-orange urine.* This symptom is harmless.
- *Confusion and hallucinations.* Provide for safety.
- *Chorea.* Means *to dance.* The person has rapid, involuntary movements that have no purpose. Flexing and extending the fingers, raising and lowering the shoulders, and grimacing may occur. Provide for safety.
- *Orthostatic hypotension.* See *Promoting Safety and Comfort: Drugs Used for Parkinson's Disease.*

DRUG CLASS: Anticholinergic Agents

There is a dopamine deficiency associated with Parkinson's disease, which leaves an excess of acetylcholine (a cholinergic neurotransmitter). Anticholinergic agents are used to reduce the overstimulation caused by excessive amounts of acetylcholine.

Anticholinergic agents are used to reduce drooling and tremors. They are more useful for persons with minor symptoms and no cognitive impairment. These agents have little effect on stiff and rigid muscles, slow movements, and stooped posture. If anticholinergic drugs are to be discontinued, it should be done gradually.

Assisting With the Nursing Process. When giving anticholinergic drugs, you will assist the nurse with the nursing process.
Assessment
- Report the person's urinary and bowel elimination patterns.
- Measure blood pressure in the supine and sitting positions.
- Measure the pulse. Note the rhythm and whether it is regular or irregular.
- Observe the person's level of alertness and orientation to person, time, and place.
Planning. See Table 15-8 for "Oral Dose Forms."
Implementation
- See Table 15-8 for "Initial Adult Dose."
- Give the drug with food or milk to prevent stomach irritation.
Evaluation. Report and record the following:
- *Constipation.* Give stool softeners if ordered (Chapter 27). Encourage fluid intake and exercise.
- *Urinary retention.* Record intake and output.

TABLE 15-8   Anticholinergic Agents Used to Treat Parkinson's Disease

Generic Name	Brand Name	Oral Dose Forms	Initial Adult Dose
benztropine mesylate	Cogentin	Tablets: 0.5, 1, 2 mg	0.5-1 mg at bedtime
diphenhydramine hydrochloride	Benadryl	Tablets: 25, 50 mg Capsules: 25, 50 mg Strips, orally disintegrating: 12.5 mg ODT: 25 mg Elixir: 12.5 mg/5 mL Syrup: 12.5 mg/5 mL	25-50 mg three or four times daily
trihexyphenidyl hydrochloride	Artane	Tablets: 2, 5 mg Elixir: 2 mg/5 mL Sustained-release capsules: 5 mg	1-2 mg daily

Modified from Willihnganz M: Clayton's Basic Pharmacology for Nurses, ed 18, St Louis, 2020, Elsevier.

- *Blurred vision.* Provide for safety if the person has blurred vision.
- *Dryness of the mouth, throat, and nose.* The nurse may allow the person to suck on hard candy or ice chips or chew gum.
- *Confusion, depression, nightmares, hallucinations.* Provide for safety.
- *Orthostatic hypotension.* See *Promoting Safety and Comfort: Drugs Used for Parkinson's Disease.*
- *Palpitations, dysrhythmias.* Alert the nurse at immediately—the nurse needs to tell the doctor.

DRUG CLASS: Monoamine Oxidase Type B Inhibitor

Monoamine oxidase Type B inhibitors (MAO-B) are also used to treat Parkinson's disease. They slow the metabolism of dopamine in the brain.

- Rasagiline (ra sa' ji leen); Azilect (az a lec' t)
- Selegiline (se le' ji leen); Eldepryl (el' da pril)
- Safinamide (sa fin' a mide); Xadago (za da' go)

The combination of MAO-B and carbidopa-levodopa improves memory and motor speed and may also increase life expectancy. MAO-B inhibitors may be used early during the treatment of Parkinson's disease to slow the progression of symptoms. Levodopa therapy can be delayed.

Assisting With the Nursing Process. When giving MAO-B inhibitors, you will assist the nurse with the nursing process.

Assessment
- Report GI symptoms.
- Measure blood pressure in the supine and sitting positions.
- Observe the person's level of alertness and orientation to person, time, and place.

Planning
- Rasagiline oral dose forms are:
  - 0.5 mg tablets
  - 1 mg tablets
- Selegilinie oral dose forms are:
  - 5 mg tablets
  - 5 mg capsules
  - 1.25 mg ODT
- Safinamide oral dose forms are:
  - 50 mg tablets
  - 100 mg tablets

Implementation
- The dosage is adjusted according to the person's response and tolerance.
- Selegilinie ODT should be taken before breakfast, without liquid. Eating or drinking should be avoided 5 minutes before and 5 minutes after taking Selegiline ODT.

Evaluation. Report and record the following:
- *Constipation, stomach upset.* Give stool softeners if ordered (Chapter 27). Encourage fluid intake and exercise.
- *Chorea, confusion, and hallucinations.* Provide for safety.
- *Orthostatic hypotension.* See *Promoting Safety and Comfort: Drugs Used for Parkinson's Disease.*

DRUGS USED FOR ALZHEIMER'S DISEASE

Alzheimer's disease (AD) is a brain disease. Nerve cells that control intellectual and social function are damaged. Memory, thinking, reasoning, judgment, language, behavior, mood, and personality are affected. The person may have problems working and performing everyday functions. Problems with family and social relationships may occur. There is a steady decline in memory and mental function.

The disease is gradual in onset and gets more severe over time. AD usually occurs after the age of 60. The risk increases with age. It is often diagnosed around the age of 80. Nearly half of all persons age 85 and older have AD.

The classic sign of AD is *gradual loss of short-term memory*. At first, forgetfulness may be the only noticeable symptom. Signs and symptoms become more apparent and severe as the disease progresses. The disease ends in death. The Alzheimer's Association describes seven stages:

- *No impairment.* The person does not show signs of memory problems.
- *Very mild decline.* The person thinks that they have memory lapses. Familiar words or names may be forgotten. The person may not know where to find keys, eyeglasses, or other commonly used objects. These problems are not apparent to family, friends, or the health team.
- *Mild decline.* Family, friends, and others begin to notice symptoms. The person may have problems with memory or concentration and with words or names. The person may lose or misplace something valuable. Functioning in social and work settings declines.

- *Moderate decline.* Memory of recent or current events declines. The person may have difficulty with simple arithmetic. As a result, problems with shopping, paying bills, and managing money may occur. The person may withdraw or be reserved in social situations. Short-term memory loss is present.
- *Moderately severe decline.* The person experiences major memory problems. There may be confusion about the current date or day of the week. They may need help choosing appropriate clothing. The person knows his or her own name, a partner's name, and children's names. Usually help is not needed with eating or elimination.
- *Severe decline.* Memory problems are worse. Personality and behavior changes develop including delusions, hallucinations, and repetitive behavior. The person needs a great deal of help with daily activities such as dressing and elimination. Names may be forgotten, but faces may still be recognized. Sleep problems, incontinence (urinary and fecal), and wandering are common. Confusion or unawareness of environment and surroundings may occur.
- *Very severe decline.* The person cannot respond to their environment, speak, or control movement. The person cannot walk without assistance. Over time, the person cannot sit up without support or someone holding their head up. Muscles become rigid and swallowing is impaired. Because the disease is a terminal illness, people in stage seven are nearing death. Drug therapy includes the use of the following:
- acetylcholinesterase inhibitors (donepezil, rivastigmine, and galantamine) and NMDA receptor inhibitors (memantine).

DRUG CLASS: Acetylcholinesterase Inhibitors

These acetylcholinesterase inhibitors are used in the treatment of AD:

- Donepezil (don ep' i zil); Aricept (ar' i sept)
- Rivastigmine (riva stig' meen); Exelon
- Galantamine (ga lanta meen); Razadyne; Razadyne ER

Donepezil (Aricept)

There is a loss of cholinergic neurons with AD, which results in memory loss and dementia. Donepezil (Aricept) inhibits acetylcholinesterase (the enzyme that metabolizes acetylcholine when released by a nerve ending). The drug enhances cholinergic function. However, its effects lessen as more neurons are lost.

The drug is used in mild to moderate dementia. The goals of therapy are to improve cognitive skills (e.g., word recall, naming objects, language, word finding, and ability to perform tasks).

Assisting With the Nursing Process. When giving donepezil (Aricept), you will assist the nurse with the nursing process.

Assessment
- Measure vital signs.
- Observe cognitive function.
- Observe for GI symptoms.

Planning
- Aricept oral dose forms are:
  - 5, 10, and 23 mg tablets
  - 5 and 10 mg ODT
- Exelon dose forms are:
  - Transdermal patch

- 4.6 mg/24 hours
- 9.5 mg/24 hours
- 13.3 mg/24 hours
- Razadyne oral dose forms are:
  - 4, 8, and 12 mg tablets
  - 4 mg/mL oral solution
  - 16 and 24 mg extended-release capsules

Implementation
- For Aricept, the initial dose is 5 mg daily at bedtime. After 4 to 6 weeks, the dosage may be increased to 10 mg daily. After 3 months, the dosage may be increased to 23 mg.
- The ODT may be helpful for patients who have difficulty swallowing.
- When using Exelon, the initial dose for 4 weeks is a 4.6 mg transdermal patch once a day. The dose may be titrated up every 4 weeks. The maximum dose is 13.3mg /24 hr patch.
- When using Razadyne, the initial dose is 4 mg two times a day (8 mg per day).

After 4 weeks, the dose is increased to 8 mg two times a day (16 mg per day).

After another 4 weeks, the dose is increased to 12 mg two times a day (24 mg per day). Extended-release initial dosage is 8 mg once daily. The dose may be titrated up every 4 weeks. The maximum dose is 24 mg once daily.

Evaluation. Report and record:
- *Nausea, vomiting, indigestion, diarrhea.* Symptoms lessen with lower doses and tend to subside after 2 to 3 weeks of therapy.
- *Bradycardia.* Alert the nurse immediately if the person's pulse is less than 60 beats per minute.

DRUG CLASS: NMDA Receptor Inhibitors
Memantine (Namenda)

Memantine (Namenda) blocks a receptor in the CNS that is activated in AD. The drug may be used alone or with other drugs to treat moderate to severe AD. Cognitive function and behaviors may be improved. The decline in activities of daily living is slower. However, the drug does not prevent or slow the progress of AD.

Assisting With the Nursing Process. When giving memantine (Namenda), you will assist the nurse with the nursing process.

Assessment
- Measure vital signs.
- Observe cognitive function.

Planning. The oral dose forms are:
- 5 and 10 mg tablets
- 7, 14, 21, and 28 mg tablets
- 2 mg/mL in 360 mL solution

Implementation
- The oral dose is 5 mg once a day.
- The dosage is increased by 5 mg every 7 days to 10 mg daily, 15 mg daily, and 20 mg daily.
- The drug is given with or without food.

Evaluation. Report and record:
- Headache, dizziness, insomnia, restlessness, increased motor activity, excitement, agitation. These tend to decline with continued therapy. The dosage may need adjustment.

REVIEW QUESTIONS

Circle the BEST answer.

1. Nerve signals or impulses are caused by:
   a. neurons
   b. synapses
   c. agonists
   d. neurotransmitters

2. Which is *not* an adrenergic agent?
   a. levodopa
   b. dopamine
   c. epinephrine
   d. norepinephrine

3. Most adrenergic agents cause:
   a. vasoconstriction
   b. vasodilation
   c. bronchospasm
   d. hypotension

4. Beta blocking agents are commonly used to treat:
   a. hypotension
   b. hypertension
   c. vasoconstriction
   d. respiratory disorders

5. When giving a beta blocker, you assist with assessment by:
   a. measuring heart rate and blood pressure
   b. observing the color of urine
   c. asking the person to use a pain rating scale
   d. observing the person's level of alertness

6. Cholinergic agents are used in the treatment of:
   a. myocardial infarction
   b. Parkinson's disease
   c. myasthenia gravis
   d. heart failure

7. Anticholinergic actions include all of the following, *except*:
   a. increasing the heart rate
   b. drying respiratory secretions
   c. increasing GI motility
   d. dilating the pupil

8. Which of the following drugs is an anticholinergic?
   a. carvedilol (Coreg)
   b. terbutaline (Brethine)
   c. bethanechol (Urecholine)
   d. glycopyrrolate (Robinul)

9. When giving an anticholinergic agent, you assist with assessment by:
   a. measuring heart rate and blood pressure
   b. observing the color of urine
   c. asking the person to use a pain rating scale
   d. observing the person's level of alertness

10. Sedative-hypnotic drugs are used to:
    a. produce sleep
    b. dry respiratory secretions before surgery
    c. decrease drooling and tremors
    d. stimulate the central nervous system

11. All of the following are barbiturates, *except*:
    a. phenobarbital (Luminal)
    b. butabarbital (Butisol)
    c. secobarbital (Seconal)
    d. flurazepam (Dalmane)

12. The benzodiazepines are used for the following reasons, *except*:
    a. to dry respiratory secretions
    b. to produce mild sedation
    c. to produce sleep
    d. for preoperative sedation

13. The following are benzodiazepines, *except*:
    a. zolpidem (Ambien)
    b. lorazepam (Ativan)
    c. temazepam (Restoril)
    d. triazolam (Halcion)

14. Which drug is *not* used to promote sleep?
    a. eszopiclone (Lunesta)
    b. diphenhydramine (Benadryl)
    c. zaleplon (Sonata)
    d. carbidopa, levodopa (Sinemet)

15. Which is a common side effect of drugs used to treat Parkinson's disease?
    a. drooling
    b. rigid, stiff muscles
    c. orthostatic hypotension
    d. tremors

16. Signs and symptoms of Parkinson's disease are caused by a deficiency of:
    a. levodopa
    b. dopamine
    c. carbidopa
    d. norepinephrine

17. The following drugs are used to treat Parkinson's disease, *except*:
    a. pramipexole (Mirapex)
    b. ropinirole (Requip)
    c. secobarbital (Seconal)
    d. selegiline (Eldepryl)

18. Drugs used to treat Parkinson's disease:
    a. depress the central nervous system
    b. increase the amount of dopamine available to brain cells
    c. cure the disease
    d. inhibit the use of dopamine

Circle T if the statement is true. Circle F if the statement is false.

19. T F Side effects of adrenergic agents resolve when the dosage is reduced.
20. T F Most body systems are affected by cholinergic drugs.
21. T F Anticholinergic agents are used preoperatively.
22. T F Sedative-hypnotics are used preoperatively.
23. T F Barbiturates stimulate the central nervous system.
24. T F Barbiturate use can lead to addiction.
25. T F Donepezil (Aricept) can stop the progress of Alzheimer's disease.
26. T F Memantine (Namenda) is given to improve cognitive function in persons with dementia.

Answers to these questions can be found on the Evolve Resources site: http://evolve.elsevier.com/Anderson/medasst/

16

Drugs Used for Mental Health Disorders

OBJECTIVES

- Define the key terms and key abbreviations used in this chapter.
- Describe the common mental health disorders.
- Describe the drugs used to treat anxiety.
- Explain how to assist with the nursing process when giving drugs to treat anxiety.

- Describe the drugs used to treat mood disorders.
- Explain how to assist with the nursing process when giving drugs to treat mood disorders.
- Describe the drugs used in alcohol rehabilitation.
- Explain how to assist with the nursing process when giving drugs used in alcohol rehabilitation.

KEY TERMS

antagonist A drug that exerts an opposite action to that of another; it may compete for the same receptor sites

antianxiety drugs Used to treat anxiety

antidepressants Several classes of drugs used to treat mood disorders

anxiety A vague, uneasy feeling in response to stress

anxiolytics Antianxiety drugs, tranquilizers

psychosis A state of severe mental impairment; the person cannot view the real or unreal correctly

tranquilizers Antianxiety drugs, anxiolytics

KEY ABBREVIATIONS

CNS Central nervous system
GI Gastrointestinal
MAOI Monoamine oxidase inhibitor
mg Milligram
mL Milliliter

OCD Obsessive-compulsive disorder
PO Per os (orally), by mouth
PTSD Post-traumatic stress disorder
SSRI Selective serotonin reuptake inhibitor
TCA Tricyclic antidepressant

Physical health problems range from mild to severe. The common cold is at one extreme and a life-threatening illness is at the other. Mental health problems have the same extremes.

Mental relates to the mind; mental health involves the health of the mind. A mentally healthy person copes with and adjusts to everyday stresses in ways accepted by society. The person with a *mental health disorder* has problems with coping with or adjusting to stress.

Causes of mental health disorders include:

- Inability to cope or adjust to stress
- Chemical imbalances
- Genetics
- Drug or substance abuse
- Social and cultural factors

Common mental health disorders are described in Box 16-1. Psychotherapy, drugs, and other treatments and therapies can be used to treat mental health disorders. Many of the drugs used can affect the central nervous system (CNS). See Chapter 15 for a review of the nervous system.

See *Delegation Guidelines: Drugs Used for Mental Health Disorders.*

DELEGATION GUIDELINES
Drugs Used for Mental Health Disorders

Some drugs used to treat mental health disorders are given parenterally (by injection). Because you do not give parenteral dose forms, they are not included in this chapter. Should a nurse delegate the administration of such to you, you must:
- Remember that parenteral dosages are often very different from dosages for other routes.
- Refuse the delegation but do not ignore the request. Make sure the nurse knows that you cannot give the drug and why.

DRUGS USED FOR ANXIETY DISORDERS

Anxiety is a vague, uneasy feeling in response to stress. The person may not know the cause. The person senses danger or harm—real or imagined. The person acts to relieve the unpleasant feeling; anxiety occurs when needs are not met.

Some anxiety is normal. Persons with mental health disorders have higher levels of anxiety. Signs and symptoms

BOX 16-1   Common Mental Health Disorders

Anxiety Disorders

Obsessive-Compulsive Disorder. An *obsession* is a recurrent, unwanted thought, idea, or image. *Compulsion* is repeating an act over and over again (i.e., a ritual). The act may not make logical sense, but the person experiences anxiety if it is not done. Common rituals include hand washing, constant checking to make sure the stove is off, cleaning, and counting things to a certain number. Such activities can take over an hour every day. They may be very distressing and affect daily life. Some persons with obsessive-compulsive disorder (OCD) also experience depression, eating disorders, substance abuse, and other anxiety disorders.

Panic Disorder. Panic is the highest level of anxiety. *Panic* is an intense and sudden feeling of fear, anxiety, terror, or dread. Onset is sudden with no obvious reason. The person cannot function. Signs and symptoms of anxiety (p.165) are severe. The person may have:

- Chest pain
- Shortness of breath
- Rapid heart rate ("heart pounding")
- Numbness and tingling in the hands
- Dizziness
- A smothering sensation
- Feeling of impending doom or loss of control

The person may feel that they are having a heart attack, losing their mind, or are on the verge of death. Attacks can occur at any time, even during sleep.

Panic attacks can last for 10 minutes or longer. They may occur often. Panic disorder can last for a few months or for many years.

Many people avoid places where past panic attacks occurred. For example, if a person had a panic attack in a shopping mall, malls are then avoided.

Phobias. *Phobia* means an intense fear. The person has an intense fear of an object, situation, or activity that has little to no actual danger. The person avoids what is feared. When faced with the fear, the person experiences high anxiety and cannot function. Common phobias include fears of:

- Being in an open, crowded, or public place (agoraphobia—*agora* means marketplace)
- Being in pain or seeing others in pain (algophobia—*algo* means pain)
- Water (aquaphobia—*aqua* means water)
- Being in or being trapped in an enclosed or narrow space (claustrophobia—*claustro* means closing)
- The slightest uncleanliness (mysophobia—*myso* means anything that is disgusting)
- Night or darkness (nyctophobia—*nycto* means night or darkness)
- Fire (pyrophobia—*pyro* means fire)
- Strangers (xenophobia—*xeno* means strange)

Mood Disorders

Bipolar Disorder. *Bipolar* means two *(bi)* poles or ends *(polar)*. The person with bipolar disorder experiences severe extremes in mood, energy, and ability to

function. There are emotional lows *(depression)* and emotional highs *(mania)*. The disorder was formerly known as manic depression. The person may:

- Be more depressed than manic
- Be more manic than depressed
- Experience symptoms of both mania and depression (mixed)
- Be between episodes

The disorder tends to run in families. It usually develops in the late teens or in early adulthood. The disorder requires lifelong management.

See Box 16-2 for the signs and symptoms of mania and depression, which can range from mild to severe. Mood changes are called "episodes." Bipolar disorder can damage relationships and affect school or work performance. Some people may be suicidal.

Major Depressive Disorder. Depression involves the body, mood, and thoughts. Symptoms (see Box 16-4) affect work, study, sleep, eating, and other activities. The person is very sad and loses interest in daily activities.

There are varying degrees of depression (mild, moderate, and severe). Depression may occur because of a stressful event such as death of a partner, parent, or child. Divorce and loss of job are also highly stressful events. Some physical disorders can cause depression (e.g., stroke, myocardial infarction [heart attack], cancer, and Parkinson's disease). Hormonal factors may cause depression in women—menstrual cycle changes, pregnancy, miscarriage, after birth (postpartum depression), and before and during menopause.

Psychotic Disorder

Schizophrenia. *Schizophrenia* means split *(schizo)* mind *(phrenia)*. It is a severe, chronic, disabling brain disorder. The person with schizophrenia has severe mental impairment *(psychosis)*. Thinking and behavior are disturbed and the person has false beliefs *(delusions) and experiences hallucinations*. That is, the person sees, hears, smells, or feels things that are not real. The person has problems relating to others and may be *paranoid*, meaning the person is suspicious about a person or situation. The person may have difficulty organizing thoughts. Responses are inappropriate. Communication is disturbed. The person may ramble or repeat what another says. Sometimes speech cannot be understood. They may make up words. The person may lack interest in others and usually are not involved with people or society.

Some persons experience regression. To *regress* means to retreat or move back to an earlier time or condition. For example, it is normal for a 5-year-old to wet the bed when there is a new baby in the home. Healthy adults do not act like infants or children.

In men, the symptoms usually begin in the late teens or early 20s. In women, symptoms usually begin in the mid-20s and early 30s. People with schizophrenia do not tend to be violent. However, if a person with paranoid schizophrenia becomes violent, it is often directed at family members. The violence usually occurs at home. Some persons with schizophrenia may attempt suicide.

---

depend on the degree of anxiety (Box 16-3). A person has an anxiety disorder when their responses to stressful situations:

- Are abnormal or irrational
- Impair normal daily function

Anxiety disorders may last at least 6 months and can worsen if untreated. Anxiety disorders commonly occur with other physical illnesses involving the cardiovascular, pulmonary, digestive, and endocrine systems. It also is a major symptom of many mental health disorders (e.g., schizophrenia, mania, depression, dementia, and substance abuse). The anxious person is evaluated to determine if the anxiety is due to a physical or mental health problem.

Antianxiety drugs are used to treat anxiety. They also are known as anxiolytics or **tranquilizers**.

DRUG CLASS: Benzodiazepines

Benzodiazepines are commonly used to treat anxiety disorders (Table 16-1). They are:

- Consistently effective
- Less likely to interact with other drugs
- Less likely to cause overdose
- Have a lower risk for abuse than barbiturates and other antianxiety drugs

These drugs stimulate the action of an inhibitory neurotransmitter. (A *neurotransmitter* is a chemical substance that transmits nerve impulses. Something that *inhibits* prevents or restricts a certain action. See Chapter 15.). They can lower

BOX 16-2 Signs and Symptoms of Bipolar Disorder

MANIA (MANIC EPISODE)

Increased energy, activity, and restlessness
Excessively "high," overly positive mood
Extreme irritability
Racing thoughts and very rapid speech
Jumping from one idea to another
Easily distracted; problems concentrating
Little sleep needed
Unrealistic beliefs in one's abilities and powers
Poor judgment
Spending sprees
A lasting period of behavior that is different from usual
Increased sexual drive
Drug abuse (particularly cocaine, alcohol, and sleeping pills)
Aggressive behavior
Denial that anything is wrong

DEPRESSION (DEPRESSIVE EPISODE)

Lasting sad, anxious, or "empty" feelings
Feelings of hopelessness
Feelings of guilt, worthlessness, or helplessness
Loss of interest or pleasure in activities the person once enjoyed
Loss of interest in sex
Decreased energy; a feeling of fatigue or being "slowed down"
Problems concentrating, remembering, or making decisions
Restlessness or irritability
Sleeping too much, or unable to sleep
Change in appetite
Unintended weight loss or gain
Chronic pain or other symptoms not caused by physical illness or injury
Thoughts of death or suicide
Suicide attempts

BOX 16-3 Signs and Symptoms of Anxiety

- A "lump" in the throat
- "Butterflies" in the stomach
- Rapid pulse or palpitations
- Rapid breathing
- Increased blood pressure
- Talking fast and excitedly
- Voice changes
- Dry mouth
- Sweating
- Nausea
- Diarrhea
- Urinary frequency and urgency
- Poor attention span; difficulty concentrating
- Difficulty following directions
- Difficulty sleeping
- Loss of appetite
- Tension or tear

TABLE 16-1 Benzodiazepines Used to Treat Anxiety

Generic Name	Brand Name	Oral Dose Forms	Initial Adult Oral Dose
alprazolam	Xanax Xanax XR	Tablets: 0.25, 0.5, 1, 2 mg Tablets, orally disintegrating: 0.25, 0.5, 1, 2 mg Tablets, extended-release: 0.5, 1, 2, 3 mg	0.25-0.5 mg three times daily 0.5-1 mg daily
chlordiaz-epoxide	Librium	Capsules: 5, 10, 25 mg	5-10 mg three or four times daily
clorazepate	Tranxene	Tablets: 3.75, 7.5, 11.25, 15 mg	10 mg one to three times daily
diazepam	Valium	Tablets: 2, 5, 10 mg Liquid: 5 mg/5 mL Rectal gel: 2.5, 10, 20 mg rectal delivery system	2-10 mg two to four times daily
lorazepam	Ativan	Tablets: 0.5, 1, 2 mg Liquid: 2 mg/mL	2-3 mg two or three times daily
oxazepam	Serax	Capsules: 10, 15, 30 mg	10-15 mg three or four times daily

Modified from Willihnganz M: Clayton's Basic Pharmacology for Nurses, ed 18, St Louis, 2020, Elsevier.

anxiety within a short time. The intent is to decrease anxiety so that:

- Coping is improved.
- Physical signs are reduced (see Box 16-3).

These drugs are usually ordered for a short time. If taken for weeks or months, drug tolerance and dependence may occur. Abuse and withdrawal symptoms are possible. The use of benzodiazepines during pregnancy should be avoided.

See *Promoting Safety and Comfort: Benzodiazepines.*

PROMOTING SAFETY AND COMFORT

Benzodiazepines

Safety

Benzodiazepines have few side effects, drowsiness and loss of coordination being the most common. Fatigue, confusion, and slower mental function may also occur. Provide for safety.

People working around machines, driving a car, pouring and giving drugs, or performing other duties that require mental alertness should not take these drugs while performing such functions.

Assisting With the Nursing Process. When giving benzodiazepines, you assist the nurse with the nursing process.

Assessment

- Measure blood pressure in the sitting and supine positions.
- Observe for signs and symptoms of anxiety.

Planning. See Table 16-1 for "Oral Dose Forms."

Implementation

- See Table 16-1 for "Initial Adult Dose."
- Long-term use may cause physical and psychological dependence. Mild withdrawal signs and symptoms can occur after taking the drug for 4 to 6 weeks. Restlessness, worsening of anxiety, insomnia, tremors, muscle tension, rapid pulse, and hearing sensitivity are common. Delirium and seizures may occur. Signs and symptoms may not appear for several days after the benzodiazepine is discontinued.

If the drug is to be discontinued, decrease the dose gradually over 1 week.
- *It is recommended that benzodiazepines not be administered during at least the first trimester of pregnancy.* Breastfeeding women should not receive benzodiazepines.
Evaluation. Report and record:
- *Drowsiness, hangover, sedation, lethargy.* Provide for safety.
- *Orthostatic hypotension.* Provide for safety. Remind the person to rise slowly from a supine or sitting position. Have the person sit or lie down if they feels faint.
- *Excessive use or abuse.* This may cause physical and psychological dependence.
- *Anorexia, nausea, vomiting, and jaundice.* These may signal liver toxicity.

OTHER ANTIANXIETY AGENTS

Other drugs used to treat anxiety disorders include:
- buspirone (byoo spy' rone) and BuSpar (byoo sphar')
- fluvoxamine (fluv ox' ah meen) and Luvox (loo' vox)
- hydroxyzine (hi drox' ee zeen) and Vistaril (vis tar' il)

Buspirone (BuSpar)

This drug causes less sedation than other antianxiety agents and does not alter psychomotor function. Improvement is seen after 7 to 10 days of treatment. The person may need 3 to 4 weeks of therapy. The risk for abuse is low.

Assisting With the Nursing Process. When giving buspirone (BuSpar), you assist the nurse with the nursing process.
Assessment. Observe for signs and symptoms of anxiety.
Planning. The oral dose forms are:
- 5, 7.5, 10, 15, and 30 mg tablets
Implementation
- The adult initial dose is 5 mg orally three times a day.
- The dosage may be increased by 5 mg every 2 to 3 days.
- The maximum daily dose is 60 mg.
Evaluation. Report and record:
- *Insomnia, nervousness, drowsiness, and light-headedness.* Provide for safety.
- *Slurred speech and dizziness.* These are signs of excess dosing.

Fluvoxamine (Luvox)

This drug is used to treat OCD. Symptoms are reduced, but obsessions and compulsions are not prevented. The person may have more control over them while taking the drug. Its purpose is to:
- Decrease anxiety
- Improve coping with obsessions
- Reduce the frequency of compulsive activity

Assisting With the Nursing Process. See p. 169 for "Selective Serotonin Reuptake Inhibitors."

Hydroxyzine (Vistaril)

This drug produces sedation and reduces anxiety. It may also be used to prevent vomiting or control allergic reactions.

Vistaril is used to:
- Decrease anxiety
- Produce sedation and relaxation before surgery
- Reduce the amount of pain relief medication needed after surgery
- Prevent vomiting
- Control itching from allergic reactions

Assisting With the Nursing Process. When giving hydroxyzine (Vistaril), you assist the nurse with the nursing process.
Assessment. Observe for signs and symptoms of anxiety.
Planning. The oral dose forms are:
- Vistaril
  - 10, 25, and 50 mg tablets
  - 25, 50, and 100 mg capsules
  - 10 mg/5 mL suspension
Implementation. For an adult, 25 to 100 mg are given orally three to four times a day.
Evaluation. Report and record:
- *Blurred vision; constipation; dryness of the mouth, nose, and throat.* Provide for safety if the person has blurred vision. Give stool softeners as ordered. The nurse may allow the person to suck on hard candy or ice chips or chew gum.
- *Sedation.* See *Promoting Safety and Comfort: Benzodiazepines.*
- *Dizziness, slurred speech.* These symptoms signal excessive dosing.

DRUGS USED FOR MOOD DISORDERS

Mood or *affect* relates to feelings and emotions. Mood (or affective) disorders involve feelings, emotions, and moods.

Before regaining full function, most persons pass through three therapy phases:
- *Acute phase.* The time from diagnosis to the first treatment response. Symptoms are reduced. This phase usually takes 6 to 8 weeks but may take longer if the person does not take prescribed drugs and follow other therapies. Some people simply stop treatment.
- *Continuation phase.* This phase involves preventing a relapse and reaching a full recovery. The person should be symptom-free for 6 months.
- *Maintenance phase.* The goal of this phase is to prevent the mood disorder from recurring.

Mood disorders are treated with several classes of drugs called **antidepressants.** They prolong the action of neurotransmitters—norepinephrine, dopamine, and serotonin. The drug classes are:
- Monoamine oxidase inhibitors (MAOIs)
- Tricyclic antidepressants (TCAs)
- Selective serotonin reuptake inhibitors (SSRIs)
- Serotonin-norepinephrine reuptake inhibitors (SNRIs)
- Other agents
See *Focus on Older Persons: Drugs Used for Mood Disorders.*

See *Promoting Safety and Comfort: Drugs Used for Mood Disorders.*

BOX 16-4 Signs and Symptoms of Depression in Older Persons

- Fatigue and lack of interest
- Inability to experience pleasure, including during sex
- Feelings of uselessness, hopelessness, and helplessness
- Increased dependency
- Anxiety, agitation, or irritability
- Appetite changes
- Aches, pains, headaches, cramps, or digestive problems
- Slow or unreliable memory
- Feeling sad, empty, or distant from others
- Focus on the past
- Thoughts of death and suicide
- Difficulty completing daily activities
- Changes in sleep patterns
- Poor personal grooming
- Withdrawal from people and interests
- Dry mouth

From Modified from Williams: *Basic Geriatric Nursing*, ed 7, St Louis, 2020, Elsevier.

FOCUS ON OLDER PERSONS
Drugs Used for Mood Disorders

Depression is common in older persons. They experience many losses—death of family and friends, loss of health, loss of body functions, loss of independence. Loneliness and the side effects of some drugs may also contribute to depression. See Box 16-4 for the signs and symptoms of depression in older persons.

Depression in older persons is often overlooked or incorrectly diagnosed. The person may be wrongly thought to have dementia. Therefore, depression is often left untreated.

PROMOTING SAFETY AND COMFORT
Drugs Used for Mood Disorders

Safety
Antidepressants may increase the risk of suicidal ideation and behavior. When started on antidepressants, observe the person carefully. Observe for agitation, changes in behavior, objects that could cause harm, writing a will, giving away belongings, and statements or comments about death. Report your observations and concerns to the nurse. Follow suicide precautions according to the care plan.

DRUG CLASS: Monoamine Oxidase Inhibitors

Monoamine oxidase inhibitors (MAOIs) are listed in Table 16-2. They prevent the breakdown of neurotransmitters (epinephrine, norepinephrine, dopamine, and serotonin). These neurotransmitters are involved in areas of the brain that control mood and emotion. Drug effects can be seen within 2 to 4 weeks. If MAOIs are to be discontinued, decrease the dose gradually over 1 week. If a dose is missed, give the drug immediately. The remaining doses should be spaced out throughout the day.

MAOIs may have serious side effects when taken with certain drugs, foods, and fluids. Doctors often initially order other antidepressants and MAOIs may be used if other drugs fail.

See *Promoting Safety and Comfort: Drug Class—Monoamine Oxidase Inhibitors.*

PROMOTING SAFETY AND COMFORT
Drug Class—Monoamine Oxidase Inhibitors

Safety
MAOIs can cause serious hypertension if taken with foods or fluids that contain tyramine. Tyramine stimulates the release of epinephrine and norepinephrine. The person taking an MAOI should avoid the following:
- Aged cheese—Camembert, Edam, Roquefort, Parmesan, Swiss, blue, cheddar
- Smoked or pickled meats, poultry, and fish—corned beef, herring, salami, pepperoni, sausage
- Aged or fermented meats—chicken or beef paté, game fish, poultry
- Meat extracts—bouillon, consommé
- Products containing yeast
- Red wines
- Beer
- Avocados
- Chicken livers
- Sauerkraut
- Fava beans

Signs and symptoms of a hypertensive crisis include severe headache, stiff neck, sweating, nausea, vomiting, and very high blood pressure.

Assisting With the Nursing Process. When giving MAOIs, you assist the nurse with the nursing process.

Assessment
- Measure pulse rate.
- Measure blood pressure in the supine and standing positions.
- Measure blood glucose.
- Ask about foods and fluids consumed during the past few days.

Planning. See Table 16-2 for "Oral Dose Forms."

Implementation
- See Table 16-2 for "Initial Adult Oral Dose" and "Daily Maintenance Dose."
- MAOIs are given two or three times a day. To prevent insomnia, the last dose is given no later than 1800 (6:00 PM).

Evaluation. Report and record:
- *Orthostatic hypotension.* This is the most common side effect of MAOIs. Dizziness and weakness may occur when the drug is started. Blood pressure is measured daily in the supine and standing positions. Provide for safety. Remind the person to rise slowly from a supine or sitting position. Have the person sit or lie down if they feel faint.
- *Drowsiness, sedation.* These tend to resolve with dosage adjustment and continued therapy. Provide for safety. Remind the person to use caution when performing tasks that require alertness.
- *Restlessness, agitation, insomnia.* These resolve when the dosage is adjusted. The last dose should be given before 1800 (6:00 PM).
- *Blurred vision; constipation; urinary retention; dryness of the mouth, nose, and throat.* Provide for safety if the person has blurred vision. Follow the care plan for constipation and urinary retention. For mouth, nose, and throat dryness, the nurse may allow the person to suck on hard candy or ice chips or chew gum.

TABLE 16-2 Antidepressants

Generic Name	Brand Name	Oral Dose Forms	Initial Adult Oral Dose	Daily Maintenance Dose (Mg)
Monoamine Oxidase Inhibitors (MAOI)				
phenelzine	Nardil	Tablets: 15 mg	15 mg three times daily	15-60
tranylcypromine	Parnate	Tablets: 10 mg	30 mg daily divided	30
isocarboxazid	Marplan	Tablets: 10 mg	10 mg twice daily	40
selegiline	Emsam	Transdermal patch: 6, 9, 12 mg/24 hr	6 mg patch daily	6
Selective Serotonin Reuptake Inhibitors (SSRI)				
citalopram	Celexa	Tablets: 10, 20, 40 mg Liquid: 10 mg/5 mL	20 mg daily	20-40
escitalopram	Lexapro	Tablets: 5, 10, 20 mg Liquid: 1 mg/1 mL	10 mg daily	10-20
fluoxetine	Prozac	Capsules: 10, 20, 40 mg Tablets: 10, 20, 60 mg Solution: 20 mg/5 mL Weekly capsule: 90 mg	20 mg every morning	20-60
fluvoxamine	Luvox	Tablets: 25, 50, 100 mg Capsules, 24 hr sustained-release: 100, 150 mg	50 mg at bedtime	50-300
paroxetine	Paxil Paxil CR	Tablets: 10, 20, 30, 40 mg Suspension: 10 mg/5 mL Sustained-release tablets: 12.5, 25, 37.5 mg	20 mg daily	20-50
sertraline	Zoloft	Tablets: 25, 50, 100 mg Oral concentrate: 20 mg/mL	50 mg daily	50-200
Serotonin-Norepinephrine Reuptake Inhibitors (SnRI)				
desvenlafaxine	Pristiq, Khedezla	Tablets, 24 hr sustained-release: 25, 50, 100 mg	50 mg daily at the same time	50-400
duloxetine	Cymbalta	Capsules, sustained-release: 20, 30, 40, 60 mg	40 mg daily	60
levomilnacipran	Fetzima	Capsules, extended-release: 20, 40, 80, 120 mg	20 mg once daily for 2 days; then 40 mg once daily	40-120
venlafaxine	Effexor	Tablets: 25, 37.5, 50, 75, 100 mg Capsules, tablets, sustained-release: 37.5, 75, 150, 225 mg	75 mg in two or three doses daily, taken with food	75-225
Tricyclic Antidepressants (TCA)				
amitriptyline		Tablets: 10, 25, 50, 75, 100, 150 mg	25-75 mg daily, divided as needed	75-200
amoxapine		Tablets: 25, 50, 100, 150 mg	50 mg two to three times daily	200-300
clomipramine	Anafranil Apo-Clomipramine	Capsules: 25, 50, 75 mg	25 mg daily	100-150
desipramine	Norpramin	Tablets: 10, 25, 50, 75, 100, 150 mg	50-75 mg daily, divided in one to four doses	75-200
doxepin	Apo-Doxepin	Capsules: 10, 25, 50, 75, 100, 150 mg Oral concentrate 10 mg/mL	25 mg three times daily	75-150
imipramine	Tofranil Impril	Tablets: 10, 25, 50 mg	30-75 mg daily in one to four divided doses	50-150
nortriptyline	Pamelor PMS-Nortriptyline	Capsules: 10, 25, 50, 75 mg Solution: 10 mg/5 mL	25-50 mg in one to four divided doses	50-75
protriptyline	Vivactil	Tablets: 5, 10 mg	5-10 mg three times daily	20-40
trimipramine	Surmontil	Capsules: 25, 50, 100 mg	25 mg three times daily	50-150

Modified from Willihnganz M: Clayton's Basic Pharmacology for Nurses, ed 18, St Louis, 2020, Elsevier.

- *Hypertension.* Many drugs, foods, and fluids can cause serious hypertension. See *Promoting Safety and Comfort: Drug Class—Monoamine Oxidase Inhibitors.*

DRUG CLASS: Selective Serotonin Reuptake Inhibitors

Selective serotonin reuptake inhibitors (SSRIs) affect serotonin. *Reuptake* means reabsorption. SSRIs block certain nerve cells from reabsorbing serotonin, leaving more serotonin available for the brain. Mood is improved because the sending of nerve impulses is improved.

SSRIs are used to improve the person's mood and reduce depression. They are the most widely used antidepressants (see Table 16-2) and are the safest class of antidepressants. People experience fewer adverse effects than with other antidepressants. Drug effects are seen within 2 to 4 weeks. SSRIs should be taken in the morning due to possible insomnia (except for fluvoxamine).

Assisting With the Nursing Process. When giving SSRIs, you assist the nurse with the nursing process.
Assessment
- Measure blood pressure in the supine and standing positions.
- Weigh the person weekly.
- Observe for insomnia, nervousness, and other CNS signs and symptoms.
- Ask the person if they have experienced any GI symptoms.
Planning. See Table 16-2 for "Oral Dose Forms."
Implementation. See Table 16-2 for "Initial Adult Oral Dose" and "Daily Maintenance Dose."
Evaluation. Report and record:
- *Restlessness, agitation, anxiety, insomnia.* These symptoms usually occur early in therapy. The drug should be given before 1800 (6:00 PM). The doctor may order a sedative-hypnotic agent.
- *Sedative effects.* Remind the person to use caution when performing tasks that require alertness.
- *GI effects.* Give the drug with food. The doctor may adjust the dose accordingly.
- *Suicidal actions.* See *Promoting Safety and Comfort: Drugs Used for Mood Disorders.*

DRUG CLASS: Serotonin-Norepinephrine Reuptake Inhibitors

Serotonin-norepinephrine reuptake inhibitors (SNRIs) affect serotonin and norepinephrine. SNRIs block certain nerve cells from reabsorbing serotonin and norepinephrine, leaving more available for the brain. Mood is improved because the sending of nerve impulses is improved. If SNRIs are to be discontinued, the dose should be decreased gradually over 1 to 2 weeks.

SNRIs are widely used antidepressants intended to improve the person's mood and reduce depression (see Table 16-2). As with other antidepressants, drug effects are seen within 2 to 4 weeks.

Assisting With the Nursing Process. When giving SNRIs, you assist the nurse with the nursing process.
Assessment
- Measure blood pressure in the supine and standing positions.

- Weigh the person weekly.
- Observe for insomnia, nervousness, and other CNS signs and symptoms.
- Ask the person about GI symptoms.
Planning. See Table 16-2 for "Oral Dose Forms."
Implementation. See Table 16-2 for "Initial Adult Oral Dose" and "Daily Maintenance Dose."
Evaluation. Report and record:
- *Restlessness, agitation, anxiety, insomnia.* These symptoms usually occur early in therapy. The drug should be given before 1800 (6:00 PM). The doctor may order a sedative-hypnotic agent.
- *Sedative effects.* Remind the person to use caution when performing tasks that require alertness.
- *GI effects.* Give the drug with food. The doctor may adjust the dose.
- *Suicidal actions.* See *Promoting Safety and Comfort: Drugs Used for Mood Disorders.*

DRUG CLASS: Tricyclic Antidepressants

Tricyclic antidepressants (TCAs) prolong the action of norepinephrine, dopamine, and serotonin. They do so by blocking the reuptake of these neurotransmitters in the synapses between the neurons.

This class of drugs produces antidepressant and tranquilizing effects. After 2 to 4 weeks of therapy, they elevate mood, improve appetite, and increase alertness.

Some TCAs also are used to treat other disorders, including:
- Phantom limb pain
- Chronic pain
- Cancer pain
- Peripheral neuropathy with pain
- Arthritic pain
- Eating disorders
- Premenstrual symptoms
- Obstructive sleep apnea

Assisting With the Nursing Process. When giving TCAs, you assist the nurse with the nursing process.
Assessment
- Ask about bowel movements. Constipation is common when taking these drugs.
- Measure blood pressure in the supine and sitting positions.
- Measure pulse rate and rhythm. Report tachycardia or an irregular pulse to the nurse.
Planning. See Table 16-2 for "Oral Dose Forms."
Implementation
- See Table 16-2 for "Initial Adult Oral Dose" and "Daily Maintenance Dose."
- Dose increases are usually started in the evening due to the drug's sedative effects.
Evaluation. Report and record:
- *Blurred vision; constipation; urinary retention; dryness of the mouth, nose, and throat.* Provide for safety if the person has blurred vision. Follow the care plan for constipation and urinary retention. If mouth, nose, or throat dryness occur, the nurse may allow the person to suck on hard candy or ice chips or chew gum.

- *Orthostatic hypotension.* All drugs in this class may cause some degree of orthostatic hypotension. The person may experience dizziness and weakness when first starting the drug. Blood pressure is measured daily in the supine and standing positions. Provide for safety. Remind the person to rise slowly from a supine or sitting position. Have the person sit or lie down if they feel faint.
- *Sedative effects.* Provide for safety.
- *Tremors, numbness, tingling, Parkinson-like symptoms.* Provide for safety.
- *Tachycardia, dysrhythmias, signs and symptoms of heart failure.* See Chapters 21 and 22.
- *Seizures.* Provide for safety. See Chapter 17.
- *Suicidal actions.* See *Promoting Safety and Comfort: Drugs Used for Mood Disorders.*

OTHER ANTIDEPRESSANTS

Other antidepressant agents include:
- bupropion hydrochloride (byoo pro' pee on); Wellbutrin (wel byoo' trihn)
- mirtazapine (mer taz' ah peen); Remeron (rem' er on)
- trazodone hydrochloride (tray' zoh doan); Desyrel (dez' er el)
- vilazodone (vil az' zo dohn); Viibryd (vy' brid)
- vortioxetine (vor tee ox' a teen); Trintellix (trin tel' ix)

Bupropion Hydrochloride (Wellbutrin)

Wellbutrin is a weak inhibitor of the reuptake of serotonin, norepinephrine, and dopamine.

The drug is used for persons who:
- Do not respond to TCAs
- Cannot tolerate the adverse effects of TCAs

Assisting With the Nursing Process. When giving bupropion (Wellbutrin), you assist the nurse with the nursing process.

Assessment. Weigh the person.

Planning. Oral dose forms are:
- 75 and 100 mg tablets
- 100, 150, and 200 mg 12-hour extended-release tablets
- 150, 174, 300, 348, and 450 mg 24-hour extended-release tablets

Implementation
- The initial adult dose is usually 100 mg twice daily and may be increased to 100 mg three times a day (at least every 6 hours) after several days of therapy.
- The maximum dose in one day is 450 mg. Avoid a dose shortly before bedtime.

Evaluation. Report and record:
- *GI effects.* Give with food. Give stool softeners as ordered for constipation.
- *Restlessness, agitation, anxiety, headache and insomnia.* Bedtime doses are avoided if the person has insomnia. The doctor may order a sedative-hypnotic.
- *Seizures.* Provide for safety. See Chapter 17.
- *Suicidal actions.* See *Promoting Safety and Comfort: Drugs Used for Mood Disorders.*

Mirtazapine (Remeron)

Remeron is a serotonin antagonist; an **antagonist** is a drug that exerts an opposite action to that of another drug, or it competes for the same receptor sites. Mirtazapine's response is like that of the TCAs. The drug elevates mood and reduces symptoms of depression.

Assisting With the Nursing Process. When giving mirtazapine (Remeron), you assist the nurse with the nursing process.

Assessment
- Measure blood pressure in the supine, sitting, and standing positions.
- Weigh the person weekly.

Planning. Oral dose forms are:
- 7.5, 15, 30, and 45 mg tablets
- 30 and 45 mg orally disintegrating tablets (Remeron SolTab)

Implementation
- The starting dose for adults is typically 15 mg daily.
- The dosage may be increased every 1 to 2 weeks up to a maximum of 45 mg daily.
- Dosage increases are usually made in the evening due to increased sedation.

Evaluation. See "Tricyclic Antidepressants".

Trazodone Hydrochloride (Desyrel)

This drug elevates mood and reduces symptoms of depression. It is useful in treating:
- Depression
- Depression associated with schizophrenia
- Depression, tremors, and anxiety associated with alcohol dependence
- Insomnia in persons with substance abuse

Assisting With the Nursing Process. When giving trazodone hydrochloride (Desyrel), you assist the nurse with the nursing process.

Assessment. Measure blood pressure in the supine, sitting, and standing positions.

Planning. Oral dose forms are 50, 100, 150, and 300 mg tablets.

Implementation
- The starting dose is 150 mg in three divided doses.
- The drug may be increased by 50 mg daily every 3 to 4 days.
- The maximum daily dose is 400 mg for outpatients and 600 mg daily for hospital patients.
- Dosage increases are usually made in the evening due to increased sedation.
- Give the drug after a meal or with a light snack to reduce adverse effects.

Evaluation. Report and record:
- *Confusion, dizziness, and light-headedness.* Provide for safety.
- *Drowsiness.* The person needs to exercise caution when working around machines, driving a car, pouring and giving drugs, or performing other duties that require mental alertness.
- *Orthostatic hypotension.* Provide for safety. Remind the person to rise slowly from a supine or sitting position. Have the person sit or lie down if they feel faint.
- *Dysrhythmias, tachycardia.* Report tachycardia or an irregular pulse to the nurse.

Vilazodone (Viibryd)

This drug acts like an SSRI and stimulates some of the serotonin receptors. The drug is used to treat depression, elevates mood, and reduce symptoms of anxiety.

Assisting With the Nursing Process. When giving vilazodone (Viibryd), you assist the nurse with the nursing process.

Assessment
- Ask about GI symptoms.
- Observe for CNS symptoms such as insomnia or nervousness.

Planning. Oral dose forms are:
- 10, 20, and 40 mg tablets

Implementation
- The daily adult dose typically starts at 10 mg daily followed by 20 mg daily for the next 7 days.
- Dosages may be increased to 40 mg daily.
- The drug should be given with food.

Evaluation. Report and record:
- *Dizziness, drowsiness, lightheadedness, and confusion.* The person needs to exercise caution when working around machines, driving a car, pouring and giving drugs, or performing other duties that require mental alertness. Provide for safety.
- *GI symptoms.* Give the drug with food. Any symptoms should resolve with continued use.
- *Suicidal actions.* See *Promoting Safety and Comfort: Drugs Used for Mood Disorders.*

Vortioxetine (Trintellix)

Trintellix acts like an SSRI and stimulates some of the serotonin receptors. The drug elevates mood and reduces symptoms of depression. If vortioxetine is to be discontinued, it should be gradually decreased over 1 to 2 weeks.

Assisting With the Nursing Process. When giving vortioxetine, you assist the nurse with the nursing process.

Assessment
- Ask about GI symptoms.
- Observe for CNS symptoms (e.g., insomnia or nervousness).

Planning. Oral dose forms are 5, 10, and 20 mg tablets.

Implementation
- The adult starting dose is 10 mg daily, followed by 20 mg daily, as tolerated.
- Give 5 mg daily to those who cannot tolerate 10 mg.
- The maximum daily dose is 20 mg.

Evaluation
- *GI symptoms.* Give the drug with food. Any symptoms should resolve with continued use.
- *Dizziness and abnormal dreams.* Provide for safety. The person needs to exercise caution when working around machines, driving a car, pouring and giving drugs, or performing other duties that require mental alertness.
- *Suicidal actions.* See *Promoting Safety and Comfort: Drugs Used for Mood Disorders.*

ANTIMANIC AGENTS

Lithium can be used to treat acute mania and prevent manic and depressive episodes that may be present in bipolar disorder.

In persons with bipolar disorder, lithium is more effective in preventing signs and symptoms of mania than those of depression. The goal of therapy is to maintain the person at an optimal level of functioning with as few mood swings as possible.

Acute antimanic effects usually occur within 5 to 7 days. Full therapeutic effect often takes 10 to 21 days.

Lithium may cause a loss of sodium. To address this, the person must:
- Maintain a normal dietary intake of sodium.
- Drink 10 to 12 eight-ounce glasses of water daily.

Assisting With the Nursing Process. When giving lithium, you assist the nurse with the nursing process.

Assessment
- Measure blood pressure in the supine, sitting, and standing positions.
- Measure weight daily.
- Record intake and output.

Planning. Oral dose forms are:
- 150, 300, and 600 mg capsules and tablets
- 300 and 450 mg slow-release tablets
- 8 mEq/5 mL solution

Implementation
- The daily adult dose is 300 to 600 mg three or four times a day.
- Give the drug with food or milk.

Evaluation. Report and record:
- *Nausea, vomiting, anorexia, abdominal cramps.* These symptoms are usually mild and tend to resolve with continued therapy. Give the drug with food or milk to prevent stomach irritation.
- *Excess thirst and urination, fine hand tremor.* These symptoms are usually mild and tend to resolve with continued therapy.
- *Vomiting, diarrhea, increased reflex reactions, lethargy, weakness.* These symptoms signal toxicity. Alert the nurse immediately. Give the next dose only with the nurse's permission.
- *Progressive fatigue, weight gain.* These symptoms are early signs of a thyroid problem.
- *Itching, ankle edema, metallic taste, hyperglycemia.* These symptoms are rare.
- *Increased or decreased urinary output.* These symptoms may signal renal toxicity.

DRUGS USED FOR PSYCHOSES

Psychosis describes a mental state in which a person is out of touch with reality. The following symptoms are common with psychosis:
- *Delusion*—a false belief (e.g., the person believes that a radio station is broadcasting their thoughts).
- *Delusion of grandeur*—an exaggerated belief about one's importance, wealth, power, or talents (e.g., a person believes they are Superman or the Queen of England).
- *Delusion of persecution*—the false belief that one is being mistreated, abused, or harassed (e.g., a person believes that someone is "out to get" them).

- *Hallucination*—seeing, hearing, smelling, or feeling something that is not real. A person may see animals, insects, or people that are not real. "Voices" are the most common type of hallucination in schizophrenia. "Voices" may comment on the person's behavior, order the person to do things, warn the person of danger, or talk to other "voices."
- *Paranoia*—The person has false beliefs (i.e., delusions) and may be suspicious about a certain person or situation. For example, a person may believe that others are cheating, harassing, poisoning, spying upon, or plotting against them.

Schizophrenia is the most common psychotic disorder. Psychotic symptoms can also occur from medical problems such as:

- *Dementia and delirium.* The underlying cause may be an infection or a metabolic or endocrine disorder.
- *Mood disorders.* Examples include major depression and bipolar disorder.
- *Drugs and substance abuse.* Examples include opiates (see Chapter 18), amphetamines, cocaine, hallucinogens, and alcohol.

Drug and non-drug therapies can be used to treat psychoses. The goal of therapy is to restore behaviors, cognitive function, and psychosocial processes and skills to as close to normal as possible. Unless the psychosis is caused by a medical problem, symptoms will reoccur for most of the person's life.

Antipsychotic drugs (Table 16-3) are classified as:

- *Typical or first-generation antipsychotic agents.* These drugs block dopamine in the central nervous system.
- *Atypical or second-generation antipsychotic agents.* These drugs inhibit dopamine receptors. To a certain degree, they also inhibit serotonin receptors.

The drugs may also affect other neurotransmitter receptors. This accounts for the many adverse effects of therapy.

The initial goals of therapy are to:

- Calm the agitated person. An agitated person may be a threat to themselves or to others.
- Begin treatment of the psychosis and thought disorder.

Therapy often combines benzodiazepines (often lorazepam; Ativan) with antipsychotic agents to lower doses of the antipsychotic agent. This reduces the risk of serious adverse effects common in higher-dose therapy. Some therapeutic effects occur within 1 week of therapy. Reduced agitation and insomnia are examples. Other symptoms, including hallucinations, delusions, and thought disorders, often require 6 to 8 weeks for full therapeutic effects. Increasing the dose of antipsychotic drugs does not reduce the response time.

The need for maintenance therapy depends on the psychotic disorder and the person's tolerance of drug side effects. Most psychotic disorders are treated with low maintenance doses. This lowers the risk of the disorder reoccurring.

Antipsychotic drugs can cause many adverse effects (Box 16-5). Other classes of drugs may be needed to control involuntary body movements and other side effects.

BOX 16-5   Adverse Effects From Antipsychotic Drugs

Involuntary Body Movements

- Tongue protrusion
- Rolling back of the eyes
- Jaw spasm
- Head turned to one side
- Parkinson-like symptoms:
  - Tremors
  - Muscle rigidity
  - Mask-like expression
  - Shuffling gait
  - Loss or weakness of motor function
- Pacing
- Rocking
- Not being able to sit or stand in one place
- Tongue movements:
  - Forward, backward, lateral
  - Thrusting
  - Rolling
  - Fly-catching
- Chewing
- Jaw movements that produce smacking noises
- Problems chewing, speaking, or swallowing
- Blinking
- Brow arching
- Grimacing
- Upward movement of the eyes

Other Adverse Effects

- Allergic reactions
- Increased appetite
- Dysrhythmias
- Changes in blood cells
- Blurred vision
- Constipation
- Drowsiness
- Dry mouth
- Endocrine disorders
- Hyperglycemia
- Hypotension
- Liver toxicity
- Sedation
- Seizures
- Sexual dysfunction
- Urinary retention
- Weight gain

DRUG CLASS: Antipsychotic Agents

Antipsychotic agents (listed in Table 16-3) work by blocking the action of dopamine in the brain. The atypical (not typical) antipsychotic agents also block serotonin receptors.

All antipsychotic agents work at different sites within the brain. Therefore, side effects are observed in different body systems. Atypical antipsychotic agents tend to be more effective and have fewer side effects than typical antipsychotic agents.

The intent of therapy is to:

- Maintain the person at an optimal level of function
- Limit reoccurrence of psychotic symptoms
- Limit adverse effects from drug therapy

Assisting With the Nursing Process. When giving antipsychotic drugs, you assist the nurse with the nursing process.

Assessment

- Measure blood pressure in the supine, sitting, and standing positions.
- Measure weight and height.
- Measure blood glucose.

Planning. See Table 16-3 for "Dose Forms."

Implementation

- See Table 16-3 for "Adult Dosage Range."
- The dosage is adjusted according to the degree of mental and emotional disturbance. It often takes several weeks for the person to show the desired improvements.

TABLE 16-3 Antipsychotic Agents

Generic Name	Brand Name	Dose Forms	Adult Dosage Range (Mg)
Typical (First-Generation) Antipsychotic Agents			
Phenothiazines			
chlorpromazine		Tablets: 10, 25, 50, 100, 200 mg	25-2000
fluphenazine		Tablets: 1, 2.5, 5, 10 mg Elixir: 2.5 mg/5 mL	0.5-40
perphenazine		Tablets: 2, 4, 8, 16 mg	12-64
prochlorperazine		Tablets: 5, 10 mg Suppository: 25 mg	15-150
thioridazine		Tablets: 10, 25, 50, 100 mg	150-800
trifluoperazine		Tablets: 1, 2, 5, 10 mg	2-40
Thioxanthenes			
thiothixene		Capsules: 1, 2, 5, 10 mg	6-60
Non-Phenothiazines			
haloperidol	Haldol	Tablets: 0.5, 1, 2, 5, 10, 20 mg Concentrate: 2 mg/mL	1-100
loxapine	Xylac	Capsules: 5, 10, 25, 50 mg	20-250
Atypical (Second-Generation) Antipsychotic Agents			
aripiprazole	Abilify	Tablets: 2, 5, 10, 15, 20, 30 mg Tablets, orally disintegrating: 10, 15 mg Solution: 1 mg/mL	10-30
asenapine	Saphris	Tablets, sublingual: 2.5, 5, 10 mg	5-20
brexpiprazole	Rexulti	Tablets: 0.25, 0.5, 1, 2, 3, 4 mg	2-4
cariprazine	Vraylar	Capsules: 1.5, 3, 4.5, 6 mg	1.5-6
clozapine	Clozaril	Tablets: 25, 50, 100, 200 mg Tablets, orally disintegrating: 12.5, 25, 100, 150, 200 mg Oral suspension: 50 mg/mL in 100 mL bottle	300-900
iloperidone	Fanapt	Tablets: 1, 2, 4, 6, 8, 10, 12 mg	2-24
lurasidone	Latuda	Tablets: 20, 40, 60, 80, 120 mg	20-160
olanzapine	Zyprexa	Tablets: 2.5, 5, 7.5, 10, 15, 20 mg Tablets, orally disintegrating: 5, 10, 15, 20 mg	5-20
paliperidone	Invega Invega Trinza Invega Sustenna	Tablets, extended-release: 1.5, 3, 6, 9 mg	3-12
quetiapine	Seroquel Seroquel XR	Tablets: 25, 100, 200, 300 mg Tablets, 24-hr extended-release: 50, 150, 200, 300, 400 mg	50-800
risperidone	Risperdal	Tablets: 0.25, 0.5, 1, 2, 3, 4 mg Tablets, orally disintegrating: 0.25, 0.5, 1, 2, 3, 4 mg Solution: 1 mg/mL	4-16
ziprasidone	Geodon	Capsules: 20, 40, 60, 80 mg	40-160

Modified from Willihnganz M: Clayton's Basic Pharmacology for Nurses, ed 18, St Louis, 2020, Elsevier.

Evaluation. Report and record:

- *Fatigue, drowsiness.* The dose is usually ordered for bedtime. The person needs to exercise caution when working around machines, driving a car, pouring and giving drugs, or performing other duties that require mental alertness.
- *Orthostatic hypotension.* Provide for safety. Remind the person to rise slowly from a supine or sitting position. Have the person sit or lie down if they feel faint.
- *Blurred vision; constipation; urinary retention, dryness of the mouth, nose, and throat.* Provide for safety if the person has blurred vision. Give stool softeners as ordered. The nurse may allow the person to suck on hard candy or ice chips or chew gum.
- *Seizures.* Provide for safety. See Chapter 17.
- *Parkinson-like symptoms.* Provide for safety.
- *Involuntary body movements* (see Box 16-5). Provide for safety.
- *Anorexia, nausea, jaundice.* These signal liver toxicity.
- *Hives, itching, rash.* These signal an allergic reaction. Immediately alert the nurse. Do not give the next dose unless approved by the nurse.

DRUGS USED FOR ALCOHOL REHABILITATION

Alcohol slows down brain activity. It affects alertness, judgment, coordination, and reaction time. Over time, heavy drinking damages the brain, central nervous system, liver, heart, kidneys, and stomach. It causes changes in the heart and blood vessels and may also cause forgetfulness and confusion.

Alcohol use disorder (AUD), more commonly known as alcoholism, is a chronic disease. It lasts throughout a person's lifetime. Lifestyle and genetics are risk factors. Some people turn to alcohol for relief from life stresses—retirement, lowered income, loss of job, failing health, loneliness, or the deaths of loved ones or friends. The craving for alcohol can be as strong as the need for food or water. An alcoholic will continue to drink despite serious family, health, or legal problems.

There is no cure, but alcoholism can be treated. Support groups, counseling, and behavior therapy should be used along with drugs to help the person stop drinking. The person must avoid all alcohol to avoid a relapse.

The following drugs are used in alcohol rehabilitation:
- acamprosate (a kamp' roh sait); Campral (kam' prahl)
- disulfiram (di sul' fi ram); Antabuse (ant' ah buse)
- naltrexone (nal trex' own); Vivitrol (viv ih trol')

The goal of therapy is that the person will no longer consume alcohol.

Acamprosate (Campral)

Acamprosate (Campral) is used for chronic alcohol patients who want to maintain a sober state by enhancing the person's ability to not drink. The drug reduces drinking rates in persons who are alcohol-dependent and are not drinking at the start of treatment. The drug does not treat withdrawal symptoms.

Assisting With the Nursing Process. When giving acamprosate (Campral), you assist the nurse with the nursing process.
  Assessment
- Observe the person's level of alertness and orientation to person, time, and place.
- Measure vital signs.
- Ask about GI symptoms.
  Planning. The oral dose form is 333 mg delayed-release tablets.
  Implementation
- The adult dose is two 333 mg tablets (666 mg) three times a day.
- Tablets may be taken without regard to meals.
  Evaluation. Report and record:
- *Diarrhea.* This is usually mild and tends to resolve with continued therapy.
- *Suicidal actions.* Observe for negative thoughts, feelings, behaviors, depression, or suicidal thinking. Report your observations and concerns to the nurse. Follow suicide precautions according to the care plan.

Disulfiram (Antabuse)

Disulfiram (Antabuse) produces a very unpleasant reaction when taken before alcohol. Nausea, severe vomiting, sweating, throbbing headache, dizziness, blurred vision, and confusion occur.

The level of reaction depends on the person and the amount of alcohol consumed. Reaction time depends on the presence of alcohol in the blood. Mild reactions may last from 30 to 60 minutes while more severe reactions may last for several hours.

Taking the drug over a prolonged period does not produce tolerance. The person becomes more sensitive to alcohol the longer they remain on therapy.

The drug is used for chronic alcohol patients who want to maintain a sober state. As little as 10 to 15 mL of alcohol may produce a reaction. The person must not drink or apply alcohol in any form. This includes over-the-counter products such as sleep aids, cough and cold products, after shave lotions, mouthwashes, and rubbing alcohol. The person must not eat sauces, vinegars, and other foods containing alcohol.

Assisting With the Nursing Process. When giving disulfiram (Antabuse), you assist the nurse with the nursing process.
  Assessment
- Observe the person's level of alertness and orientation to person, time, and place.
- Measure vital signs.
- Ask about GI symptoms.
  Planning. The oral dose forms are 250 or 500 mg tablets.
  Implementation
- The adult initial dose is 500 mg once a day for 1 to 2 weeks.
- The maintenance dose ranges from 125 to 500 mg daily. The maximum daily dose is 500 mg.
- The drug is never given to persons who are intoxicated.
- The drug is given when the person has not used alcohol for at least 12 hours.
  Evaluation. Report and record:
- *Drowsiness, fatigue, headache, impotence, metallic taste.* These are usually mild and tend to resolve with continued therapy.

- *Anorexia, nausea, vomiting, jaundice.* These may signal liver toxicity.
- *Hives, rash, itching.* These signal an allergic reaction. Immediately alert the nurse. Do not give the next dose unless approved by the nurse.

Naltrexone (Vivitrol)

Naltrexone (Vivitrol) blocks the effects of opioids by competing for binding sites at opioid receptors (Chapter 18). It may also be used to treat patients with alcoholism by diminishing the craving for alcohol. It must be used with supplemental treatment forms such as group and behavioral therapy.

Assisting With the Nursing Process. When giving naltrexone (Vivitrol), you assist the nurse with the nursing process.

Assessment
- Observe the person's level of alertness and orientation to person, time, and place.
- Measure vital signs.
- Ask about GI symptoms.
  Planning. The oral dose form is 50 mg tablets.
  Implementation
- The adult initial dose is 50 mg daily.
  Evaluation. Report and record:
- *Headache.* These are usually mild and tend to resolve with continued therapy.
- *Anorexia, nausea, vomiting, jaundice.* These may signal liver toxicity.

REVIEW QUESTIONS

Circle the BEST answer.

1. Many of the drugs used to treat mental health disorders affect the:
   a. central nervous system
   b. endocrine system
   c. respiratory system
   d. cardiovascular system
2. Which of the following are used to treat anxiety?
   a. benzodiazepines
   b. monoamine oxidase inhibitors
   c. selective serotonin reuptake inhibitors
   d. antimanic agents
3. The following drugs are used to treat anxiety, *except:*
   a. alprazolam (Xanax)
   b. diazepam (Valium)
   c. clorazepate (Tranxene)
   d. fluoxetine (Prozac)
4. The following drugs are used to treat anxiety, *except:*
   a. hydroxyzine (Vistaril)
   b. paroxetine (Paxil)
   c. doxepin (Apo-Doxepin)
   d. fluvoxamine (Luvox)
5. Which of the following is used to produce sedation before surgery?
   a. hydroxyzine (Vistaril)
   b. chlordiazepoxide (Librium)
   c. lorazepam (Ativan)
   d. clorazepate (Tranxene)
6. Mood disorders are treated with:
   a. antianxiety drugs
   b. antidepressant drugs
   c. antipsychotic drugs
   d. sedative-hypnotics
7. Which of the following have severe side effects when taken with aged cheese and other foods?
   a. monoamine oxidase inhibitors
   b. tricyclic antidepressants
   c. selective serotonin reuptake inhibitors
   d. benzodiazepines

8. The last dose of an MAOI is usually given no later than:
   a. 1400
   b. 1600
   c. 1800
   d. 2000
9. What is the most common side effect of an MAOI?
   a. orthostatic hypotension
   b. sedation
   c. insomnia
   d. mouth dryness
10. Which of the following is an MAOI?
    a. doxepin (Apo-Doxepin)
    b. fluoxetine (Prozac)
    c. sertraline (Zoloft)
    d. phenelzine (Nardil)
11. Selective serotonin reuptake inhibitors are used to treat:
    a. anxiety
    b. depression
    c. bipolar disorder
    d. schizophrenia
12. How long does it usually take to see the effects of SSRIs?
    a. 1 week
    b. 1 to 2 weeks
    c. 2 to 4 weeks
    d. 4 to 6 weeks
13. Which is an SNRI?
    a. duloxetine (Cymbalta)
    b. amitriptyline hydrochloride
    c. selegeline (Emsam)
    d. escitalopram (Lexapro)
14. Which is *not* an antidepressant?
    a. vilazodone (Viibryd)
    b. mirtazapine (Remeron)
    c. buspirone (BuSpar)
    d. trazodone hydrochloride (Desyrel)
15. Which is an antimanic agent?
    a. lithium carbonate (Lithium)
    b. paroxetine (Paxil)
    c. clozapine (Clozaril)
    d. aripiprazole (Abilify)

16. Antimanic agents are used to treat:
    a. psychosis
    b. bipolar disorder
    c. anxiety
    d. depression
17. The full effect of antimanic agents is usually seen within:
    a. 5 to 7 days
    b. 7 to 14 days
    c. 10 to 21 days
    d. 6 months
18. Lithium can cause a loss of:
    a. sodium
    b. calories
    c. protein
    d. potassium
19. When a person is out of touch with reality, this is called:
    a. anxiety
    b. depression
    c. a mood disorder
    d. psychosis
20. The most common psychotic disorder is:
    a. hallucinations
    b. delusions
    c. schizophrenia
    d. post-traumatic stress disorder

21. Antipsychotic drugs often cause:
    a. involuntary body movements
    b. severe hypertension
    c. suicidal actions
    d. sedation
22. The following are antipsychotic agents, *except*:
    a. vortioxetine (Trintellix)
    b. chlorpromazine (Thorazine)
    c. prochlorperazine (Compazine)
    d. haloperidol (Haldol)

Circle T if the statement is true. Circle F if the statement is false.

23. T   F   Drugs used to treat anxiety can lead to dependence.
24. T   F   Drowsiness is a common side effect of anxiolytics.
25. T   F   Serotonin-norepinephrine reuptake inhibitors can cause severe hypotension.
26. T   F   Tricyclic antidepressants have tranquilizing effects.
27. T   F   Acamprosate (Campral) can cause a reaction when mixed with as little as 10 mL of alcohol.
28. T   F   The person taking naltrexone (Vivitrol) can use this alone in the treatment of alcoholism.

Answers to these questions can be found on the Evolve Resources site: http://evolve.elsevier.com/Anderson/medasst/

17

Drugs Used for Seizure Disorders

OBJECTIVES

- Define the key terms and key abbreviations used in this chapter.
- Describe the causes and types of seizure disorders.
- Describe the major types of seizures.
- Identify the factors that affect the antiepileptic drug therapy ordered for a person.
- Describe the drugs used to control seizures.
- Explain how to assist with the nursing process when giving drugs to control seizures.

KEY TERMS

anticonvulsants Drugs used to prevent or reduce seizures; antiepileptic drugs (AEDs)

antiepileptic drugs Drugs used to prevent or reduce seizures; anticonvulsants

epilepsy A brain disorder in which clusters of nerve cells sometimes signal abnormally

seizure Violent and sudden contractions or tremors of muscle groups; convulsion

KEY ABBREVIATIONS

AED antiepileptic drug
kg Kilogram

mg Milligram
mL Milliliter

A **seizure** is abnormal electrical activity in brain neurons involving the nerves. Movements are uncontrolled and may be convulsive (often violent, involuntary muscle movements). Sometimes they are nonconvulsive. The person may lose consciousness or have a change in behavior. Causes include head injury during birth or from trauma, high fever, brain tumors, poisoning, low blood sugar, drug overdose or withdrawal, and nervous system disorders.

Epilepsy is a brain disorder in which clusters of nerve cells sometimes signal abnormally. There are brief, sudden changes in the brain's electrical function. The person may experience strange sensations, emotions, and behaviors. Sometimes there are seizures, muscle spasms, and loss of consciousness. A single seizure does not mean the person has epilepsy. In epilepsy, seizures recur. The person with this disorder has a permanent brain injury or defect.

Children and young adults are commonly affected. However, epilepsy can develop at any time in a person's life. It can occur alongside any problem affecting the brain. Such causes include:

- Brain injury before, during, or after birth
- Problems with brain development before birth
- The mother having an injury or infection during pregnancy
- Head injury (e.g., accidents, gunshot wounds, sports injuries, falls, blows to the head)
- Poor nutrition
- Brain tumor
- Childhood fevers
- Poison (e.g., lead and alcohol)
- Infection (e.g., meningitis and encephalitis)
- Stroke

There is currently no cure for seizure disorders. Doctors order drugs to help prevent seizures. While the drugs controls seizures in many people, drug therapy may not work in others.

When controlled, epilepsy usually does not affect learning and activities of daily living. Activity and job limits occur in severe cases. For example, a person has seizures at any time. The person may not be allowed to drive, which may limit job choices. Also, the person is at risk for accidents and injuries. Safety measures are needed for the home, workplace, transportation, and recreation.

The major types of seizures are.

- *Focal* (partial) onset seizure. Only one part of the brain is involved. A body part may jerk involuntarily or the person may have a hearing or vision problem or stomach discomfort. The person does not lose consciousness. Focal seizures may turn into generalized seizures. There are two types of focal seizures:
  - *Simple motor seizures.* A single body part is involved. A finger, arm, or leg may start jerking. Examples include turning the head, smacking the lips, and drooling.
  - *Complex seizures.* Many different symptoms may occur, such as wandering aimlessly or unusual movements when chewing or swallowing. The person may also appear normal. They may be confused or be in a dream-like state. They do not remember having these seizures.
- *Generalized onset.* Both sides of the brain are involved. There are three types of generalized seizures:
  - *Tonic-clonic seizures.* In the *tonic phase,* the person loses consciousness. If standing or sitting, the person falls to the floor. The body is rigid because all muscles contract at once. The *clonic phase* follows in which muscle groups

contract and relax. This causes jerking and twitching movements and possible urinary and fecal incontinence. A deep sleep is common after the seizure. Confusion and headache may occur on awakening.

- *Atonic seizures (drop attack).* Abrupt loss of muscle tone where the person suddenly falls. A person seated may slump forward violently while remaining conscious. Protective head gear must be worn to protect the person.
- *Myoclonic seizures.* Lightning-like repetitive contractions of the face, trunk, arms, and legs. The person remains conscious. These occur most often at night right before falling asleep.
- *Nonconvulsive seizures.* The most common of this type is *absence* seizures. These occur mostly in children and disappear at puberty. Attacks may last 5-20 seconds long with altered consciousness. They appear to be staring into space with a few rhythmic movements of the eyes or head, lip smacking, mumbling, chewing, or swallowing movements. They have no memory of the events.

ANTICONVULSANT THERAPY

Seizure treatment must include the cause. If caused by an infection, the infection is treated. If seizures continue after treating the cause, anticonvulsant therapy is the main treatment.

Anticonvulsants are used to prevent or reduce seizures. They are commonly referred to as **antiepileptic drugs** (AEDs). The goals of therapy are to:

- Improve the person's quality of life
- Reduce the frequency of seizures
- Reduce injury from seizure activity
- Have few adverse effects from therapy

The drug ordered for a person depends on:
- The type of seizure
- The person's age and sex
- Other health problems
- Potential adverse effects from the drugs

The ordered drug is discontinued, and another is ordered, if the first drug does not control seizures. The process continues until a drug or a combination of drugs controls seizure activity.

AEDs control seizures by:
- Inhibiting the processes that excite the neurons
- Enhancing the processes that inhibit the neurons
- Preventing the seizure from spreading to other neurons

See *Delegation Guidelines: Antiepileptic Drug Therapy.*

DELEGATION GUIDELINES
Antiepileptic Drug Therapy

Some antiepileptic drugs are given parenterally. Because you do not give parenteral dose forms, they are not included in this chapter. Should a nurse delegate the administration of such to you, you must:
- Remember that parenteral dosages are often very different from dosages for other routes.
- Refuse the delegation but do not ignore the request. Make sure the nurse knows that you cannot give the drug and why.

DRUG CLASS: Benzodiazepines

The benzodiazepines used for AED therapy are listed in Table 17-1. How they control seizures is not fully understood. They might inhibit neurotransmission.

TABLE 17.1   Antiepileptic Drugs

Generic Name	Brand Name	Dose Forms	Adult Dosage Range
Benzodiazepines			
clobazam	Onfi	Tablets: 10, 20 mg Oral suspension: 2.5 mg/mL (120 mL)	Up to 40 mg/day
clonazepam	Klonopin	Tablets: 0.5, 1, 2 mg Tablets, orally disintegrating: 0.125, 0.25, 0.5, 1, 2 mg	Up to 20 mg/day
clorazepate	Tranxene	Tablets: 3.75, 7.5, 11.25, 15, 22.5 mg	Up to 90 mg/day
diazepam	Valium	Tablets: 2, 5, 10 mg Liquid: 1, 5 mg/mL Gel, rectal: 2.5, 5, 10, 15, 20 mg	Initially 5-10 mg, up to 30 mg
lorazepam	Ativan	Tablets: 0.5, 1, 2 mg Oral solution: 2 mg/mL	If the person is seizing, the nurse will give this drug intravenously.
Hydantoins			
ethotoin	Peganone	Tablets: 250 mg	2-3 g/day
phenytoin	Dilantin	Tablets: 50 mg Capsules: 30, 100 mg Suspension: 125 mg/5 mL	300-600 mg/day
Succinimides			
ethosuximide	Zarontin	Capsules: 250 mg Syrup: 250 mg/5 mL	1000-1250 mg/day
methsuximide	Celontin	Capsules: 150, 300 mg	900-1200 mg/day

Modified from Willihnganz M: Clayton's Basic Pharmacology for Nurses, ed 18, St Louis, 2020, Elsevier.

Assisting With the Nursing Process. When giving benzodiaz-epines for AED therapy, you assist the nurse with the nursing process.

> *Assessment*
> * Observe the person's:
>   * Speech pattern
>   * Degree of alertness
>   * Orientation to person, time, and place
>
> *Planning.* See Table 17-1 for oral and rectal "Dose Forms."
> *Implementation*

* See Table 17-1 for "Adult Dosage Range."
* Rapidly discontinuing these drugs after long-term use may cause symptoms similar to alcohol withdrawal. These can vary from weakness and anxiety to delirium and seizures. Symptoms may not appear for several days after the drug is discontinued. Benzodiazepines are safely withdrawn over 2 to 4 weeks.

> *Evaluation.* Report and record:

* *Sedation, drowsiness, dizziness, blurred vision, fatigue, lethargy.* These resolve with dosage adjustment or when the drug is discontinued. Provide for safety. The person must use caution when working around machines, driving a car, pouring and giving drugs, or performing other duties that require mental alertness.
* *Behavior disturbances.* The person may be aggressive and agitated. Provide for safety.
* *Sore throat, fever, weakness.* These may signal changes in red blood cells and white blood cells.
* *Anorexia, nausea, vomiting, jaundice.* These may signal liver toxicity.

DRUG CLASS: Hydantoins

Hydantoins work in the part of the brain where it can stop the spread of seizure activity.

Assisting With the Nursing Process. When giving hydanto-ins, you assist the nurse with the nursing process.

> *Assessment*
> * Measure blood glucose.
> * Observe the person's:
>   * Speech pattern
>   * Degree of alertness
>   * Orientation to person, time, and place
>
> *Planning.* See Table 17-1 for oral "Dose Forms."
> *Implementation*

* See Table 17-1 for "Adult Dosage Range."
* Give the drug with food or milk to reduce stomach irritation.
* If an oral suspension is ordered, shake the container well and use an oral syringe to measure the dose.

> *Evaluation.* Report and record:

* *Nausea, vomiting, indigestion.* Give the drug with food or milk.
* *Sedation, drowsiness, dizziness, blurred vision, fatigue, lethargy.* These resolve with dosage adjustment or when the drug is discontinued. Provide for safety. The person must use caution when working around machines, driving a car, pouring and giving drugs, or performing other duties that require mental alertness.
* *Confusion.* Provide for safety.
* *Gum overgrowth.* Provide good oral hygiene.
* *Hyperglycemia.* Measure blood glucose.

* *Sore throat, fever, jaundice, weakness.* These may signal changes in red blood cells and white blood cells.
* *Anorexia, nausea, vomiting, jaundice.* These may signal liver toxicity.
* *Rash, itching.* These may signal an allergic reaction. Immediately notify the nurse. Do not give the next dose unless approved by the nurse.

DRUG CLASS: Succinimides

Succinimides slow the electrical activity in the brain. They are used to treat absence seizures.

Assisting With the Nursing Process. When giving succin-imides, you assist the nurse with the nursing process.

> *Assessment*
> * Observe the person's:
>   * Speech pattern
>   * Degree of alertness
>   * Orientation to person, time, and place
>
> *Planning.* See Table 17-1 for oral "Dose Forms."
> *Implementation.* See Table 17-1 for "Adult Dosage Range."
> *Evaluation.* Report and record:

* *Nausea, vomiting, indigestion.* Give the drug with food or milk.
* *Sedation, drowsiness, dizziness, fatigue, lethargy.* Provide for safety. The person must use caution when working around machines, driving a car, pouring and giving drugs, or performing other duties that require mental alertness.

OTHER ANTIEPILEPTIC DRUGS

The following are also AED agents:
* Carbamazepine (kar bah maz' e peen); Tegretol (teg' reh tol)
* Gabapentin (gah bah pen' tin); Neurontin (nuhr on' tin)
* Lamotrigine (lah mot' rah geen); Lamictal (lah mik' tahl)
* Levetiracetam (lehv et tihr see' tahm); Keppra (kep' rah)
* Oxcarbazepine (ox karb az' e peen); Trileptal (tri lehp' tahl)
* Phenobarbital (fee' no barb' it al)
* Pregabalin (prĕ GĂB ă lĭn); Lyrica (LĬR ĭ kă)
* Primidone (prih' mih doan); Mysoline (my' so leen)
* Tiagabine (tee ag' ah bean); Gabitril (gab' ah tril)
* Topiramate (toh peer' ah mate); Topamax (toh' pah max)
* Valproic acid (val proe' ik ah' sid); Depakene (dep' ah keen)
* Zonisamide (zoh nis' am eyd); Zonegran (zoh' negh grahn)
  See Table 17-2 for a list of newer antiepileptic drugs.

Carbamazepine (Tegretol)

This drug blocks the reuptake of norepinephrine and the release of norepinephrine. It also affects dopamine. The drug is often used with other AEDs to control generalized tonic-clonic and focal seizures.

Assisting With the Nursing Process. When giving carbamaze-pine (Tegretol), you assist the nurse with the nursing process.

> *Assessment*
> * Measure blood pressure in the supine and standing positions.
> * Measure weight daily.
> * Measure intake and output.

TABLE 17.2   Other Antiepileptic Drugs

Generic Name	Brand Name	Availability	Adult Dosage Range	Use For Seizure
brivaracetam	Briviact	Oral solution: 10 mg/mL (300 mL) Tablets: 10, 25, 50, 75, 100 mg	50-200 mg/day	Focal seizures
eslicarbazepine	Aptiom	Tablets: 200, 400, 600, 800 mg	Up to 1600 mg/day	Focal seizures
lacosamide	Vimpat	Oral solution: 10 mg/mL (200, 465 mL) Tablets: 50, 100, 150, 200 mg	200-400 mg/day	Simple or complex focal seizures
perampanel	Fycompa	Oral suspension: 0.5 mg/mL (340 mL) Table ts: 2, 4, 6, 8, 10, 12 mg	2-12 mg/day	Focal and generalized seizures

Modified from Willihnganz M: Clayton's Basic Pharmacology for Nurses, ed 18, St Louis, 2020, Elsevier.

- Observe the person's:
  - Speech pattern
  - Degree of alertness
  - Orientation to person, time, and place
  - *Planning.* Oral dose forms are:
- 200 mg tablets
- 100 mg chewable tablets
- 100, 200, and 400 mg 12-hr extended-release tablets
- 100, 200, and 300 mg 24-hr extended-release tablets
- 100 mg/5 mL oral solution
  Implementation
- The initial adult dose is 200 mg two times a day during the first day.
- The drug is gradually increased by 200 mg/day in divided doses every 6 to 8 hours.
- Total daily dosage should not exceed 1600 mg.
  Evaluation. Report and record:
- *Nausea, vomiting, drowsiness, dizziness.* Provide for safety. The person must use caution when working around machines, driving a car, pouring and giving drugs, or performing other duties that require mental alertness.
- *Hypertension, orthostatic hypotension.* Provide for safety. Remind the person to rise slowly from a supine or sitting position. Have the person sit or lie down if they feel faint.
- *Dyspnea, edema.* Measure intake and output.
- *Kidney toxicity.* Check urine color.
- *Sore throat, fever, jaundice, weakness.* These may signal changes in red blood cells and white blood cells.
- *Anorexia, nausea, vomiting, jaundice.* These may signal liver toxicity.
- *Rash, itching.* These may signal an allergic reaction. Tell the nurse at once. Do not give the next dose unless approved by the nurse.

Gabapentin (Neurontin)

This drug is usually used with other AEDs to reduce the frequency of focal seizures.

Assisting With the Nursing Process. When giving gabapentin (Neurontin), you assist the nurse with the nursing process.
Assessment
- Observe the person's:
  - Speech pattern
  - Degree of alertness
  - Orientation to person, time, and place

Planning. Oral dose forms are:
- 100, 300, and 400 mg capsules
- 300, 600, and 800 mg tablets
- 25 mg/mL, 250 mg/5 mL, and 300 mg/6 mL oral solution
Implementation
- The adult dosage is 900 to 1800 mg daily.
- The dosage is usually adjusted as follows:
  - Day 1 at bedtime: 300 mg
  - Day 2: 300 mg two times a day
  - Day 3: 300 mg three times a day
- The dosage is increased to no more than 1800 mg daily in three divided doses. Doses of up to 3600 mg have been administered for short periods of time with no adverse effects.
- If antacids (Chapter 26) are ordered for the person, give the gabapentin (Neurontin) at least 2 hours after the last dose of antacid. Antacids reduce the absorption of the drug.
Evaluation. Report and record:
- *Sedation, drowsiness, dizziness, blurred vision.* These resolve with dosage adjustment or when the drug is discontinued. Provide for safety. The person must use caution when working around machines, driving a car, pouring and giving drugs, or performing other duties that require mental alertness.
- *Speech, alertness, and orientation to person, time, and place.* Observe for changes.

Lamotrigine (Lamictal)

This drug stabilizes neuron membranes. It inhibits the release of some excitatory neurotransmitters and is used in combination with other AEDs to treat focal and generalized seizures.

Assisting With the Nursing Process. When giving lamotrigine (Lamictal), you assist the nurse with the nursing process.
Assessment
- Observe the person's:
  - Speech pattern
  - Degree of alertness
  - Orientation to person, time, and place
  Planning. Oral dose forms are:
- 25, 100, 150, 200, and 250 mg tablets
- 5 and 25 mg chewable tablets
- 25, 50, 100, and 200 mg orally disintegrating tablets
- 25, 50, 100, 200, 250, and 300 mg 24-hr extended-release tablets

Implementation

- The adult dosage is started at 25 mg once a day for 2 weeks. It is followed by 50 mg twice a day for 2 weeks. The dose may be increased by 50 mg per day every 1 to 2 weeks until the maintenance dose is reached.
- The usual maintenance dose is 225 to 375 mg per day in two divided doses.

Evaluation. Report and record:

- *Nausea, vomiting, indigestion.* Give the drug with food or milk.
- *Sedation, drowsiness, dizziness, blurred vision.* These resolve with dosage adjustment or when the drug is discontinued. Provide for safety. The person must use caution when working around machines, driving a car, pouring and giving drugs, or performing other duties that require mental alertness.
- *Rash, itching.* Slower increases in dosage adjustment may resolve this problem. Rash and itching may signal an allergic reaction. Tell the nurse at once. Do not give the next dose unless approved by the nurse.

Levetiracetam (Keppra)

This drug is used in combination with other AEDs to treat focal seizures.

Assisting With the Nursing Process. When giving levetiracetam (Keppra), you assist the nurse with the nursing process.

Assessment

- Observe the person's:
  - Speech pattern
  - Degree of alertness
  - Orientation to person, time, and place

Planning. Oral dose forms are:

- 250, 500, 750, and 1000 mg tablets
- 250, 500, 750, 1000 mg disintegrating tablets
- 500 and 750 mg 24-hr extended-release tablets
- 100 mg/mL oral solution

Implementation

- The initial adult dose is 500 mg two times a day.
- Dosage may be increased every 2 weeks by 500 mg two times a day.
- The maximum daily dose is 3000 mg in divided doses.

Evaluation. Report and record:

- *Weakness, drowsiness, dizziness.* These are usually mild and resolve with continued therapy. Provide for safety. The person must use caution when working around machines, driving a car, pouring and giving drugs, or performing other duties that require mental alertness.
- *Speech, alertness, and orientation to person, time, and place.* Observe for changes.

Oxcarbazepine (Trileptal)

This drug stabilizes neurons. It prevents repeated firing of electrical impulses thought to produce seizures. The drug is used alone or in combination with other AEDs to treat focal seizures.

Assisting With the Nursing Process. When giving oxcarbazepine (Trileptal), you assist the nurse with the nursing process.

Assessment

- Observe the person's:
  - Speech pattern
  - Degree of alertness
  - Orientation to person, time, and place

Planning. Oral dose forms are:

- 150, 300, and 600 mg tablets
- 300 mg/5 mL suspension

Implementation

- The adult initial dosage is 300 mg two times a day for the first 3 days.
- The dosage may be increased by 300 mg per day every 3 days to a dosage of 1200 mg per day.
- Dosages of 2400 mg a day are effective in some persons.

Evaluation. Report and record:

- *Confusion, poor coordination, drowsiness, dizziness.* These are usually mild and resolve with continued therapy. Provide for safety. The person must use caution when working around machines, driving a car, pouring and giving drugs, or performing other duties that require mental alertness.
- *Speech, alertness, and orientation to person, time, and place.* Observe for changes.
- *Nausea, headache, lethargy, confusion, reduced level of consciousness, weakness.* These are signs of low sodium.
- *Sore throat, fever, jaundice, weakness.* These may signal changes in red blood cells and white blood cells.

Phenobarbital

This drug is a long-acting barbiturate (Chapter 15) that prevents the spread of seizure activity. The drug is used in combination with other AEDs to treat focal and generalized seizures.

The drug has sedative effects. Therefore, it is used when non-sedating AEDs do not control seizures.

Assisting With the Nursing Process. See Chapter 16.

Pregabalin (Lyrica)

This drug is related to gabapentin. The drug is used in combination with other AEDs to treat focal seizures. It has the potential for abuse and dependence. It is a Schedule V controlled substance (Chapter 3, pg. 20).

Assisting With the Nursing Process. When giving pregabalin (Lyrica), you assist the nurse with the nursing process.

Assessment

- Observe the person's:
  - Speech pattern
  - Degree of alertness
  - Orientation to person, time, and place

Planning

- 25, 50, 75, 100, 150, 200, 225, and 300 mg capsules
- 82.5, 165, 330 mg 24-hr extended-release tablets
- 20 mg/mL oral solution

Implementation

- The adult dosage is 50 mg three times daily or 75 mg twice daily.
- The daily dosage is 600 mg daily in divided doses.

Evaluation. Report and record:

- *Sedation, drowsiness, dizziness, blurred vision.* These resolve with continued therapy or with dosage adjustment. Provide for safety. The person must use caution when working around machines, driving a car, pouring and giving drugs, or performing other duties that require mental alertness.
- *Speech, alertness, and orientation to person, time, and place.* Observe for changes.

Primidone (Mysoline)

This drug is related to the barbiturates. The drug is used in combination with other AEDs to treat focal and generalized seizures.

Assisting With the Nursing Process. When giving primidone (Mysoline), you assist the nurse with the nursing process.

Assessment
- Observe the person's:
  - Speech pattern
  - Degree of alertness
  - Orientation to person, time, and place

Planning. The oral dose forms are 50 and 250 mg tablets.

Implementation
- For an adult, the drug is ordered as follows:
  - Days 1, 2, and 3 at bedtime: 100 to 125 mg daily.
  - Days 4, 5, and 6: the dosage is increased to 100 to 125 mg two times a day.
  - Days 7, 8, and 9: the dosage is increased to 100 to 125 mg three times a day.
  - Every 3 or 4 days: the dosage is increased by 100 to 125 mg until the person responds, or tolerance develops.
- The typical dosage is 750 to 1500 mg in one day. The dosage should not exceed 2000 mg in one day.

Evaluation. Report and record:

- *Sedation, drowsiness, dizziness, blurred vision.* These resolve with continued therapy or dosage adjustment. Provide for safety. The person must use caution when working around machines, driving a car, pouring and giving drugs, or performing other duties that require mental alertness.
- *Sore throat, fever, jaundice, weakness.* These may signal changes in red blood cells and white blood cells.

Tiagabine (Gabitril)

This drug is used in combination with other AEDs to treat focal seizures.

Assisting With the Nursing Process. When giving tiagabine (Gabitril), you assist the nurse with the nursing process.

Assessment
- Observe the person's:
  - Speech pattern
  - Degree of alertness
  - Orientation to person, time, and place

Planning. The oral dose forms are 2, 4, 12, and 16 mg tablets.

Implementation
- Initially, 4 mg are given daily for an adult. The daily dosage is increased by 4 to 8 mg every week until:
  - The person responds.

- A total daily dose of 56 mg is given. A total daily dosage of 32 to 56 mg may be given in 2 to 4 divided doses.

Evaluation. Report and record:

- *Sedation, drowsiness, dizziness.* These resolve with continued therapy or with dosage adjustment. Provide for safety. The person must use caution when working around machines, driving a car, pouring and giving drugs, or performing other duties that require mental alertness.
- *Speech, alertness, memory loss, and orientation to person, time, and place.* Observe for changes.

Topiramate (Topamax)

This drug is used in combination with other AEDs to treat focal and generalized seizures.

Assisting With the Nursing Process. When giving topiramate (Topamax), you assist the nurse with the nursing process.

Assessment
- Observe the person's:
  - Speech pattern
  - Degree of alertness
  - Orientation to person, time, and place
- Measure weight.
- Measure intake and output.
- Ask about headaches.

Planning. Oral dose forms are:

- 25, 50, 100, and 200 mg tablets
- 15 and 25 mg sprinkle capsules
- 25, 50, 100, 150, and 200 mg 24-hr extended-release sprinkle capsules

Implementation
- The adult initial dose is 25 mg twice a day.
- The daily dosage is increased by 50 mg at weekly intervals until the person responds.
- The usually daily dosage is 400 mg two times a day.
- Note the following when giving this drug:
  - Tablets should not be broken. They taste bitter.
  - Sprinkle capsules can be swallowed whole. If they are not swallowed whole, open the capsule carefully and sprinkle the entire contents on a teaspoon of soft food. Ask the person to swallow the drug/food mixture at once. Tell the person not to chew the drug/food mixture.

Evaluation. Report and record:

- *Sedation, drowsiness, dizziness.* These resolve with continued therapy or with dosage adjustment. Provide for safety. The person must use caution when working around machines, driving a car, pouring and giving drugs, or performing other duties that require mental alertness.
- *Speech, alertness, and orientation to person, time, and place.* Observe for changes.
- *Decreased sweating, overheating.* These may occur with vigorous activity or exposure to warm or hot temperatures. Be sure to keep the person hydrated.

Valproic Acid (Depakene)

The action of this drug is not known. It may inhibit neurotransmitter activity. The drug is used to treat focal and generalized seizures.

Assisting With the Nursing Process. When giving valproic acid (Depakene), you assist the nurse with the nursing process.

Assessment
- Observe the person's:
  - Speech pattern
  - Degree of alertness
  - Orientation to person, time, and place

Planning. Oral dose forms are:
- 250 mg capsules
- 125 mg capsules containing coated particles
- 125, 250, and 500 mg 24-hr sustained-release tablets
- 250 mg/5 mL syrup

Implementation
- The adult dosage is based on the person's body weight and ranges from 10 to 15 mg/kg two to three times a day.
- The dosage is increased by 5 to 10 mg/kg at weekly intervals. Maximum daily dosage is 60 mg/kg.
- Give the drug with food or milk to reduce gastric irritation.

Evaluation. Report and record:
- *Sedation, drowsiness, dizziness, blurred vision.* These resolve with continued therapy or with dosage adjustment. Provide for safety. The person must use caution when working around machines, driving a car, pouring and giving drugs, or performing other duties that require mental alertness.
- *Nausea, vomiting, and indigestion.* Give the drug with food or milk.
- *Sore throat, fever, jaundice, weakness.* These may signal changes in red blood cells and white blood cells.
- *Anorexia, nausea, vomiting, jaundice.* These may signal liver toxicity.
- *Abdominal pain, nausea, vomiting, anorexia.* These are symptoms of pancreatitis.

Zonisamide (Zonegran)

This drug is used in combination with other AEDs to treat focal seizures.

Assisting With the Nursing Process. When giving zonisamide (Zonegran), you assist the nurse with the nursing process.

Assessment
- Observe the person's:
  - Speech pattern
  - Degree of alertness
  - Orientation to person, time, and place
- Measure vital signs.

Planning. The oral dose forms are 25, 50, and 100 mg capsules.

Implementation
- The initial adult dose is 100 mg daily.
- After 2 weeks, the dosage may be increased to 200 mg a day for at least 2 weeks. The 200 mg may be taken at the same time.
- The dosage can be increased up to 600 mg per day. Two weeks should pass between dosage changes.
- Note the following when giving this drug:
  - It may be taken with or without food.
  - Due to sedative effects, it may be taken at bedtime.
  - The person should drink six to eight glasses of water each day.

Evaluation. Report and record:
- *Sedation, drowsiness, dizziness.* These resolve with continued therapy or with dosage adjustment. Provide for safety. The person must use caution when working around machines, driving a car, pouring and giving drugs, or performing other duties that require mental alertness.
- *Speech, alertness, and orientation to person, time, and place.* Observe for changes.
- *Back pain, abdominal pain, pain during urination.* These may signal kidney problems.
- *Sore throat, fever, jaundice, weakness.* These may signal changes in red blood cells and white blood cells.
- *Rash, itching.* Slower increases in dosage adjustment may resolve the problem. Rash and itching may signal an allergic reaction. Alert the nurse at once. Do not give the next dose unless approved by the nurse.

REVIEW QUESTIONS

Circle the BEST answer.

1. A body part may jerk. The person does not lose consciousness. This is:
   a. epilepsy
   b. a focal (partial) onset seizure
   c. a generalized seizure
   d. a petit mal seizure
2. Seizure treatment must always include:
   a. antiepileptic drug therapy
   b. benzodiazepines
   c. the cause of the seizures
   d. treatment of epilepsy
3. Antiepileptic drugs control seizures by affecting:
   a. neurons in the brain
   b. nerves in the central nervous system
   c. voluntary muscles
   d. involuntary muscles
4. Which is a benzodiazepine?
   a. clobazam (Onfi)
   b. ethotoin (Peganone)
   c. perampanel (Fycompa)
   d. ethosuximide (Zarontin)
5. When giving a benzodiazepine, you must:
   a. give the drug with food or milk
   b. provide for safety
   c. provide good oral hygiene
   d. measure blood pressure
6. Which is a hydantoin?
   a. lacosamide (Vimpat)
   b. tiagabine (Gabitril)
   c. phenytoin (Dilantin)
   d. methsuximide (Celontin)

7. Succinimides are given:
   a. with food or milk
   b. at bedtime
   c. before meals
   d. after meals
8. Before giving carbamazepine (Tegretol), you:
   a. measure blood glucose
   b. provide good oral hygiene
   c. measure weight
   d. give the person food
9. When giving most AEDs, you observe the following, *except*:
   a. the person's speech pattern
   b. the person's urine color
   c. the person's degree of alertness
   d. the person's orientation to person, time, and place
10. The first dose of gabapentin (Neurontin) is given:
    a. with food or milk
    b. at bedtime
    c. before meals
    d. after meals
11. Which is a barbiturate?
    a. phenobarbital
    b. lorazepam (Ativan)
    c. phenytoin (Dilantin)
    d. ethosuximide (Zarontin)
12. Before giving topiramate (Topamax), you:
    a. observe urine color
    b. provide good oral hygiene
    c. measure weight
    d. measure blood pressure

13. Which drug's dosage is based on the person's body weight?
    a. valproic acid (Depakene)
    b. pregabalin (Lyrica)
    c. oxcarbazepine (Trileptal)
    d. zonisamide (Zonegran)
14. Before giving zonisamide (Zonegran), you:
    a. provide food or milk
    b. provide good oral hygiene
    c. measure weight
    d. measure vital signs

Circle T if the statement is true. Circle F if the statement is false.

15. T F   Many antiepileptic drugs cause sedation.
16. T F   Phenytoin (Dilantin) is given with food or milk.
17. T F   The person with a seizure disorder can take only one antiepileptic.
18. T F   Lamotrigine (Lamictal) is given before meals.
19. T F   The first doses of primidone (Mysoline) are given in the morning.
20. T F   Sprinkle capsules are a dose form of topiramate (Topamax). The person can chew the capsule contents.

Answers to these questions can be found on the Evolve Resources site: http://evolve.elsevier.com/Anderson/medasst/

Drugs Used to Manage Pain

OBJECTIVES

- Define the key terms and key abbreviations used in this chapter.
- Explain how to assist the nurse in assessing a person's pain.
- Describe the different types of pain.
- Describe the factors that affect a person's reaction to pain.
- Describe the drugs used for pain management.
- Explain how to assist with the nursing process when giving drugs for pain management.

KEY TERMS

analgesic A drug that relieves pain; *an* means *without* and *algesic* means *pain*

drug tolerance When a person needs increasingly higher doses of a drug to treat their pain

euphoria An exaggerated feeling or state of physical or mental well-being

opiate A drug that contains opium, is derived from opium, or has opium-like activity

opioids Drugs that provide pain relief; they come from opium or are man-made.

pain To ache, hurt, or be sore; discomfort

semi-synthetic A natural substance that has been partially altered by chemicals

synthetic A substance that is made rather than naturally occurring

KEY ABBREVIATIONS

CNS Central nervous system
g Gram
GI Gastrointestinal
h Hour
MAR Medication administration record
mcg Microgram
mg Milligram
MI Myocardial infarction

mL Milliliter
NSAID Non-steroidal anti-inflammatory drug
PG Prostaglandin
PO Per os (orally)
PRN When necessary, as needed
q Every
STAT At once, immediately

Pain *(discomfort)* means to ache, hurt, or be sore. It is unpleasant. Pain is subjective (Chapter 4), meaning you cannot see, hear, touch, or smell pain. You must rely on what the person says. Report complaints to the nurse. The information is used for the nursing process.

Pain is personal and differs for each person. What *hurts* to one person may *ache* to another. What one person calls *sore* another may call *aching*. If a person complains of pain, the person *has* pain. You must believe the person. You cannot see, hear, feel, or smell the pain.

Pain is a warning from the body. It means there is tissue damage. Pain often causes the person to seek health care.

There are different types of pain. The doctor references the type of pain when diagnosing and ordering drugs for pain relief. The nurse uses it for the nursing process.

- *Acute pain* is felt suddenly from injury, disease, trauma, or surgery. There is tissue damage. Acute pain lasts a short time, usually less than 6 months. It lessens with healing.
- *Chronic pain* lasts longer than 3 months. There is no longer tissue damage, and the pain remains long after healing.

Arthritis and cancer are common causes. Chronic pain may be constant or occur off and on.

- *Radiating pain* is felt at the site of tissue damage and in nearby areas. For example, pain from a heart attack is often felt in the left chest, left jaw, left shoulder, and left arm. Gallbladder disease can cause pain in the right upper abdomen, the back, and the right shoulder.
- *Phantom pain* is felt in a body part that is no longer there. For example, a person with an amputated leg may still sense leg pain.

A person may handle pain well one time and poorly the next time. Many factors affect reactions to pain.

- *Past experience.* We learn from past experiences; they help us know what to do or what to expect. A person may have had pain before. The severity of pain, its cause, how long it lasted, and if relief occurred all affect the person's current response to pain. Knowing what to expect can help or hinder how the person handles pain. Some people have not had pain and may experience fear and anxiety when it occurs. Fear and anxiety can make pain worse.

- *Anxiety.* Anxiety relates to feelings of fear, dread, worry, and concern. The person is uneasy and tense. The person may feel troubled or threatened. Pain and anxiety are related. Pain can cause anxiety, which increases how much pain the person feels. Reducing anxiety helps lessen pain. For example, when the nurse explains to Mr. Smith that he will have pain after surgery, the nurse also explains that he will receive drugs for pain relief. Mr. Smith knows the cause of the pain and he knows what to expect. This helps reduce his anxiety and therefore may decrease the amount of pain felt.
- *Rest and sleep.* Rest and sleep restore energy. They reduce body demands, and the body repairs itself. Lack of needed rest and sleep affects thinking and coping with daily life. Sleep and rest should be increased with illness and injury. Pain may seem worse when the person is tired or restless. Also, the person tends to focus on pain when tired and unable to rest or sleep.
- *Attention.* The more a person thinks about the pain, the worse it seems. Sometimes severe pain is all the person thinks about. However, even mild pain can seem worse if the person thinks about it all the time. Pain often seems worse at night. Activity is less, and it is quieter than during the day. There are no visitors. The radio or TV is off. Others are asleep. When unable to sleep, the person has extra time to think about the pain.
- *Personal and family duties.* Pain is often ignored when there are children to whom care must be provided. Some people may go to work with pain and others may deny pain if they fear a serious illness. The illness can interfere with job performance, going to school, or caring for children, a partner, or ill parents.
- *The value or meaning of pain.* To some people, pain is a sign of weakness. It may mean a serious illness and the need for painful tests and treatments. Therefore, pain may be ignored or denied. Sometimes, pain gives pleasure. The pain of childbirth is one example. For some persons, pain means not having to work or assume daily routines. Pain is sometimes used to avoid certain people or things. The pain may be useful. Some people like doting and pampering by others. Therefore, the person values and wants such attention.
- *Support from others.* Dealing with pain is often easier when family and friends offer comfort and support. Physical touch by a valued person is very comforting. Just having a loved one nearby also helps. Some people do not have caring family or friends and therefore deal with pain alone. Being alone may increase anxiety; the person has more time to think about the pain.
- *Culture.* Culture affects pain responses. In some cultures, the person in pain is *stoic.* To be stoic means to show no reaction to joy, sorrow, pleasure, or pain. Strong verbal and nonverbal reactions to pain are seen in other cultures. Non-English speaking persons may have problems describing pain. The agency must be aware of which persons require someone to interpret and translate the person's needs. All persons have the right to be comfortable and as pain-free as possible.
- *Illness.* Some diseases cause decreased pain sensations (e.g., central nervous system [CNS] disorders). The person may not feel pain, or it may not feel severe. The person is at risk for undetected disease or injury. Pain occurs with tissue damage and serves as an alert to illness or injury. If pain is not felt, the person does not know to seek care.
- *Age.* Children may not understand pain. They simply know it feels bad. They have fewer pain experiences and they do not know what to expect. Children do not know how to relieve their own pain. They rely on adults for help. Adults must be alert to behaviors and situations that signal a child's pain. Infants cry, fuss, and are restless. Toddlers and preschoolers may not have the words to express pain. See *Focus on Older Persons: Factors Affecting Pain.*

FOCUS ON OLDER PERSONS

Factors Affecting Pain

Older persons may have decreased pain sensations. They may not feel pain, or it may not feel severe. The person is at risk for undetected disease or injury. Pain occurs with tissue damage and signals illness or injury. If pain is not felt, the person does not know to seek care.

Some older persons may have multiple painful health problems. Chronic pain may mask new pain. Older persons may ignore or deny new pain—they may think it relates to a known health problem. Older persons may also deny or ignore pain for fear of what that pain may mean.

Thinking and reasoning are affected in some older persons. Some cannot verbally communicate pain. Changes in usual behavior may signal pain. For example, a person who normally moans and groans may become quiet and withdrawn, or a person who is friendly and outgoing may become agitated and aggressive. Someone who is normally nonverbal and quiet may become restless and cry easily. Loss of appetite also signals pain.

Report any changes in a person's usual behavior to the nurse. All persons have the right to correct pain management. The nurse needs to do a pain assessment when the person's behavior changes.

You cannot see, hear, feel, or smell the person's pain. You must rely on what the person tells you and promptly report any pain-related information you have collected. Write down what the person says—use the person's exact words when reporting and recording. The nurse needs this information to accurately assess the person's pain:

- *Location.* Where is the pain? Ask the person to point to the area of pain. Because pain can radiate, ask the person if the pain is anywhere else and to point to those areas.
- *Onset and duration.* When did the pain start? How long has it lasted?
- *Intensity.* Does the person complain of mild, moderate, or severe pain? Ask the person to rate the pain on a scale of 0 to 10, with 10 as the most severe (Fig. 18-1), or use the Wong-Baker Faces Pain Rating Scale (Fig. 18-2). Although designed for children, the scale is useful for persons of all ages. To use the scale, tell the person that each face shows how a person is feeling. Read the description for each face. Then ask the person to choose the face that best describes how they feel.
- *Description.* Ask the person to describe the pain. If the person cannot describe the pain, offer some of the words listed in Box 18-1.
- *Factors causing pain.* These are called *precipitating* factors. *To precipitate* means *to cause.* Such factors include moving or

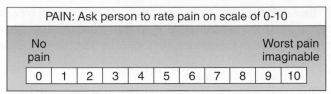

PAIN: Ask person to rate pain on scale of 0-10

No pain										Worst pain imaginable
0	1	2	3	4	5	6	7	8	9	10

Fig. 18-1 Pain rating scale. (Modified from deWit SC: *Fundamental concepts and skills for nursing,* ed 5, Philadelphia, 2018, Saunders.)

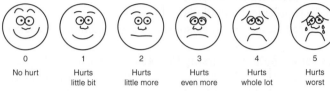

0	1	2	3	4	5
No hurt	Hurts little bit	Hurts little more	Hurts even more	Hurts whole lot	Hurts worst

Fig. 18-2 Wong-Baker Faces Pain Rating Scale. (From Hockenberry MJ, Wilson D: *Wong's nursing care of infants and children,* ed 10, St Louis, 2015, Mosby.)

BOX 18-1 Words Used to Describe Pain

- Aching
- Burning
- Cramping
- Crushing
- Dull
- Gnawing
- Knife-like
- Piercing
- Pressure
- Sharp
- Sore
- Squeezing
- Stabbing
- Throbbing
- Vise-like

turning in bed, coughing or deep breathing, and exercise. Ask what the person was doing before the pain started and when it started.

- *Factors affecting pain.* Ask the person what seems to make the pain better and what makes it worse.
- *Vital signs.* Measure the person's pulse, respirations, and blood pressure. Increases in these vital signs often occur with acute pain. Vital signs may be normal with chronic pain.
- *Other signs and symptoms.* Does the person have other symptoms? These may include dizziness, nausea, vomiting, weakness, numbness, or tingling. Box 18-2 lists the signs and symptoms that often occur with pain.

See Promoting Safety and Comfort: Nonverbal Observations.

PROMOTING SAFETY AND COMFORT

Nonverbal Observations

Comfort

Some people are unable to communicate verbally. Common signs a person is experiencing pain include:

- Facial grimacing
- Crying
- Holding or protecting a body part
- Resisting movement of a body part
- Anxiety or fear
- Inability to sleep
- Restlessness

Report any of these observations to the nurse immediately.

BOX 18-2 Signs and Symptoms of Pain

Body Responses

- Appetite: changes in
- Dizziness
- Nausea
- Numbness
- Pulse, respirations, and blood pressure: increased
- Skin: pale (pallor)
- Sleep: difficulty with
- Sweating (diaphoresis)
- Tingling
- Vomiting
- Weakness

Behaviors

- Crying
- Gasping
- Grimacing
- Groaning
- Grunting
- Holding the affected body part (splinting; guarding)
- Irritability
- Moaning
- Mood: changes in
- Positioning: maintaining one position; refusing to move
- Quietness
- Restlessness
- Rubbing
- Screaming
- Speech: slow or rapid; loud or quiet

PAIN MANAGEMENT

An **analgesic** is a drug that relieves pain. (*An* means *without; algesic* means *pain.*). The goals of pain management are to:

- Relieve the intensity of pain and how long the person is in pain.
- Prevent the pain from becoming chronic.
- Prevent suffering and disability associated with pain.
- Prevent psychologic and socioeconomic consequences resulting from inadequate pain management.
- Control the side effects of pain management.
- Improve the person's ability to perform typical daily activities at an optimal level.

Pain is transmitted from the site of injury to the brain. First, pain receptors are stimulated at the site of damage. Neurotransmitters then send nerve impulses from the site of damage to the spinal cord. The impulses travel up the spinal cord to various areas of the brain.

Opiate receptors within the CNS control pain. When opiates stimulate these receptors, pain sensation is blocked. An **opiate** is a drug that either contains opium, is derived from opium, or has opium-like activity. Opiate comes from the Greek word *opion,* which means *poppy juice. Opium* is the milky substance from unripe poppy seed pods. **Opioids** in general come from opium or are man-made. They are a group of drugs that are analgesics and provide relief from pain by binding to opiate receptors in the brain.

Opioids are divided into the following classes:

- Opiate agonists
- Opiate partial agonists
- Opiate antagonists

When cells are damaged, other chemicals are released that stimulate pain receptors. Other drugs block the release of such chemicals and stop pain. These drugs fall into two other classes:

- Prostaglandin inhibitors
- Nonsteroidal antiinflammatory drugs (NSAIDs)

Most drugs for pain management are given PRN (when necessary; as needed). *The nurse decides when a PRN drug is needed.*

See Delegation Guidelines: Pain Management.

See Delegation Guidelines: PRN Drugs.

BOX 18-3 Signs and Symptoms of Opiate Withdrawal

- Restlessness
- Perspiration
- Gooseflesh
- Tears
- Nose: runny
- Pupils: dilated
- Muscle spasms
- Pain: severe back, abdominal, and leg
- Cramps: muscle and abdominal

- Flashes: hot and cold
- Insomnia
- Nausea
- Vomiting
- Diarrhea
- Sneezing: severe
- Vital signs: increased temperature, heart rate, respiratory rate, and blood pressure

ADDICTION AND DRUG TOLERANCE

Opiate agonists and opiate partial agonists can produce addiction. They are considered controlled substances under the Federal Controlled Substances Act of 1970. If used for recreational purposes, addiction may develop after 3 to 6 weeks of continuous use. The addicted person has the signs and symptoms listed in Box 18-3 when the drug is withdrawn. The symptoms become increasingly severe and peak within 36 to 72 hours and then disappear over the next 5 to 14 days.

Drug tolerance occurs when a person needs increasingly higher doses of a drug to treat their pain. If a person develops a tolerance to one opiate, they usually need higher doses of other opiates as well.

DRUG CLASS: Opiate Agonists

Opiate agonists are a group of semisynthetic or synthetic drugs that can relieve severe pain without causing loss of consciousness. A **synthetic** is a substance that is made rather than naturally occurring. A **semi-synthetic** is a natural substance that has been partially altered by chemicals.

Morphine and heroine (a morphine-like drug) are major examples of opiate agonists. Other analgesics unrelated to morphine act at the same sites in the brain. Opiate agonists are listed in Table 18-1.

DELEGATION GUIDELINES
Pain Management

Some drugs used for pain management are given parenterally—by subcutaneous, intramuscular, or intravenous injection. Because you do not give parenteral dose forms, they are not included in this chapter. Should a nurse delegate the administration of this task to you, you must:
- Remember that parenteral dosages are often very different from doses for other routes.
- Refuse the delegation but do not ignore the request. Make sure the nurse knows that you cannot give the drug and why.

DELEGATION GUIDELINES
PRN Drugs

Many states and agencies do not let MA-Cs give PRN drugs, including controlled substances, by any route. Others let MA-Cs give oral, rectal, and transdermal dose forms. You must know and follow the policy of your state and agency before administering PRN drugs.

Remember, an *agonist* is a drug that acts on a certain type of cell to produce a predictable response (Chapter 15). They stimulate opiate receptors in the CNS. A list of their effects are found in Box 18-4.

Opiate agonists are used:
- To relieve acute or chronic moderate to severe pain. Examples include pain resulting from acute injury, surgery, renal or biliary colic, myocardial infarction (MI), or cancer.
- For preoperative sedation
- To supplement anesthesia
- To reduce anxiety in persons with acute pulmonary edema

Assisting With the Nursing Process. *Many states and agencies do not let MA-Cs give PRN drugs, including controlled substances, by any route. Others let MA-Cs give oral, rectal, and transdermal dose forms. You must know and follow the policy of your state and agency.*

Opiate agonists are given PRN for pain relief. They may be given as a STAT order (at once, immediately) to treat such conditions as MI or pulmonary edema. They may also be given as a one-time order (e.g., for preoperative sedation). Oral dose forms are usually PRN.

When a person receives an opiate agonist, you assist the nurse with the nursing process.
Assessment
- Observe the person's speech pattern, degree of alertness, and orientation to person, time, and place.
- Measure vital signs. Tell the nurse at once if the person's respirations are below 12 per minute.
- Ask the person to rate their pain using a pain rating scale.
- Check the medication administration record (MAR) to see when the person last received an analgesic.
  Planning. See Table 18-1 for "Dose Forms."
- Many opiate agonists are available for subcutaneous, intramuscular, or intravenous injection. You do not give drugs by those routes. See *Delegation Guidelines: Pain Management.*
  Implementation. See Table 18-1 for "Initial Adult Dose."
  Evaluation. Report and record:
- *Light-headedness, dizziness, sedation, nausea, vomiting, sweating.* These tend to occur with the first dose. The supine position helps reduce these symptoms. Provide for safety.
- *Confusion, disorientation.* Observe the person's alertness and orientation to person, time, and place. Provide for safety.
- *Orthostatic hypotension.* The person may have dizziness and weakness with the first dose. Provide for safety. Measure blood pressure. Do not allow the person to sit up.
- *Constipation.* This may occur from continued use. Follow the care plan for fluid intake and diet. Give stool softeners or laxatives as ordered (see Chapter 27).
- *Respiratory depression.* Tell the nurse at once if the person's respiratory rate is below 12 per minute. Also observe the depth of respirations. Alert the nurse immediately if the person has shallow breathing.

TABLE 18-1 Opiate Agonists

Generic Name	Brand Name	Dose Forms	Initial Adult Dose
Morphine and Morphine-Like Derivatives			
codeine	Codeine Sulfate Codeine Phosphate	Tablets: 15, 30, 60 mg	Analgesic: 15-60 mg q4-6h Antitussive: 10-20 mg q4-6h

hydrocodone	Zohydro ER
	Hysingla ER
		Capsule, 12-hr extended-release: 10, 15, 20, 30, 40,
		  50 mg
		Tablet, 24-hr extended-release abuse deterrent: 20, 30,
		  40, 60, 80, 100, 120 mg	

hydromorphone	Dilaudid	Tablets: 2, 4, 8 mg Liquid: 1 mg/mL Suppositories: 3 mg Tablets, 24-hr extended-release abuse deterrent: 8, 12, 16, 32 mg	PO: 2 mg q4-6h Rectal: 3 mg q6-8h
levorphanol		Tablets: 2 mg	2 mg q6-8h
morphine	Morphine Sulfate	Tablets: 15, 30 mg Oral Solution: 10, 20, 100 mg/5 mL; 20 mg/mL Suppositories: 5, 10, 20, 30 mg	PO: 10-30 mg q4h Rectal: 10-20 mg q4h
	Morphine Sulfate CR MS Contin Kadian	Tablets, 12-hr sustained-release: 15, 30, 60, 100, 200 mg Capsules, 24-hr extended-release: 10, 20, 30, 40, 50, 60, 80, 100, 200 mg	

morphine sulfate/naltrexone	Embedab	Capsules, extended-release: morphine (mg)/naltrexone
		  (mg): 20/0.8, 30/1.2, 50/2, 60/2.4, 80/3.2, 100/4
			PO: Start with lowest dosage; dose no
			  more frequently than q12h. Requires
			  individual patient adjustment.

oxycodone	Roxicodone Oxycontin	Tablets: 5, 10, 15, 20, 30 mg Tablets, 12-hr controlled-release abuse deterrent: 10, 15, 20, 30, 40, 60, 80 mg	5 mg q6h PO:10-160 mg q12h (controlled-release)
	Oxycodone	Capsules: 5 mg Oral solution: 5 mg/5 mL Oral Concentrate: 100 mg/5 mL	
	Xtampza ER	Capsules, 12-hr extended-release abuse deterrent: 9, 13.5, 18, 27, 36 mg	
	Oxaydo	Tablets, abuse deterrent, oral: 5, 7.5 mg	

oxymorphone	Opana,
	Opana ER 12 Hour Abuse-
	  Deterrent
		Tablets: 5, 10 mg
		Tablets, 12-hr sustained-release: 5, 7.5, 10, 15, 20,
		  30, 40 mg
			PO: 10-20 mg q4-6h
			PO: 5-10 mg q12h (sustained-release)

Meperidine-Like Derivatives			
fentanyl	Fentora Actiq Duragesic	Lozenges: 200, 400, 600, 800, 1200, 1600 mcg Buccal: 100, 200, 300, 400, 600, 800 mcg Transdermal patch: 12, 25, 50, 75, 100 mcg/hour	Buccal: 200 mcg Upper torso: 25 mcg/hour every 72 hours
meperidine	Demerol	Tablets: 50, 100 mg Syrup: 50 mg/5 mL	50-150 mg q3-4h
Methadone-Like Derivatives			
methadone	Methadone, Dolophine	Tablets: 5, 10 mg Orally disintegrating tablets: 40 mg Oral solution: 5, 10 mg/5 mL Oral concentrate: 10 mg/mL	Analgesia: 2.5-10 mg q8-12h Maintenance: 20-40 mg; up to 120 mg daily
Other Opiate Agonists			
tramadol	Ultram ConZip	Tablets: 50 mg Tablets, 24-hr extended-release:100, 200, 300 mg Capsules, 24-hr extended-release: 100, 150, 200, 300 mg	PO: 50-100 mg PO: 100 mg every 24 hours, adjust every 5 days as needed
tapentadol	Nucynta Nucynta ER	Tablets: 50, 75, 100 mg Tablets, 12-hr extended-release: 50, 100, 150, 200, 250 mg	PO: 50-100 mg

Modified from Willihnganz M: Clayton's Basic Pharmacology for Nurses, ed 18, St Louis, 2020, Elsevier.

BOX 18-4   Effects of Opioid Agonists

- Analgesia
- Respiratory depression
- Cough reflex suppression
- Drowsiness
- Sedation
- Mental clouding
- Euphoria (an exaggerated feeling or state of physical or mental well-being)
- Nausea and vomiting

- *Urinary retention.* Opiate agonists can cause ureter and bladder spasms. Urine is retained; the person may have problems starting a urine stream. Measure intake and output and ask about problems urinating. Follow the care plan to promote urination.
- *Excess use or abuse.* The person often complains of pain or requests a drug for pain relief. The report of pain may occur well before the next dose can be given. Always report complaints of pain or drug requests to the nurse at once. See Box 18-3 for signs and symptoms of withdrawal.

DRUG CLASS: Opiate Partial Agonists

Opiate partial agonists work well if the person has not used or has not developed a drug tolerance to opiate agonists. If the person has developed a drug tolerance to opiate agonists, higher doses of opiate partial agonists are needed to provide the same relief. This class of drug works well only for a few weeks and increasing the dose does not provide more pain relief.

Opiate partial agonists are listed in Table 18-2.

Opiate partial agonists are used for:

- Short-term (up to 3 weeks) pain relief from cancer, burns, and renal colic
- Preoperative sedation
- Surgical anesthesia
- Obstetric procedures

Assisting With the Nursing Process. *Many states and agencies do not let MA-Cs give PRN drugs, including controlled substances, by any route. Others let MA-Cs give oral, rectal, and transdermal dose forms. Know and follow state and agency policies.*

Opiate partial agonists are also given PRN for pain relief. Oral dose forms are usually PRN.

When a person receives an opiate partial agonist, you assist the nurse with the nursing process.

Assessment
- Observe the person's speech pattern, degree of alertness, and orientation to person, time, and place.
- Measure vital signs. Tell the nurse at once if the person's respiratory rate is below 12 per minute.
- Ask the person to rate their pain using a pain rating scale.
- Check the medication administration record (MAR) for when the person last received an analgesic.

Planning. See Table 18-2 for "Dose Forms."
- Many opiate partial agonists are available for subcutaneous, intramuscular, or intravenous injection. You do not give drugs by those routes. See *Delegation Guidelines: Pain Management.*

Implementation. See Table 18-2 for "Adult Dosage Range."

Evaluation. Report and record:
- *Clamminess, dizziness, sedation, nausea, vomiting, sweating, dry mouth.* These tend to occur with the first dose. The supine position helps reduce these symptoms. Provide for safety.
- *Confusion, disorientation, hallucinations.* Observe the person's alertness and orientation to person, time, and place. Provide for safety.
- *Orthostatic hypotension.* The person may have dizziness and weakness with the first dose. Provide for safety. Measure blood pressure. Do not allow the person to sit up.
- *Constipation.* This may occur from continued use. Follow the care plan for fluid intake and diet. Give stool softeners or laxatives as ordered (Chapter 27).
- *Respiratory depression.* Tell the nurse at once if the person's respiratory rate is under 12 per minute. Also observe the depth of respirations. Alert the nurse at once if the person has shallow breathing.
- *Excess use or abuse.* The person often complains of pain or requests a drug for pain relief. The report of pain may be well before the next dose can be given. Always report complaints of pain or drug requests to the nurse at once. See Box 18-3 for signs and symptoms of withdrawal.

DRUG CLASS: Opiate Antagonists

Opiate antagonists include:
- naloxone (nal ox' own); Narcan (nar' kan)
- naltrexone (nal trex' own); Vivitrol (viv ih trol')

TABLE 18-2   Opiate Partial Agonists

Generic Name	Brand Name	Dose Forms	Adult Dosage Range
buprenorphine	Buprenex	Tablets, sublingual: 2, 8 mg	0.3 mg q 6-8h
	Butrans	Patch (weekly): 5, 7.5, 10, 15, 20 mcg/hr	75 mcg daily, may increase every 4 days
	Belbuca	Buccal Film: 75, 150, 300, 450, 600, 750, 900 mcg	
buprenorphine/naloxone	Suboxone	Sublingual Film: 2/0.5, 4/1, 8/2, 12/3 mg buprenorphine/naloxone	2/0.5 mg q2h
	Bunavail	Buccal Film: 2.1/0.3, 4.2/0.7, 6.3/1 mg buprenorphine/naloxone	2.1/0.3 mg q2h
	Zubsolv	Tablets, sublingual: 0.7/0.18, 1.4/0.36, 2.9/0.71, 5.7/1.4, 8.6/2.1, 11.4/2.9 mg buprenorphine/naloxone	1.4/0.36 mg q1.5-2h
butorphanol		Nasal spray: 10 mg/mL	Nasal: 1 spray in each nostril repeated in 3-4 hrs as needed
pentazocine	Talwin	Tablets (with naloxone 0.5 mg): 50 mg	PO: 50-100 mg q3-4h; maximum 600 mg daily

Modified from Willihnganz M: Clayton's Basic Pharmacology for Nurses, ed 18, St Louis, 2020, Elsevier.

Opiate antagonists reverse the CNS depression that can occur when taking opiate agonists and opiate partial agonists. The person may experience respiratory depression if given too much opiate agonists and opiate partial agonists.

- Many opiate partial agonists are available for subcutaneous, intramuscular, or intravenous injection. You do not give drugs by those routes. See *Delegation Guidelines: Pain Management.*

Naloxone (Narcan)

This is the drug of choice for treatment of respiratory depression when excessive doses of opiate agonists or opiate partial agonists have been given, or if the cause is unknown.

Assisting With the Nursing Process. *Many states and agencies do not let MA-Cs give PRN drugs, including controlled substances by any route. Others let MA-Cs give oral, rectal, and transdermal dose forms. You must know and follow the policy of your state and agency.*

When a person receives Narcan, you assist the nurse with the nursing process.

Assessment
- Observe the person's speech pattern, degree of alertness, and orientation to person, time, and place.
- Measure vital signs. Tell the nurse at once if the person's respirations are below 12 per minute.

Planning
- Nasal solution dose:
- 4 mg/0.1 mL

Implementation
- 1 nasal spray (4 mg) in one nostril.
- May repeat every 2 to 3 minutes alternating nostrils.

Evaluation. Report and record:
- *Nausea, vomiting, sweating, and tachycardia.* These tend to occur if the effects of opiates are reversed early. Keep the person supine. Provide for safety.
- *Suicidal actions, depression.* Observe for negative thoughts, feelings, behaviors, depression, or suicidal thinking. Report your observations and concerns to the nurse. Follow suicide precautions according to the care plan.
- *Tachycardia and dysrhythmias.* See Chapter 21.

Naltrexone (Vivitrol)

This drug is similar to Narcan; however, it is active after orally administration and its action lasts much longer than Narcan. Naltrexone blocks the effects of opiates and may lessen or eliminate opiate-seeking behavior by blocking the feeling of euphoria from opiates. It is also used to treat alcoholism. See Chapter 16 (pg. 175).

For treatment of opiate agonist dependence:
- Give 25 mg for the first dose.
- Give 50 mg on day two.
- Maintenance dose is 50 mg daily.
- 100 mg every other day or 150 mg every third day can help improve adherence during a behavior modification program.

DRUG CLASS: Prostaglandin Inhibitors

Prostaglandin inhibitors include:
- Acetaminophen (a seat a min' o fen); Tylenol (ty' le nol)
- Salicylates (sal i sil' ates)

Prostaglandin (PG) is a chemical released by the body during trauma and contributes to pain. Prostaglandin inhibitors block this chemical.

Acetaminophen (Tylenol)

Acetaminophen is a synthetic non-opiate analgesic. It is an effective analgesic and antipyretic drug that has no anti-inflammatory activity. Its analgesic-antipyretic effects are useful to treat fever and discomfort from bacterial and viral infections. It is also useful for headaches and musculoskeletal pain.

Assisting With the Nursing Process. *Many states and agencies do not let MA-Cs give PRN drugs by any route. Others let MA-Cs give oral, rectal, and transdermal dose forms. You must know and follow state and agency policy.*

When a person receives acetaminophen, you assist the nurse with the nursing process.

Assessment
- Measure vital signs.
- Ask the person to rate their pain using a pain rating scale.
- Check the MAR for when the person last received the ordered drug.

Planning
- Oral dose forms:
- 650 mg extended-release tablets
- 80 and 160 mg chewable tablets
- 325 and 500 mg capsules, caplets, and tablets
- 80 and 160 mg dispersible tablets
- 80 mg/0.8 mL, 160 mg/5 mL, 500 mg/15 mL, and 650 mg/20.3 mL liquid
- Rectal dose forms:
- 80, 120, 325, and 650 mg suppositories

Implementation
- The usual adult oral dose is 325 to 650 mg every 4 to 6 hours.
- The maximum adult dose is 4 g (4000 mg) per day. People with liver disease should take no more than 2 g (2000 mg) per day. Older adults should take no more than 3 g (3000 mg) per day.

Evaluation. Report and record:
- *Stomach irritation.* Give the drug with food, milk, or large amounts of water.
- *Anorexia, nausea, vomiting, low blood pressure, drowsiness, confusion, abdominal pain, jaundice.* These signal liver toxicity.

Salicylates

Salicylates are the most often used analgesics to treat slight to moderate pain. See Table 18-3. Drugs in this class inhibit the production of prostaglandins (PGs) and cause the following effects:
- *Analgesic effect.* Salicylates inhibit the formation of PGs affecting pain receptors.
- *Anti-inflammatory effect.* Salicylates inhibit PGs that produce signs and symptoms of inflammation (e.g., redness, swelling, or unusual warmth).
- *Anti-pyretic effect.* Anti means against. Pyretic comes from the Greek word that means fever. Salicylates inhibit the formation and release of PGs in the brain that cause body temperature to rise. An anti-pyretic is a drug given to reduce fever.

Drugs in this class do not dull alertness, cause mental sluggishness, or affect memory. They do not cause hallucinations, euphoria, or sedation.

Aspirin

Aspirin is a PG that inhibits platelet activity (Chapter 24). Platelets are needed for blood clotting. Aspirin reduces blood clotting by inhibiting platelet activity. Therefore, aspirin is used to:
- Reduce the risk of transient ischemic attacks or stroke in men
- Reduce the risk of MI in persons with previous MI or unstable angina

Assisting With the Nursing Process. When a person receives salicylates, you assist the nurse with the nursing process.
Assessment
- Observe the person's speech pattern, degree of alertness, and orientation to person, time, and place.
- Measure vital signs.
- Ask the person to rate their pain using a pain rating scale.
- Check the MAR for when the person last received the ordered drug.
Planning. See Table 18-3 for "Dose Forms."
Implementation. See Table 18-3 for "Uses and Adult Dosages."
Evaluation. Report and record:
- *Stomach irritation.* Give the drug with food, milk, or large amounts of water. If antacids (Chapter 26) are ordered, they are given 1 hour later. Enteric drug forms are often ordered to reduce stomach irritation.
- *GI bleeding.* Vomitus that may resemble coffee grounds ("coffee ground emesis"), red vomitus, and black or dark, tarry stools are signs of GI bleeding. Test stool for occult blood as directed by the nurse and care plan.
- *Tinnitus (ringing in the ears), impaired hearing, dimmed vision, sweating, fever, lethargy, dizziness, confusion, nausea, vomiting.* These signal salicylate toxicity, which can occur from continuous use of high doses. The condition resolves when the dose is reduced.

DRUG CLASS: Non-Steroidal Anti-Inflammatory Drugs

Non-steroidal anti-inflammatory drugs (NSAIDs) are known as "aspirin-like" drugs. They are prostaglandin inhibitors and have varying degrees of analgesic, anti-inflammatory, and antipyretic effects.

NSAIDs are used to reduce pain, inflammation, and fever. Over-the-counter NSAIDs are used to:
- Reduce fever
- Relieve minor aches and pains from the common cold
- Relieve pain and inflammation from rheumatoid arthritis, osteoarthritis, ankylosing spondylitis (arthritis in the spine), and gout
- Relieve headaches, toothaches, muscle aches, and menstrual cramps

Side effects tend to be less severe than those from the salicylates. However, there is a risk of MI, stroke, and life-threatening GI bleeding from NSAIDs.

NSAIDs are not given to persons allergic to aspirin.

Assisting With the Nursing Process. When a person receives NSAIDs, you assist the nurse with the nursing process.
Assessment
- Observe the person's speech pattern, degree of alertness, and orientation to person, time, and place.
- Measure vital signs.
- Ask the person to rate their pain using a pain rating scale.
Planning. See Table 18-4 for "Dose Forms."
Implementation. See Table 18-4 for "Uses and Adult Dosages."
Evaluation. Report and record:
- *Stomach irritation.* Give the drug with food or milk.
- *Constipation.* This may occur from continued use. Follow the care plan for fluid intake and diet. Give stool softeners or laxatives as ordered.
- *GI bleeding.* Vomitus that resembles coffee grounds ("coffee ground emesis"), red vomitus, and black or dark, tarry stools are signs of GI bleeding. Test stools for occult blood as directed by the nurse and care plan.
- *Confusion.* Observe the person's alertness and orientation to person, time, and place. Provide for safety.
- *Rash, hives, itching.* These may signal an allergic reaction. Alert the nurse at once. Do not give the next dose unless approved by the nurse.
- *Decreased urine output, red or smoky-colored urine.* These signal kidney problems.

TABLE 18-3   Salicylates

Generic Name	Brand Name	Dose Forms	Uses and Adult Dosages
aspirin	Ecotrin, St. Joseph	Tablets: 81, 325, 500 mg Sustained-release tablets: 81, 162, 325, 500 mg Chewable tablets: 81 mg Suppositories: 60, 120, 200, 300, 600 mg	Minor aches and pains: 325-600 mg q4h Arthritis: 2.6-5.2 g/day in divided doses Acute rheumatic fever: 7.8 g/day Myocardial infarction prophylaxis: 75-325 mg daily Ischemic stroke: 50-325 mg daily
diflunisal		Tablets: 500 mg	Mild to moderate pain: Initially, 1000 mg, then 500 mg q8h Osteoarthritis and rheumatoid arthritis: 250-500 mg twice daily
magnesium salicylate	Doan's	Tablets: 325, 580 mg	Mild aches and pains: 580-650 mg three or four times daily
salsalate		Tablets: 500, 750 mg	Mild pain: 500-750 mg four to six times daily

Modified from Willihnganz M: Clayton's Basic Pharmacology for Nurses, ed 18, St Louis, 2020, Elsevier.

TABLE 18-4 Non-Steroidal Anti-Inflammatory Agents

Generic Name	Brand Name	Dose Forms	Uses and Adult Dosages
celecoxib	Celebrex	Capsules: 50, 100, 200, 400 mg	Rheumatoid and osteoarthritis: 100-200 mg twice daily Ankylosing spondylitis: 200-400 mg daily Acute pain and primary dysmenorrhea: 400 mg initially, followed by 200 mg on the first day, then 200 mg twice daily
diclofenac	Cataflam, Voltaren Flector Voltaren	Tablets: 50 mg Tablets, 24-hr delayed-release: 25, 50, 75, 100 mg Capsules: 18, 25, 35 mg Patch, transdermal: 1.3% Gel, transdermal: 3% Gel, transdermal: 1%	Rheumatoid and osteoarthritis, ankylosing spondylitis: 25-50 mg two or three times daily Primary dysmenorrhea: 50 mg three times daily Apply to pain site twice daily. Do not apply to broken skin. For actinic keratoses: Apply twice daily. Avoid direct sun exposure. Osteoarthritis: Apply to affected arm, hand, foot, and knee joints four times daily. Do not apply to spine, hips, or shoulders.
etodolac		Capsules: 200, 300 mg Tablets: 400, 500 mg Tablets, extended-release: 400, 500, 600 mg	Osteoarthritis, pain: 300-400 mg three or four times daily
fenoprofen	Nalfon	Capsules: 200, 400 mg Tablets: 600 mg	Rheumatoid and osteoarthritis: 300-600 mg three or four times daily Mild to moderate pain: 200 mg q4-6h
flurbiprofen		Tablets: 50, 100 mg	Rheumatoid and osteoarthritis: 50-100 mg two or three times daily
ibuprofen	Motrin, Advil	Tablets: 100, 200, 400, 600, 800 mg Tablets, chewable: 100 mg Capsules: 200 mg Oral suspension: 40 mg/mL, 50 mg/1.25 mL; 100 mg/5 mL	Rheumatoid and osteoarthritis: 300-600 mg three or four times daily Mild to moderate pain: 400 mg q4-6h Primary dysmenorrhea: 400 mg q4h
indomethacin	Indocin	Capsules: 25, 50 mg Capsules, sustained-release: 75 mg Oral suspension: 25 mg/5 mL Suppository: 50 mg	Rheumatoid and osteoarthritis, ankylosing spondylitis: 25-50 mg three or four times daily Acute painful shoulder: 25-50 mg two or three times daily Acute gouty arthritis: 50 mg three times daily
ketoprofen		Capsules: 25, 50, 75 mg Capsules, extended-release: 200 mg	Rheumatoid and osteoarthritis: Initially 75 mg three times daily or 50 mg four times daily; reduce initial dose by $\frac{1}{2}$ to $\frac{1}{3}$ in elderly patients or those with impaired renal function Mild pain, primary dysmenorrhea: 25-50 mg three or four times daily
ketorolac	Toradol	Tablets: 10 mg	Analgesic: 40 mg or less per 24 hours; do not exceed 5 days of therapy
meclofenamate		Capsules: 50, 100 mg	Rheumatoid and osteoarthritis: 200-400 mg daily in 3 or 4 equal doses Mild to moderate pain: 50-100 mg three or four times daily Primary dysmenorrhea: 100 mg three times daily
mefenamic acid		Capsules: 250 mg	Moderate pain or primary dysmenorrhea: Initially 500 mg daily, then 250 mg q6h; do not exceed 7 days of therapy
meloxicam	Mobic	Tablets: 7.5, 15 mg Capsules: 5, 10 mg	Osteoarthritis: 7.5-15 mg daily
nabumetone		Tablets: 500, 750 mg	Rheumatoid and osteoarthritis: 1000-1500 mg daily in 1 or 2 doses
naproxen	Naprosyn, Aleve, Anaprox DS	Tablets: 220, 250, 275, 375, 500, 550 mg Tablets, extended-release: 375, 500, 750 mg Capsules: 220 mg Oral suspension: 125 mg/5 mL	Rheumatoid and osteoarthritis, ankylosing spondylitis: 250-375 mg twice daily Rheumatoid arthritis, osteoarthritis, ankylosing spondylitis: 250-375 mg twice daily Acute gout: 750-825 mg initially, followed by 250-275 mg q8h Moderate pain, primary dysmenorrhea, acute tendonitis, bursitis: 500-550 mg followed by 250-275 mg
oxaprozin	Daypro	Caplets: 600 mg	Rheumatoid arthritis, osteoarthritis: 1200 mg once daily
piroxicam	Feldene	Capsules: 10, 20 mg	Rheumatoid and osteoarthritis: 20 mg once daily
sulindac		Tablets: 150, 200 mg	Rheumatoid and osteoarthritis, ankylosing spondylitis: 150 mg twice daily Acute painful shoulder: 200 mg twice daily
tolmetin		Tablets: 200, 600 mg Capsules: 400 mg	Rheumatoid and osteoarthritis: 400-600 mg three times daily

Modified from Willihnganz M: Clayton's Basic Pharmacology for Nurses, ed 18, St Louis, 2020, Elsevier.

TABLE 18-5   Selected Analgesic Combination Products

Product	NON-CONTROLLED SUBSTANCE			CONTROLLED SUBSTANCE	
	Aspirin (Mg)	Acetaminophen (Mg)	Other (Mg)	Codeine (Mg)	Other (Mg)
Anacin caplets and tablets	400		caffeine, 32		
Anacin Maximum Strength	500		caffeine, 32		
BC Powder Arthritis Strength	742		caffeine, 38 salicylamide, 222		
Excedrin Extra-strength	250	250	caffeine, 65		
Fioricet		300	caffeine, 40		butalbital, 50
Fiorinal	325		caffeine, 40		butalbital, 50
Fiorinal w/Codeine	325		caffeine, 40	30	butalbital, 50
Lortab HD		325			hydrocodone, 10
Norco		325			hydrocodone, 10
Percocet 7.5		325			oxycodone, 7.5
Percogesic		325	Diphenhydramine, 12.5		
Tylenol Codeine #3 Codeine #4		300 300		30 60	
Vicodin		300			hydrocodone, 5
Vicodin ES		300			hydrocodone, 7.5
Vicodin HP		300			hydrocodone, 10

Modified from Willihnganz M: Clayton's Basic Pharmacology for Nurses, ed 18, St Louis, 2020, Elsevier.

- *Anorexia, nausea, vomiting, jaundice.* These may signal liver toxicity.
- *Sore throat, fever, jaundice, weakness.* These may signal changes in red blood cells and white blood cells.

OTHER ANALGESIC AGENTS

Other drugs may also be used to relieve pain. Many are combination products. In most cases, these drugs combine a non-controlled substance, such as aspirin, acetaminophen (Tylenol), or caffeine with a controlled substance, such as codeine or hydrocodone. See Table 18-5 for a list of combination drugs. When giving combination drugs, assist the nurse with the nursing process based on the patient's drugs combinations.

▮ REVIEW QUESTIONS

Circle the BEST answer.

1. A person complains of pain. What should you do?
   a. Ask to see the pain.
   b. Tell the nurse.
   c. Give an analgesic.
   d. Decide if the pain is acute or chronic.
2. A pain rating scale is used:
   a. to describe pain
   b. for the location of pain
   c. for the intensity of pain
   d. to describe the duration of pain
3. Who decides when you should give an analgesic?
   a. the patient or resident
   b. the nurse
   c. the doctor
   d. you
4. An opiate acts as an analgesic by:
   a. transmitting pain to the brain
   b. releasing chemicals that stimulate pain receptors
   c. blocking the pain sensation
   d. producing sleep

5. Opiate agonists can cause euphoria. Euphoria is:
   a. an exaggerated feeling of well-being
   b. drowsiness and sedation
   c. mental clouding
   d. addiction
6. Opiate partial agonists are given:
   a. to treat chronic pain
   b. to treat short-term moderate to severe pain
   c. to reverse the effects of opiates
   d. to treat fevers
7. Which of the following are given to reduce fever?
   a. opiate agonists
   b. prostaglandin inhibitors
   c. methadone-like derivatives
   d. opiate partial agonists
8. Which of the following signals respiratory depression?
   a. a respiratory rate of 12 per minute or less
   b. a respiratory rate of 14 per minute
   c. a respiratory rate of 16 per minute
   d. a respiratory rate of 18 per minute

9. The following are opiate agonists, *except*:
   a. codeine and morphine sulfate
   b. Oxycontin and Actiq
   c. Talwin and Suboxone
   d. Dilaudid and Demerol
10. Tylenol is good for the following people, except:
    a. those with bleeding problems
    b. those who cannot take aspirin because of allergic reactions
    c. those with gastric ulcers
    d. those with pain from rheumatoid arthritis
11. Salicylates have the following effects, *except*:
    a. analgesia
    b. anti-inflammatory
    c. antipyretic
    d. dulling alertness
12. Combination products usually include all the following, *except*:
    a. Aleve
    b. Tylenol
    c. hydrocodone
    d. aspirin
13. To prevent stomach irritation from salicylates or NSAIDs, you should give the drug:
    a. with food or milk
    b. before meals
    c. after meals
    d. at bedtime

14. NSAIDS are given for the following reasons, *except* to reduce:
    a. pain
    b. inflammation
    c. fever
    d. euphoria
15. Which has the strongest analgesic effect?
    a. Ultram
    b. aspirin
    c. Motrin
    d. Tylenol

Circle T if the statement is true. Circle F if the statement is false.

16. T   F   Anxiety can increase a person's pain.
17. T   F   Vital signs often decrease when the person feels pain.
18. T   F   Older persons feel pain at the same intensity as younger persons do.
19. T   F   Naloxone is the drug of choice for treatment of respiratory depression caused by opiates.
20. T   F   Addiction from the use of opiates for pain management is a common problem.
21. T   F   A person was given an opiate partial agonist. You must provide for safety.
22. T   F   Acetaminophen has an anti-inflammatory effect.

Answers to these questions can be found on the Evolve Resources site: http://evolve.elsevier.com/Anderson/medasst/

Drugs Used to Lower Lipids

OBJECTIVES

- Define the key terms and key abbreviations used in this chapter.
- Identify the main lipids in the blood.
- Explain how lipids can cause coronary artery disease.
- Explain the difference between low-density and high-density lipoproteins.
- Describe the drugs used to lower blood lipid levels.
- Explain how to assist with the nursing process when giving drugs to reduce blood lipid levels.

KEY TERMS

cholesterol A waxy, fat-like substance found in all body cells

dyslipidemia An abnormality of one or more of the blood fats (lipids)

hyperlipidemia Excess *(hyper)* lipids *(fats)* in the blood *(emia)*

lipids Fats

triglycerides Fatty compounds that come from animal and vegetable fats

KEY ABBREVIATIONS

CAD   Coronary artery disease
g   Gram
HDL   High-density lipoprotein

LDL   Low-density lipoprotein
mg   Milligram
MI   Myocardial infarction

Lipids are fats. (*Lipos* is the Greek work meaning *fat.*) **Hyperlipidemia** (hi per lip' id e' mi ah) means excess *(hyper)* lipids *(fats)* in the blood *(emia).* The main lipids in the blood are:

- **Cholesterol** is a waxy, fat-like substance found in all body cells. The body produces the cholesterol it needs to make hormones, vitamin D, and substances used for food digestion. Cholesterol is also found in foods from animal sources—egg yolks, meat, and cheese. The body converts excess dietary fat into cholesterol.
- **Triglycerides** are fatty compounds that come from animal and vegetable fats. A source of energy, they are stored in the body's fatty tissues.

When there are too many lipids in the blood, fat can build up on the walls of arteries and arterioles throughout the body. This is called *atherosclerosis.* (*Athero* means an *abnormal mass of fat or lipids. Sclerosis* means *hardening.*) Often called "hardening of the arteries," atherosclerosis blocks blood flow (Fig. 19-1). When it occurs in the heart's coronary arteries, it causes coronary artery disease (CAD). CAD can lead to angina or myocardial infarction (MI). CAD is a leading cause of death in the United States in men and women.

Blood is a liquid. Lipids are fatty. Liquids and fat do not mix. To travel in the bloodstream, fats are carried in the blood by lipoproteins. *Lipoproteins* are made up of fat *(lipo)* and proteins.

- *Low-density lipoprotein (LDL) cholesterol.* This is often called "bad cholesterol." It leads to the build-up of plaque in the arteries. The higher the LDL level, the greater the risk of CAD.

- *High-density lipoprotein (HDL) cholesterol.* This is often called "good cholesterol." HDL carries cholesterol from other body parts to the liver. The liver removes it from the body. The higher the HDL level, the lower the risk of CAD.

Dyslipidemia (dis lip' id e' me ah) is an abnormality of one or more blood fats (lipids). Causes include:

- *Heredity.* High blood cholesterol can run in families.
- *A diet high in fat, cholesterol, carbohydrates, calories, and alcohol.*
- *Weight gain and being overweight.* Losing weight can lower LDL ("bad cholesterol"). It can raise HDL ("good cholesterol").
- *Lack of regular exercise.* Regular exercise can lower LDL ("bad cholesterol") and raise HDL ("good cholesterol").
- *Age and gender.* According to the National Heart, Lung, and Blood Institute, men have lower levels of HDL ("good cholesterol") than women. As men and women age, LDL levels ("bad cholesterol") rise. Younger women have lower LDL levels than men. After age 55, women have higher LDL levels than men.

DRUG THERAPY FOR HYPERLIPIDEMIA

Lifestyle management helps in treating hyperlipidemia. This involves losing weight, regular exercise, avoiding tobacco products, and a diet low in cholesterol and fat. For some persons, lifestyle changes and drug therapy are needed. *Antilipemic drugs* are used to reduce *(anti)* fats *(lip)* in the blood *(emic).* The drug is intended to decrease cholesterol levels and reduce the risk of

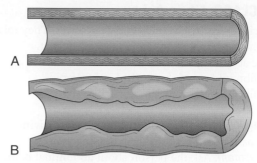

Fig. 19-1 A, Normal artery. **B,** Plaque on the artery wall in atherosclerosis.

atherosclerosis leading to CAD. They are used only if diet, exercise, and weight loss do not lower LDL ("bad cholesterol").

DRUG CLASS: Bile Acid-Binding Resins

Bile is a yellow-green liver secretion stored in the gallbladder. It is released into the duodenum to prepare fats for digestion. *Bile acid* is produced when cholesterol is metabolized. *Resins* are solid or semi-solid substances.

Bile acid-binding resins interrupt the normal circulation of bile acids between the liver and intestines. More bile acids are excreted into the feces. The liver produces bile acids from cholesterol. Because there are fewer bile acids, the liver takes more LDL cholesterol from the blood to replace them. Therefore, LDL cholesterol levels in the blood decrease and HDL levels increase.

Bile acid-binding resins may be used along with statins to lower LDL. The bile acid-binding resins are:

- Cholestyramine (koe less teer' a meen); Questran (quest' tran)
- Colestipol (koe les' ti pole); Colestid (co lest' tid)
- Colesevelam (koh leh sev' eh lam); Welchol (wel' coal)

Assisting With the Nursing Process. When giving bile acid-binding resins, you assist the nurse with the nursing process.

Assessment. Ask the person about abdominal pain, nausea, and flatus.

Planning. Oral dose forms are:

- Cholestyramine (Questran):
  - 4 g powder packets
- Colestipol (Colestid) forms include:
  - 1 g tablets
  - 5 g granule packets
- Colesevelam (Welchol):
  - 625 mg tablets
  - 3.75 mg packets

Implementation. The adult dosages are:

- Cholestyramine (Questran):
  - 4 g one to six times daily.
  - The initial dose is 4 g daily.
  - The maintenance dose is 8 to 16 g daily.
  - The maximum daily dose is 24 g.
- Colestipol (Colestid):
  - Granules: 5 to 30 g per day in divided doses. The initial dose is 5 g one or two times a day.
  - Tablets: 2 to 16 g per day. The initial dose is 2 g one or two times a day.

- Colesevelam (Welchol):
  - 6 tablets once a day or in two divided doses.
  - The drug is given with liquid at meals.

Preparing and giving these drugs:

- Do not give the person dry powder to swallow.
- Mix granules or powder with 2 to 6 ounces of water, juice, soup, applesauce, or crushed pineapple, as the person prefers. Stir well until mixed. The powder will not dissolve. Allow it to stand for a few minutes. After the person drinks the mixture, fill the glass with water. Have the person drink all the water. This ensures that the person receives the full dose.
- Have the person swallow tablets whole. Do not crush or cut them. The person must not chew the tablet.
- Doses are usually given with meals. Other drugs are given 1 hour before or at least 4 hours after giving bile acid-binding resins.

Evaluation. Report and record:

Constipation, abdominal pain, bloating, fullness, nausea, flatulence. These side effects can be reduced by:

- Starting with a low dose
- Mixing the drug with non-carbonated drinks, pulpy juices, or sauces
- Having the person swallow without gulping air
- Drinking several glasses of water or other liquids throughout the day
- Having a diet adequate in fiber

DRUG CLASS: Niacin

Niacin (nicotinic acid) is vitamin B_3. Niacin limits the liver's ability to produce LDL cholesterol. Niacin can be used with bile acid–producing resins or statins to lower cholesterol and triglyceride levels. Niacin also causes vasodilation and increases blood flow.

Assisting With the Nursing Process. When giving niacin, you assist the nurse with the nursing process.

Assessment

- Measure blood pressure and heart rate.
- Ask the person about abdominal pain, nausea, and flatus.

Planning. Oral dose forms are:

- 50, 100, 250, and 500 mg tablets
- 250 and 500 mg timed-release capsules
- 250, 500, 750, 1000 mg timed-release tablets

Implementation

- The initial adult dose is 500 mg at bedtime during weeks 1 to 4.
- During weeks 5 to 8, give 1000 mg at bedtime.
- After week 8, increase to 1500 mg at bedtime if 1000 mg is ineffective.
- If 1500 mg is ineffective, the dose can be increased to 2000 mg.

Evaluation. Report and record:

- *Flushing, itching, rash, tingling, headache.* These are common when therapy is started.
- *Nausea, gas, abdominal discomfort, pain.* Give all doses with food.
- *Dizziness, faintness, hypotension.* Provide for safety. The person must use caution when working around machines, driving a car, pouring and giving drugs, or performing other duties that require mental alertness.

- *Fatigue, anorexia, nausea, malaise, jaundice.* These may signal liver toxicity.
- *Muscle aches, soreness, weakness.* These may signal changes in muscle tissue.

DRUG CLASS: Statins

Statins are the strongest antilipemic drugs available. They block the enzyme the liver needs to produce cholesterol. This reduces the amount of cholesterol in the liver. Therefore, the liver must remove cholesterol from the blood. The goal of therapy is to reduce LDL and lower total cholesterol levels.

Statins combined with other drugs are also available (see Table 19-1). Atorvastatin (a lipid-lowering agent) and amlodipine (an antihypertensive agent) are combined into one drug. Vytorin is made up of two lipid-lowering agents: simvastatin and ezetimibe.

Statins also reduce inflammation and blood clotting. This helps to reduce the risk of MI and stroke.

Assisting With the Nursing Process. When giving statins, you assist the nurse with the nursing process.

Assessment. Ask the person about abdominal pain, nausea, and flatus.

Planning. See Table 19-1 for "Oral Dose Forms."

Implementation. See Table 19-1 for "Daily Adult Dose."
- Do not give the drug with grapefruit juice. Grapefruit juice inhibits the metabolism of some statins.

Evaluation. Report and record:
- *Headache, nausea, gas, abdominal bloating.* Symptoms should resolve with continued use.
- *Fatigue, anorexia, nausea, malaise, jaundice.* These may signal liver problems.
- *Muscle aches, soreness, weakness.* These may signal changes in muscle tissue.

DRUG CLASS: Fibric Acids

Fibric acids lower triglyceride and LDL levels. They raise HDL levels. They are used together with a healthy diet.

Fibric acid drugs are:
- Gemfibrozil (gem fi' broe zil); Lopid (lo pid)
- Fenofibrate (fen oh fye' brate); Tricor (tri' cor)

Assisting With the Nursing Process. When giving fibric acids, you assist the nurse with the nursing process.

Assessment. Ask the person about abdominal pain, nausea, and flatus.

Planning. Oral dose forms are:
- Gemfibrozil (Lopid):
  - 600 mg tablets
- Fenofibrate (Tricor):
  - 35, 40, 48, 54, 105, 120, 145, and 160 mg tablets
  - 30, 43, 50, 67, 90, 130, 134, 150, and 200 mg capsules
  - 45 and 135 mg delayed-release capsules

Implementation. The adult dosages are:
- Gemfibrozil (Lopid):
  - 1200 mg per day in two divided doses.
  - The drug is given 30 minutes before morning and evening meals.
- Fenofibrate (Tricor):
  - The initial dose is 45 to 160 mg per day.
  - The dosage is increased every 4 to 8 weeks up to 160 mg daily.
  - The drug is given with meals.

Evaluation. Report and record:
- *Nausea, diarrhea, flatulence, bloating, abdominal distress.* These are common. A lower dose taken between meals may reduce these effects.
- *Fatigue, anorexia, nausea, malaise, jaundice.* These signal gallbladder disease and liver toxicity.

TABLE 19-1	Statins			
Generic Name	**Brand Name**	**Oral Dose Forms**		**Daily Adult Dose**
HMG-CoA Reductase Inhibitors (Statins)				
atorvastatin	Lipitor	Tablets: 10, 20, 40, 80 mg		10-40 mg daily at any time
fluvastatin	Lescol XL	Capsules: 20, 40 mg Tablets, extended-release: 80 mg		20-80 mg at bedtime
lovastatin	Altoprev	Tablets: 10, 20, 40 mg Tablets, extended-release: 20, 40, 60 mg		20-40 mg with evening meal or 10-60 mg daily at bedtime
pitavastatin	Livalo	Tablets: 1, 2, 4 mg		2 mg daily at anytime
pravastatin	Pravachol	Tablets: 10, 20, 40, 80 mg		40 mg daily at anytime
rosuvastatin	Crestor	Tablets: 5, 10, 20, 40 mg		5-40 mg daily at any time
simvastatin	Zocor	Tablets: 5, 10, 20, 40, 80 mg Oral suspension: 20, 40 mg/5 mL in 150-mL bottles		5-40 mg daily at bedtime
HMG-CoA Reductase Inhibitor Combination Products				
atorvastatin-amlodipine	Caduet	10-40 mg atorvastatin and 2.5 mg amlodipine 10-80 mg atorvastatin and 5 mg amlodipine 10-80 mg atorvastatin and 10 mg amlodipine		maximum daily dose for atorvastatin is 80 mg and 10 mg of amlodipine
simvastatin-ezetimibe	Vytorin	10-80 mg simvastatin and 10 mg ezetimibe		maximum daily dose for simvastatin is 80 mg and 10 mg of ezetimibe

- *Muscle aches, soreness, weakness.* These may signal changes in muscle tissue.

OTHER ANTILIPEMIC DRUGS

Other antilipemic drugs are:
- Ezetimibe (ehz et' tih meeb'); Zetia (zeh te' ah)
- Omega-3 fatty acids; Lovaza (lo vah' za)

Ezetimibe (Zetia)

The small intestine absorbs dietary cholesterol and releases it into the blood. Cholesterol absorption inhibitors block the absorption of cholesterol from the small intestine, thus lowering cholesterol levels. The drug may be used with statins. The drug should be used while sticking to a healthy diet.

Assisting With the Nursing Process. When giving ezetimibe (Zetia), you assist the nurse with the nursing process.
Assessment
- Ask the person about abdominal pain, nausea, and flatus.
Planning
- The oral dose form is 10 mg tablets.
Implementation
- The usual adult dose is 10 mg once a day. It may be taken with or without meals.
Evaluation. Report and record:
- *Abdominal pain, diarrhea.* These are generally mild and do not affect therapy.

Omega-3 Fatty Acids (Lovaza)

Lovaza contains fatty acids that are sometimes called "fish oils." The drug reduces the synthesis of triglycerides in the liver. It lowers triglyceride levels and causes small increases in HDL.

BOX 19-1 Side Effects of Lovaza

Report the following at once:
- Arm, back, or jaw pain
- Chest pain or discomfort
- Chest tightness or heaviness
- Breathing: difficult or labored, shortness of breath
- Heartbeat: fast or irregular
- Nausea
- Sweating
- Wheezing

Other side effects:
- Appetite: loss of
- Belching
- Bloating
- Chills
- Cough
- Diarrhea
- Fever

- Discomfort
- Headache
- Hoarseness
- Joint pain
- Pain: lower back, side
- Muscles: aches and pains
- Urination: difficulty or painful
- Rash
- Runny nose
- Shivering
- Sore throat
- Sweating
- Sleep problems
- Taste: unusual or unpleasant, change in
- Tiredness
- Weakness
- Vomiting

Assisting With the Nursing Process. When giving Lovaza, you assist the nurse with the nursing process.
Assessment. Ask the person about abdominal pain, nausea, and flatus.
Planning
- The oral dose form is 1 g capsules.
Implementation
- The adult dose is 4 g once a day or 2 g two times a day.
Evaluation. Report and record the side effects listed in Box 19-1.

REVIEW QUESTIONS

Circle the BEST answer.

1. These statements are about cholesterol. Which is *false?*
   a. Cholesterol is found in all body cells.
   b. The body produces cholesterol.
   c. Cholesterol is needed by the body.
   d. Cholesterol is a source of energy.
2. Triglycerides are stored in the body's:
   a. muscle tissue
   b. fatty tissue
   c. bones
   d. nerve cells
3. Foods high in cholesterol include the following, *except:*
   a. vegetables
   b. egg yolks
   c. meat
   d. cheese
4. Which is called "bad cholesterol?"
   a. atherosclerosis
   b. bile
   c. low-density lipoprotein (LDL)
   d. high-density lipoprotein (HDL)
5. Which are the strongest antilipemic drugs?
   a. bile acid-binding resins
   b. fibric acids
   c. statins
   d. Zetia and Lovaza
6. You are giving a bile acid resin in powdered form. What should you do?
   a. give the person the dry powder to swallow
   b. mix the powder with 2 to 6 ounces of water or juice
   c. give the drug before meals
   d. give the drug after meals
7. You are giving a bile acid resin in tablet form. Which is *true?*
   a. The tablet must be swallowed whole.
   b. You can cut the tablet.
   c. You can crush the tablet.
   d. The person can chew the tablet.
8. Niacin acts as an antilipemic because it:
   a. excretes bile acids into the feces
   b. limits the liver's ability to produce LDL
   c. blocks the enzyme needed to produce cholesterol
   d. lowers triglyceride levels

9. Niacin can cause hypotension because of:
   a. vasoconstriction
   b. vasodilation
   c. atherosclerosis
   d. coronary artery disease
10. Statins lower LDL and total cholesterol levels because they:
    a. excrete bile acids into the feces
    b. limit the liver's ability to produce LDL
    c. block the enzyme needed to produce cholesterol
    d. block the absorption of cholesterol from the small intestine
11. The following are statins, *except*:
    a. fenofibrate (Tricor)
    b. atorvastatin (Lipitor)
    c. simvastatin (Zocor)
    d. fluvastatin (Lescol XL)

12. A common side effect of antilipemic drugs is:
    a. chest pain
    b. nausea
    c. hypotension
    d. dizziness

Circle T if the statement is true. Circle F if the statement is false.
13. T F Niacin is given with food.
14. T F Statins reduce inflammation and blood clotting.
15. T F Statins are given with grapefruit juice.

Answers to these questions can be found on the Evolve Resources site: http://evolve.elsevier.com/Anderson/medasst/

20

Drugs Used to Treat Hypertension

OBJECTIVES

- Define the key terms and key abbreviations used in this chapter.
- Identify the five blood pressure categories.
- Explain the factors that affect blood pressure.
- Explain the factors that cause high blood pressure.
- Describe the drugs used to treat hypertension.
- Explain how to assist with the nursing process when giving drugs to treat hypertension.

KEY TERMS

aldosterone A substance that causes the kidneys to retain sodium

angiotensin A substance that causes vasoconstriction, increased blood pressure, and the release of aldosterone

antihypertensive agents Drugs that reduce blood pressure

blood pressure The amount of force exerted against the walls of an artery by the blood

diuretic A drug that promotes the formation and excretion of urine; *dia* means through; *ur* means urine

hypertension The systolic pressure is 140 mm Hg or higher *(hyper)*, or the diastolic pressure is 90 mm Hg or higher; high blood pressure

renin An enzyme that affects blood pressure

KEY ABBREVIATIONS

ACE Angiotensin-converting enzyme

ARB Angiotensin II receptor blocker

g Gram

mg Milligram

MI Myocardial infarction

mm Hg Millimeters of mercury

PO Per os (orally)

Blood pressure is the amount of force exerted against the walls of an artery by the blood (Chapter 4). Blood pressure is controlled by:

- The force of heart contractions
- The amount of blood pumped with each heartbeat
- How easily blood flows through the blood vessels

Blood pressure can change from minute to minute. Factors affecting blood pressure are listed in Box 20-1. Because it can vary so easily, blood pressure has normal ranges:

- Systolic pressure—less than 120 mm Hg (millimeters of mercury)
- Diastolic pressure—less than 80 mm Hg

Blood pressures are divided into five categories. These categories can be seen here in Fig. 20-1.

With **hypertension** (high blood pressure), the blood pressure is too high. The systolic pressure is 130 mm Hg or higher (hyper), or the diastolic pressure is 80 mm Hg or higher. Such measurements must occur several times to establish hypertension.

Blood Pressure Categories

BLOOD PRESSURE CATEGORY	SYSTOLIC mm Hg (upper number)		DIASTOLIC mm Hg (lower number)
NORMAL	LESS THAN 120	and	LESS THAN 80
ELEVATED	120 – 129	and	LESS THAN 80
HIGH BLOOD PRESSURE (HYPERTENSION) STAGE 1	130 – 139	or	80 – 89
HIGH BLOOD PRESSURE (HYPERTENSION) STAGE 2	140 OR HIGHER	or	90 OR HIGHER
HYPERTENSIVE CRISIS (consult your doctor immediately)	HIGHER THAN 180	and/or	HIGHER THAN 120

©American Heart Association

heart.org/bplevels

Fig. 20-1 Blood pressure categories (From: American Heart Association: Understanding Blood Pressure Readings, 2017).

BOX 20-1   Factors Affecting Blood Pressure

- *Age.* Blood pressure increases with age. It is lowest in infancy and childhood and highest in adulthood.
- *Gender (male or female).* Women usually have lower blood pressures than men. Blood pressures rise in women after menopause.
- *Blood volume.* This is the amount of blood in the system. Severe bleeding lowers blood volume. Therefore, blood pressure lowers. Giving intravenous fluids rapidly increases the blood volume. The blood pressure rises.
- *Stress.* Stress includes anxiety, fear, and strong emotions. Blood pressure increases as the body responds to stress.
- *Pain.* Pain generally increases blood pressure. However, severe pain can cause *shock.* Blood pressure is seriously low in the state of shock.
- *Exercise.* Blood pressure increases. Do not measure blood pressure right after exercise.
- *Weight.* Blood pressure is higher in overweight persons. It lowers with weight loss.
- *Race.* Black persons generally have higher blood pressures than White persons do.
- *Diet.* A high-sodium diet increases the amount of water in the body. The extra fluid volume increases blood pressure.
- *Drugs.* Drugs can be given to raise or lower blood pressure. Other drugs have side effects of high or low blood pressure.
- *Position.* Blood pressure is lower when lying down. It is higher in the standing position. Sudden changes in position can cause a sudden drop in blood pressure (orthostatic hypotension). When standing suddenly, the person may have a sudden drop in blood pressure. Dizziness and fainting can occur.
- *Smoking.* Blood pressure increases. Nicotine in cigarettes causes blood vessels to narrow. The heart must work harder to pump blood through narrowed vessels.
- *Alcohol.* Excessive alcohol intake can raise blood pressure.

BOX 20-2   Risk Factors for Hypertension

Factors You *Cannot* Change
- Age—45 years or older for men; 55 years or older for women
- Gender—younger men are at greater risk than younger women; the risk increases for women after menopause
- Race—Black persons are at greater risk than White persons
- Family history—tends to run in families

Factors You *Can* Change
- Being overweight—related to diet, lack of exercise, and atherosclerosis
- Stress—increased sympathetic nervous system activity
- Tobacco use—nicotine narrows blood vessels
- High-salt diet—sodium causes fluid retention; increased fluid raises blood volume
- Excessive alcohol—increases chemical substances in the body that increase blood pressure
- Lack of exercise—increases the risk of being overweight
- Atherosclerosis—arteries narrow because of fatty buildup in the vessels
- Elevated blood pressure—blood pressure can be controlled with lifestyle changes and drugs

---

Risk factors for hypertension include those that you can change and those you cannot change. A risk factor that you can change would be lack of exercise. A risk factor you cannot change would be your age. Box 20-2 lists additional risk factors from both categories.

Narrowed blood vessels are a common cause of hypertension. The heart must pump with more force to move blood through narrowed vessels. Kidney disorders, head injuries, some pregnancy problems, and adrenal gland tumors are causes of narrowed blood vessels.

A person can have high blood pressure for many years without knowing it, earning hypertension the moniker "the silent killer." Hypertension is usually found when blood pressure is measured. Signs and symptoms develop over time. Headache, blurred vision, dizziness, and nose bleeds may occur. Hypertension can lead to stroke, hardening of the arteries, myocardial infarction (MI), heart failure, kidney failure, and blindness.

Lifestyle changes can sometimes help lower blood pressure. A diet low in fat and salt, a healthy weight, and regular exercise are needed. No smoking is allowed. Alcohol and caffeine are limited. Managing stress and sleeping well also lower blood pressure.

DRUG THERAPY FOR HYPERTENSION

Drug therapy is not necessary if lifestyle changes control blood pressure. Even if lifestyle changes do not adequately control hypertension, they may reduce the number and doses of drugs needed. Once drug therapy is started, it may take months to control hypertension. The dosage may be increased, another drug may be tried, or a second one may be added. Many people require two or more antihypertensive agents. Some can take a combination product containing two drugs (See Table 20-6). This simplifies drug therapy for the person.

Antihypertensive agents are drugs that reduce blood pressure. Drug therapy depends on the person's:
- Age
- Gender
- Race
- Other health problems
- Risk factors
- Previous therapy—what has or has not worked
- Drug therapy for other health problems
- Cost

See Delegation Guidelines: Drugs Used to Treat Hypertension.

DELEGATION GUIDELINES

Drugs Used to Treat Hypertension

Some drugs used to treat hypertension are given parenterally. Because you do not give parenteral dose forms, they are not included in this chapter. Should a nurse delegate the administration of such to you, you must:
- Remember that parenteral dosages are often very different from dosages for other routes.
- Refuse the delegation but do not ignore the request. Make sure the nurse knows that you cannot give the drug and why.

DRUG CLASS: DIURETICS

A **diuretic** is a drug that promotes the formation and excretion of urine. (*Dia* means *through. Ur* means *urine.*) Diuretics:
- Reduce the amount of extracellular fluid
- Promote sodium excretion
- Cause vasodilation (widening) of peripheral arterioles

Diuretics are the most commonly prescribed antihypertensive agent. They may be prescribed alone or with other antihypertensive drugs to treat hypertension. The risk of adverse effects is low and they are less expensive than other antihypertensive drugs.

Diuretics are discussed in Chapter 23.

DRUG CLASS: Beta-Adrenergic Blocking Agents

Beta-adrenergic blocking agents (beta blockers) inhibit the heart's response to sympathetic nerve stimulation (Chapter 15) by blocking beta receptors. Beta receptors increase the heart rate. By blocking the beta receptors, the heart rate and blood pressure are reduced.

Beta blockers also block renin release from the kidneys. **Renin** is an enzyme that increases blood pressure through:

- Vasoconstriction, which narrows blood vessels
- Sodium retention, which causes the body to retain water

Assisting With the Nursing Process. When giving beta blockers, you assist the nurse with the nursing process.

Assessment

- Use the apical pulse to measure heart rate and rhythm.
- Measure blood pressure.
- See "Assisting with the Nursing Process" for dysrhythmic therapy (Chapter 21)

Planning. See Table 15-2 in Chapter 15 for "Oral Dose Forms."

Implementation

- See Table 15-2 in Chapter 15 for "Adult Dosage Range."
- The onset of action is rapid. However, it may take several days or weeks to reach the desired level of improvement and to stabilize on the lowest dose needed.
- Angina and MI are risks if the drug is suddenly discontinued. To discontinue the drug, the doctor reduces the dosage over 1 to 2 weeks.

Evaluation. Most adverse effects from beta blockers are dose-related and therefore resolve when the dosage is adjusted. Report and record:

- *Bradycardia, peripheral vasoconstriction (purple, mottled skin).* The nurse may tell you to withhold the next dose until the doctor can evaluate the person.
- *Bronchospasm, wheezing.* The nurse may tell you to withhold the next dose until the doctor can evaluate the person.
- *Headache, weakness, decreased coordination, general apprehension, sweating, hunger, or blurred or double vision.* These signal hypoglycemia.
- *Edema, dyspnea, bradycardia, and orthopnea.* Observe persons with heart failure.

DRUG CLASS: Angiotensin-Converting Enzyme Inhibitors

Angiotensin-converting enzyme (ACE) inhibitors reduce blood pressure by affecting the renin-angiotensin-aldosterone system.

- Renin is secreted by the kidneys when blood pressure, sodium levels, or kidney blood flow is reduced. Renin causes vasoconstriction and sodium retention.
- **Angiotensin** is a substance that causes vasoconstriction, increased blood pressure, and the release of aldosterone.
- **Aldosterone** is a substance that causes the kidneys to retain sodium.

The renin-angiotensin-aldosterone system regulates blood pressure as follows:

- Renin is secreted by the kidneys when blood pressure, sodium levels, or kidney blood flow is reduced. Renin causes vasoconstriction and sodium retention, both of which increase blood pressure.
- Angiotensinogen is secreted by the liver. Renin converts (changes) angiotensinogen to angiotensin I.
- The angiotensin-converting enzyme then converts (changes) angiotensin I to angiotensin II.
- Angiotensin II:
  - Acts on receptors in the blood vessels to produce strong vasoconstriction. Narrowing of the blood vessels increases blood pressure.
  - Promotes aldosterone secretion. This causes sodium retention. Increased sodium causes the body to retain water. This increases blood pressure.

ACE inhibitors affect the angiotensin-converting enzyme. Therefore, the conversion (change) of angiotensin I to angiotensin II is inhibited. When ACE inhibitors are used:

- Blood levels of angiotensin II are reduced. There is less vasoconstriction. This lowers blood pressure.
- Aldosterone levels are lower. Less sodium and less water is retained. This lowers blood pressure.

ACE inhibitors may be used alone to control blood pressure. However, they are more effective when combined with diuretic therapy.

Assisting With the Nursing Process. When giving ACE inhibitors, you assist the nurse with the nursing process.

Assessment

- Use the apical pulse to measure heart rate and rhythm.
- Measure blood pressure in the supine and standing positions.
- Measure intake and output.
- Measure weight daily.
- Ask about bowel elimination.
- Ask if the person has a cough.

Planning. See Table 20-1 for "Oral Dose Forms."

Implementation. See Table 20-1 for "Adult Dosage Range."

- ACE inhibitors can be given twice daily, but should not exceed the maximum daily dose.

Evaluation. Report and record:

- *Hypotension with dizziness, tachycardia, fainting.* These may occur within the first 3 hours after the first several doses. They are more common in persons who also receive diuretics. Check the person often until blood pressure is stable. Measure blood pressure in the supine and standing positions. Provide for safety. Remind the person to rise slowly from a supine or sitting position. Have the person sit or lie down if symptoms develop.
- *Nausea, fatigue, headache, diarrhea.* These are usually mild and tend to resolve with continued therapy.
- *Swelling of the face, eyes, lips, tongue; difficulty breathing.* These may signal a drug allergy. Tell the nurse at once. Do not give the next dose unless approved by the nurse.
- *Sore throat, fever, jaundice, weakness.* These may signal changes in white blood cells.
- *Intake and output.* These are used to monitor kidney function.
- *Changes in alertness, disorientation, confusion.* Provide for safety. These may signal changes in potassium levels.
- *Changes in muscle strength, muscle cramps, tremors, nausea, drowsiness, anxiety, lethargy.* These may signal changes in potassium levels.

TABLE 20-1   Angiotensin-Converting Enzyme (ACE) Inhibitors

Generic Name	Brand Name	Oral Dose Forms	Adult Dosage Range
benazepril	Lotensin	Tablets: 5, 10, 20, 40 mg	Initial—10 mg once daily Maintenance—20-40 mg daily

captopril		Tablets: 12.5, 25, 50, 100 mg	Initial—12.5-25 mg two or three times daily,
			    1 hour before meals
			Maintenance—50-450 mg daily in two to three divided
			    doses, 1 hour before meals

enalapril	Vasotec	Tablets: 2.5, 5, 10, 20 mg Oral solution: 1 mg/mL in 150 mL bottle	Initial—2.5-5 mg once daily Maintenance—10-40 mg daily
fosinopril		Tablets: 10, 20, 40 mg	Initial—10 mg once daily Maintenance—20-80 mg daily
lisinopril	Prinivil, Zestril	Tablets: 2.5, 5, 10, 20, 30, 40 mg Oral solution: 1 mg/mL in 150 mL bottle	Initial—5-10 mg once daily Maintenance—20-80 mg daily
moexipril		Tablets: 7.5, 15 mg	Initial—with diuretic, 3.75 mg; without diuretic, 7.5 mg Maintenance—7.5-30 mg in one or two divided doses, 1 hour before meals
perindopril		Tablets: 2, 4, 8 mg	Initial—4 mg daily Maintenance—4-16 mg daily
quinapril	Accupril	Tablets: 5, 10, 20, 40 mg	Initial—with diuretic, 5 mg; without diuretic, 10-20 mg daily Maintenance—20-80 mg daily
ramipril	Altace	Capsules: 1.25, 2.5, 5, 10 mg	Initial—1.25-2.5 mg daily Maintenance—2.5-20 mg daily
trandolapril		Tablets: 1, 2, 4, mg	Initial—1 mg daily Maintenance—2-4 mg daily

Modified from Willihnganz M: Clayton's Basic Pharmacology for Nurses, ed 18, St Louis, 2020, Elsevier.

- *Chronic, dry, nonproductive, persistent cough.* This may appear 1 week to 6 months after the start of therapy.

DRUG CLASS: Angiotensin II Receptor Blockers

Angiotensin II receptor blockers (ARBs) bind to angiotensin II receptor sites. Therefore, they block angiotensin II from binding to the receptor sites. Such sites are in the blood vessels, brain, heart, kidneys, and adrenal glands. By blocking angiotensin II receptor sites, ARBs lower blood pressure because:

- Vasoconstriction does not occur. Blood vessels do not narrow.
- Aldosterone secretion is blocked. This prevents sodium retention. The body does not retain excess water.

ARBs may be used alone to control blood pressure. The blood pressure-lowering effect is seen within 1 week. It may take 3 to 6 weeks for the full therapeutic effect. Sometimes a low-dose diuretic is needed. They should not be given at the same time as ACE inhibitors.

Assisting With the Nursing Process. When giving ARBs, you assist the nurse with the nursing process.

Assessment
- Use the apical pulse to measure heart rate and rhythm.
- Measure blood pressure in the supine and standing positions.
- Measure intake and output.
- Measure weight daily.
- Ask about bowel elimination patterns.
- Ask about gastrointestinal symptoms.

Planning. See Table 20-2 for "Oral Dose Forms."
Implementation. See Table 20-2 for "Adult Dosage Range."
Evaluation. Report and record:

- *Headache, heartburn, indigestion, cramps, diarrhea.* These are mild and tend to resolve with continued therapy.
- *Hypotension, dizziness, weakness, fainting.* These may occur within the first 3 hours after the first several doses. They are more common in persons who also receive diuretics. Check the person often until blood pressure is stable. Measure blood pressure in the supine and standing positions. Provide for safety. Remind the person to rise slowly from a supine or sitting position. Have the person sit or lie down if symptoms develop.
- *Changes in alertness, disorientation, confusion.* Provide for safety. These may signal changes in potassium levels.
- *Changes in muscle strength, muscle cramps, tremors, nausea, drowsiness, anxiety, lethargy.* These may signal changes in potassium levels.

DRUG CLASS: Direct Renin Inhibitor

Renin is discussed in this chapter on page 203. It plays a part in the conversion (change) of angiotensinogen into a potent vasoconstrictor, which increases blood pressure. Direct renin inhibitors block this process.

- Aliskiren (a lis keer' en); Tekturna (tek' turn a)

Assisting With the Nursing Process. When giving aliskiren (Tekturna), you assist the nurse with the nursing process.

TABLE 20-2   Angiotensin II Receptor Blockers (ARBs)

Generic Name	Brand Name	Oral Dose Forms	Adult Dosage Range
azilsartan	Edarbi	Tablets: 20, 40 mg	Initial— with diuretic, 40 mg daily; without diuretic, 80 mg daily
candesartan	Atacand	Tablets: 4, 8, 16, 32 mg	Initial—16 mg once daily; adjust over 4-6 weeks with total daily dose from 8-32 mg Dose may be administered once or twice daily for optimal control
eprosartan	Teveten	Tablets: 600 mg	Initial—600 mg once daily; adjust over 2-3 weeks with total daily dose of 800 mg Dose may be administered once or twice daily for optimal control
irbesartan	Avapro	Tablets: 75, 150, 300 mg	Initial—150 mg once daily; adjust over 3-4 weeks with a total daily dose of 300 mg
losartan	Cozaar	Tablets: 25, 50, 100 mg	Initial—50 mg once daily; adjust over 4-6 weeks with a total daily dose from 25-100 mg Dose may be administered once or twice daily for optimal control
olmesartan	Benicar	Tablets: 5, 20, 40 mg	Initial—20 mg once daily; adjust over 2 weeks with total daily dose from 20-40 mg Twice daily dosing offers no benefit
telmisartan	Micardis	Tablets: 20, 40, 80 mg	Initial—40 mg once daily; adjust over 4-6 weeks with total daily dose from 20-80 mg
valsartan	Diovan	Capsules: 40, 80, 160, 320 mg	Initial—80 mg once daily; adjust over 4-6 weeks with total daily dose from 80-320 mg

Modified from Willihnganz M: Clayton's Basic Pharmacology for Nurses, ed 18, St Louis, 2020, Elsevier.

Assessment
- Use the apical pulse to measure heart rate and rhythm.
- Measure blood pressure in the supine and standing positions.
- Measure intake and output.
- Measure weight daily.
- Ask about bowel elimination patterns.

Planning
- Oral dose forms are 150 and 300 mg tablets.

Implementation
- The initial dose is 150 mg daily.
- If blood pressure is not controlled after a few weeks, increase to 300 mg daily.

Evaluation. Report and record:
- *Headache, heartburn, indigestion, cramps, diarrhea.* These are mild and tend to resolve with continued therapy.
- *Hypotension, dizziness, weakness, fainting.* These may occur within the first 3 hours after the first several doses. They are more common in persons who also receive diuretics. Check the person often until blood pressure is stable. Measure blood pressure in the supine and standing positions. Provide for safety. Remind the person to rise slowly from a supine or sitting position. Have the person sit or lie down if symptoms develop.
- *Changes in alertness, disorientation, confusion.* Provide for safety. These may signal changes in potassium levels.
- *Changes in muscle strength, muscle cramps, tremors, nausea, drowsiness, anxiety, lethargy.* These may signal changes in potassium levels.

DRUG CLASS: Aldosterone Receptor Blocking Agent

The renin-angiotensin-aldosterone system regulates blood pressure as follows:
- Renin is secreted by the kidneys when blood pressure, sodium levels, or kidney blood flow is reduced. Renin causes vasoconstriction and sodium retention, both of which increase blood pressure.
- Angiotensinogen is secreted by the liver. Renin converts (changes) angiotensinogen to angiotensin I.
- The angiotensin-converting enzyme then converts (changes) angiotensin I to angiotensin II.
- Angiotensin II:
  - Acts on receptors in the blood vessels to produce strong vasoconstriction. Narrowing of the blood vessels increases blood pressure.
  - Promotes aldosterone secretion. This causes sodium retention. Increased sodium causes the body to retain water. This increases blood pressure.

The aldosterone receptor-blocking agent blocks aldosterone receptors. This prevents sodium from being reabsorbed. The following is an aldosterone receptor-blocking agent used alone. Or it is used with other antihypertensive drugs.
- Eplerenone (ep lehr' en own); Inspra (in' sprah)

Assisting With the Nursing Process. When giving eplerenone (Inspra), you assist the nurse with the nursing process.

Assessment
- Measure blood pressure in the supine and standing positions.

- Measure intake and output.
- Measure weight daily.
- Ask about bowel elimination patterns.
  Planning. Oral dose forms are 25 and 50 mg tablets.
  Implementation
- The initial dose is 50 mg daily with or without food.
- The full therapeutic effect should be seen within 4 weeks.
- If necessary, the dosage may be increased to 50 mg two times a day.
  Evaluation. Report and record:
- *Nausea, fatigue, headache, diarrhea.* These tend to be mild and resolve with continued therapy.
- *Hypotension, dizziness, weakness, fainting.* These are more common in persons who also receive diuretics. Check the person often until blood pressure is stable. Measure blood pressure in the supine and standing positions. Provide for safety. Remind the person to rise slowly from a supine or sitting position. Have the person sit or lie down if symptoms develop.
- *Changes in alertness, disorientation, confusion.* Provide for safety. These may signal changes in potassium levels.
- *Changes in muscle strength, muscle cramps, tremors, nausea, drowsiness, anxiety, lethargy.* These may signal changes in potassium levels.
- *Intake and output.* These are used to monitor kidney function.
- *Anorexia, nausea, vomiting, jaundice.* These may signal liver toxicity.

DRUG CLASS: Calcium Channel Blockers

To understand how calcium ion antagonists lower blood pressure, you need to know these terms:

- Ion—an atom with an electrical charge.
- Atom—the smallest part of an element.

- Element—a simple substance that cannot be broken down into another substance.
- Calcium—an element. The body needs calcium ions for the transmission of nerve impulses, muscle contractions, blood clotting, and heart functions.
- Calcium channel—the way calcium ions pass through the cell membrane.
- Antagonist—a drug that exerts an opposite action to that of another or competes for the same receptor sites.

Calcium channel blockers stop the movement of calcium ions across a cell membrane. They also are called calcium antagonists and calcium ion antagonists. These drugs relax the smooth muscle of blood vessels. That results in vasodilation (widening of blood vessels) and reduced blood pressure. These drugs are also used to treat dysrhythmias (Chapter 21) and angina (Chapter 22).

Assisting With the Nursing Process. When giving calcium ion antagonists, you assist the nurse with the nursing process.
  Assessment
- Use the apical pulse to measure heart rate and rhythm.
- Measure blood pressure in the supine and standing positions.
- Measure intake and output.
- Measure weight daily.
  Planning. See Table 20-3 for "Oral Dose Forms."
  Implementation. See Table 20-3 for "Adult Dosage Range."
  Evaluation. Report and record:
- *Hypotension and fainting.* These may occur during the first week. They decline once the dosage is stabilized. Provide for safety. Remind the person to rise slowly from a supine or sitting position. Have the person sit or lie down if he or she feels faint.
- *Edema.* Measure weight daily. Measure intake and output.

TABLE 20-3   Calcium Channel Blockers Used to Treat Hypertension

Generic Name	Brand Name	Oral Dose Forms	Adult Dosage Range
amlodipine	Norvasc	Tablets: 2.5, 5, 10 mg	Initial—5 mg daily; adjust over 7-14 days to a maximum of 10 mg daily
diltiazem	Cardizem Cardizem LA Cardizem CD	Tablets: 30, 60, 90, 120 mg Tablets, 24-hr extended-release: 120, 180, 240, 300, 360, 420 mg Capsules, 24-hr sustained-release: 120, 180, 240, 300, 360, 420 mg	Initial—60-120 mg sustained-release capsule twice daily; adjust as needed after 14 days Maintenance—240-360 mg daily Maximum—480 mg once daily
felodipine		Tablets, 24-hr extended-release: 2.5, 5, 10 mg	Initial—5 mg daily; adjust after 14 days Maintenance—2.5-10 mg daily Maximum—10 mg daily
isradipine		Capsules: 2.5, 5 mg	Initial—2.5 mg twice daily Maximal response may require 2-4 weeks Maintenance—10 mg daily Maximum—20 mg daily
nicardipine	Cardene	Capsules: 20, 30 mg Capsules, extended-release: 30, 45 mg	Initial—20 mg three times daily; extended-release: 30 mg two times daily Maximal response may require 2 weeks of therapy Adjust dose by measuring blood pressure about 8 hours after last dose Peak effect is determined by measuring blood pressure 1-2 hours after dosage administration Maintenance—20-40 mg three times daily Maximum—120 mg daily

TABLE 20-3   Calcium Channel Blockers Used to Treat Hypertension—cont'd

Generic Name	Brand Name	Oral Dose Forms	Adult Dosage Range
nifedipine	Procardia	Capsules: 10, 20 mg Tablets, 24-hr sustained-release: 30, 60, 90 mg	Initial—sustained-release: 30-60 mg once daily; immediate release not used to treat hypertension Maximum—sustained-release tablets: 120 mg daily
nisoldipine	Sular	Tablets: 24-hr sustained-release: 8.5, 17, 25.5, 34 mg Tablets: 24-hr extended-release: 10, 20, 30, 40 mg	Initial—sustained-release: 17 mg once daily Maintenance—17-34 mg once daily Initial—extended-release: 20 mg once daily Maintenance—20-60 mg once daily
verapamil	Calan	Tablets: 40, 80, 120 mg Tablets, 24-hr sustained-release: 120, 180, 240 mg Capsules, 24-hr sustained-release: 100, 120, 180, 200, 240, 300, 360 mg	Initial—80 mg three or four times daily Sustained-release tablets and capsules: 120-240 mg once daily in the morning Maintenance—240-480 mg daily Administer with food

Modified from Willihnganz M: Clayton's Basic Pharmacology for Nurses, ed 18, St Louis, 2020, Elsevier.

TABLE 20-4   Alpha-1 Adrenergic Blocking Agents

Generic Name	Brand Name	Oral Dose Forms	Adult Dosage Range
doxazosin	Cardura	Tablets: 1, 2, 4, 8 mg Tablets: 24-hr extended-release: 4, 8 mg	Hypertension: Initial—1 mg daily am or pm; hypotensive effects most likely occur within 2-6 hours; monitor standing blood pressure Maintenance—increase to 2 mg, then (if needed) 4, 8, and 16 mg to achieve desired reduction in blood pressure
prazosin	Minipress	Capsules: 1, 2, 5 mg	Hypertension: Initial—1 mg two or three times daily with first dose at bedtime to reduce syncopal episodes Maintenance—6-15 mg daily in two or three divided doses Maximum dose—40 mg daily
terazosin		Capsules: 1, 2, 5, 10 mg	Hypertension: Initial—1 mg at bedtime; measure blood pressure 2-3 hours after dosing and evaluate for symptoms of dizziness or tachycardia; if response is substantially diminished at 24 hours, increase dosage Maintenance—1-5 mg daily Maximum dose—20 mg daily

Modified from Willihnganz M: Clayton's Basic Pharmacology for Nurses, ed 18, St Louis, 2020, Elsevier.

DRUG CLASS: Alpha-1 Adrenergic Blocking Agents

Alpha-1 receptors in the nervous system cause blood vessels to constrict (Chapter 15). Alpha-1 adrenergic blocking agents (alpha-1 blockers) block alpha-1 receptors. By blocking receptors that cause blood vessels to constrict (narrow), the blood vessels dilate (widen). Such vasodilation reduces blood pressure.

Alpha-1 blockers may be used alone or with other antihypertensive drugs.

Alpha-1 blockers also are used to treat benign prostatic hyperplasia (Chapter 30). They relax the smooth muscles of the bladder and prostate.

Assisting With the Nursing Process. When giving alpha-1 blockers, you assist the nurse with the nursing process.

Assessment
- Use the apical pulse to measure heart rate and rhythm.
- Measure blood pressure in the supine and standing positions.

Planning. See Table 20-4 for "Oral Dose Forms."
Implementation. See Table 20-4 for "Adult Dosage Range."
Evaluation. Report and record:
- *Hypotension with dizziness, tachycardia, fainting.* These may occur within 15 to 90 minutes after the first several doses. They are more common in persons who also receive diuretics. Check the person often until blood pressure is stable. Measure blood pressure in the supine and standing positions. Provide for safety. Remind the person to rise slowly from a supine or sitting position. Have the person sit or lie down if symptoms develop.
- *Drowsiness, headache, dizziness, weakness, lethargy.* These may resolve with continued therapy.

DRUG CLASS: Central-Acting Alpha-2 Agonists

Alpha-2 receptors prevent the further release of norepinephrine (Chapter 15). Norepinephrine stimulates the sympathetic nervous system. The sympathetic nervous system speeds up body functions.

TABLE 20-5 Central-Acting Alpha-2 Agonists

Generic Name	Brand Name	Dose Forms	Adult Dosage Range
clonidine	Catapres Catapres-TTS Kapvay	Tablets: 0.1, 0.2, 0.3 mg Transdermal patch: • TTS-1: 0.1 mg/24 hrs • TTS-2: 0.2 mg/24 hrs • TTS-3: 0.3 mg/24 hrs Tablets: 12-hr extended release: 0.1 mg	PO: Initial—0.1 mg twice daily Maintenance—0.2-0.8 mg daily in two or three divided doses Maximum—2.4 mg daily Transdermal—apply to a hairless area of intact skin on upper arm or torso once every 7 days; use a different site each week Initial—TTS-1: Adjust dosage weekly Maximum—Two TTS-3 patches weekly Note: Antihypertensive effect starts 2-3 days after initiation of therapy
guanfacine		Tablets: 1, 2 mg	Initial—1 mg daily at bedtime Maintenance—1-2 mg daily Maximum—3 mg daily
methyldopa		Tablets: 250, 500 mg	Initial—250 mg two or three times daily Maintenance—500 mg to 3 g daily in two to four divided doses

Modified from Willihnganz M: Clayton's Basic Pharmacology for Nurses, ed 18, St Louis, 2020, Elsevier.

An agonist is a drug that acts on a certain type of cell. It produces a predictable response. Central-acting alpha-2 agonists stimulate the alpha-adrenergic receptors in the brainstem. This reduces sympathetic nervous system activity. Heart rate and peripheral vascular resistance are reduced, resulting in lower systolic and diastolic blood pressures.

Alpha-2 agonists are used in combination with other antihypertensive agents.

Assisting With the Nursing Process. When giving alpha-2 agonists, you assist the nurse with the nursing process.
>   *Assessment*
> * Use the apical pulse to measure heart rate and rhythm.
> * Measure blood pressure in the supine and standing positions.
>   * Observe for signs and symptoms of depression (Chapter 16).
>   * Observe the person's sleep patterns (Chapter 15).
>   **Planning.** See Table 20-5, for "Dose Forms."
>   **Implementation.** See Table 20-5, for "Adult Dosage Range."
> * If a transdermal patch becomes loose, apply the adhesive overlay directly over the patch.
>   **Evaluation.** Report and record:
> * *Drowsiness, dizziness, dry mouth.* These tend to resolve with continued therapy. Provide for safety. Provide oral hygiene and offer fluids as directed by the nurse and the care plan.
> * *Dark urine.* This is harmless.
> * *Depression.* See Chapter 16 for the signs and symptoms of depression.
> * *Rash.* This may occur at the site of a transdermal patch.

DRUG CLASS: Direct Vasodilators

Direct vasodilators act directly on the smooth muscles of arterioles. The arterioles relax. This reduces peripheral vascular resistance. Blood pressure lowers.
* Hydralazine (hy dral' ah zeen)

Hydralazine causes the smooth muscles of arterioles to relax. This reduces peripheral vascular resistance causing lower blood pressure. However, the following increase:
* Cardiac output
* Renin release (p. 203)
* Sodium and water retention
   Hydralazine is used in combination with diuretics and other drugs.

Assisting With the Nursing Process. When giving hydralazine, you assist the nurse with the nursing process.
>   *Assessment*
> * Use the apical pulse to measure heart rate and rhythm.
> * Measure blood pressure in the supine and standing positions.
> * Measure daily weight.
> * Measure intake and output.
>   *Planning*
> * The oral dose forms are 10, 25, 50, and 100 mg tablets.
>   *Implementation*
> * The initial adult dose is 10 mg four times a day for the first 2 to 4 days. Then, 25 mg are given four times a day.
> * During the second week, the dosage is increased to 50 mg four times a day as blood pressure is brought under control.
>   *Evaluation.* Report and record:
> * *Nausea, dizziness, tachycardia, numbness and tingling in the legs, nasal congestion.* The dosage may need adjustment.
> * *Orthostatic hypotension.* Blood pressure is measured in the supine and standing positions. Provide for safety. Remind the person to rise slowly from a supine or sitting position. Have the person sit or lie down if feeling faint.
> * *Fever, chills, joint and muscle pain, skin problems.* These may signal changes in white blood cells.

COMBINATION DRUGS

Some persons take more than one antihypertensive drug; the second is often a diuretic. A combination drug may be ordered for simple and easy use. See Table 20-6.

TABLE 20-6 Combination Drugs Used to Treat Hypertension

Combination Type	Brand Name
ACEIs and CCBs	Lotrel
	Lexxel
	Tarka
CCB and statin	Caduet
CCBs and ARBs	Exforge
	Azor
	Twynsta
CCBs/diuretic/ARBs	Exforge HCT
	Tribenzor
ACEIs and diuretics	Lotensin HCT
	Vaseretic
	Zestoretic
	Accuretic
ARBs and diuretics	Edarbyclor
	Atacand HCT
	Avalide
	Hyzaar
	Benicar HCT
	Micardis HCT
	Diovan HCT
BBs and diuretics	Tenoretic
	Ziac
	Lopressor HCT
	Corzide
Direct renin inhibitor combination products	Tekturna HCT
Diuretic and diuretic combination	Aldactazide
	Dyazide
	Maxzide

ACEI, Angiotensin-converting enzyme inhibitor; *ARB*, angiotensin receptor blocker; *BB*, beta blocker; *CCB*, calcium channel blocker.
Modified from Willihnganz M: Clayton's Basic Pharmacology for Nurses, ed 18, St Louis, 2020, Elsevier.

REVIEW QUESTIONS

Circle the BEST answer.

1. Which lowers blood pressure?
   a. vasoconstriction
   b. vasodilation
   c. cardiac output
   d. heart rhythm

2. Lifestyle changes to lower blood pressure include the following, *except:*
   a. drug therapy
   b. a low-fat, low-salt diet
   c. a healthy weight
   d. regular exercise

3. When a person requires two or more antihypertensive drugs, one drug is usually:
   a. a beta blocker
   b. a calcium channel
   c. an ACE inhibitor
   d. a diuretic

4. Which promote the formation and excretion of urine?
   a. beta blockers
   b. calcium channel blockers
   c. ACE inhibitors
   d. diuretics

5. Beta blockers lower blood pressure because:
   a. heart rate and cardiac output are reduced
   b. aldosterone levels increase
   c. vasoconstriction occurs
   d. the body retains sodium and water

6. Which is a beta blocker?
   a. carvedilol (Coreg)
   b. enalapril (Vasotec)
   c. quinapril (Accupril)
   d. benazepril (Lotensin)

7. Before giving any antihypertensive drug, you should:
   a. give the person food
   b. measure the person's blood pressure
   c. ask the person to void
   d. ask about bowel elimination patterns
8. Which produces strong vasoconstriction?
   a. renin
   b. angiotensin I
   c. angiotensin II
   d. aldosterone
9. ACE inhibitors affect the conversion of:
   a. angiotensin I to angiotensin II
   b. renin to angiotensin I
   c. renin to aldosterone
   d. aldosterone to angiotensin II
10. Which ACE inhibitor is given before meals?
    a. benazepril (Lotensin)
    b. captopril (Capoten)
    c. enalapril (Vasotec)
    d. quinapril (Accupril)
11. Hypotension as a side effect from ACE inhibitors:
    a. may occur within the first 3 hours after therapy starts
    b. is seen after several weeks of therapy
    c. can be prevented with diuretics
    d. is not a concern
12. Besides preventing vasoconstriction, angiotensin II receptor blockers prevent:
    a. sodium retention
    b. the release of renin
    c. decreased cardiac output
    d. abnormal heart rhythms
13. Hypotension as a side effect from angiotensin II receptor blockers:
    a. may occur within the first 3 hours after therapy starts
    b. is seen after several weeks of therapy
    c. can be prevented with diuretics
    d. is not a concern
14. Which is a direct renin inhibitor agent?
    a. hydralazine
    b. aliskiren (Tekturna)
    c. losartan (Cozaar)
    d. quinapril (Accupril)
15. Which is an aldosterone receptor blocking agent?
    a. amlodipine (Norvasc)
    b. terazosin
    c. lisinopril (Prinivil)
    d. eplerenone (Inspra)
16. Calcium channel blockers lower blood pressure because they:
    a. lower the heart rate
    b. increase cardiac output
    c. increase aldosterone levels
    d. relax the smooth muscle of blood vessels

17. Hypotension and fainting from calcium channel blockers may occur:
    a. within the first 15 to 90 minutes after therapy starts
    b. within the first 3 hours after therapy starts
    c. during the first week
    d. after several weeks
18. Which is a calcium channel blocker?
    A. irbesartan (Avapro)
    b. olmesartan (Benicar)
    c. amlodipine (Norvasc)
    d. nitroprusside sodium (Nitropress)
19. Alpha-1 adrenergic blocking agents lower blood pressure by:
    a. slowing the heart rate
    b. increasing cardiac output
    c. causing vasodilation
    d. relaxing the smooth muscle of blood vessels
20. When giving an Alpha-1 adrenergic blocking agent, you assist the nurse with the nursing process by checking the following, *except*:
    a. the blood pressure while standing
    b. the amount of urine output
    c. the apical heart rate
    d. the blood pressure while laying down
21. Central-acting alpha-2 agonists prevent the release of:
    a. norepinephrine
    b. renin
    c. angiotensin II
    d. aldosterone
22. Central-acting alpha-2 agonists stimulate receptors in the:
    a. brainstem
    b. kidneys
    c. liver
    d. heart
23. Which central-acting alpha-2 agonist comes in a transdermal patch?
    a. clonidine (Catapres)
    b. doxazosin (Cardura)
    c. guanfacine
    d. methyldopa
24. Direct vasodilators lower blood pressure because they:
    a. prevent the release of norepinephrine
    b. cause arterioles to relax
    c. prevent the release of renin
    d. increase cardiac output

Circle T if the statement is true. Circle F if the statement is false.
25. T F Renin causes vasodilation.
26. T F Renin causes sodium retention.
27. T F Aldosterone causes the kidneys to excrete water and sodium.
28. T F Calcium channel blockers are used to treat angina.

Answers to these questions can be found on the Evolve Resources site: http://evolve.elsevier.com/Anderson/medasst/

21

Drugs Used to Treat Dysrhythmias

OBJECTIVES

- Define the key terms and key abbreviations used in this chapter.
- Identify the classification of drugs used to treat dysrhythmias.
- Describe the drugs used to treat dysrhythmias.
- Explain how to assist with the nursing process when giving drugs to treat dysrhythmias.

KEY TERMS

antidysrhythmic agents Drugs used to prevent or correct abnormal heart rhythms

arrhythmia Without *(a)* a rhythm *(rhythmia)*; dysrhythmia

diastole The resting phase of the heartbeat; heart chambers fill with blood

dysrhythmia An abnormal *(dys)* rhythm *(rhythmia)*; arrhythmia

systole The working phase of the heartbeat; the heart contracts and pumps blood through the blood vessels

KEY ABBREVIATIONS

ECG Electrocardiogram
GI Gastrointestinal

mcg Microgram
mg Milligram

The heart pumps blood to itself through the coronary arteries and to the rest of the body's tissues. There are two phases of heart action. During diastole, the resting phase, heart chambers fill with blood. The heart relaxes during this phase. During systole, the working phase, the heart contracts. Blood is pumped through the blood vessels when the heart contracts. Systole and diastole make up the cardiac cycle.

The conduction system (electrical system) controls the cardiac cycle. The heart muscle must relax (fill with blood) and contract (pump blood) in a coordinated fashion. Otherwise, cells do not get enough blood and oxygen. A disturbance in the normal electrical conduction is called an **arrhythmia**, meaning without *(a)* a rhythm *(rhythmia)*. Another term for arrhythmia is **dysrhythmia**—an abnormal *(dys)* rhythm *(rhythmia)*.

An arrhythmia causes:
- An abnormal heart muscle contraction
- An abnormal heart rate

An electrocardiogram (ECG) records the electrical activity of the conduction system. The electrical activity is recorded in waves. By studying the ECG, the doctor determines the site of the problem in the conduction system or the area of heart muscle damage.

DRUG THERAPY FOR DYSRHYTHMIAS

Antidysrhythmic agents are drugs used to prevent or correct abnormal heart rhythms. They are classified based on their effects on the electrical conduction system. The classes include:
- Class I—these drugs disrupt the movement of sodium.

- Class II—these are beta-adrenergic blocking agents (beta blockers) (see Chapter 15).
- Class III—these drugs block potassium channels.
- Class IV—these drugs block calcium channels (calcium channel blockers) (see Chapter 20).
- Miscellaneous—these drugs work differently from those in Classes I-IV.

See *Delegation Guidelines: Drug Therapy for Dysrhythmias.*

DELEGATION GUIDELINES

Drug Therapy for Dysrhythmias

Some drugs used to treat dysrhythmias are given parenterally—by intramuscular or intravenous injection. Because you do not give parenteral dose forms, they are not included in this chapter. Should a nurse delegate the administration of such to you, you must:

- Remember that parenteral dosages are often very different from dosages for other routes.
- Refuse the delegation but do not ignore the request. Make sure the nurse knows that you cannot give the drug and why.

DRUG CLASS: Class I Antidysrhythmic Agents

These drugs disrupt the movement of sodium.
- Quinidine (kwin' i deen)
- Flecainide acetate (fleh kayn' ayd); Tambocor (tam boh' kor)
- Propafenone (pro pah' fen own); Rythmol (rith' mohl)

Quinidine

Quinidine slows the heart rate and changes a rapid, irregular pulse to a slow, regular pulse.

Assisting With the Nursing Process. When giving quinidine, you assist the nurse with the nursing process.

Assessment
- Observe for dyspnea, chest pain, fatigue, edema, fainting, palpitations (the person may describe palpitations as "my heart skips some beats" or "my heart is racing").
- Measure blood pressure, apical pulse (for 1 minute), and respirations.
- Ask about bowel elimination.

Planning. The oral dose forms are:
- Quinidine sulfate:
  - 200 and 300 mg tablets
- Quinidine gluconate:
  - 324 mg sustained-release tablets

Implementation. The adult dosages are:
- Quinidine sulfate:
  - 200 to 300 mg orally every 6 to 8 hours. Higher doses may be used.
  - The maximum single dose should not exceed 600 mg.
  - Give with food or milk.
- Quinidine gluconate:
  - 648 mg every 8 hours.
  - Give with food or milk.

Evaluation. Report and record:
- *Diarrhea.* This is common when therapy is started. It usually subsides. Note the frequency and consistency of stools.
- *Dizziness, faintness.* These usually subside within a few days. Provide for safety. Remind the person to rise slowly from a supine or sitting position. Have the person sit or lie down if feeling faint.
- *Hearing loss, headache, tinnitus (ringing in the ears), increasing mental confusion, rash, chills, fever.* These result from excess quinidine.
- *Hypotension.* This may occur if the person also takes diuretics or antihypertensive agents. Provide for safety. Remind the person to rise slowly from a supine or sitting position. Have the person sit or lie down if feeling faint.

Flecainide Acetate (Tambocor)

Flecainide acetate (Tambocor) slows the conduction rate through the atria and ventricles.

Assisting With the Nursing Process. When giving flecainide acetate (Tambocor), you assist the nurse with the nursing process.

Assessment
- Observe for dyspnea, chest pain, fatigue, edema, fainting, palpitations (the person may describe palpitations as "my heart skips some beats" or "my heart is racing").
- Measure blood pressure, apical pulse (for 1 minute), and respirations.
- Observe for signs and symptoms of heart failure (Chapter 22).

Planning
- Oral dose forms are 50, 100, and 150 mg tablets.

Implementation
- The initial adult dose is 50 mg every 12 hours. It is increased by 50 mg twice a day every 4 days.
- The usual dose is 150 mg twice a day.
- The maximum daily dose is 400 mg.

Evaluation. Report and record:
- *Dizziness, headache, constipation, nausea.* These are mild and tend to resolve with continued therapy.
- *Vision disturbances.* Provide for safety. The person should avoid tasks that require good vision (driving, operating machines). Remind the person not to forcefully rub his or her eyes when tearing.
- *Signs and symptoms of heart failure (Chapter 21).* This drug may cause heart failure or cause existing heart failure to worsen.
- *Dysrhythmias.* The drug may cause dysrhythmias or cause existing dysrhythmias to worsen.

Propafenone (Rythmol)

Propafenone (Rythmol) slows the conduction rate between the atria and ventricles. Because it can cause other dysrhythmias, it is used when the benefits are greater than the risks. This drug should not be given to people with asthma.

Assisting With the Nursing Process. When giving propafenone (Rythmol), you assist the nurse with the nursing process.

Assessment
- Observe for dyspnea, chest pain, fatigue, edema, fainting, palpitations (the person may describe palpitations as "my heart skips some beats" or "my heart is racing").
- Measure blood pressure, apical pulse (for 1 minute), and respirations.
- Ask about GI symptoms.

Planning
- Oral dose forms:
  - 150, 225, and 300 mg tablets
  - 225, 325, and 425 mg 12-hour extended-release capsules

Implementation
- The initial adult dose is 150 mg every 8 hours.
- Every 3 to 4 days, the dosage may be increased to 225 mg every 8 hours, then 300 mg every 8 hours (900 mg daily).
- If a dose is missed, the next dose should not be doubled. (Check with the nurse. The nurse tells you what to do when a dose is missed.)

Evaluation. Report and record:
- *Dizziness.* Provide for safety. Remind the person to rise slowly from a supine or sitting position. Have the person sit or lie down if feeling faint.
- *Nausea, vomiting, constipation.* Give the drug with food or milk to prevent nausea.
- *Dysrhythmias.* The drug may cause dysrhythmias or cause existing dysrhythmias to worsen.

DRUG CLASS: Class II Antidysrhythmic Agents

Class II antidysrhythmic agents are beta-adrenergic blocking agents (beta blockers). They are widely used as antidysrhythmic agents (Chapter 15). By blocking beta receptors, they block the heart's response to sympathetic nerve stimulation. Heart rate, blood pressure, and cardiac output are reduced.

See Table 15-2 (Chapter 15) for a list of beta blockers.

DRUG CLASS: Class III Antidysrhythmic Agents

These drugs disrupt the movement of potassium.
- Amiodarone hydrochloride (am e o' dahr own); Pacerone (pace' er own)
- Dofetilide (doe fet' i lide); Tikosyn (tik' o sin)

Amiodarone Hydrochloride (Pacerone)

Amiodarone hydrochloride (Pacerone) slows the rate of electrical conduction. It also increases the time between contractions.

Assisting With the Nursing Process. When giving amiodarone (Pacerone), you assist the nurse with the nursing process.
Assessment
- Observe for dyspnea, chest pain, fatigue, edema, fainting, palpitations (the person may describe palpitations as "my heart skips some beats" or "my heart is racing").
- Measure blood pressure, apical pulse (for 1 minute), and respirations.
- Ask about GI symptoms.
- Monitor sleep pattern.
Planning
- Oral dose forms are 100, 200, and 400 mg tablets.
Implementation
- The initial adult dose is 800 to 1600 mg daily in divided doses for 1 to 3 weeks. Then a dosage of 600 to 800 mg daily is given for about 1 month.
- The lowest effective dose should be used, usually 400 mg.
Evaluation. Report and record:
- *Fatigue, tremors, involuntary muscle movements, sleep problems, numbness and tingling, coordination problems, dizziness, confusion.* Many of these may resolve when the dose is reduced, or the drug is discontinued. Provide for safety. Remind the person to rise slowly from a supine or sitting position. Have the person sit or lie down if feeling faint.
- *Dyspnea on exertion, nonproductive cough, chest pain with breathing.* Symptoms gradually resolve when the drug is discontinued.
- *Blurred vision, narrowed peripheral vision, halos.* Provide for safety. Remind the person not to forcefully rub his or her eyes when tearing. These symptoms resolve when the drug is discontinued.
- *Nausea, vomiting, constipation, abdominal pain, anorexia.* These are common with high dosages. They resolve with lower doses or divided doses.
- *Dysrhythmias.* The drug may cause dysrhythmias or cause existing dysrhythmias to worsen.
- *Skin reactions: rash, burning, tingling, redness, and blistering.* These are from exposure to sunlight (photosensitivity). The person should use sunscreens, wear long-sleeve shirts and pants, and avoid sunlamps.
- *Anorexia, nausea, vomiting, jaundice.* These may signal liver toxicity.

Dofetilide (Tikosyn)

Dofetilide (Tikosyn) slows the rate of electrical conduction. It also increases the time between contractions.

Assisting With the Nursing Process. When giving dofetilide (Tikosyn), you assist the nurse with the nursing process.
Assessment
- Measure blood pressure in the supine and standing positions.
Planning
- Oral dose forms are 125, 250, and 500 mcg capsules.
Implementation
- The dosage of this drug is based on the persons kidney function and ECG monitoring. The dose can range between 125 mg daily up to 500 mcg twice a day.

Evaluation. Report and record:
- *Dysrhythmias.* The drug may cause dysrhythmias or cause existing dysrhythmias to worsen.
- *Headache, dizziness, insomnia, and rash.* These usually resolve with continued therapy.
- *Nausea abdominal pain, diarrhea.* These usually resolve with continued therapy.

DRUG CLASS: Class IV Antidysrhythmic Agents

Class IV antidysrhythmic agents are calcium channel blocking agents (calcium channel blockers). They are widely used as antidysrhythmic agents (Chapter 20). These drugs block the calcium channels found in the heart. This results in a reduced heart rate.

See Table 20-3 (Chapter 20) for a list of calcium channel blockers.

DRUG CLASS: Miscellaneous Antidysrhythmic Agents

These drugs are not related to other antidysrhythmic agents.
- Digoxin (di joks' in); Lanoxin (lah noks' in)

Digoxin (Lanoxin)

Digoxin (Lanoxin) slows the heart rate. It also helps the heart pump harder. This allows the heart to fill and empty blood out more completely. Lanoxin is also used to treat heart failure (Chapter 22).

Assisting With the Nursing Process. When giving digoxin (Lanoxin), you assist the nurse with the nursing process.
Assessment
- Observe for dyspnea, chest pain, fatigue, edema, fainting, palpitations (the person may describe palpitations as "my heart skips some beats" or "my heart is racing").
- Measure vital signs: blood pressure, the apical pulse for 1 minute, and respirations.
- Measure daily weight.
- Measure intake and output.
Planning
- Adult oral dose forms are 0.0625, 0.125, 0.187.5 and 0.25 mg tablets.
Implementation
- The adult digitalizing dose is 0.5 to 0.75 mg. It is followed by 0.125 to 0.375 mg every 6 to 8 hours until adequate digitalization is achieved. Digitalization is discussed further in Chapter 22.
- The maintenance dose is 0.125 to 0.25 mg daily. Some people need 0.375 to 0.5 mg daily.
- *Measure the apical pulse for 1 minute before giving the drug.* Follow agency policy for withholding the drug. The drug is not usually given if the pulse is less than 60 or greater than 100 beats per minute.
- The drug is given in very small amounts. If you are allowed to do dose calculations, have a nurse check your calculation. If a pharmacist or nurse did the dose calculation, ask another nurse to check the calculation.
- Give the drug after meals to reduce stomach irritation.
Evaluation. Report and record:
- *Signs and symptoms of digoxin toxicity.* See Chapter 22, Box 22-4.
- *Nausea, vomiting, diarrhea, excessive urinary output.* The person is at risk for low serum potassium levels (hypokalemia).

REVIEW QUESTIONS

Circle the BEST answer.

1. Another term for dysrhythmia is:
   a. anrhythmia
   b. bradyrhythmia
   c. arrhythmia
   d. tachyrhythmia
2. All of the following are actions of antidysrhythmic drugs, *except*:
   a. blocking potassium channels
   b. blocking glucose channels
   c. blocking sodium channels
   d. blocking calcium channels
3. Which of the following drugs is not a Class I antidysrhythmic agent?
   a. quinidine
   b. flecainide acetate
   c. digoxin (Lanoxin)
   d. propafenone (Rythmol)
4. Diarrhea is common when which drug is started?
   a. amiodarone hydrochloride (Pacerone)
   b. digoxin (Lanoxin)
   c. quinidine
   d. propafenone (Rythmol)
5. Flecainide acetate (Tambocor) is used to:
   a. increase the heart rate
   b. slow the heart rate
   c. decrease the time between contractions
   d. increase the rate of electrical conduction
6. Class II antidysrhythmic agents are also called:
   a. potassium channel blockers
   b. calcium channel blockers
   c. ACE inhibitors
   d. beta-adrenergic blocking agents
7. Which is not a Class II antidysrhythmic agent?
   a. metoprolol (Lopressor)
   b. atenolol (Tenormin)
   c. sotalol (Betapace)
   d. amiodarone (Pacerone)
8. Beta blockers are used to:
   a. increase the heart rate
   b. slow the heart rate
   c. decrease the time between contractions
   d. increase the rate of electrical conduction
9. Before giving any antidysrhythmic drug, you should do all the following, *except*:
   a. observe for dyspnea, chest pain, and palpitations
   b. observe for fatigue and fainting
   c. measure blood pressure
   d. measure the radial pulse and respirations
10. Before giving any antidysrhythmic agent, the pulse is measured:
    a. for 30 seconds
    b. for 1 minute
    c. by ECG
    d. every 6 hours

11. Most antidysrhythmic drugs can cause:
    a. diarrhea
    b. gastrointestinal bleeding
    c. increased urinary output
    d. other dysrhythmias
12. What is the action of a Class III antidysrhythmic drug?
    a. These drugs block sodium channels.
    b. These drugs block potassium channels.
    c. These drugs block calcium channels.
    d. These drugs are beta blockers.
13. Amiodarone hydrochloride (Pacerone) is given to:
    a. increase the heart rate
    b. slow the heart rate
    c. decrease the time between contractions
    d. increase the rate of electrical conduction
14. Which drug dosage is calculated based on the person's kidney function?
    a. quinidine
    b. amiodarone (Pacerone)
    c. dofetilide (Tikosyn)
    d. flecainide acetate
15. Class IV antidysrhythmic drugs work by:
    a. attaching to the heart muscles
    b. attaching to potassium channels
    c. blocking sodium channels
    d. blocking calcium channels
16. Which drug helps the heart fill and empty blood more completely?
    a. propafenone (Rythmol)
    b. metoprolol (Lopressor)
    c. digoxin (Lanoxin)
    d. amlodipine (Norvasc)
17. Before you give digoxin, what should you do first?
    a. Measure the person's height and weight.
    b. Measure the apical pulse for 1 full minute.
    c. Check the person's oral temperature.
    d. Ask about the person's sleep pattern.

Circle T if the statement is true. Circle F if the statement is false.

18. T F During diastole, the resting phase, heart chambers fill with blood.
19. T F During systole, the working phase, the heart contracts.
20. T F An electrocardiogram (ECG) records the electrical activity of the conduction system within the heart.
21. T F Quinidine increases the heart rate.

Answers to these questions can be found on the Evolve Resources site: http://evolve.elsevier.com/Anderson/medasst/

Drugs Used to Treat Angina, Peripheral Vascular Disease, and Heart Failure

OBJECTIVES

- Define the key terms and key abbreviations used in this chapter.
- Describe the causes, signs and symptoms, and treatment of angina.
- Describe the drugs used to treat angina.
- Explain how to assist with the nursing process when giving drugs to treat angina.
- Describe the causes, signs and symptoms, and treatment of peripheral vascular disease.

- Describe the drugs used to treat peripheral vascular disease.
- Explain how to assist with the nursing process when giving drugs to treat peripheral vascular disease.
- Describe the causes, signs and symptoms, and treatment of heart failure.
- Describe the drugs used to treat heart failure.
- Explain how to assist with the nursing process when giving drugs to treat heart failure.

KEY TERMS

digitalization Giving a larger dose of digoxin for the first 24 hours, then giving the person a daily dose

hemorrheologic agent A drug that prevents the clumping of red blood cells and platelets: hemorrheologic relates to the science (logic) of blood (hemo) flow (rrheo)

inotropic agents Drugs that stimulate the heart to increase the force of contractions

intermittent claudication A pain pattern usually described as aching, cramping, tightness, or weakness in the calves, usually during walking; it is relieved with rest

platelet aggregation inhibitor A drug that prevents platelets from clumping together and causes vasodilation

vasodilators Drugs that widen blood vessels to increase blood flow

vasospasm A sudden contraction of a blood vessel causing vasoconstriction

KEY ABBREVIATIONS

ACE   Angiotensin-converting enzyme
CAD   Coronary artery disease
CHF   Congestive heart failure
h   Hour
MAR   Medication administration record
mg   Milligram

MI   Myocardial infarction
mL   Milliliter
PO   Per os (orally)
PVD   Peripheral vascular disease
q   Every

Cardiovascular system disorders are leading causes of death in the United States. Many people have these disorders. Examples of cardiovascular system disorders include angina, peripheral vascular disease, and heart failure.

DRUG THERAPY FOR ANGINA

The coronary arteries are in the heart. They supply the heart with blood. In coronary artery disease (CAD), the coronary arteries become hardened and narrow. One or all arteries can be affected. Therefore, the heart muscle gets less blood and oxygen.

The most common cause of CAD is atherosclerosis (Chapter 19). Plaque—made up of fat, cholesterol, and other substances—collects on the arterial walls. The narrowed arteries block blood flow.

Blockage may be total or partial. Blood clots also can form along the plaque and block blood flow.

The major complications of CAD are angina (also called chest pain), myocardial infarction (MI) (or heart attack), dysrhythmias (or arrhythmias), and sudden death. The more risk factors, the greater the chance of CAD and its complications. Risk factors are listed in Box 22-1.

Angina (pain) means *chest pain*. It is from reduced blood flow to part of the heart muscle (myocardium). It occurs when the heart needs more oxygen. Normally blood flow to the heart increases when the need for oxygen increases. Exertion, a heavy meal, stress, and excitement increase the heart's need for oxygen. Smoking and exposure to very hot or cold temperatures also increase the heart's need for oxygen. In CAD, narrowed vessels prevent increased blood flow.

BOX 22-1 Risk Factors for Coronary Artery Disease

RISK FACTORS THAT *CANNOT* BE CONTROLLED

- Gender—men are at greater risk than women
- Age—in men, the risk increases after age 45; in women, the risk increases after age 55
- Family history
- Race—African Americans are at greater risk than other groups

RISK FACTORS THAT *CAN* BE CONTROLLED

- Being overweight
- Lack of exercise
- High blood cholesterol
- Hypertension
- Smoking
- Diabetes
- Stress (anger, worry, arguing)

Chest pain is described as a tightness, pressure, squeezing, or burning in the chest (Fig. 22-1). Pain can occur in the shoulders, arms, neck, jaw, or back. Pain in the jaw, neck, and down one or both arms is common. The person may be pale, feel faint, and perspire. Dyspnea is common. Nausea, fatigue, and weakness may occur. Some persons complain of "gas" or indigestion. Rest often relieves symptoms in 3 to 15 minutes. Rest reduces the heart's need for oxygen. Therefore, normal blood flow is achieved. Heart damage is prevented.

DELEGATION GUIDELINES

Drugs Used to Treat Angina, Peripheral Vascular Disease, and Heart Failure

Some drugs used to treat angina, peripheral vascular disease, and heart failure are given parenterally—by subcutaneous, intramuscular, or intravenous injection. Because you do not give parenteral dose forms, they are not included in this chapter. Should a nurse delegate the administration of such to you, you must:

- Remember that parenteral dosages are often very different from dosages for other routes.
- Refuse the delegation but do not just ignore the request. Make sure the nurse knows that you cannot give the drug and why.

Things that cause angina are avoided. These include overexertion, heavy meals and overeating, and emotional stress. The person needs to stay indoors during cold weather or during hot, humid weather. Exercise programs are helpful. They are supervised by the doctor.

Some persons need drugs to decrease the heart's workload and relieve symptoms. Other drugs are given to prevent an MI or sudden death. Drugs also can delay the need for medical and surgical procedures that open or bypass diseased arteries (Fig. 22-2). The goal is to increase blood flow to the heart. Doing so may prevent or lower the risk of heart attack and death.

With angina, the coronary arteries cannot deliver enough oxygen to meet the heart's demands. Seven groups of drugs may be used to treat angina:

- Nitrates
- Beta-adrenergic blocking agents (beta blockers)
- Angiotensin-converting enzyme (ACE) inhibitors
- Calcium ion antagonists (calcium channel blockers)
- Statins (Chapter 19)
- Platelet-active agents (Chapter 24)
- Myocardial cell sodium channel blockers

See *Delegation Guidelines: Drugs Used to Treat Angina, Peripheral Vascular Disease, and Heart Failure.*

DRUG CLASS: Nitrates

Nitrates are the oldest effective therapy for angina. They relieve angina by:

- *Relaxing peripheral vascular smooth muscles.* Arteries and veins dilate (widen). This reduces venous blood flow to the heart. It also decreases oxygen demands on the heart.
- *Dilating coronary arteries.* This enhances blood flow and myocardial oxygen supply.

Nitroglycerin is the drug of choice in the treatment of angina. Various dose forms are available to meet the person's needs. The goals of nitrate therapy are to:

- Relieve the pain of angina during an attack
- Reduce the frequency and severity of anginal attacks (prophylaxis)
- Increase activity and exercise tolerance

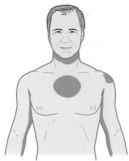

- Mid sternum
- Left shoulder and down both arms
- Neck and arms

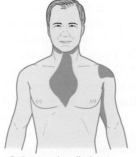

- Substernal radiating to neck and jaw
- Substernal radiating down left arm

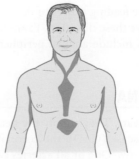

- Epigastric
- Epigastric radiating to neck, jaw, and arms

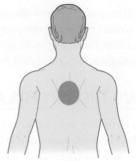

- Intrascapular

Fig. 22-1 Common locations and patterns of pain during angina or myocardial infarction. (From Lewis SM and others: *Medical-surgical nursing: assessment and management of clinical problems,* ed 10, St Louis, 2017, Mosby).

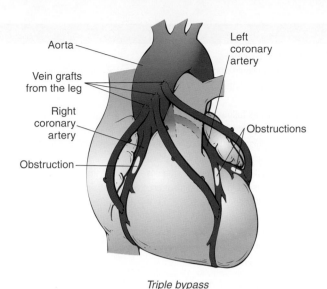

Fig. 22-2 Coronary artery bypass surgery. (Modified from Thibodeau GA, Patton KT: *The human body in health and disease,* ed 4, St Louis, 2005, Mosby.)

Assisting With the Nursing Process. When a person receives nitrates, you assist the nurse with the nursing process.

Assessment
- Ask about the severity, location, duration, intensity, and pattern of pain.
- Ask when the last dose of nitrates was taken.
- Ask if relief was obtained from the nitrate.
- Measure blood pressure.
  Planning. See Table 22-1 for "Dose Forms."
  Implementation. See Table 22-1 for "Adult Dosage Range." See Box 22-2, for the administration of nitrate dose forms.
  Evaluation. Report and record:
- *Hypotension, dizziness, nausea, flushing, fainting.* The dosage may need adjustment.

- *Headache.* This is the most common side effect. It can range from a feeling of mild fullness in the head to an intense and severe headache. Most people develop tolerance within a few weeks. The dosage may need adjustment.
- *Tolerance (increasing dosage to attain relief).* Tolerance to nitrate dosages can develop rapidly, particularly if large doses are given often. It can appear within a few days and may be well established within a few weeks. The smallest dose for a satisfactory result should be used. To break tolerance, the doctor withdraws the drug for a short time.

DRUG CLASS: Beta-Adrenergic Blocking Agents

Beta-adrenergic blocking agents (beta blockers) block the beta-adrenergic receptors in the heart. This prevents stimulation from norepinephrine and epinephrine (Chapter 15). Normally such stimulation would increase the heart rate and increase myocardial oxygen demands. Heart rate, oxygen demand, and blood pressure are reduced by blocking the receptors.

All beta blockers are effective in treating angina. The goals of therapy are to:
- Reduce the number of angina attacks
- Reduce nitroglycerin use
- Improve activity and exercise tolerance

Assisting With the Nursing Process. When giving beta blockers to treat angina, you assist the nurse with the nursing process.

Assessment
- Measure blood pressure in the supine and standing positions.
- Ask about respiratory signs and symptoms.
- Measure blood glucose if the person has diabetes.
  Planning. See Chapter 15.
  Implementation. See Chapter 15.
  Evaluation. See Chapter 15.

TABLE 22-1	**Nitrates**		
Generic Name	**Brand Name**	**Dose Forms**	**Adult Dosage Range**
isosorbide dinitrate	Isordil	Tablets: 5, 10, 20, 30, 40 mg Sustained-release tablets and capsules: 40 mg	PO: 5-40 mg two to three times daily on empty stomach PO: 40-160 mg a day
isosorbide mononitrate		Tablets: 10, 20 mg 24-hr sustained-release tablets: 30, 60, 120 mg	PO: 20 mg twice daily, 7 hours apart PO: 30-240 mg once daily; do not crush or chew tablets
nitroglycerin	Nitrostat	Sublingual tablets: 0.3, 0.4, 0.6 mg Sustained-release capsules: 2.5, 6.5, 9 mg	Sublingual: 0.3-0.6 mg for prophylactic use before activity that may induce angina or at time of acute attack PO: 2.5-9 mg two to four times daily for prophylaxis
	Nitro-Bid	Ointment: 2%	Topical: 0.5-2 inches of ointment using special applicator q6h
	Nitro-Dur	Transdermal: 0.1, 0.2, 0.3, 0.4, 0.6, 0.8 mg/hour patches	Topical: Initial 0.2 to 0.4 mg/hr. patch applied for 12 hours. Titrate dose to response. Wait 12 hours after removing old patch before applying new patch
	Nitrolingual Pumpspray	Translingual: 0.4 mg metered spray	Spray: one to two sprays onto or under tongue for acute attack; repeat if needed in 3-5 minutes; may be used prophylactically 5-10 minutes before exercise

Modified from Willihnganz M: Clayton's Basic Pharmacology for Nurses, ed 18, St Louis, 2020, Elsevier.

BOX 22-2 Administration of Nitrate Dose Forms

Sublingual Tablets

- Remind the person to sit or lie down at the first sign of an anginal attack.
- Remind the person to:
  - Place a tablet under the tongue.
  - Let the tablet dissolve.
  - Not to swallow saliva immediately.
  - Tell the nurse at once:
  - When the person takes a sublingual tablet.
  - If the person does not obtain relief of chest pain within 5 minutes, assist the nurse as directed.
- Remind the person to tell the nursing team if they take one or two tablets before activities that may cause an angina attack.
- Remind the person that sublingual tablets deteriorate within a few months.
  - The drug should produce a slight stinging or burning sensation. This means that the drug is still potent.
  - The person should have the prescription refilled every 3 months.
  - The person should discard unused tablets.
- Store nitroglycerin in the original, dark-colored glass container. Make sure the lid is tight.
- Make sure the drug is within the person's reach.
  - Home settings: The person should always carry nitroglycerin. It should not be carried in a pocket directly next to the person's body. Heat speeds up deterioration of the drug.
  - Health care settings: Nitroglycerin is kept at the bedside. Remind the person to tell the nursing team at once when taking a nitroglycerin tablet.

Sustained-Release Tablets

- Give sustained-release nitroglycerin tablets as ordered. They are usually taken on an empty stomach every 8 to 12 hours.
- Give the drug with food if gastritis develops. Check with the nurse and the MAR.

Transmucosal Tablets

- Place the tablet under the upper lip or buccal pouch. The drug is absorbed by the oral mucosa over 3 to 5 hours.
- Remind the person that they may eat, drink, and talk while the tablet is in place.
- Give the drug as ordered. The usual initial dose is one tablet three times a day:
  - On arising
  - After lunch
  - After the evening meal
- Do not give more than one tablet every 2 hours.

Translingual Spray

- *Do not use the spray where it can ignite. The spray is highly flammable.*
- Do not shake the container. Bubbles may form which can slow the release of the drug.
- Give the spray as follows:
  - Position the person in a sitting position.
  - Hold the canister vertically so the valve head is uppermost. Hold the spray opening as close to the mouth as possible.
  - Press the button firmly to spray the dose onto or under the tongue.
  - Have the person close the mouth at once after each dose. *The spray should not be swallowed or inhaled.*
- Tell the nurse at once:
  - When the person uses a translingual spray.
  - If the person does not obtain relief of chest pain within 5 minutes. Assist the nurse as directed.

Topical Ointment

- See Chapter 12 for applying topical ointment.
- Rotate application sites to prevent skin irritation. Do not use a site with signs of irritation.
- Close the tube tightly. Store it in a cool place according to agency policy.

Transdermal Disk

- Remember the following:
  - This dose form provides controlled release of the drug for 24 hours when applied to intact skin.
  - The dosage released depends on the surface area of the disk.
  - Therapeutic effect can be observed about 30 minutes after application. It continues for about 30 minutes after removal.
  - The person may need sublingual nitroglycerin for anginal attacks.
- Practice hand washing before applying and after removing a patch.
- See Chapter 12 for applying a transdermal disk.
- Rotate the application site daily. The best sites are the upper chest, pelvis, and inner side of the upper arm. Avoid scars, skinfolds, and wounds.
- Remove and discard a patch that has become partly dislodged. Apply a new disk.
- Keep discarded patches out of the reach of children. Discarded patches still contain enough active drug to be dangerous to children.

DRUG CLASS: Calcium Channel Blockers

Calcium channel blockers inhibit the movement of calcium ions across a cell membrane (Chapter 20). They do the following:

- Decrease myocardial oxygen demand.
- Dilate coronary arteries, which improves blood flow. This increases myocardial blood supply.
- Dilate peripheral vessels. This decreases resistance to blood flow, which reduces the heart's workload.
  The goals of therapy are to:
- Decrease the frequency of angina attacks
- Decrease the severity of angina attacks
- Increase activity and exercise tolerance

Assisting With the Nursing Process. When giving calcium channel blockers to treat angina, you assist the nurse with the nursing process.

Assessment

- Measure blood pressure in the supine and standing positions.
- Observe for signs and symptoms of heart failure (p. 221).
  Planning. See Table 22-2 for "Oral Dose Forms."
  Implementation. See Table 22-2 for "Adult Dosage Range."
  Evaluation. See Chapter 20.

DRUG CLASS: Angiotensin-Converting Enzyme Inhibitors

Angiotensin-converting enzyme (ACE) inhibitors have a significant effect on the coronary arteries. By preventing vasoconstriction, the blood vessels dilate. The drugs also prevent blood clots from forming. See Chapter 20 for a discussion of ACE inhibitors.

ACE inhibitors are used to prevent MI.

TABLE 22-2	Calcium Channel Blockers Used to Treat Angina		
Generic Name	**Brand Name**	**Oral Dose Forms**	**Adult Dosage Range**
amlodipine	Norvasc	Tablets: 2.5, 5, 10 mg Oral suspension: 1 mg/mL in 120-mL bottle	Initial—5 mg once daily; adjust over 7-14 days to a maximum of 10 mg/day
diltiazem	Cardizem	Tablets: 30, 60, 90, 120 mg	Initial—30 mg four times daily, gradually increasing dosage to 180-360 mg in three or four divided doses
	Cardizem LA, Cardizem CD	Tablets and capsules, 24-hr extended-release: 120, 180, 240, 300, 360, 420 mg	Initial—120-180 mg sustained-release capsule once daily; adjust as needed after 14 days Maximum—480 mg daily
nicardipine		Capsules: 20, 30 mg	Initial—20 mg three times daily Maximal response may require 2 weeks of therapy Allow at least 3 days between dosage adjustments Maintenance—20-40 mg three times daily
nifedipine	Procardia, Adalat CC Procardia XL	Capsules: 10, 20 mg Sustained-release tablets: 30, 60, 90 mg	Initial—10 mg three times daily; adjust over 7-14 days to balance antianginal and hypotensive activity Sustained-release tablets: 30-60 mg once daily Maximum—capsules: 180 mg daily; sustained-release tablets: 120 mg daily
verapamil	Calan Calan SR	Tablets: 40, 80, 120 mg 24-hr sustained-release tablets and capsules: 100, 120, 180, 200, 240, 300, 360 mg	Immediate-release: Initial—40-120 mg three times daily Sustained-release: Initial—180 mg once daily at bedtime Maintenance—120-480 mg daily Administer with food

Modified from Willihnganz M: Clayton's Basic Pharmacology for Nurses, ed 18, St Louis, 2020, Elsevier.

Assisting With the Nursing Process. When giving ACE inhibitors to prevent MI, you assist the nurse with the nursing process.

Assessment
- Measure blood pressure in the supine and standing positions.
- Use the apical pulse to measure heart rate and rhythm for 1 minute.
- Ask about bowel elimination.
- Ask if the person has a cough.
  Planning. See Table 20-1 (Chapter 20) for "Oral Dose Forms."
  Implementation. See Table 20-1 (Chapter 20) for "Adult Dosage Range."
- Captopril (Capoten) is given two to three times daily 1 hour before or 2 hours after meals. All other ACE inhibitors are given one or two times a day.
  Evaluation. See Chapter 20.

DRUG CLASS: Myocardial Cell Sodium Channel Blocker

A myocardial cell sodium channel blocker produces myocardial relaxation. The oxygen demand is reduced, and symptoms of angina are also reduced.

The following drug is a myocardial cell sodium channel blocker:
- Ranolazine (ran oh' lah zeen); Ranexa (ran ex' ah)
  Ranexa does not affect blood pressure or heart rate. It is used with a calcium channel blocker, a beta blocker, or nitrates. The goals of therapy are to:
- Decrease the frequency of angina attacks
- Decrease the severity of angina attacks
- Increase activity and exercise tolerance

- Reduce the use of nitroglycerin in anginal attacks
- Ranexa should only be used in people who have not experienced anginal relief using other antianginal drugs.

Assisting With the Nursing Process. When giving ranolazine (Ranexa), you assist the nurse with the nursing process.
  Assessment. Ask the nurse if measurements are needed.
  Planning. The oral dose forms are 500 and 1000 mg 12-hour extended-release tablets.
  Implementation
- The usual adult dose is 500 mg twice daily. It may be increased to 1000 mg twice daily.
- The drug may be taken with or without meals.
- Tablets should be swallowed whole. They should not be broken, crushed, or chewed.
  Evaluation. Report and record:
- *Dizziness, headache, constipation, nausea.* These are usually mild. The person should not drive, operate machines, or engage in activities that require mental alertness until it is known how they will react to the drug.

DRUG THERAPY FOR PERIPHERAL VASCULAR DISEASE

Peripheral vascular disease (PVD) involves the blood vessels outside of the heart, particularly in the arms and legs (extremities). They can be arterial or venous in origin.
- *Deep vein thrombosis.* This is a venous disorder. See Chapter 24.

- *Arteriosclerosis obliterans.* *Arterio* means *artery.* *Sclerosis* means *hardening.* *Obliterans* means *to narrow or close.* It results from atherosclerosis (Chapter 19) of the lower aorta and major arteries supplying the legs. There is gradual narrowing of the arteries with thrombus (clot) formation. Cholesterol, hypertension, smoking, and diabetes are causes. Symptoms occur when there is significant narrowing (75% or more) of the major arteries and arterioles in the legs. Blood flow is obstructed and tissues do not get needed oxygen. The pain pattern is usually described as aching, cramping, tightness, or weakness in the calves, usually during walking. It is relieved with rest. This is called **intermittent claudication.** *Intermittent* means *to come and go.* *Claudication* means *limping.* As the disease progresses, the person may have pain at rest, numbness, and tingling. Gangrene is a risk.
- *Raynaud's disease.* Exposure to strong emotions or cold trigger blood vessel spasms—vasospasms. A **vasospasm** is a sudden contraction of a blood vessel causing vasoconstriction. In Raynaud's disease, vasospasms obstruct blood flow to fingers, toes, ears, and the nose. The disease is more common in women than in men. Risk factors include arterial diseases, repeated trauma (such as vibrations caused by typing, playing the piano, using air hammers), some drugs, strong emotions, and exposure to cold. The fingers, toes, ears, or nose become white from the lack of blood flow. Then they turn blue—tiny blood vessels dilate to allow more blood to stay in the tissues. When blood flow returns, the area becomes red. Later it returns to normal color. Swelling, tingling, and painful throbbing may occur. Attacks can last from minutes to hours. As the disease progresses, the fingers become thin and tapered with smooth, shiny skin. Ulcers and gangrene may occur if an artery becomes completely blocked.

See Box 22-3 for the treatment of arteriosclerosis obliterans and Raynaud's disease. Some persons need drug therapy. The goals of treatment are to:
- Reverse disease progression
- Improve blood flow

BOX 22-3 **Treatment of Peripheral Vascular Disease**

Arteriosclerosis Obliterans
- Control of existing diseases (diabetes, hypertension, angina, high cholesterol)
- Weight control
- Daily exercise (usually walking)
- Proper foot care:
  - Feet are kept warm and dry
  - Shoes fit properly
- Avoiding cold
- Raising the head of the bed 12 to 16 inches
- Medical or surgical procedures to improve blood flow

Raynaud's Disease
- Avoiding cold temperatures
- Avoiding emotional stress
- Avoiding tobacco use
- Keeping the hands and feet warm with gloves and socks
- Using foam "wraparounds" when handling iced beverages

- Provide pain relief
- Prevent skin ulcers and gangrene

DRUG CLASS: Hemorrheologic Agent

Hemorrheologic relates to the science *(logic)* of blood *(hemo)* flow *(rrheo).* A **hemorrheologic agent** prevents the clumping of red blood cells and platelets. Blood flow to small vessels increases. They receive more oxygen.

The following drug is a hemorrheologic agent:
- Pentoxifylline (pen tox e' fi leen)

Pentoxifylline is used to treat intermittent claudication. It is used along with the measures listed in Box 22-3. The goals of therapy are to:
- Improve the blood and oxygen supply to tissues
- Reduce the frequency of pain
- Improve exercise tolerance
- Improve pulses in the legs

Assisting With the Nursing Process. When giving pentoxifylline, you assist the nurse with the nursing process.

Assessment
- Ask about nausea, vomiting, indigestion, or poor tolerance to caffeine products (coffee, tea, chocolate, colas).
- Ask about dizziness or headache.
- Ask about cardiac symptoms.
- Ask the person to rate his or her pain using a pain rating scale. (See Chapter 18.)

Planning
- The oral dose form is 400 mg extended-release tablets.

Implementation
- The usual adult dose is 400 mg three times a day.
- If adverse effects occur, the dosage is reduced, or the drug is discontinued.
- Give the drug with food or milk if directed to do so by the nurse or the MAR.

Evaluation. Report and record:
- *Nausea, vomiting, indigestion.* These are usually mild and tend to resolve with continued therapy.
- *Dizziness, headache.* These are usually mild and tend to resolve with continued therapy. Provide for safety. Have the person sit or lie down if feeling faint.
- *Chest pain, dysrhythmias, shortness of breath.* These signal a cardiac event. Tell the nurse at once.
- *Tachycardia.* This may signal intolerance to other drugs or caffeine.

DRUG CLASS: Platelet Aggregation Inhibitor

Platelets are needed for blood clotting. To aggregate means to clump. A **platelet aggregation inhibitor** prevents platelets from clumping together. It also causes vasodilation.

The following drug is a platelet aggregation inhibitor:
- Cilostazol (sigh lo stay' zohl)

Cilostazol is used in the treatment of intermittent claudication. It is used along with the measures listed in Box 22-3. The goals of therapy are to:
- Improve the blood and oxygen supply to tissues
- Reduce the frequency of pain

- Improve exercise tolerance
- Improve pulses in the legs

Assisting With the Nursing Process. When giving cilostazol, you assist the nurse with the nursing process.

Assessment
- Ask about dizziness and headache.
- Ask the person to rate his or her pain using a pain rating scale. (See Chapter 18.)
- Ask about cardiac symptoms.

Planning
- The oral dose forms are 50 and 100 mg tablets.

Implementation
- The usual adult dose is 100 mg two times a day.
- The dose is given 30 minutes before or 2 hours after breakfast and dinner.
- Symptom relief may start within 2 to 4 weeks. However, it may take 12 weeks to achieve the full effect.

Evaluation. Report and record:
- *Indigestion, diarrhea.* These are usually mild and tend to resolve with continued therapy.
- *Dizziness, headache.* These are usually mild and tend to resolve with continued therapy. Provide for safety. Remind the person to rise slowly from a supine or sitting position. Have the person sit or lie down if feeling faint.
- *Chest pain, palpitations, dysrhythmias, shortness of breath.* These signal a cardiac event. Tell the nurse at once.

DRUG THERAPY FOR HEART FAILURE

Heart failure (previously known as congestive heart failure [CHF]) occurs when the heart is weakened and cannot pump normally. Blood backs up. Tissue congestion occurs.

When the left side of the heart cannot pump blood normally, blood backs up into the lungs. Respiratory congestion occurs. The person has dyspnea (difficulty breathing), increased sputum, cough, and gurgling sounds in the lungs. The rest of the body does not get enough blood. Signs and symptoms occur from the effects on other organs. Poor blood flow to the brain causes confusion, dizziness, and fainting. The kidneys produce less urine. The skin is pale. Blood pressure falls.

Blood backs up into the venous system when the right side of the heart cannot pump blood normally. Feet and ankles swell. This swelling is called edema. Neck veins bulge. Liver congestion affects liver function. The abdomen becomes congested with fluid. The right side of the heart pumps less blood to the lungs. Normal blood flow does not occur from the lungs to the left side of the heart. The left side has less blood to pump to the body. As with left-sided heart failure, organs receive less blood. The signs and symptoms occur as described for when the left side fails.

A very severe form of heart failure is *pulmonary edema* (fluid in the lungs). It is an emergency. The person can die.

A damaged or weakened heart usually causes heart failure. CAD, MI, hypertension, age, diabetes, and dysrhythmias (Chapter 21) are common causes. Damaged heart valves and kidney disease are also common causes. Treatment depends on the cause of the heart failure. Drug therapy is common. The goals of therapy are to:
- Reduce signs and symptoms
- Increase exercise tolerance
- Prolong life

Heart failure is treated with a combination of vasodilator, inotropic, and diuretic therapy. If failure is acute, most drugs are given intravenously. Other drugs, such as ACE inhibitors, ARBs, and beta blockers, are also used in treating heart failure.

- **Vasodilators** widen blood vessels. This reduces the heart's workload. Tissues receive more blood and oxygen. Vasodilators also reduce the amount of blood returning to the heart. This decreases lung congestion. The person can breathe more easily.
- **Inotropic** (in oh troh' pik) **agents** stimulate the heart to increase the force of contractions. This increases the amount of blood pumped with each heartbeat. Digitalis glycosides are inotropic agents.
- Diuretics are given to increase sodium and water excretion (Chapter 23). This relieves congestion and the heart's workload.

DRUG CLASS: Digitalis Glycosides

Digitalis glycosides are among the oldest agents used to treat heart failure. The only digitalis glycoside currently available for use in the United States is:
- Digoxin (di joks' in); Lanoxin (lah noks' in)

Digoxin (Lanoxin) increases the force of heart muscle contraction. It also slows the heart rate. The heart can fill and empty more completely. This improves circulation, resulting in reduced swelling in the lungs and tissues. Heart size returns to normal. Edema lessens because of improved circulation to the kidneys.

The drug is used to treat heart failure that does not respond to diuretics, beta blockers, or ACE inhibitors. It is also used to treat dysrhythmias (Chapter 21).

Digitalization is giving a larger dose of digoxin for the first 24 hours. The person is then given a daily dose.

Assisting With the Nursing Process. When giving digoxin (Lanoxin), you assist the nurse with the nursing process.

Assessment
- Observe for dyspnea, chest pain, fatigue, edema, fainting, palpitations (the person may describe palpitations as "my heart skips some beats" or "my heart is racing").
- Measure vital signs: blood pressure, the apical pulse for 1 minute, and respirations.
- Measure daily weight.
- Measure intake and output.

Planning
- Oral dose forms are:
- 0.0625, 0.125, 0.1875 and 0.25 mg tablets

Implementation. The adult digitalizing dose is 0.5 to 0.75 mg. It is followed by 0.125 to 0.375 mg every 6 to 8 hours until adequate digitalization is achieved.
- The maintenance dose is 0.125 to 0.25 mg daily. Some people need 0.375 to 0.5 mg daily.

BOX 22-4   Signs and Symptoms of Digoxin Toxicity

- Bradycardia
- Tachycardia
- Anorexia
- Nausea
- Vomiting
- Diarrhea
- Fatigue: extreme
- Weakness: arm and leg
- Nightmares
- Agitation
- Listlessness
- Hallucinations
- Vision problems: hazy or blurred vision, problems reading, problems seeing red and green

---

- *Measure the apical pulse for 1 minute before giving the drug.* Follow agency policy for withholding the drug. The drug is not usually given if the pulse is less than 60 or greater than 100 beats per minute.
- The drug is given in very small amounts. If you are allowed to do dose calculations, have a nurse check your calculation. If a pharmacist or nurse did the dose calculation, ask another nurse to check the calculation.
- Give the drug after meals to reduce stomach irritation.
  Evaluation. Report and record:
- *Signs and symptoms of digoxin toxicity.* See Box 22-4.
- *Nausea, vomiting, diarrhea, excessive urinary output.* The person is at risk for low serum potassium levels (hypokalemia).

DRUG CLASS: Angiotensin-Converting Enzyme Inhibitors

Angiotensin-converting enzyme (ACE) inhibitors are discussed in Chapter 20. They are useful in the treatment of heart failure because they:
- Prevent vasoconstriction. Blood pressure is reduced.
- Inhibit aldosterone secretion. Blood volume is reduced.

Assisting With the Nursing Process. See Chapter 20.

DRUG CLASS: Angiotensin II Receptor Blockers

Angiotensin II receptor blockers (ARBs) are discussed in Chapter 20. They are useful in the treatment of heart failure because they:
- Block angiotensin II from binding to the receptor sites. This prevents vasoconstriction. Blood pressure is reduced.
- Inhibit aldosterone secretion. The body does not retain excess water.

Assisting With the Nursing Process. See Chapter 20.

DRUG CLASS: Beta-Adrenergic Blocking Agents

Beta-adrenergic blocking agents (beta blockers) are discussed in Chapters 15 and 20. They are useful in the treatment of heart failure because they:
- Lower the heart rate
- Reduce cardiac output
- Lower blood pressure
- Prevent sodium and water retention by blocking renin release

Assisting With the Nursing Process. See Chapter 20.

DRUG CLASS: Miscellaneous Agent

Ivabradine (eye vab' ra deen); Corlanor (cor' la nor)

Corlanor helps people with heart failure stay out of the hospital. It interrupts some of the electrical activity of the heart which helps keep the heart from racing. It helps decrease the heart rate.

Assisting With the Nursing Process. When giving ivabradine (Corlanor), you assist the nurse with the nursing process.
  Assessment
- Observe for dyspnea, chest pain, fatigue, edema, fainting, palpitations (the person may describe palpitations as "my heart skips some beats" or "my heart is racing").
- Measure vital signs: blood pressure, the apical pulse for 1 minute, and respirations.
- Measure daily weight.
- Measure intake and output.
  Planning
- Oral dose forms are 5 and 7.5 mg tablets
  Implementation
- Initially, start with 5 mg twice daily. If the heart rate is already slow, start with 2.5 mg twice daily.
- The maximum dose is 7.5 mg twice daily based on the person's heart rate.
- Take with meals. Avoid grapefruit juice while taking this drug.
  Evaluation. Report and record:
- *Hypotension or hypertension.* Provide for safety. Remind the person to rise slowly from a supine or sitting position. Have the person sit or lie down if feeling faint. Monitor blood pressure regularly and notify the nurse immediately of any changes.
- *Vision changes, halos, colored bright lights.* Provide for safety. These symptoms start within the first 2 months and may suddenly improve during treatment.
- *Dysrhythmias, slow heart rate, or fast heart rate.* These signal a cardiac event. Tell the nurse at once.

REVIEW QUESTIONS

Circle the BEST answer.

1. Nitrates relieve angina by:
   a. dilating the coronary arteries
   b. lowering the heart rate
   c. lowering blood pressure
   d. increasing oxygen use

2. Which is the *most* common side effect from nitrates?
   a. dizziness
   b. flushing
   c. fainting
   d. headache

3. Tell the nurse at once after the person takes:
   a. 1 dose of sublingual nitroglycerin
   b. 2 doses of sublingual nitroglycerin
   c. 3 doses of sublingual nitroglycerin
   d. 4 doses of sublingual nitroglycerin

4. Sustained-released nitroglycerin tablets are taken:
   a. in the morning before breakfast
   b. on an empty stomach every 8 to 12 hours
   c. with meals
   d. at bedtime

5. The application sites for transdermal disks are rotated:
   a. daily
   b. every 8 hours
   c. every other day
   d. weekly

6. A transdermal nitroglycerin disk is dislodged. What should you do?
   a. Remove the disk and apply a new one.
   b. Reapply the disk.
   c. Leave the disk as is until the next ordered dose.
   d. Tape the disk in place.

7. Beta blockers are used to treat angina because they:
   a. dilate coronary arteries
   b. reduce oxygen demands
   c. raise blood pressure
   d. prevent the clumping of platelets

8. Before giving a beta blocker for angina, you need to measure the person's:
   a. weight
   b. intake and output
   c. blood pressure in the supine and standing positions
   d. apical pulse for 30 seconds

9. Calcium channel blockers are used in the treatment of angina. They do all the following, *except*:
   a. decrease myocardial oxygen demand
   b. dilate the coronary arteries
   c. dilate peripheral vessels
   d. prevent the clumping of platelets

10. ACE inhibitors are used to prevent:
    a. CAD
    b. PVD
    c. MI
    d. peripheral vascular disease

11. Before giving a drug for peripheral vascular disease, you should ask the person:
    a. to void
    b. to rate their pain
    c. if you may take the apical pulse for 1 minute
    d. what application site they prefer

12. Besides dilating blood vessels, ACE inhibitors prevent:
    a. peripheral vascular disease
    b. blood clots
    c. atherosclerosis
    d. vasodilation

13. Intermittent claudication occurs with:
    a. deep vein thrombosis
    b. arteriosclerosis obliterans
    c. Raynaud's disease
    d. heart failure

14. Pentoxifylline is used to treat intermittent claudication. The drug:
    a. prevents the clumping of red blood cells and platelets
    b. reduces oxygen needs
    c. dilates blood vessels
    d. constricts blood vessels

15. A person taking pentoxifylline complains of chest pain and shortness of breath. What should you do?
    a. Tell the nurse at once.
    b. Have the person take a nitroglycerin tablet.
    c. Measure blood pressure in the supine and standing positions.
    d. Have the person rest.

16. A platelet aggregation inhibitor prevents:
    a. platelet production
    b. platelets from clumping
    c. the destruction of platelets
    d. platelets from splitting

17. Heart failure can be treated with the following drug classes, *except*:
    a. nitrates
    b. ACE inhibitors
    c. beta blockers
    d. ARBs

18. Digoxin (Lanoxin) is used in the treatment of heart failure. It:
    a. prevents vasoconstriction
    b. promotes sodium excretion
    c. increases the force of heart muscle contraction
    d. decreases blood flow to the kidneys

19. The maintenance dose of digoxin (Lanoxin) is usually:
    a. 0.125 to 0.25 mg daily
    b. 0.25 to 0.5 mg daily
    c. 1.25 to 2.5 mg daily
    d. 2.5 to 5 mg daily

20. ACE inhibitors are used in the treatment of heart failure because they:
    a. reduce blood pressure and blood volume
    b. increase sodium and water retention
    c. lower the heart rate
    d. increase cardiac output

21. Beta blockers are used in the treatment of heart failure. They do all the following, *except*:
    a. reduce blood pressure
    b. increase sodium and water retention
    c. lower the heart rate
    d. reduce cardiac output

22. Ivabradine (Corlanor) does all the following, *except*:
    a. keep people stay out of the hospital
    b. interrupt some of the electrical activity
    c. lower the heart rate
    d. increase the force of heart muscle contraction

Circle T if the statement is true. Circle F if the statement is false.

23. **T   F**   Sublingual nitroglycerin should produce a slight stinging or burning sensation.

24. **T   F**   Sublingual nitroglycerin is stored in a clear container.

25. **T   F**   Sublingual nitroglycerin should be kept within the person's reach.

26. **T   F**   The person can eat, drink, and talk with a transmucosal tablet in place.

27. **T   F**   Translingual nitroglycerin spray is highly flammable.

28. **T   F**   Vasodilators are used to treat peripheral vascular disease.

29. **T   F**   Pentoxifylline should be given with caffeine products.

30. **T   F**   Before giving digoxin (Lanoxin) you need to measure the apical pulse for 1 minute.

31. **T   F**   Diuretics are used in the treatment of heart failure.

Answers to these questions can be found on the Evolve Resources site: http://evolve.elsevier.com/Anderson/medasst/

Drugs Used for Diuresis

OBJECTIVES

- Define the key terms and key abbreviations used in this chapter.
- Describe the drugs that promote diuresis.
- Explain how to assist with the nursing process when giving drugs to promote diuresis.

KEY TERMS

diuresis The increased formation and excretion of urine; *dia* means *through*, *ur* means *urine*

diuretic A drug that promotes the formation and excretion of urine

KEY ABBREVIATIONS

mg Milligram

mL Milliliter

Diuresis is the increased formation and excretion of urine. (*Dia* means *through*. *Ur* means *urine*.) A **diuretic** is a drug that promotes the formation and excretion of urine. Diuretics increase the flow of urine. Their purpose is to increase the loss of water from the body. They do so by increasing the excretion of sodium.

DRUGS USED FOR DIURESIS

Diuretics are used in the treatment of hypertension and heart failure. They may also be used in the treatment of cerebral edema, glaucoma, and liver disease.

See Box 23-1 for a review of the urinary system.

See *Delegation Guidelines: Drugs Used for Diuresis*.

DELEGATION GUIDELINES

Drugs Used for Diuresis

Some drugs used for diuresis are given parenterally—by intramuscular or intravenous injection. Because you do not give parenteral dose forms, they are not included in this chapter. Should a nurse delegate the administration of such to you, you must:

- Remember that parenteral dosages are often very different from dosages for other routes.
- Refuse the delegation but do not ignore the request. Make sure the nurse knows that you cannot give the drug and why.

DRUG CLASS: Loop Diuretics

The *loop of Henle* is the U-shaped part of a renal tubule (see Fig. 23-2). It has a thin descending limb and a thick ascending limb. Loop diuretics inhibit the reabsorption of sodium and chloride from the ascending loop of Henle.

The goals of therapy are to:

- Promote diuresis
- Reduce edema
- Improve symptoms related to excess fluid in tissues

BOX 23-1 The Urinary System: Body Structure and Function

The urinary system (Fig. 23-1):

- Removes waste products from the blood
- Maintains water balance within the body

The *kidneys* are two bean-shaped organs in the upper abdomen. They lie against the back muscles on each side of the spine. They are protected by the lower edge of the rib cage.

Each kidney has over a million tiny *nephrons* (Fig. 23-2). Each nephron is the basic working unit of the kidney. Each nephron has a *convoluted tubule*, which is a tiny coiled tubule. Each convoluted tubule has a *Bowman's capsule* at one end. The capsule partly surrounds a cluster of capillaries called a *glomerulus*. Blood passes through the glomerulus and is filtered by the capillaries. The fluid part of the blood is squeezed into the Bowman's capsule. The fluid then passes into the tubule. Most of the water and other needed substances are reabsorbed by the blood. The rest of the fluid and the waste products form *urine* in the tubule. Urine flows through the tubule to a *collecting tubule*. All collecting tubules drain into the *renal pelvis* in the kidney.

A tube, called the *ureter*, is attached to the renal pelvis of the kidney. Each ureter is about 10 to 12 inches long. The ureters carry urine from the kidneys to the *bladder*. The bladder is a hollow, muscular sac toward the front of the lower part of the abdominal cavity.

Urine is stored in the bladder until the need to urinate is felt. This usually occurs when there is about a half pint (250 mL) of urine in the bladder. Urine passes from the bladder through the *urethra*. The opening at the end of the urethra is the *meatus*. Urine passes from the body through the meatus. Urine is a clear, yellowish fluid.

Assisting With the Nursing Process. When giving loop diuretics, you assist the nurse with the nursing process.

Assessment

- Measure vital signs.
- Measure weight daily.
- Measure intake and output.
- Observe alertness and orientation to person, time, and place.
- Observe for confusion.

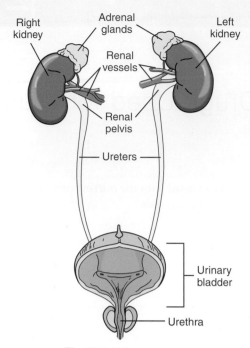

Fig. 23-1 Urinary system.

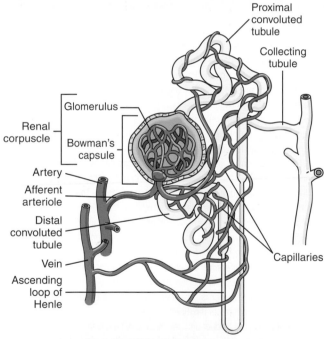

Fig. 23-2 A nephron.

- Observe muscle strength.
- Observe for tremors.
- Ask about muscle cramps.
- Ask about nausea.
- Measure blood glucose if the person has diabetes.
  Planning. See Table 23-1 for "Oral Dose Forms."
  Implementation. See Table 23-1 "Adult Dosage Range."
  Evaluation. Report and record:
- *Oral irritation, dry mouth.* Give oral hygiene as directed by the nurse and the care plan. The nurse may allow the person to suck on ice chips or hard candy.

TABLE 23-1	Loop Diuretics		
Generic Name	**Brand Name**	**Oral Dose Forms**	**Adult Dosage Range**
bumetanide		Tablets: 0.5, 1, 2 mg	0.5-10 mg daily
ethycrynic acid	Edecrin	Tablets: 25 mg	50-200 mg daily
Furosemide	Lasix	Tablets: 20, 40, 80 mg
Oral solution: 8, 10 mg/mL	20-600 mg daily
torsemide	Demadex	Tablets: 5, 10, 20, and 100 mg	5-200 mg daily

Modified from Willihnganz M: Clayton's Basic Pharmacology for Nurses, ed 18, St Louis, 2020, Elsevier.

- *Orthostatic hypotension, dizziness, weakness, fainting.* Blood pressure is measured daily in the supine and standing positions. Provide for safety. Remind the person to rise slowly from a supine or sitting position. Have the person sit or lie down if feeling faint.
- *Stomach irritation, abdominal pain.* Give the drug with food or milk.
- *Changes in alertness and orientation to person, time, and place; confusion; muscle cramps; nausea; diarrhea.* These may signal dehydration or electrolyte imbalance (potassium, sodium, and chloride).
- *"Coffee ground" vomitus; dark, tarry stools.* These signal gastrointestinal bleeding.
- *Deafness, tinnitus, changes in hearing and balance.* These may signal impaired kidney function.
- *Hyperglycemia.* This may occur in persons with diabetes or persons at risk for diabetes.
- *Hives, rash, itching.* These may signal an allergic reaction. Tell the nurse at once. Do not give the next dose unless approved by the nurse.

DRUG CLASS: Thiazide Diuretics

Thiazide diuretics act on the distal tubules to block the reabsorption of sodium and chloride. The sodium and chloride that are not reabsorbed take water with them. This results in diuresis.

Thiazides are used in the treatment of edema due to:
- Heart failure
- Kidney disease
- Liver disease
- Pregnancy
- Obesity
- Premenstrual syndrome
- The administration of corticosteroids (Chapter 29)

Thiazides also have antihypertensive effects. They cause vasodilation of peripheral arterioles.

The goals of therapy are to:
- Promote diuresis
- Reduce edema
- Improve symptoms related to excess fluid in tissues
- Reduce blood pressure

Assisting With the Nursing Process. When giving thiazides, you assist the nurse with the nursing process.

Assessment
- Measure vital signs.
- Measure weight daily.
- Measure intake and output.
- Observe alertness and orientation to person, time, and place.
- Observe for confusion.
- Observe muscle strength.
- Observe for tremors.
- Ask about muscle cramps.
- Ask about nausea.
- Measure blood glucose if the person has diabetes.
- Observe for signs of hearing loss.
  Planning. See Tables 23-2 and 23-3 for "Oral Dose Forms."
  Implementation. See Tables 23-2 and 23-3 for "Adult Dosage Range."
- Give the drug before midafternoon. This prevents nocturia.
- For hypertension, most of the diuretics listed are given in divided doses.
- For edema, most of the diuretics listed are given in single daily doses.
  Evaluation. Report and record:
- *Oral irritation, dry mouth.* Give oral hygiene as directed by the nurse and the care plan. The nurse may allow the person to suck on ice chips or hard candy.
- *Orthostatic hypotension, dizziness, weakness, fainting.* Blood pressure is measured daily in the supine and standing positions. Provide for safety. Remind the person to rise slowly from a supine or sitting position. Have the person sit or lie down if feeling faint.

TABLE 23-2   Thiazide Diuretics

Generic Name	Brand Name	Oral Dose Forms	Adult Dosage Range
Chlorothiazide	Diuril	Tablets: 250, 500 mg Oral suspension: 250 mg/5 mL	500-1000 mg once or twice daily
Hydrochlorothiazide		Tablets: 12.5, 25, 50 mg Capsules: 12.5 mg	12.5-200 mg daily

Modified from Willihnganz M: Clayton's Basic Pharmacology for Nurses, ed 18, St Louis, 2020, Elsevier.

TABLE 23-3   Thiazide-Related Diuretics

Generic Name	Brand Name	Oral Dose Forms	Adult Dosage Range
Chlorthalidone		Tablets: 25, 50 mg	50-200 mg daily
Indapamide		Tablets: 1.25, 2.5 mg	1.25-5 mg daily
Metolazone	Zaroxolyn	Tablets: 2.5, 5, 10 mg	2.5-20 mg daily

Modified from Willihnganz M: Clayton's Basic Pharmacology for Nurses, ed 18, St Louis, 2020, Elsevier.

- *Stomach irritation, nausea, vomiting, constipation.* Give the drug with food or milk if stomach irritation occurs.
- *Changes in alertness and orientation to person, time, and place; confusion; muscle cramps; nausea.* These may signal dehydration or electrolyte imbalance (potassium, sodium, and chloride).
- *Hyperglycemia.* This may occur in persons with diabetes or persons at risk for diabetes.
- *Hives, rash, itching.* These may signal an allergic reaction. Tell the nurse at once. Do not give the next dose unless approved by the nurse.

DRUG CLASS: Potassium-Sparing Diuretics

Potassium-sparing diuretics excrete sodium but retain potassium. The following are potassium-sparing diuretics:
- Amiloride (ah mihl' or eyd); Midamor (my' da mor)
- Spironolactone (spy ro no lak' tone); Aldactone (al dak' tone)
- Triamterene (try am' ter een); Dyrenium (dy reen' ee um)

Amiloride (Midamor). Amiloride (Midamor) acts on the distal renal tubule to retain potassium and excrete sodium. Diuresis is mild. The drug has weak antihypertensive effects.

The drug is used with other diuretics to treat hypertension or heart failure. The goals of therapy are to:
- Reduce edema
- Improve symptoms related to excess fluid in tissues

Assisting With the Nursing Process. When giving amiloride (Midamor), you assist the nurse with the nursing process.
  Assessment
- Measure vital signs.
- Measure weight daily.
- Measure intake and output.
- Observe alertness and orientation to person, time, and place.
- Observe for confusion.
- Observe muscle strength.
- Observe for tremors.
- Ask about muscle cramps.
- Ask about nausea.
  Planning
- The oral dose form is 5 mg tablets.
  Implementation
- The initial adult dose is 5 mg daily.
- Dosages may be increased by 5 mg to achieve a maximum daily dose of 20 mg.
- Give the drug with food or milk to reduce stomachirritation.
- Give the drug before midafternoon. This prevents nocturia.
  Evaluation. Report and record:
- *Anorexia, nausea, vomiting, flatulence.* These should be mild if the drug is given with food.
- *Headache.* Measure blood pressure.
- *Changes in alertness and orientation to person, time, and place; confusion; muscle cramps; nausea.* These may signal dehydration or electrolyte imbalance (potassium, sodium, and chloride).

Spironolactone (Aldactone)

Spironolactone (Aldactone) blocks the sodium-retaining properties of aldosterone. It blocks potassium and magnesium excretion caused by aldosterone. Sodium and water are excreted.

The drug is useful in relieving edema and ascites that do not respond to the usual diuretics. The drug may be given with other diuretics. The goals of therapy are to:
- Reduce edema
- Improve symptoms related to excess fluid in tissues
- Improve symptoms from heart failure

Assisting With the Nursing Process. When giving spironolactone (Aldactone), you assist the nurse with the nursing process.
    Assessment
- Measure vital signs.
- Measure weight daily.
- Measure intake and output.
- Observe alertness and orientation to person, time, and place.
- Observe for confusion.
- Observe muscle strength.
- Observe for tremors.
- Ask about muscle cramps.
- Ask about nausea.
    Planning
- Oral dose forms are:
    - 25, 50, and 100 mg tablets.
    - 25 mg/5 mL in 118 and 473 mL bottles of oral suspension.
    Implementation
- The initial adult dose is 100 mg daily.
- The maintenance dose is usually 25 to 200 mg daily. Some persons need up to 400 mg daily.
- Give the drug with food or milk to reduce stomach irritation.
- Give the drug before midafternoon. This prevents nocturia.
    Evaluation. Report and record:
- *Headache.* Measure blood pressure.
- *Diarrhea.* Note the number and consistency of stools.
- *Changes in alertness and orientation to person, time, and place; confusion; muscle cramps; nausea.* These may signal dehydration or electrolyte imbalance (potassium, sodium, and chloride).
- *Breasts may enlarge in men; breast tenderness and menstrual irregularities may occur in women.* These reverse when therapy is discontinued.

Triamterene (Dyrenium)

Triamterene (Dyrenium) is a mild diuretic. It blocks the exchange of potassium for sodium in the distal tubules. Potassium is retained while sodium and water are excreted through the urine.

The drug is used with potassium-excreting diuretics (thiazides and loop diuretics). The goals of therapy are to:
- Cause diuresis
- Improve symptoms related to excess fluid in tissues

Assisting With the Nursing Process. When giving triamterene (Dyrenium), you assist the nurse with the nursing process.
    Assessment
- Measure vital signs.
- Measure weight daily.
- Measure intake and output.
- Observe alertness and orientation to person, time, and place.
- Observe for confusion.
- Observe muscle strength.
- Observe for tremors.
- Ask about muscle cramps.
- Ask about nausea.
    Planning
- The oral dose forms are 50 and 100 mg tablets.
    Implementation
- The adult dose is 100 to 300 mg one or two times a day.
- Maximum dose is 300 mg daily.
    Evaluation. Report and record:
- *Changes in alertness and orientation to person, time, and place; confusion; muscle cramps; nausea; vomiting.* These may signal dehydration or electrolyte imbalance (potassium, sodium, and chloride).
- *Hives, rash, itching.* These may signal an allergic reaction. Tell the nurse at once. Do not give the next dose unless approved by the nurse.

DRUG CLASS: Combination Diuretic Products

Low potassium (hypokalemia) is a common problem with thiazide diuretics. Several products contain a potassium-sparing diuretic with a thiazide diuretic (Table 23-4). The goal is to promote diuresis and antihypertensive effects while maintaining normal potassium levels.

Persons receiving a combination product are at risk for side effects from each of the drugs in the product. High potassium and low sodium levels have been reported.

TABLE 23-4   Combination Diuretics

Generic Name	Brand Name	Adult Dosage Range
spironolactone 25 mg, hydrochlorothiazide 25 mg	Aldactazide	1-8 tablets daily
spironolactone 50 mg, hydrochlorothiazide 50 mg	Aldactazide	1-4 tablets daily
triamterene 37.5 mg, hydrochlorothiazide 25 mg	Dyazide	1 or 2 capsules once daily
triamterene 37.5 mg, hydrochlorothiazide 25 mg	Maxzide-25	1 or 2 capsules once daily
triamterene 50 mg, hydrochlorothiazide 55 mg	-	1 or 2 capsules once daily
triamterene 75 mg, hydrochlorothiazide 50 mg	Maxzide	1 tablet daily
amiloride 5 mg, hydrochlorothiazide 50 mg		1 or 2 tablets daily with meals

Modified from Willihnganz M: Clayton's Basic Pharmacology for Nurses, ed 18, St Louis, 2020, Elsevier.

REVIEW QUESTIONS

Circle the BEST answer.

1. Diuretics increase water loss from the body by:
   a. increasing sodium excretion
   b. increasing sodium retention
   c. decreasing potassium excretion
   d. increasing potassium retention

2. Ascites occurs from:
   a. kidney disease
   b. liver disease
   c. cerebral edema
   d. hypertension

3. Loop diuretics inhibit the reabsorption of:
   a. sodium
   b. potassium
   c. aldosterone
   d. renin

4. Which is *not* a loop diuretic?
   a. furosemide (Lasix)
   b. ethacrynic acid (Edecrin)
   c. bumetanide
   d. chlorthalidone

5. Which is *not* a thiazide or thiazide-related diuretic?
   a. chlorothiazide (Diuril)
   b. hydrochlorothiazide
   c. metolazone (Zaroxolyn)
   d. spironolactone (Aldactone)

6. The effects of loop diuretics last about:
   a. 30 minutes
   b. 1 hour
   c. 4 hours
   d. 6 hours

7. Which diuretics are used in the treatment of obesity, pregnancy, and premenstrual syndrome?
   a. loop diuretics
   b. thiazide diuretics
   c. potassium-sparing diuretics
   d. combination diuretic products

8. Diuretics are given:
   a. at 0500
   b. before lunch
   c. before midafternoon
   d. at bedtime

9. Which may signal dehydration and electrolyte imbalance from diuretics?
   a. stomach irritation
   b. changes in alertness and confusion
   c. dry mouth
   d. orthostatic hypotension

10. Potassium-sparing diuretics:
    a. retain potassium
    b. excrete potassium
    c. retain sodium
    d. excrete aldosterone

11. Which is *not* a potassium-sparing diuretic?
    a. amiloride (Midamor)
    b. spironolactone (Aldactone)
    c. triamterene (Dyrenium)
    d. spironolactone, hydrochlorothiazide (Aldactazide)

12. Which is a combination diuretic?
    a. Dyazide
    b. Dyrenium
    c. Aldactone
    d. Edecrin

Answers to these questions can be found on the Evolve Resources site: http://evolve.elsevier.com/Anderson/medasst/

24

Drugs Used to Treat Thromboembolic Diseases

OBJECTIVES

- Define the key terms and key abbreviations listed in this chapter.
- Describe thromboembolic diseases.
- Describe the drugs used to treat thromboembolic diseases.
- Explain how to assist with the nursing process when giving drugs to treat thromboembolic diseases.

KEY TERMS

anticoagulants Drugs that prevent arterial and venous thrombi; "blood thinners"

embolus A small part of a thrombus that breaks off and travels through the vascular system until it lodges in a blood vessel

infarction A local area of tissue death

ischemia A decreased supply of oxygenated blood to a body part

platelet inhibitors Drugs that prevent platelet aggregation (clumping)

thrombosis The process of clot formation

thromboembolic diseases Diseases associated with abnormal clotting within blood vessels

thrombus A blood clot

KEY ABBREVIATIONS

DVT	Deep vein thrombosis
GI	Gastrointestinal
IV	Intravenous
mg	Milligram

MI	Myocardial infarction
PE	Pulmonary embolism
TED hose	Thromboembolic disease hose
TIA	Transient ischemic attack

Thrombosis is the process of clot formation. A **thrombus** is a blood clot (Fig. 24-1, *A*). An **embolus** is a small part of a thrombus that breaks off and travels through the vascular system until it lodges in a blood vessel (Fig. 24-1, *B*). Pulmonary embolism (PE) and cerebral embolism are examples. An embolus causes ischemia or infarction to the area below the obstruction:

- **Ischemia** is a decreased supply of oxygenated blood to a body part. The person has pain. Involved organs and tissues cannot function properly.
- **Infarction** is a local area of tissue death (Fig. 24-2).

Diseases associated with abnormal clotting within blood vessels are known as **thromboembolic diseases**. Major causes of thrombosis are:

- Immobility with venous stasis (slowed blood flow through a vein)
- Surgery and the postoperative period
- Leg trauma
- Heart failure
- Vasospasm
- Cancer—lung, prostate, stomach, and pancreas
- Pregnancy
- Contraceptive agents (Chapter 30)
- Heredity

Diseases caused by clotting within blood vessels are major causes of death. They include:

- Deep vein thrombosis (DVT)
- Myocardial infarction (MI)
- Dysrhythmias with clot formation

- Coronary artery spasm leading to clot formation
- See Box 24-1 for the methods used to treat thromboembolic disease.

See *Delegation Guidelines: Drugs Used to Treat Thromboembolic Disorders.*

DRUG THERAPY FOR THROMBOEMBOLIC DISEASES

The goals of drug therapy are to:

- Stop the formation of clots in the veins and arteries
- Dissolve clots that have already formed

Drugs used to dissolve clots are given parenterally and are not given by MA-Cs and are not discussed in this chapter.

DELEGATION GUIDELINES

Drugs Used to Treat Thromboembolic Disorders

Some drugs used to treat thromboembolic disorders are given parenterally—by subcutaneous or intravenous injection. Because you do not give parenteral dose forms, they are not included in this chapter. Should a nurse delegate the administration of such to you, you must:

- Remember that parenteral dosages are often very different from dosages for other routes.
- Refuse the delegation but do not ignore the request. Make sure the nurse knows that you cannot give the drug and why.

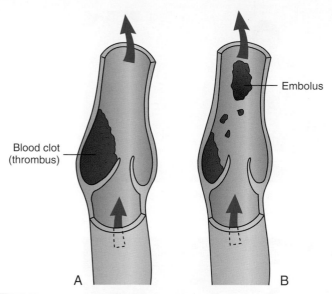

Fig. 24-1 **A,** A blood clot is attached to the wall of a vein. The arrow shows the direction of blood flow. **B,** Part of the thrombus breaks off and becomes an embolus. The embolus travels in the bloodstream until it lodges in a distant vessel.

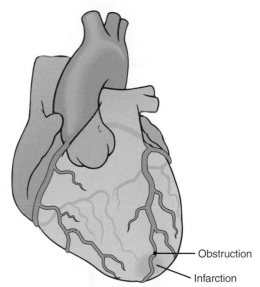

Fig. 24-2 Myocardial infarction. (Modified from Lewis SM and others: *Medical-surgical nursing: assessment and management of clinical problems,* ed 10, St Louis, 2017, Mosby.)

DRUG CLASS: Platelet Inhibitors

Platelet inhibitors prevent platelet aggregation (clumping). They are used to reduce arterial clot formation. The following are platelet inhibitors:
- Aspirin (as' per in)
- Clopidogrel (clo pid' oh grel); Plavix (plah' vix)
- Prasugrel (pra' su grel); Effient (ef' ee ent)
- Ticagrelor (tye ka' gre lor); Brilinta (bri lin' ta)

Aspirin

Aspirin is used to relieve pain, fever, and inflammation (Chapter 18). It also inhibits platelet clumping and prolongs bleeding time. The

---

BOX 24-1 Treatment of Thromboembolic Diseases

Prevention
- Leg exercises (Fig. 24-3).
- Leg elevation.
- Early ambulation after surgery.
- Turning and repositioning at least every 2 hours.
- No standing or sitting for prolonged periods.
- Thromboembolic disease hose (TED hose). See Fig. 24-4.
- Sequential compression device (Fig. 24-5). This device is wrapped around the leg and is secured in place with Velcro. The device is attached to a pump. The pump inflates the device with air, promoting venous blood flow to the heart by causing pressure on the veins. The pump then deflates the device. After deflation, the device is inflated again. The inflation-to-deflation sequence is repeated as ordered by the doctor.

Procedures to Reopen the Blood Vessel
- Thrombolytic agents. *Thrombo* means *clot. Lytic* means *to produce decomposition.* Thrombolytic agents are used to dissolve the clot.
- Angioplasty. *Angio* means *blood vessel. Plasty* means *to mold.* A balloon-tipped catheter is inserted into a coronary artery. The balloon is repeatedly inflated and deflated to stretch and open the artery.
- Stents. A *stent* is a wire-mesh tube inserted after angioplasty. It is placed to keep obstructed areas open. The stent stays in the artery.
- Coronary artery bypass graft (Fig. 24-6). A leg vein or an artery from the chest is used to bypass the obstructed area (commonly known as "bypass surgery").

Drug Therapy
- Platelet inhibitors.
- Factor Xa inhibitors.
- Anticoagulants.
- Thrombin inhibitors.

---

platelet loses its ability to clump and form clots for the duration of its lifetime. Platelets live 7 to 10 days.

Aspirin is used to reduce the risk of MI in persons with a previous MI or persons who have angina (Chapter 22). It also is used to reduce the risk of recurrent transient ischemic attacks and stroke caused by blood clots.
- *Transient ischemic attack (TIA). Transient* means temporary or short-term. *Ischemic* means to hold back *(ischein)* blood *(hemic).* Blood supply to the brain is interrupted for a short time. A TIA may sometimes occur before a stroke.
- *Stroke.* Stroke is a disease that affects the arteries that supply blood to the brain. It occurs when a blood clot blocks blood flow to the brain. Another cause is when a blood vessel in the brain bursts. Bleeding occurs in the brain (cerebral hemorrhage) and brain cells in the affected area do not get enough oxygen and nutrients. Brain cells die, brain damage occurs, and functions controlled by that part of the brain are lost.

The goals of therapy are to:
- Reduce the frequency of TIA
- Reduce the frequency of stroke
- Reduce the frequency of MI

Assisting With the Nursing Process. When giving aspirin, you assist the nurse with the nursing process.

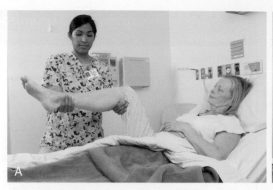
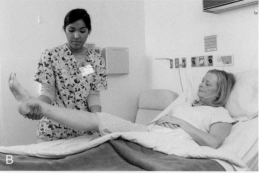

Fig. 24-3 Leg exercises to stimulate circulation. **A,** The knee is flexed and then extended. **B,** The leg is raised and lowered.

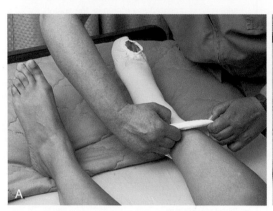
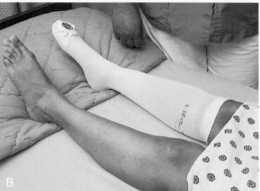

Fig. 24-4 Applying TED hose. **A,** The stocking is slipped over the toes, foot, and heel. **B,** The stocking turns right side out as it is pulled up over the leg.

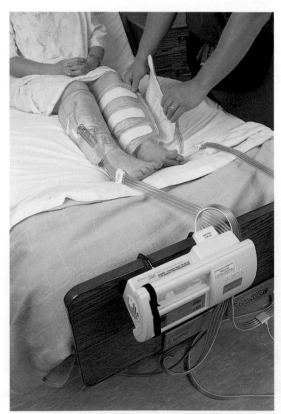

Fig. 24-5 Sequential compression device. (From deWit SC: *Fundamental concepts and skills for nursing*, ed 5, Philadelphia, 2014, Saunders.)

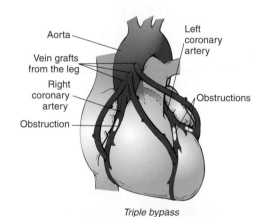

Triple bypass

Fig. 24-6 Coronary artery bypass graft. (Modified from Thibodeau GA, Patton KT: *The human body in health and disease*, ed 6, St Louis, 2014, Mosby.)

Assessment

- Observe alertness and orientation to person, time, and place.
- Observe the person's balance.
- Observe the person's hearing.
- Observe hand strength.
- Test stools for occult blood.
- Ask about gastrointestinal (GI) symptoms.
  Planning. See Table 18-2 (Chapter 18).
  Implementation
- To prevent blood clots, the oral adult dose is usually 81 to 325 mg daily.

- Larger doses may be given. They are usually divided into 325 mg in two, three, or four doses daily.
- The dose depends on the person's history of clot formation and other drugs the person is taking.
- Give the drug with meals to prevent stomach irritation.
  Evaluation. See Chapter 18.

Clopidogrel (Plavix)

Clopidogrel (Plavix) helps prevent harmful blood clots. It is used to prevent strokes and MIs in persons at risk for such problems.

Assisting With the Nursing Process. When giving clopidogrel (Plavix), you assist the nurse with the nursing process.
  Assessment
- Measure vital signs.
- Ask about gastrointestinal (GI) symptoms.
  Planning
- The oral dose forms are 75 and 300 mg tablets.
  Implementation
- The initial adult dose for MIs, angioplasty, or stents is 600 mg once a day.
- The maintenance dose is 75 mg once a day.
- The drug is given with food or on an empty stomach.
  Evaluation. Report and record:
- *Nausea, vomiting, anorexia, diarrhea.* These tend to occur with early doses and resolve with continued therapy over the next 2 weeks. Give the drug with food.
- *Sore throat, fever, fatigue.* These may signal changes in white blood cells.
- *Bleeding.* This includes nosebleeds, easy bruising, bright red or "coffee ground" emesis, blood in the urine (hematuria), dark tarry stools.

Prasugrel (Effient)

Prasugrel (Effient) is similar to clopidogrel, except it starts working faster.

Assisting With the Nursing Process. When giving prasugrel (Effient), you assist the nurse with the nursing process.
  Assessment. Measure vital signs.
  Planning
- The oral dose forms are 5 and 10 mg tablets.
  Implementation
- The initial adult dose is 60 mg.
- The maintenance dose is 10 mg once a day. If the person weighs less than 60 kg, 5 mg is recommended.
- Aspirin therapy should be continued when taking this drug.
  Evaluation. Report and record:
- *Bleeding.* This includes nosebleeds, easy bruising, bright red or "coffee ground" emesis, blood in the urine (hematuria), dark tarry stools.

Ticagrelor (Brilinta)

Ticagrelor (Brilinta) reduces the rate of cardiovascular death, MI, and stroke in people with heart disease. It also reduces the rate of clot formation in stents.

Assisting With the Nursing Process. When giving ticagrelor (Brilinta), you assist the nurse with the nursing process.
  Assessment
- Measure vital signs.
  Planning
- The oral dose forms are 60 and 90 mg tablets.
  Implementation
- The initial adult dose is 180 mg of ticagrelor with 325 mg of aspirin, followed by 90 mg ticagrelor with 75 to 100 mg aspirin daily for 1 year.
- After 1 year, ticagrelor 60 mg twice a day with 75 to 100 mg of aspirin.
- The drug is given with meals.
  Evaluation. Report and record:
- *Difficulty breathing.* This tends to resolve with continued therapy.
- *Bleeding.* This includes nosebleeds, easy bruising, bright red or "coffee ground" emesis, blood in urine (hematuria), dark tarry stools.

DRUG CLASS: Factor Xa Inhibitors

Factor Xa inhibitors prevent the formation of thromboemboli in people with certain dysrhythmias (Chapter 21). They are also used for the treatment of DVTs and PEs.

Assisting With the Nursing Process. When giving factor Xa inhibitors, you assist the nurse with the nursing process.
  Assessment
- Measure vital signs.
- Check for bleeding. This includes nosebleeds, bleeding gums, bruises, bright red or "coffee ground" emesis, blood in urine (hematuria), dark tarry stools.
  Planning. See Table 24-1 for "Oral Dose Forms."
  Implementation. See Table 24-1 for "Adult Dosage Range."
  Evaluation. Report and record:
- *Bleeding.* This includes nosebleeds, easy bruising, bright red or "coffee ground" emesis, blood in urine (hematuria), dark tarry stools.

DRUG CLASS: Anticoagulants

Anticoagulants are used to prevent arterial and venous thrombi. They are often called "blood thinners." The intent is to prevent blood clots from forming or growing larger. They cannot dissolve an existing clot.

Common anticoagulant drugs are:
- Heparin (hep' ahr in). *Heparin is only given subcutaneously and intravenously (IV). You do not give subcutaneous or IV drugs.*
- Warfarin (war' fah rin); Coumadin (koo' mah din).

Warfarin (Coumadin)

Warfarin (Coumadin) is a very strong anticoagulant. It inhibits the activity of vitamin K, which is needed for blood clotting. The drug is used to prevent:
- Venous thrombosis
- Embolism associated with atrial fibrillation
- Embolism associated with heart valve replacement
- Pulmonary embolism
- MI

TABLE 24-1	**Factor Xa Inhibitors**		
Generic Name	**Brand Name**	**Oral Dose Forms**	**Adult Dosage Range**
apixaban	Eliquis	Tablets: 2.5, 5 mg	*DVT and PE:* *Treatment:* 10 mg twice daily for 7 days followed by 5 mg twice daily *Reduction in the risk of recurrence:* 2.5 mg twice daily after at least 6 months of treatment for DVT or PE Dysrhythmias with clot formation *(to prevent stroke and systemic embolism):* 5 mg twice daily unless patient has any two of the following: Age ≥80 years, body weight ≤60 kg, or kidney dysfunction; then reduce dose to 2.5 mg twice daily *Prophylaxis of DVT and PE:* *Hip replacement surgery:* 2.5 mg twice daily beginning 12-24 hours postoperatively; duration: 35 days *Knee replacement surgery:* 2.5 mg twice daily beginning 12-24 hours postoperatively; duration: 12 days
betrixaban	Bevyxxa	Capsules: 40, 80 mg	Initially 160 mg, followed by 80 mg once daily, taken with food for 35-42 days
edoxaban	Savaysa	Tablets: 15, 30, 60 mg	*Treatment for DVT and PE:* 60 mg once daily after 5-10 days of initial therapy with a parenteral anticoagulant Dysrhythmias with clot formation *(to prevent stroke and systemic embolism):* 60 mg once daily
rivaroxaban	Xarelto	Tablets: 10, 15, 20 mg	*DVT and PE:* *Treatment:* 15 mg twice daily with food for the first 21 days *Reduction in the risk of recurrence:* 10 mg orally once daily with or without food, after at least 6 months of standard anticoagulant therapy Dysrhythmias with clot formation *(to prevent stroke and systemic embolism):* 20 mg once daily with the evening meal *Prophylaxis of DVT and PE:* *Hip replacement surgery:* 10 mg once daily beginning at least 6-10 hours after surgery; total duration of therapy: 35 days *Knee replacement surgery:* 10 mg once daily beginning at least 6-10 hours after surgery; recommended total duration of therapy: 12 days

Modified from Willihnganz M: Clayton's Basic Pharmacology for Nurses, ed 18, St Louis, 2020, Elsevier.

Assisting With the Nursing Process. When giving warfarin (Coumadin), you assist the nurse with the nursing process.

Assessment
- Measure vital signs.
- Check for bleeding. This includes nosebleeds, bleeding gums, bruises, bright red or "coffee ground" emesis, blood in urine (hematuria), dark tarry stools.
- Ask about GI symptoms.

Planning
- The oral dose forms are 1, 2, 2.5, 3, 4, 5, 6, 7.5, and 10 mg tablets.

Implementation
- Give the dose only if the nurse instructs you to do so. The nurse checks laboratory prothrombin times before the drug is given.
- The oral dose is usually 2 to 5 mg daily. The dosage is adjusted every few days.
- The maintenance dose is usually 2 to 10 mg daily.

Evaluation. Report and record:
- *Bleeding.* This includes nosebleeds, bleeding gums, easy bruising, bright red or "coffee ground" emesis, blood in urine (hematuria), dark tarry stools.
- *Low blood pressure; rapid pulse; cold, clammy skin; faintness; changes in alertness.* These may signal internal bleeding.

DRUG CLASS: Thrombin Inhibitors

Thrombin inhibitors block certain clotting factors from forming a thrombus (blood clot).

One thrombin inhibitor drug is:
- Dabigatran (da big' a tran); Pradaxa (pra dak' sa)

Assisting With the Nursing Process. When giving dabigatran (Pradaxa), you assist the nurse with the nursing process.

Assessment
- Measure blood pressure while laying and sitting.
- Check bowel elimination patters and ask about GI symptoms.

Planning
- The oral dose forms are 75, 110, and 150 mg tablets.

Implementation
- The dosage depends on what the drug is being used to treat. For some dysrhythmias, thromboses, and emboli, the initial dosage is 150 mg two times daily.
- Give 110 mg 1 to 4 hours after hip surgery. Maintenance dose is 220 mg once daily for 28 to 35 days.
- After knee surgery, 150 or 220 mg is given daily for 10 to 35 days. A half-dose is given 1 to 4 hours after surgery.

- Capsules are sensitive to moisture, and the bottle must be resealed quickly after taking a capsule out. Capsule must be swallowed whole with a full glass of water. Do not open or crush the capsule. A severe overdose can occur.

Evaluation. Report and record:
- *Bleeding.* This includes nosebleeds, easy bruising, bright red or "coffee ground" emesis, blood in urine (hematuria), dark tarry stools.

REVIEW QUESTIONS

Circle the BEST answer.

1. A blood clot is called:
   a. ischemia
   b. an embolus
   c. thrombosis
   d. a thrombus
2. A part of a blood clot breaks off and travels in the vascular system. This is called:
   a. ischemia
   b. an embolus
   c. thrombosis
   d. a thrombus
3. Which drug is not a platelet inhibitor?
   a. Coumadin
   b. aspirin
   c. Effient
   d. Plavix
4. Aspirin is used to reduce the frequency of the following, *except*:
   a. TIA
   b. MI
   c. stroke
   d. dysrhythmias
5. Aspirin is given:
   a. before meals
   b. with meals
   c. after meals
   d. at bedtime
6. Clopidogrel (Plavix) is given to prevent:
   a. stroke and MI
   b. angina
   c. dysrhythmias
   d. heart failure
7. The adult dose of clopidogrel (Plavix) is:
   a. 75 mg
   b. 80 mg
   c. 100 mg
   d. 250 mg
8. Which drug reduces the rate of clot formation in stents?
   a. rivaroxaban (Xarelto)
   b. ticagrelor (Brilinta)
   c. clopidogrel (Plavix)
   d. dabigatran (Pradaxa)

9. Which drug is not a factor Xa inhibitor?
   a. aspirin
   b. apixaban (Eliquis)
   c. edoxaban (Savaysa)
   d. betrixaban (Bevyxxa)
10. Anticoagulant drugs:
    a. dissolve clots
    b. destroy clots
    c. prevent new clots
    d. prevent dysrhythmias
11. Coumadin inhibits:
    a. red blood cell formation
    b. vitamin K activity
    c. vitamin C activity
    d. platelet formation
12. Which drug class is Pradaxa?
    a. anticoagulant
    b. factor Xa inhibitor
    c. thrombin inhibitor
    d. platelet inhibitor

Circle T if the statement is true. Circle F if the statement is false.

13. T F You need to observe for bleeding when a person is receiving aspirin.
14. T F You need to observe for bleeding when a person is receiving clopidogrel (Plavix).
15. T F Clopidogrel (Plavix) is given with food or on an empty stomach.
16. T F Anticoagulants are often called "blood thinners."
17. T F You can give heparin.
18. T F The nurse tells you when to give warfarin (Coumadin).
19. T F A person on warfarin (Coumadin) has high blood pressure. This is a sign of internal bleeding.
20. T F For a person taking dabigatran (Pradaxa), you must close the bottle quickly after removing the drug.

Answers to these questions can be found on the Evolve Resources site: http://evolve.elsevier.com/Anderson/medasst/

25

Drugs Used to Treat Respiratory Diseases

OBJECTIVES

- Define the key terms and key abbreviations used in this chapter.
- Describe the common respiratory diseases.
- Describe the drugs used to treat upper respiratory diseases.
- Explain how to assist with the nursing process when giving drugs to treat upper respiratory diseases.
- Describe the drugs used to treat lower respiratory diseases.
- Explain how to assist with the nursing process when giving drugs to treat lower respiratory diseases.

KEY TERMS

antihistamines Drugs that compete with released histamine for receptor sites in the arterioles, capillaries, and glands in mucous membranes

antitussives Drugs that suppress the cough center in the brain; cough suppressants

bronchodilators Drugs that relax the smooth muscles of the tracheobronchial tree

cough suppressants See "antitussives"

decongestants Drugs that cause vasoconstriction of the nasal mucosa

expectorants Drugs that liquefy mucus to promote the ejection of mucus from the lungs and tracheobronchial tree

histamine A substance released in response to allergic reactions and tissue damage from trauma or infection

intranasal Within *(intra)* the nose *(nasal)*

mucolytic agents Drugs that reduce the stickiness and thickness of pulmonary secretions

rhinitis medicamentosa Drug-induced congestion

rhinorrhea Nasal discharge (*rhino* means *nose*; *rrhea* means *discharge*); runny nose

tracheobronchial tree The trachea, bronchi, and bronchioles

KEY ABBREVIATIONS

cAMP   cyclic adenosine monophosphate
CO_2 Carbon dioxide
COPD   Chronic obstructive pulmonary disease
g   Gram
GI   Gastrointestinal
h   Hour
kg   Kilogram

mcg   Microgram
mg   Milligram
mL   Milliliter
O_2 Oxygen
PDE-4   Phosphodiesterase-4
PO   Per os (orally)
q   Every

The respiratory system is a series of airways that start with the nose and mouth and end at the alveoli in the lungs (Fig. 25-1). The respiratory system is divided into the:

- Upper respiratory tract—the nose, sinuses, nasopharynx, pharynx, tonsils, eustachian tubes, and larynx (Fig. 25-2).
- Lower respiratory tract—larynx, trachea, bronchi, bronchioles, and alveoli (Fig. 25-3). The tracheobronchial tree is made up of the trachea, bronchi, and bronchioles.
- See Box 25-1 for common respiratory disorders.

See *Delegation Guidelines: Drugs Used to Treat Respiratory Diseases.*

DELEGATION GUIDELINES

Drugs Used to Treat Respiratory Diseases

Some drugs used to treat respiratory diseases are given parenterally—by subcutaneous, intramuscular, or intravenous injection. Because you do not give parenteral dose forms, they are not included in this chapter. Should a nurse delegate the administration of such to you, you must:

- Remember that parenteral dosages are often very different from dosages for other routes.
- Refuse the delegation but do not ignore the request. Make sure the nurse knows that you cannot give the drug and why.

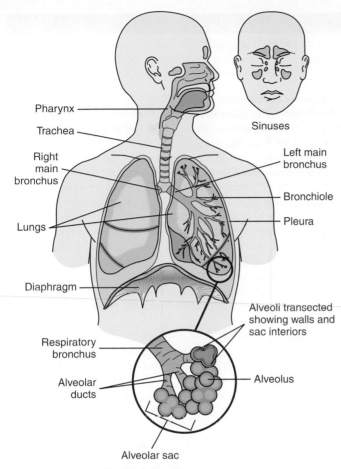

Fig. 25-1 Respiratory system.

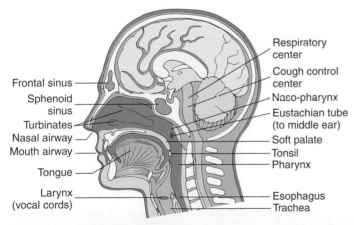

Fig. 25-2 The upper respiratory tract.

DRUG THERAPY FOR UPPER RESPIRATORY DISEASES

Antihistamines are the drugs of choice for allergic rhinitis. They are given orally and distributed throughout the body. They reduce the symptoms of nasal itching, sneezing, rhinorrhea, tearing, and itchy eyes. Antihistamines do not reduce nasal congestion.

Decongestants cause vasoconstriction of the nasal mucosa. This greatly reduces nasal congestion.

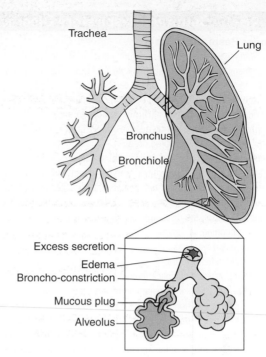

Fig. 25-3 Lower respiratory tract. Mucous plug formed in alveoli.

Antiinflammatory agents are used to treat nasal symptoms caused by mild to moderate allergic rhinitis. They are not used to treat cold symptoms. Cold symptoms start to resolve before the antiinflammatory agents become effective.

DRUG CLASS: Sympathomimetic Decongestants

Sympathomimetic nasal decongestants stimulate the alpha-adrenergic receptors of the nasal mucous membranes, causing vasoconstriction. Blood flow is reduced in the swollen nasal area. Turbinates and mucous membranes shrink. Sinus drainage is promoted. Feelings of stuffiness and obstruction are relieved.

Decongestants are the drugs of choice for relieving congestion from rhinitis and the common cold. To treat allergic rhinitis, decongestants are often given with antihistamines to:
* Reduce nasal congestion
* Reduce sedation caused by many antihistamines

Oral and topical dose forms are available (Table 25-1). Topical dose forms are nasal sprays or drops. Topical drugs have no systemic effects and they do not relieve other symptoms. They can cause rhinitis medicamentosa.

Nasal decongestants provide temporary symptom relief. At first, stuffiness is relieved. Swelling and congestion then reappear when the vasoconstrictor effect wears off. Rhinitis medicamentosa is a risk from misuse. Always follow label directions.

Drugs in this class can stimulate receptors in other body sites. Caution is needed when oral drugs are taken by persons who have hypertension, hyperthyroidism, diabetes, heart disease, glaucoma, and prostate enlargement.

The goals of therapy are to:
* Reduce nasal congestion
* Ease breathing

BOX 25-1   Common Respiratory Disorders

The Upper Respiratory Tract

Rhinitis. *Rhin* means *nose. Itis* means *inflammation.* Rhinitis is inflammation of the mucous membranes of the nose. Signs and symptoms include sneezing, nasal discharge, and nasal congestion. Rhinitis can be acute or chronic. The most common causes of acute rhinitis are the common cold, bacterial infection, a foreign body, and drug-induced congestion (**rhinitis medicamentosa**). Common causes of chronic rhinitis are allergies, non-allergic rhinitis, chronic sinusitis, and a deviated septum (broken nose, fractured nose).

Common cold. The common cold is a viral infection of the upper respiratory tissues. It usually occurs in mid-winter, spring, and early fall. Viruses are spread from person to person by way of direct contact and sneezing. Early symptoms are a clear, watery nasal discharge and sneezing. Nasal congestion quickly follows. Over the next 48 hours, the discharge becomes cloudy and thicker. Other symptoms include coughing, a "scratchy" or mildly sore throat, and hoarseness. Headache, malaise, fever, and chills may occur. Some persons may have a fever. Symptoms should subside within 5 to 7 days. Sinusitis and otitis media (middle ear infection) are possible complications.

Allergic rhinitis. This is inflammation of the mucous membranes of the nose caused by an allergic reaction. After exposure to an allergen, the person develops antibodies to the antigen. Common allergens are pollens, grasses, and house dust mites. An antigen-antibody reaction occurs when a person inhales the allergen, causing inflammation and swelling of the nasal passages. A major cause of symptoms is the release of histamine during the antigen-antibody reaction. **Histamine** is a substance released in response to allergic reactions and tissue damage from trauma or infection. Histamine is stored in most body tissues. When histamine is released in the area of tissue damage or the site of an antigen-antibody reaction, these reactions take place:

- Arterioles and capillaries in the region dilate. This allows increased blood flow to the area causing redness.
- Capillaries allow fluid to leak into extracellular spaces. This causes:
- Edema (congestion) of nasal mucous membranes and turbinates.
- The release of nasal and bronchial secretions. These result in nasal discharge (**rhinorrhea**). *Rhino* means *nose; rrhea* means *discharge.* Rhinorrhea is commonly called "runny nose." Watery eyes also occur.
- Itching of the palate, eyes, and ears.

Large amounts of histamine are released in a severe allergic reaction. Hypotension results from extensive dilation of the arterioles. Edema is severe. The skin becomes flushed with severe itching. Constriction and spasm of bronchiole tubes cause dyspnea. Large amounts of pulmonary and gastric secretions are released.

Rhinitis medicamentosa. This is inflammation *(itis)* of the mucous membranes of the nose *(rhin)* caused by a drug *(medica).* The drug causes excess vasoconstriction and irritation of the nasal membranes. When the vasoconstrictor effect wears off, swelling and congestion reappear. The nose feels stuffier and more congested than before treatment. More frequent use of the topical decongestant is needed to relieve the nasal passage of swelling and obstruction.

The Lower Respiratory Tract

Chronic obstructive pulmonary disease. Three disorders are grouped under chronic obstructive pulmonary disease (COPD). They interfere with O_2 and CO_2 exchange in the lungs. They obstruct airflow. COPD affects the airways and alveoli. Less air gets into the lungs; less air goes out of the lungs.

- **Chronic bronchitis.** Chronic bronchitis occurs after repeated episodes of bronchitis. *Bronchitis* means inflammation *(itis)* of the bronchi *(bronch).* Smoking is the major cause. Infection, air pollution, and industrial dusts are risk factors. *Smoker's cough* in the morning is often the first symptom. At first the cough is dry. Over time, the person coughs up mucus. Mucus may contain pus. The cough becomes more frequent. The person has difficulty breathing and tires easily. Mucus and inflamed breathing passages obstruct airflow into the lungs. The body cannot get normal amounts of oxygen. The person must stop smoking. Oxygen therapy and breathing exercises are often ordered. Respiratory tract infections are prevented. If one occurs, the person needs prompt treatment.
- **Emphysema.** In emphysema, the alveoli enlarge and become less elastic. They do not expand and shrink normally with breathing in and out. As a result, some air is trapped in the alveoli when exhaling. Trapped air is not exhaled. Over time, more alveoli are involved. O_2 and CO_2 exchange cannot occur in affected alveoli. The person develops a *barrel chest* (Fig. 25-4) as more air is trapped in the lungs. Smoking is the most common cause. Air pollution and industrial dusts are risk factors. The person has shortness of breath and a cough. At first, shortness of breath occurs with exertion. Over time, it occurs at rest. Sputum may contain pus. Fatigue is common. The person works hard to breathe in and out and the body does not get enough oxygen. Breathing is easier when the person sits upright and slightly forward. The person must stop smoking. Respiratory therapy, breathing exercises, oxygen, and drug therapy are ordered.
- **Asthma.** The airway becomes inflamed and narrow. Extra mucus is produced. Dyspnea results. Wheezing and coughing are common, as are pain and tightening in the chest. Symptoms are mild to severe. Asthma is usually triggered by allergies. Other triggers include air pollutants and irritants, smoking and secondhand smoke, respiratory infections, exertion, and cold air. When sudden attacks *(asthma attacks)* occur, there is wheezing, coughing, rapid pulse, sweating, cyanosis, and shortness of breath. The person gasps for air and may be very frightened. Fear makes the attack worse. Asthma is treated with drugs.

TABLE 25-1   Nasal Decongestants

Generic Name	Brand Name	Dose Forms	Adult Dosage Range
oxymetazoline	Afrin, Dristan Spray	Solution: 0.05%	Nasal: Two or three drops or sprays twice daily; use less than 3 days
phenylephrine	Neo-Synephrine Cold and Sinus Sudafed Sudafed 12 hr Sudafed 24 hr Sudafed PE Congestion	Solution: 0.25%, 0.5%, 1% Tablets: 30, 60 mg Liquid: 15, 30 mg/5 mL Syrup: 30 mg/mL 120 mg 240 mg Tablets: 10 mg Oral solution: 2.5 mg/5 mL Oral liquid: 2.5 mg/ mL	Nasal: Two or three drops or sprays twice daily; use less than 3 days PO: 30-60 mg q4-6h; do not exceed 240 mg/24 hours Oral: 10 to 20 mg q4h

Modified from Willihnganz M: *Clayton's Basic Pharmacology for Nurses,* ed 18, St Louis, 2020, Elsevier.

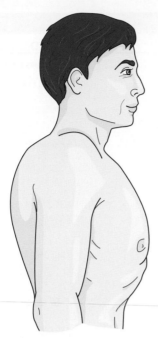

Fig. 25-4 Barrel chest from emphysema.

Assisting With the Nursing Process. When a person takes nasal decongestants, you assist the nurse with the nursing process.

Assessment
- Measure vital signs.
- Measure intake and output.
- Measure blood glucose if the person has diabetes.
  Planning. See Table 25-1 for "Dose Forms."
  Implementation. See Table 25-1 for "Adult Dosage Range."
  See Chapter 13 for how to apply topical nose medications.
  Evaluation. Report and record:
- *Burning or stinging of the nasal membranes.* A weaker solution may be needed.
- *Hypertension.* This may occur from excessive use. Measure blood pressure.
- *Hyperglycemia.* This may occur in persons with diabetes or persons at risk for diabetes.
- *Urinary retention.* Some people, particularly males, develop an obstruction or have difficulty starting a stream of urine. This adverse effect can be eliminated by switching to a topical decongestant.

DRUG CLASS: Antihistamines

Antihistamines compete with released histamine for receptor sites in the arterioles, capillaries, and glands in mucous membranes. Antihistamines do not prevent histamine release. They reduce the symptoms of an allergic reaction if the amount of antihistamine is greater than the amount of histamine. Therefore, antihistamines are more effective if taken:
- Before histamine is released
- When symptoms first appear

Antihistamines are the drugs of choice for the treatment of allergic rhinitis and conjunctivitis. The *conjunctiva* is the mucous membrane lining the inner surfaces of the eyelids and outer part of the sclera. *Conjunctivitis* is the inflammation of the conjunctiva. It is caused by bacterial or viral infections, allergies, or environmental factors. Signs and symptoms include red eyelids, itching, thick discharge, and sticky eyelids in the morning.

The drugs reduce rhinorrhea, tearing, eye itching, and sneezing. They do not stop nasal congestion. They are best taken on a schedule for allergies. They are more effective if taken before exposure to the allergen. For example, they are taken 45 to 60 minutes before going outside during the pollen season.

All antihistamines have anticholinergic side effects:
- Dilation of the pupil with increased intraocular pressure in persons with glaucoma
- Dry, thick secretions of the mouth, nose, throat, and bronchi
- Decreased secretions and motility of the gastrointestinal (GI) tract
- Increased heart rate
- Decreased sweating

Therefore, persons with asthma, prostate enlargement, or glaucoma should take antihistamines only with medical supervision.

The goals of therapy are to reduce the signs and symptoms from allergic rhinitis.

Assisting With the Nursing Process. When a person takes nasal decongestants, you assist the nurse with the nursing process.

Assessment
- Observe for nasal congestion.
- Measure intake and output.
  Planning. See Table 25-2 for "Dose Forms."
  Implementation. See Table 25-2 for "Adult Dosage Range."
  Evaluation. Report and record:
- *Sedation, cognitive impairment, memory problems, coordination problems.* Sedation is the most common side effect from antihistamines. Tolerance may develop over time. Provide for safety. People working around machines, driving a car, pouring and giving drugs, or performing other duties that require mental alertness should not take these drugs while working.
- *Drying effects.* Observe the person's cough and sputum production. Because of drying effects, antihistamines may impair expectoration.
- *Blurred vision; constipation; mouth, throat, nose dryness.* These are caused by the drying effects of antihistamines. The nurse may allow the person to chew gum or suck on ice chips or hard candy. Provide for safety if the person has blurred vision. Follow the care plan for constipation.
- *Urinary retention.* Some people, particularly males, develop an obstruction or have difficulty starting a stream of urine. This adverse effect can be eliminated by switching to a topical antihistamine.

DRUG CLASS: Respiratory Antiinflammatory Agents

Antiinflammatory agents used to treat upper respiratory diseases are:
- intranasal corticosteroids
- cromolyn sodium (kro' mo lin); Nasalcrom (nay zal krom')

Intranasal Corticosteroids

Intranasal means within *(intra)* the nose *(nasal)*. Corticosteroids (Chapter 29) are given to reduce inflammation. Persons

TABLE 25-2   Antihistamines[a]

Generic Name	Brand Name	Dose Forms	Adult Dosage Range
Azelastine	Astepro	Nasal spray: 0.1, 0.15 %; 137 mcg/spray	Two sprays per nostril twice daily
Cetirizine	Zyrtec Allergy	Tablets: 5, 10 mg Oral solution: 5 mg/5 mL Tablets, chewable: 5, 10 mg Orally disintegrating tablet: 10 mg	5-10 mg once daily
chlorpheniramine maleate	Chlor-Trimeton	Tablets: 4 mg Tablets, extended-release (12 hr): 12 mg Liquid: 2 mg/mL in 60 mL bottle Syrup: 2 mg/5 mL in 118, 473 mL bottles	4 mg q4-6h
clemastine fumarate	Tavist Allergy	Tablets: 1.34, 2.68 mg	1.34-2.68 mg two to three times daily
cyproheptadine hydrochloride		Tablets: 4 mg Syrup: 2 mg/5 mL in 473 mL bottle	4 mg three times daily
desloratadine	Clarinex	Tablets: 5 mg Syrup: 0.5 mg/mL in 473 mL bottle Orally disintegrating tablets: 2.5, 5 mg	5 mg once daily
diphenhydramine hydrochloride	Benadryl Allergy	Capsules: 25, 50 mg Tablets: 25, 50 mg Syrup: 12.5 mg/5 mL Elixir: 12.5 mg/5 mL	25-50 mg q4-8h daily
Fexofenadine	Allegra	Tablets: 60, 180 mg Oral suspension: 30 mg/5 mL in 120- and 240-mL bottle Orally disintegrating tablets: 30 mg	60 mg twice daily
Levocetirizine	Xyzal Allergy 24	Tablets: 5 mg Oral solution: 2.5 mg/5 mL	2.5-5 mg once daily in the evening
Loratadine	Claritin	Tablets: 10 mg Tablets, chewable: 5 mg Tablets, disintegrating: 5 mg, 10 mg Capsules: 10 mg Syrup: 5 mg/mL Oral solution: 5 mg/mL	10 mg daily
Olopatadine	Patanase	Nasal spray; 0.6%	Two sprays per nostril two times daily
promethazine hydrochloride[b]	Phenergan	Tablets: 12.5, 25, 50 mg Syrup: 6.25 mg/5 mL Oral solution: 6.25 mg/5 mL Suppository: 12.5, 25, 50 mg	6.25-12.5 mg three times daily

[a]Many of these antihistamines are also available in combination with decongestants.
[b]Promethazine is a phenothiazine with antihistaminic properties.
Modified from Willihnganz M: Clayton's Basic Pharmacology for Nurses, ed 18, St Louis, 2020, Elsevier.

with allergic rhinitis who do not respond to sympathomimetic and antihistamine drugs may be given corticosteroids to relieve allergy symptoms.

Intranasal corticosteroids control nasal symptoms associated with mild to moderate allergic rhinitis. They are used in short courses of therapy for acute seasonal allergies.

The goals of therapy are to reduce:
- Rhinorrhea
- Rhinitis
- Itching
- Sneezing

Assisting With the Nursing Process. When a person takes intranasal corticosteroids, you assist the nurse with the nursing process.

Assessment
- Observe for nasal congestion.
  Planning. See Table 25-3 for "Dose Forms."
  Implementation. See Table 25-3 for "Adult Dosage Range."
- Full therapeutic effect requires regular use. It is usually evident within a few days. Some persons require up to 3 weeks to achieve maximum benefit.
- Advise the person to clear nasal passages of secretions before a topical application.
- A decongestant may be ordered for use right before a topical corticosteroid. This promotes adequate penetration.
- See Chapter 13 for how to apply topical nose medications.
  Evaluation. Report and record:
- *Nasal burning.* This is usually mild and tends to resolve with continued therapy.

TABLE 25-3 Intranasal Corticosteroids

Generic Name	Brand Name	Dose Forms	Adult Dosage Range
beclomethasone dipropionate, monohydrate	Beconase AQ	Nasal spray: 40, 42 mcg/spray	One or two sprays (42-84 mcg) in each nostril twice daily
Budesonide	Rhinocort Allergy	Nasal aerosol: 120 doses/canister (32 mcg/spray)	One to four sprays in each nostril once daily
Ciclesonide	Omnaris Zetonna	Nasal spray: 50 mcg/spray Nasal spray: 37 mcg/spray	Two sprays in each nostril daily One spray in each nostril daily
Fluticasone	Flonase Sensimist	Nasal spray: 27.5 mcg/spray; 60, 120 metered-dose bottles	Up to two sprays (55 mcg) per nostril daily
Mometasone	Nasonex	Nasal spray: 120 sprays/bottle; 50 mcg/spray	Two sprays (100 mcg) in each nostril once daily
triamcinolone	Nasacort Allergy 24 Hr	Nasal spray: 55 mcg/spray	Two sprays (110 mcg each) in each nostril once daily; maximum daily dosage is two sprays in each nostril in 24 hr

Modified from Willihnganz M: Clayton's Basic Pharmacology for Nurses, ed 18, St Louis, 2020, Elsevier.

Cromolyn Sodium (Nasalcrom)

Cromolyn sodium (Nasalcrom) is an antiinflammatory agent. It inhibits the release of histamine and other substances of inflammation. To be effective, it must be used before the body receives a stimulus to release histamine.

Cromolyn sodium (Nasalcrom) is used with other drugs that prevent the release of histamine. It does not relieve nasal congestion. An antihistamine or nasal decongestant may be needed when treatment is started. A 2- to 4-week course of therapy is usually needed for a clinical response. Treatment is continued only if there is a decrease in symptoms.

The goals of therapy are to reduce:
- Rhinorrhea
- Itching
- Sneezing

Assisting With the Nursing Process. When a person takes cromolyn sodium (Nasalcrom), you assist the nurse with the nursing process.

Assessment
- Observe for nasal congestion.

Planning. Dose forms are:
- Nasal spray: 5.2 mg/spray in 13 mL (gives 100 sprays) and 26 mL (gives 200 sprays)
- Oral concentrate: 100 mg/5 mL

Implementation
- The adult dose is one spray in each nostril three or four times daily at regular intervals. Maximum dose is six sprays in each nostril daily.
- Full therapeutic effect requires regular use. It is usually evident within 2 to 4 weeks.
- Advise the person to clear nasal passages of secretions before a topical application.
- See Chapter 13 for how to apply topical nose medications.

Evaluation. Report and record:
- Nasal irritation—sneezing, itching, burning, stuffiness. Tolerance usually develops.

DRUG THERAPY FOR LOWER RESPIRATORY DISEASES

Lower respiratory diseases are treated with the following drugs:
- Expectorants
- Antitussives (cough suppressants)
- Bronchodilators such as beta-adrenergic bronchodilating agents and anticholinergic bronchodilating agents.
- Antiinflammatory agents such as corticosteroids, antileukotriene agents, and phosphodiesterase-4 inhibitors (PDE-4).
- Mucolytic agents—drugs that reduce the stickiness and thickness of pulmonary secretions. They act directly on mucous plugs to cause them to dissolve. This eases the removal of secretions by cough, postural drainage, and suction. These agents are used to treat acute and chronic respiratory disorders, before and after bronchoscopy, after chest surgery, and as part of tracheostomy care. Mucomyst (acetylcysteine) is often given by nebulizer (Fig. 25-5). A *nebulizer* is a device that produces a fine spray. See *Delegation Guidelines: Drug Therapy for Lower Respiratory Diseases.*

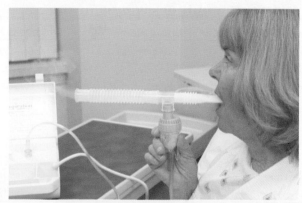

Fig. 25-5 Nebulizer. (From Perry AG, Potter PA: Clinical skills and nursing techniques, ed 6, St Louis, 2006, Mosby.)

DRUG CLASS: Expectorants

Expectorants liquefy mucus to promote the ejection of mucus from the lungs and tracheobronchial tree. They stimulate the secretion of natural fluids from the serous glands. The flow of serous fluids helps liquefy thick mucous plugs that may narrow bronchioles. Coughing helps expel the phlegm from the respiratory system. Expectorants are used to treat nonproductive cough, bronchitis, and pneumonia.

The following expectorant is used to treat lower respiratory diseases:

- Guaifenesin (gwi feh' neh sin); Robitussin (row bih tus' sin)

    Guaifenesin (Robitussin) is an expectorant that enhances the output of respiratory tract fluid. The increased flow of secretions decreases mucus thickness. This promotes the movement of the mucus out of the respiratory tract.

    The drug is used to relieve a dry, nonproductive cough and to remove mucous plugs. The drug is often used with bronchodilators, decongestants, antihistamines, or antitussive agents to make a nonproductive cough productive.

    The goals of therapy are to:

- Reduce the frequency of nonproductive cough
- Thin out the secretions in the respiratory tract

Assisting With the Nursing Process. When a person takes guaifenesin (Robitussin), you assist the nurse with the nursing process.

Assessment. Note the person's cough:

- Is it productive or nonproductive?
- What is the color, consistency, amount, and appearance of sputum?

    Planning. Oral dose forms are:

- 200 and 400 mg tablets

- 600 and 1200 mg extended-release tablets
- 100 mg/packet oral granules
- 100 mg/5 mL liquid and syrup

    Implementation

- The adult dose is 100 to 400 mg every 4 to 6 hours.
- The dose should not exceed 2400 mg per day.
- The person should drink eight to twelve 8-ounce glasses of water daily.

    Evaluation. Report and record:

- *GI upset, nausea, vomiting.* These side effects are rare.

DRUG CLASS: Antitussives

Antitussives (cough suppressants) depress the cough center in the brain. They are used when a person has a dry, hacking, nonproductive cough. These agents should decrease the frequency and suppress severe spasms that affect sleep.

The goal of therapy is to reduce the frequency of a nonproductive cough.

Assisting With the Nursing Process. When a person takes antitussives, you assist the nurse with the nursing process.

Assessment. Note the person's cough:

- Is it productive or nonproductive?
- What is the color, consistency, amount, and appearance of sputum?

    Planning. See Table 25-4 for "Oral Dose Forms."

    Implementation. See Table 25-4 for "Adult Oral Dosage Range."

- Benzonatate (Tessalon Perles) must be swallowed whole. The drug numbs the tongue if chewed or crushed. This creates a choking hazard.
- Codeine is an effective cough suppressant. Low-dose, short-term use for a cough should not produce addiction. Dependence may develop after long-term use.
- Diphenhydramine has significant sedative properties and should not be taken if the person must be mentally alert. It is excellent for suppressing cough during sleep.

    Evaluation. Report and record:

- *Drowsiness, sedation.* Provide for safety. Remind the person to use caution when performing tasks that require alertness.

TABLE 25-4	Antitussive Agents			
Generic Name	**Brand Name**	**Dose Forms**		**Adult Dosage Range**
Benzonatate	Tessalon Perles	Capsules: 100, 150, 200 mg		100-200 mg three times daily
codeine*		Tablets: 15, 30, 60 mg[a]		10-20 mg q4-6h[a]
dextromethorphan	Robitussin 12 Hour Cough Delsym	Lozenges: 5, 7.5 mg Capsules: 15 mg Syrup: 5, 7.5, 10 mg/5 mL Liquid: 7.5, 10, 12.5, 15 mg/5 mL Gel: 7.5 mg/5 mL Suspension, extended-release: 30 mg/5 mL		10-20 mg q4h or 30 mg q6-8h; 60 mg q12h (sustained-release); do not exceed 120 mg/24 hr
diphenhydramine	Diphen Allergy Relief	Syrup, liquid. 12.5 mg/5 mL Capsules and tablets: 25, 50 mg		25 to 50 mg every 4 to 6 hr; maximum dose: 300 mg/day

[a]Often an ingredient in combination antitussive products. A controlled substance. May be habit-forming.
Modified from Willihnganz M: Clayton's Basic Pharmacology for Nurses, ed 18, St Louis, 2020, Elsevier.

- *Constipation.* Codeine is the most constipating of the antitussives. Give stool softeners as ordered. Follow the care plan for fluid intake.

DRUG CLASS: Beta-Adrenergic Bronchodilating Agents

Beta-adrenergic bronchodilating agents relax the smooth muscles of the tracheobronchial tree. This opens airways to greater amounts of air. These drugs are used to reverse airway constriction caused by acute and chronic asthma, bronchitis, and emphysema.

The drugs have many side effects. This is because they also stimulate receptors in the heart, blood vessels, uterus, and gastrointestinal, urinary, and central nervous systems. Those given by inhalation usually have fewer side effects. With inhalation, the drug is placed at the site of action. Lower doses are used.

The goals of therapy are to:
- Ease breathing
- Reduce wheezing

Assisting With the Nursing Process. When giving a person beta-adrenergic bronchodilating agents, you assist the nurse with the nursing process.

Assessment
- Measure vital signs.
- Note the pulse rate and rhythm.
- Observe for confusion and orientation to person, time, and place.
  Planning. See Table 25-5, for "Dose Forms."
  Implementation. See Table 25-5, for "Adult Dosage Range."
- The person waits at least 10 minutes between inhalations. This allows the drug to dilate the bronchioles. The second dose can be inhaled more deeply into the lungs.
- Follow the manufacturer's instructions.
  Evaluation. Report and record:
- *Tachycardia, palpitations.* These are dose related. Measure heart rate and note the rhythm. Report an increase of 20 beats or more per minute after a treatment. Report dysrhythmias and palpitations.
- *Tremors.* The dosage may need adjustment.

TABLE 25-5 Bronchodilators

Generic Name	Brand Name	Dose Forms	Adult Dosage Range
Beta-Adrenergic Agonists			
albuterol	Proventil-HFA Ventolin-HFA	Tablets: 2, 4 mg; Syrup: 2 mg/5 mL; Tablets, 12 hr extended-release: 4, 8 mg; Aerosol: 90 mcg; Solution for inhalation	PO: 2-4 mg three or four times daily; maximum dose 32 mg daily; PO: Extended-release: 8 mg q12h; maximum dose 32 mg/24 hr; Inhale: Two inhalations q4-6h; maximum dose 12 inhalations/24 hr; See manufacturer's recommendations
arformoterol	Brovana	Solution for inhalation: 15 mcg/2 mL	Inhale: 15 mcg twice daily
formoterol	Perforomist	Solution for inhalation: 20 mcg/2 mL	Nebulizer: 20 mcg q12h
indacaterol	Arcapta Neohaler	Inhalation powder: 75 mcg	Inhale: One capsule q24h using Neohaler inhaler at same time daily
levalbuterol	Xopenex Xopenex HFA	Solution for inhalation: 0.31, 0.63, 1.25 mg/3 mL; 1.25 mcg/0.5 mL; Aerosol: 45 mcg/spray	0.31-1.25 mg q8h; Inhale: One to two inhalations q4-6h
metaproterenol		Tablets: 10, 20 mg; Syrup: 10 mg/5 mL	PO: 10-20 mg three or four times daily
olodaterol	Striverdi Respimat	Aerosol: 2.5 mcg/spray	Two sprays once daily at the same time of the day
salmeterol	Serevent Diskus	Powder for inhalation: 50 mcg/inhalation	Inhale: 1 inhalation q12h
terbutaline		Tablets: 2.5, 5 mg	PO: 5 mg q6h
Inhaled Anticholinergic Bronchodilators			
aclidinium	Tudorza Pressair	Powder for inhalation: 400 mcg/spray	Inhale: One inhalation twice daily
ycopyrrolate	Seebri Neohaler	Powder for inhalation: 15.6 mg/inhalation	Inhale: One capsule twice daily using Neohaler
	Lonhala Magnair	Inhalation Solution: 25 mcg/mL in 1 mL vial	Nebulize: One vial (25 mcg) inhaled twice daily; using only Magnair
ipratropium	Atrovent HFA	Aerosol: 17 mcg/spray; Inhalation Solution: 0.2%/2.5 mL vial	Inhale: Two inhalations four times daily; maximum dose: 12 inhalations per 24 hr; Nebulize: One unit-dose vial q6-8h
tiotropium	Spiriva HandiHaler Spiriva Respimat	18-mcg capsule: 1.25 mcg and 2.5 mcg per spray	Handihaler–Inhaler: One capsule once daily (to ensure drug delivery, the contents of each capsule should be inhaled twice); COPD: Two inhalations (5 mcg) once daily; Asthma: Two inhalations (2.5 mcg) once daily
umeclidinium	Incruse Ellipta	Powder for inhalation: 62.5 mcg/spray	Inhale: One inhalation once daily

Modified from Willihnganz M: Clayton's Basic Pharmacology for Nurses, ed 18, St Louis, 2020, Elsevier.

- *Nervousness, anxiety, restlessness, headache.*
- *Nausea, vomiting.* Give the drug with food and a full glass of water.
- *Dizziness.* Provide for safety.

DRUG CLASS: Anticholinergic Bronchodilating Agents

Anticholinergic bronchodilating agents relax the smooth muscles of the tracheobronchial tree. This opens airways to greater amounts of air. These drugs are used to reverse bronchoconstriction in the respiratory tract caused by asthma, bronchitis, and emphysema.

The drugs have many side effects because they also stimulate receptors in the heart, blood vessels, uterus, and gastrointestinal, urinary, and central nervous systems. Those given by inhalation usually have fewer side effects. With inhalation, the drug is placed at the site of action. Lower doses are used.

The goals of therapy are to:
- Ease breathing
- Reduce wheezing

Assisting With the Nursing Process. When a person takes anticholinergic bronchodilating agents, you assist the nurse with the nursing process.
   Assessment
- Measure vital signs.
- Measure intake and output.
   Planning. See Table 25-5 for "Dose Forms."
   Implementation. See Table 25-5 for "Adult Dosage Range."
- Use with caution in people with certain types of glaucoma (Chapter 32), prostatic hyperplasia (Chapter 30), and bladder obstruction.
   Evaluation. Report and record:
- *Mouth dryness, throat irritation.* These are usually mild and tend to resolve with continued therapy. Provide oral hygiene. The nurse may allow the person to suck on ice chips or hard candy.
- *Tachycardia, urinary retention, worsening of respiratory symptoms.*

DRUG CLASS: Respiratory Antiinflammatory Agents

Corticosteroids are given to reduce inflammation (Chapter 29). They are highly effective in treating COPD and asthma. They are commonly given by inhalation. The drug is placed at the site of inflammation with few side effects. They:
- Relax smooth muscles
- Enhance the effect of beta-adrenergic bronchodilators
- Inhibit inflammatory responses that may cause bronchoconstriction

These agents may be added to a drug therapy program if the person does not respond to other bronchodilators.

The goals of therapy are:
- Decreased pulmonary inflammation
- Easier breathing with less effort

Assisting With the Nursing Process. When a person uses inhalant corticosteroids, you assist the nurse with the nursing process.

   Assessment
- Observe the mouth for signs and symptoms of infection.
   Planning. See Table 25-6 for "Inhalant Dose Forms."
   Implementation. See Table 25-6 for "Adult Dosage Range."
- Full therapeutic effect requires regular use. It is usually evident within a few days. Some persons require up to 4 weeks to achieve maximum benefit.
- Persons receiving bronchodilators by inhalation should use them before the corticosteroid inhalant because doing so enhances penetration of the corticosteroid into the bronchial tree. Wait several minutes before the corticosteroid is inhaled to allow time for the bronchodilator to relax the smooth muscle.
   Evaluation. Report and record:
- *Hoarseness, dry mouth.* These are usually mild and tend to resolve with continued therapy.
- *Signs and symptoms of a mouth infection.* Provide oral hygiene. Follow the care plan for using a mouthwash.

DRUG CLASS: Antileukotriene Agents

Antileukotriene agents are also antiinflammatory agents. *Leukotrienes* are substances in white blood cells. White blood cells are called *leukocytes*. (*Leuko* means *white*. *Cyte* means *cell*.) Leukotrienes produce allergic and inflammatory reactions similar to those of histamine. They produce many of the signs and symptoms of asthma (see Box 25-1).

The following is an antileukotriene agent:
- Montelukast (mon teh lu' cast); Singular (sing' yu lair')

Montelukast (Singulair) competes for the receptor sites that trigger symptoms of asthma. It has been shown to reduce:
- Bronchoconstriction
- Daytime asthma symptoms
- Nighttime awakening

The goal of therapy is fewer episodes of acute asthma symptoms.

Assisting With the Nursing Process. When giving a person montelukast (Singulair), you assist the nurse with the nursing process.
   Assessment
- Measure vital signs.
   Planning
- Oral dose forms are:
- 10 mg tablets
- 4 and 5 mg chewable tablets
- 4 mg granules
   Implementation. The adult dose is 10 mg taken once daily in the evening.
   Evaluation. Report and record:
- *Headache, nausea, indigestion.* These are usually mild and resolve with continued therapy. Give the drug with food or milk to lessen discomfort.

DRUG CLASS: Phosphodiesterase-4 Inhibitor (PDE-4)

Cyclic adenosine monophosphate (cAMP) blocks inflammation throughout the body. Phosphodiesterase-4 is an enzyme

TABLE 25-6 Inhalant Corticosteroids

Generic Name	Brand Name	Inhalant Dose Forms	Adult Dosage Range
Inhalant Corticosteroids			
beclomethasone dipropionate	Qvar Redihaler	Aerosol: 40, 80 mcg/spray; 100 doses/inhaler	Inhale: One or two inhalations (80 mcg) twice daily; maximum 640 mcg daily
ciclesonide	Alvesco	Aerosol solution: 80, 160 mcg/spray	80-160 mcg twice daily
flunisolide	Aerospan	80 mcg/spray	320 mcg twice daily
fluticasone propionate	Flovent HFA	Aerosol: 44, 110, 220 mcg/spray	88-440 mcg twice daily
	Flovent Diskus	Powder for inhalation: 50, 100, 250 mcg/dose	100-500 mcg twice daily
fluticasone furoate	Arnuity Ellipta	Powder for inhalation: 50, 100, 200 mcg/inhalation	50-200 mcg daily
mometasone furoate	Asmanex HFA	Powder for inhalation: 100, 200 mcg/inhalation	200-400 mcg twice daily
	Asmanex Metered doses	Powder, breath activated: 110, 220 mcg/inhalation	
Inhalant Corticosteroid Beta-Adrenergic Bronchodilator			
budesonide/formoterol	Symbicort	Aerosol: 80 mcg budesonide and 4.5 mcg formoterol/spray; 160 mcg budesonide and 4.5 mcg formoterol/spray	Inhale: Two inhalations twice daily for maintenance on a regularly scheduled basis; not for acute bronchospasm
fluticasone/salmeterol	Advair Diskus	Powder for inhalation: 100 mcg fluticasone and 50 mcg salmeterol; 250 mcg fluticasone and 50 mcg salmeterol; 500 mcg fluticasone and 50 mcg salmeterol	Inhale: One to two inhalations twice daily for maintenance therapy on regularly scheduled basis; not for acute bronchospasm
	Advair HFA	Aerosol inhalation: 45 mcg fluticasone and 21 mcg salmeterol; 115 mcg fluticasone and 21 mcg salmeterol; 230 mcg fluticasone and 21 mcg salmeterol	Inhale: Two inhalations twice daily for maintenance therapy on regularly scheduled basis; not for acute bronchospasm
fluticasone/vilanterol	Breo Ellipta	Aerosol inhalation: 100 mcg fluticasone and 25 mcg vilanterol; 200 mcg fluticasone and 25 mcg vilanterol	Inhale: One inhalation once daily
mometasone/formoterol	Dulera	Aerosol inhalation: 100 mcg mometasone and 5 mcg formoterol/spray, 200 mcg mometasone and 5 mcg formoterol/spray	Inhale: Two inhalations twice daily for maintenance on regularly scheduled basis; not for acute bronchospasm
Inhalant Corticosteroid Beta-Adrenergic Anticholinergic Bronchodilator			
fluticasone/vilanterol/ umeclidinium	Trelegy Ellipta	Fluticasone 100 mcg/ Vilanterol 25 mcg/ umeclidinium 62.5 mcg per spray	Inhale: One inhalation once daily

Modified from Willihnganz M: Clayton's Basic Pharmacology for Nurses, ed 18, St Louis, 2020, Elsevier.

found in the lungs. It removes cAMP from the body. PDE-4 inhibitors allow cAMP to build up in the body which helps reduce inflammation.

The following is a PDE-4 agent:

- Roflumilast (ro flu' mi last); Daliresp (da li resp')

Assisting With the Nursing Process

- When giving a person roflumilast (Daliresp), you assist the nurse with the nursing process.

Assessment

- Measure vital signs.
- Measure weight weekly.
- Ask about bowel elimination and GI symptoms.
- Ask about dizziness, headache, and insomnia.
- Observe for anxiety.

Planning

- Oral dose forms are 250 and 500 mcg tablets

Implementation

- Initially, 250 mcg once daily for 4 weeks. Maintenance dose is 500 mcg once daily with or without food.

Evaluation. Report and record:

- *Nausea, vomiting, epigastric pain, abdominal cramps.* These occur from irritation caused by the stimulation of gastric acid secretion. Give the drug with food or milk.
- *Weight loss.* Watch for unexplained or significant weight loss.
- *Headache.* This usually resolves with continued therapy.
- *Insomnia, anxiety, depression.* Watch for *these and other mood changes. Provide for safety.*
- *Suicidal actions.* Observe for negative thoughts, feelings, behaviors, depression, or suicidal thinking. Report your observations and concerns to the nurse. Follow suicide precautions according to the care plan.

REVIEW QUESTIONS

Circle the BEST answer.

1. Which are the drugs of choice for allergic rhinitis?
   a. antihistamines
   b. antiinflammatory agents
   c. antitussives
   d. decongestants
2. Decongestants cause:
   a. vasodilation of the nasal mucosa
   b. vasoconstriction of the nasal mucosa
   c. vasodilation of the tracheobronchial tree
   d. vasoconstriction of the tracheobronchial tree
3. Decongestants are used to treat the following, *except:*
   a. allergic rhinitis
   b. asthma
   c. the common cold
   d. rhinitis
4. Decongestants are often used with antihistamines to:
   a. liquefy secretions
   b. ease breathing
   c. reduce sedation
   d. reduce inflammation
5. Topical dose forms of nasal decongestants:
   a. are drops or sprays
   b. have systemic side effects
   c. relieve other symptoms
   d. prevent rhinitis medicamentosa
6. Which is a nasal decongestant?
   a. Benadryl Allergy
   b. Chlor-Trimeton
   c. Phenergan
   d. Sudafed
7. These statements are about antihistamines. Which is *false?*
   a. They prevent histamine release.
   b. They are more effective if taken before histamine is released.
   c. They are more effective if taken when symptoms first appear.
   d. Sedation is the most common side effect.
8. Antihistamines are the drugs of choice for the treatment of:
   a. the common cold
   b. rhinitis
   c. allergic rhinitis
   d. rhinitis medicamentosa
9. Antihistamines cause:
   a. diarrhea
   b. decreased heart rate
   c. increased sweating
   d. dry, thick secretions of the mouth, nose, throat, and bronchi
10. Intranasal corticosteroids are given to:
    a. liquefy secretions
    b. ease breathing
    c. reduce sedation
    d. reduce inflammation

11. Intranasal corticosteroids are given to treat:
    a. the common cold
    b. emphysema
    c. allergic rhinitis
    d. rhinitis medicamentosa
12. Intranasal corticosteroids are given to reduce the following, *except:*
    a. nasal burning
    b. itching
    c. rhinorrhea
    d. sneezing
13. Cromolyn sodium (Nasalcrom):
    a. competes for histamine receptor sites
    b. prevents the release of histamine
    c. relieves nasal congestion
    d. increases rhinorrhea
14. Cromolyn sodium (Nasalcrom) is sprayed into each nostril:
    a. as needed
    b. once daily
    c. at bedtime
    d. three or four times a day at regular intervals
15. Which liquefy mucus?
    a. antiinflammatory agents
    b. antitussives
    c. bronchodilators
    d. expectorants
16. Which are cough suppressants?
    a. antiinflammatory agents
    b. antitussives
    c. bronchodilators
    d. expectorants
17. Guaifenesin (Robitussin) is a:
    a. antiinflammatory agent
    b. antitussive
    c. bronchodilator
    d. expectorant
18. Bronchodilators are given to:
    a. promote a productive cough
    b. ease breathing
    c. liquefy secretions
    d. dry secretions
19. When anticholinergic bronchodilators are given by metered-dose inhaler, the goal of therapy is to:
    a. prevent COPD
    b. reduce rhinorrhea
    c. relieve symptoms of allergic rhinitis
    d. ease breathing
20. These statements about corticosteroids are true, *except:*
    a. They relax smooth muscles.
    b. They enhance the effect of beta-adrenergic bronchodilators.
    c. They liquefy mucus.
    d. They inhibit inflammatory responses that may cause bronchoconstriction.

21. Tiotropium bromide (Spiriva) is:
    a. a tablet taken orally
    b. a dry powder taken with an inhaler
    c. a nasal spray
    d. an aerosol
22. These statements are about montelukast (Singulair). Which is *false?*
    a. It is an antileukotriene.
    b. It is used to treat asthma.
    c. It is inhaled.
    d. The dose is taken once a day in the evening.
23. Phosphodiesterase-4 (PDE-4) inhibitors work by:
    a. removing cAMP from the body
    b. allowing cAMP to build up in the body
    c. vasoconstriction
    d. vasodilation

Circle T if the statement is true. Circle F if the statement is false.
24. T F Antihistamines reduce nasal congestion.

25. T F Antiinflammatory agents are given to treat the common cold.
26. T F A nasal decongestant and an intranasal corticosteroid are ordered. The nasal decongestant is taken first.
27. T F Cromolyn sodium (Nasalcrom) is an intranasal corticosteroid.
28. T F Codeine is an antitussive.
29. T F Antitussives can cause drowsiness.
30. T F When given orally, bronchodilators can cause systemic side effects. Tachycardia, tremors, and nervousness are examples.
31. T F Persons taking inhalant corticosteroids need good oral hygiene.
32. T F A bronchodilator inhalant and a corticosteroid inhalant are ordered. The corticosteroid is taken first.

Answers to these questions can be found on the Evolve Resources site: http://evolve.elsevier.com/Anderson/medasst/

26

Drugs Used to Treat Gastroesophageal Reflux and Peptic Ulcer Diseases

OBJECTIVES

- Define the key terms and key abbreviations used in this chapter.
- Describe gastroesophageal reflux disease.
- Describe peptic ulcer disease.
- Describe the drugs used to treat gastroesophageal reflux disease and peptic ulcer disease.
- Explain how to assist with the nursing process when drugs are used to treat gastroesophageal reflux disease and peptic ulcer disease.

KEY TERMS

antacids Drugs that buffer, neutralize, or absorb hydrochloric acid in the stomach; *ant* means *against, acid* means *sour*

antagonist A drug that has the opposite action of another drug or competes for the same receptor sites

coating agents Drugs that form a substance that adheres to the crater of an ulcer

gastrointestinal prostaglandins Drugs that inhibit gastric acid secretion

histamine A substance released in response to allergic reactions and tissue damage from trauma or infection

histamine (H$_2$)-receptor antagonists Drugs that block the action of histamine; histamine blockers

peptic Pertains to digestion or the enzymes and secretions needed for digestion

peptic ulcer An ulcer in the stomach, duodenum, or other part of the GI system exposed to gastric juices

prokinetic agents Drugs that stimulate movement or motility

proton pump inhibitors Drugs that inhibit the gastric acid pump of the parietal cells

ulcer A shallow or deep crater-like sore of a mucous membrane

KEY ABBREVIATIONS

g Gram
GERD Gastroesophageal reflux disease
GI Gastrointestinal
MAR Medication administration record
mcg Microgram

mg Milligram
mL Milliliter
NSAID Non-steroidal anti-inflammatory drug
PPI Proton pump inhibitor
PUD Peptic ulcer disease

The digestive system involves the *alimentary canal (GI tract)* and the accessory organs of digestion (Fig. 26-1). The alimentary canal is a long tube extending from the mouth to the anus. Its major components are the mouth, pharynx, esophagus, stomach, small intestine, and large intestine. Accessory organs are the teeth, tongue, salivary glands, liver, gallbladder, and pancreas. See Box 26-1.

DRUG THERAPY FOR GASTROESOPHOGEAL REFLUX DISEASE AND PEPTIC ULCER DISEASES

Gastroesophageal reflux disease (GERD) is a common stomach disorder. With peptic ulcer disease (PUD), there are ulcerations in the gastrointestinal (GI) tract such as the stomach and intestines. See Box 26-1 and Box 26-2.

The goals of drug therapy for GERD and PUD are to:
- Relieve symptoms
- Promote healing
- Prevent recurrence

See *Delegation Guidelines: Drugs Used to Treat Gastroesophageal Reflux and Peptic Ulcer Diseases.*

DELEGATION GUIDELINES

Drugs Used to Treat Gastroesophageal Reflux and Peptic Ulcer Diseases

Some drugs used to treat GERD and PUD are given parenterally—by subcutaneous, intramuscular, or intravenous injection. Because you do not give parenteral dose forms, they are not included in this chapter. Should a nurse delegate the administration of such to you, you must:
- Remember that parenteral dosages are often very different from dosages for other routes.
- Refuse the delegation but do not just ignore the request. Make sure the nurse knows that you cannot give the drug and why.

DRUG CLASS: Antacids

Antacids are drugs that buffer, neutralize, or absorb hydrochloric acid in the stomach. (*Ant* means *against. Acid* means *sour.*) The pH of hydrochloric acid is 1 or 2. Antacids raise the pH to 3 or 4. The gastric juice loses its corrosive effect.

BOX 26-1   The Upper Digestive System: Structure and Function

The digestive system breaks down food physically and chemically so it can be absorbed for use by the cells. This process is called *digestion*. The digestive system is also called the *gastrointestinal (GI) system*. The system also removes solid wastes from the body.

Digestion begins in the *mouth*. The mouth also is called the *oral cavity*. It receives food and prepares it for digestion. Using chewing motions, the *teeth* cut, chop, and grind food into small particles for digestion and swallowing. The *tongue* aids in chewing and swallowing. Taste buds on the tongue's surface contain nerve endings. Taste buds allow sweet, sour, bitter, and salty tastes to be sensed. *Salivary glands* in the mouth secrete *saliva*. Saliva moistens food particles to ease swallowing and begin digestion. During swallowing, the tongue pushes food into the *pharynx*.

The *pharynx* (throat) is a muscular tube. Swallowing continues as the pharynx contracts. Contraction of the pharynx pushes food into the *esophagus*. The

esophagus is a muscular tube about 10 inches long extending from the pharynx to the *stomach*. Involuntary muscle contractions called *peristalsis* move food down the esophagus through the alimentary canal.

The stomach is a muscular, pouch-like sac. It is in the upper left part of the abdominal cavity. Strong stomach muscles stir and churn food to break it up into even smaller particles. A mucous membrane lines the stomach. It contains glands that secrete *gastric juices*. Food is mixed and churned with the gastric juices to form a semi-liquid substance called *chyme*. Through peristalsis, the chyme is pushed from the stomach into the small intestine. The *duodenum* is the first part of the small intestine.

BOX 26-2   Gastroesophageal Reflux and Peptic Ulcer Diseases

Gastroesophageal reflux disease (GERD). Gastroesophageal reflux disease is a disease in which stomach contents flow back *(reflux)* from the stomach *(gastro)* into the esophagus *(esophageal)*. It is commonly called heartburn, acid indigestion, and sour stomach.

The stomach contents contain acid. The acid can cause irritation and inflammation of the lining of the esophagus. This is called *esophagitis* (inflammation *[itis]* of the esophagus).

Heartburn (a burning sensation in the chest and sometimes the throat) is the most common symptom of GERD. The person may have a sour taste in the back of the mouth. Occasional heartburn is not a problem. If it occurs more than twice a week, the person may have GERD. Other signs and symptoms of GERD include:

- Chest pain (often when lying down)
- Hoarseness in the morning
- Dysphagia
- Choking sensation
- Feeling like food is stuck in the throat
- Feeling like the throat is tight
- Dry cough
- Sore throat
- Bad breath

Large meals and laying down after eating can cause gastric reflux, as can certain foods—citrus fruits, chocolate, caffeine drinks, fried and fatty foods, garlic, onions, spicy foods, tomato-based foods (e.g., pasta sauce, chili, pizza).

Most cases of GERD pass quickly with only mild discomfort. Frequent or prolonged bouts of acid reflux cause inflammation, tissue erosion, and ulcerations in the lower esophagus.

The doctor may order drugs to prevent stomach acid production. Some drugs promote emptying of the stomach. Surgery may be needed if drugs and lifestyle changes do not work. Lifestyle changes include:

- No smoking
- Not drinking alcohol

- Losing weight
- Eating small meals
- Wearing loose belts and loose-fitting clothes
- Not lying down until 3 hours after a meal
- Raising the head of the bed 6 to 8 inches. Blocks of cement or wood can be placed under the legs at the head of the bed.

Peptic ulcer disease (PUD). **Peptic** pertains to digestion or the enzymes and secretions needed for digestion. (*Peptic* means *to digest*.) An **ulcer** is a shallow or deep crater-like sore of a mucous membrane. A **peptic ulcer** is an ulcer in the stomach, duodenum, or other part of the GI system exposed to gastric juices.

PUD results from an imbalance between acidic stomach contents and the body's normal defense barriers that protect the stomach wall. Ulcers occur in the stomach (gastric ulcer) and duodenum (duodenal ulcer).

Epigastric pain is often the only symptom. It may be described as burning, gnawing, or aching. The pain is most often noted when the stomach is empty (usually at night or between meals) and can be relieved by food or antacids. Other symptoms include bloating, nausea, vomiting, and anorexia.

Ulcers appear to be caused by:

- Oversecretion of hydrochloric acid
- Injury to the mucosal barrier
- Infection of the mucosal wall

Risk factors include:

- A family history of PUD
- Stress
- Cigarette smoking
- Nonsteroidal antiinflammatory drugs (NSAIDs) (Chapter 17)
- Spicy foods
- Alcohol

Assisting With the Nursing Process. When giving a person antacids, you assist the nurse with the nursing process.

Assessment

- Ask about constipation or diarrhea.
- Measure blood pressure if the person has hypertension. Some antacids are high in sodium.

- Observe for edema and signs and symptoms of heart failure (Chapter 21). Some antacids are high in sodium.
- Observe for "coffee ground" vomitus and bloody or tarry stools. These signal GI bleeding.
- Ask the person to describe the onset, duration, and location of pain or discomfort.

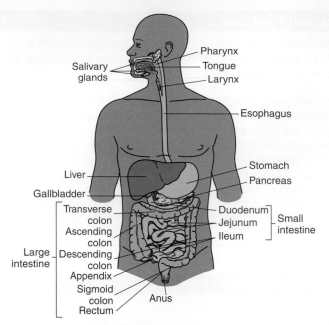

Fig. 26-1 Digestive system.

TABLE 26-1   Commonly Used Antacids

Product	Dose Forms
Gelusil	Tablets
Mylanta Advanced Maximum Strength	Suspension
Phillips' Milk of Magnesia	Tablets, suspension
Riopan Plus	Tablets, suspension
Rolaids	Tablets
Tums	Tablets

Planning. See Table 26-1 for "Dose Forms."
Implementation
- Follow directions on the MAR and product container.
- Give other drugs 1 hour before or 2 hours after giving antacids.
Evaluation. Report and record:
- *Chalky taste.* This is a common problem. The brand or flavor may need to be changed. The form may need to be changed from liquid to tablets.
- *Diarrhea, constipation.* Some products cause diarrhea. Others cause constipation. The drug order may alternate products.

DRUG CLASS: Histamine (H₂)-Receptor Antagonists

Histamine is a substance released in response to allergic reactions and tissue damage from trauma or infection. An antagonist is a drug that has the opposite action of another drug or competes for the same receptor sites.

Histamine causes an increase in the secretion of gastric juices. Histamine (H_2)-receptor antagonists block the action of histamine. Histamine (H_2)-receptor antagonists are also called *histamine blockers.* They bind to the H_2 receptor. This results in decreased amounts of gastric juices. The pH of stomach contents rises (the pH is less acidic).

These drugs are used to treat GERD, duodenal ulcers, and stress ulcers. A *stress ulcer* is a gastric or duodenal ulcer that develops in persons under severe stress. For example, a severe burn can cause a stress ulcer.

Assisting With the Nursing Process. When giving a person a histamine blocker, you assist the nurse with the nursing process.
Assessment
- Observe for confusion and orientation to person, time, and place.
Planning. See Table 26-2 for "Oral Dose Forms."
Implementation. See Table 26-2 for "Adult Dosage Range."
- The drug can be given with or without food.
- Give antacids (if ordered) 1 hour before or 2 hours after a histamine blocker.
Evaluation. Report and record:
- *Dizziness, headache, sleepiness.* These are usually mild and resolve with continued therapy. Provide for safety. Remind the person to use caution when driving or using machines.
- *Diarrhea, constipation.* Give drugs as ordered for diarrhea or constipation. Follow the care plan for fluid intake and diet.
- *Confusion, slurred speech, disorientation, hallucinations.* These may occur in persons with liver or kidney diseases and in persons over 50 years of age. They resolve over 3 or 4 days after therapy is discontinued. Provide for safety.
- *Anorexia, nausea, vomiting, jaundice.* These may signal liver toxicity.

DRUG CLASS: Gastrointestinal Prostaglandins

Prostaglandins are fatty acids. They are normally present in the GI tract. They inhibit gastric juice secretion—gastric acid and pepsin. This protects the stomach and duodenal lining from ulcers. Gastrointestinal prostaglandins inhibit gastric acid secretion. The following drug is a gastrointestinal prostaglandin:
- Misoprostol (mis oh pros' tohl); Cytotec (site' oh tek)

The drug is used to prevent and treat gastric ulcers caused by NSAIDs and aspirin (Chapter 17).

Assisting With the Nursing Process. When giving a person misoprostol (Cytotec), you assist the nurse with the nursing process.
Assessment
- Ask about diarrhea.
Planning
- The oral dose forms are 100 and 200 mcg tablets.
Implementation
- The adult dose is 100 to 200 mcg tablets four times a day.
- Give the drug with food during NSAID therapy.
Evaluation. Report and record:
- *Diarrhea.* This is dose-related, usually developing after about 2 weeks of therapy. It often resolves after about 8 days. It may be lessened by giving the drug with meals and at bedtime. Follow the care plan for fluid intake and diet.

DRUG CLASS: Proton Pump Inhibitors

Parietal cells in the stomach secrete gastric acid (hydrochloric acid). Proton pump inhibitors (PPIs) inhibit the

TABLE 26-2	Histamine (H$_2$)-Receptor Antagonists		
Generic Name	**Brand Name**	**Oral Dose Forms**	**Adult Dosage Range**
cimetidine	Tagamet HB	Tablets: 200, 300, 400, 800 mg Suspension: 300 mg/5 mL	Duodenal and gastric ulcers—800-1600 mg at bedtime, 400 mg twice daily, or 300 mg four times daily GERD—800 mg twice daily or 400 mg four times daily
famotidine	Pepcid	Tablets: 10, 20, 40 mg Suspension: 40 mg/5 mL	Duodenal and gastric ulcers—40 mg once daily at bedtime or 20 mg twice daily GERD—20 mg twice daily
nizatidine		Capsules: 150, 300 mg Oral solution: 15 mg/mL	Duodenal and gastric ulcers—300 mg at bedtime or 150 mg twice daily GERD—150 mg twice daily
ranitidine	Zantac; Zantac 75, 150	Tablets: 75, 150, 300 mg Capsules: 150, 300 mg Syrup: 15 mg/mL Suspension: 22.4 mg/mL in 250 mL bottle	Duodenal and gastric ulcers—300 mg at bedtime or 150 mg twice daily GERD—150 mg twice daily

gastric acid pump of the parietal cells. They block gastric acid production.

PPIs are used to treat severe esophagitis (inflammation of the esophagus), GERD, and gastric and duodenal ulcers. They may be used with antibiotics if infection is the cause of PUD.

Assisting With the Nursing Process. When giving PPIs, you assist the nurse with the nursing process.

Assessment
- Ask about diarrhea.
  Planning. See Table 26-3 for "Oral Dose Forms."
  Implementation. See Table 26-3 for "Adult Dosage Range."
- Capsules and tablets should be swallowed whole. They should not be opened, crushed, or chewed.
  Evaluation. Report and record:
- *Diarrhea, headache, muscle pain, fatigue.* These are usually mild. Follow the care plan for fluid intake and diet.
- *Rash.* This may signal an allergic reaction. Do not give the next dose unless approved by the nurse.
- *Muscle cramps, tremors, seizures.* These may signal a magnesium deficiency.

DRUG CLASS: Coating Agents

Coating agents form a substance that adheres to the crater of an ulcer. The agent protects the ulcer from gastric juices. It does not inhibit gastric secretions or change gastric pH. The following coating agent is used to treat duodenal ulcers:
- Sucralfate (sook rahl fate); Carafate (kair ah fate)
  This drug protects the ulcer from acids, enzymes, and bile salts. It can heal an ulcer, but will not prevent future ulcers from forming.

Assisting With the Nursing Process. When giving a person sucralfate (Carafate), you assist the nurse with the nursing process.

Assessment
- Ask about constipation.

Planning. The oral dose forms are:
- 1 g tablets
- 1 g/10 mL suspension
Implementation
- The adult dose is one tablet four times a day. Take 1 hour before each meal and at bedtime.
- The drug is given on an empty stomach.
- Antacids (if ordered) are given at least 30 minutes before or after sucralfate (Carafate).
Evaluation. Report and record:
- *Constipation.* This is usually mild and tends to resolve with continued therapy. Follow the care plan for fluid intake and diet.
- *Dry mouth.* Provide oral hygiene. This is usually mild and tends to resolve with continued therapy. The nurse may allow the person to suck on ice chips or hard candy.
- *Dizziness.* This is usually mild and tends to resolve with continued therapy. Provide for safety.

DRUG CLASS: Prokinetic Agents

Prokinetic agents are drugs that stimulate movement or motility. *Pro* means *forward. Kinetic* means *motion* or *movement.* The following is a prokinetic agent that is a gastric stimulant:
- Metoclopramide (met oh klo' prah myd); Reglan (reg' lan)
  The drug is used to:
- Lower esophageal sphincter pressure. This reduces acid reflux.
- Increase stomach contractions. This empties the stomach faster.
- Relax the pyloric valve. This allows stomach contents to empty into the duodenum faster.
- Increase GI peristalsis. This increases the rate of stomach emptying. The drug also moves chyme and feces faster through the intestinal tract.
- Prevent vomiting during cancer therapy.

Assisting With the Nursing Process. When giving a person metoclopramide (Reglan), you assist the nurse with the nursing process.

TABLE 26-3   Proton Pump Inhibitors

Generic Name	Brand Name	Oral Dose Forms	Adult Dosage Range
dexlansoprazole	Dexilant	Capsules: 30, 60 mg	Initial—60 mg once daily for 4 to 8 weeks Maintenance—30 mg once daily
esomeprazole	Nexium	Tablets, 24-hr delayed-release: 20 mg Capsules, 24-hr sustained-release: 20, 40, 49.3 mg Powder for suspension: 2.5, 5, 10, 20, 40 mg unit dose	Initial—20-40 mg once daily for 4 to 8 weeks Maintenance—20 mg daily
lansoprazole	Prevacid	Capsules, 24-hr sustained-release: 15, 30 mg Tablets, dispersible: 15, 30 mg Suspension: 3 mg/mL in 90, 150, 300 mL bottles	Initial—15-30 mg once daily 30 minutes before a meal for 4 weeks Maintenance—15 mg once daily Maximum—30 mg once daily before a meal
omeprazole	Prilosec	Capsules, sustained-release: 10, 20, 40 mg Tablets, sustained-release: 20 mg Powder: 2.5, 10 mg Suspension: 2 mg/mL in 90, 150, and 300 mL bottles	Initial—20 mg once daily for 4 weeks Maintenance—20 mg daily Maximum—120 mg three times daily for Zollinger-Ellison syndrome (a rare disorder causing pancreatic and duodenal tumors and gastric and duodenal ulcers)
pantoprazole	Protonix	Tablets, delayed-release: 20, 40 mg Powder for oral suspension: 40 mg	Initial—40 mg once daily for 8 weeks Maintenance—40 mg daily
rabeprazole	Aciphex, Aciphex Sprinkle	Tablets, delayed-release: 20 mg Capsules, sprinkle: 5, 10 mg	Initial—20 mg daily after morning meal for up to 4 weeks Maintenance—20 mg once daily Maximum—60 mg twice daily

Assessment

- Observe for GI bleeding.
- Ask about abdominal pain or discomfort.
- Observe for restlessness, involuntary movements, facial grimacing, abnormal tongue movements.
- Measure blood glucose if the person has diabetes.

Planning

- The oral dose forms are:
- 5 and 10 mg tablets
- 5 and 10 mg disintegrating tablets
- 5 mg/5 mL syrup

Implementation

- The adult oral dose is 10 to 15 mg four times a day. Take them thirty minutes before meals and at bedtime.

Evaluation. Report and record:

- *Drowsiness, fatigue, lethargy, dizziness, nausea.* These are usually mild and tend to resolve with continued therapy. Provide for safety. Remind the person to use caution when driving or using machines.
- *Restlessness, involuntary movements, facial grimacing, abnormal tongue movements.* Provide for safety.

■ REVIEW QUESTIONS

Circle the BEST answer.

1. Antacids:
   a. form a substance that adheres to the crater of an ulcer
   b. stimulate GI movement and motility
   c. block the action of histamine
   d. buffer, neutralize, or absorb hydrochloric acid in the stomach

2. A person has other drugs ordered. The drugs are given:
   a. with the antacids
   b. 30 minutes before the antacids
   c. 30 minutes after the antacids
   d. 1 hour before or 2 hours after the antacids

3. Antacids can cause:
   a. diarrhea or constipation
   b. orthostatic hypotension
   c. tachycardia
   d. blurred vision

4. An antacid is high in sodium. You should observe for signs and symptoms of:
   a. heart failure
   b. diabetes
   c. asthma
   d. urinary retention

5. Which can cause a chalky taste in the mouth?
   a. antacids
   b. coating agents
   c. proton pump inhibitors
   d. gastrointestinal prostaglandins

6. Histamine (H_2)-receptor antagonists result in:
   a. decreased amounts of gastric juices
   b. a low pH of stomach contents
   c. increased GI motility
   d. decreased GI motility

7. Histamine (H₂)-receptor antagonists are given:
   a. with food or milk
   b. on an empty stomach
   c. with antacids
   d. after meals

8. Which is a (H₂)-receptor antagonist?
   a. Tagamet HB
   b. Protonix
   c. Rolaids
   d. Phillips' Milk of Magnesia

9. Gastrointestinal prostaglandins:
   a. form a substance that adheres to the crater of an ulcer
   b. stimulate GI movement and motility
   c. block the action of histamine
   d. inhibit gastric acid secretion

10. Which drug is a gastrointestinal prostaglandin?
    a. Pepcid
    b. cimetidine
    c. Cytotec
    d. Carafate

11. Which drug is *not* a proton pump inhibitor?
    a. Pepcid
    b. Nexium
    c. Prilosec
    d. Prevacid

12. When giving a proton pump inhibitor, the dose form:
    a. should be swallowed whole
    b. should be opened
    c. should be crushed
    d. should be chewed

13. A person on PPIs should be monitored for muscle cramps, tremors, seizures. These may signal:
    a. liver toxicity
    b. a magnesium deficiency
    c. an allergic reaction
    d. constipation

14. Coating agents can cause:
    a. diarrhea
    b. heartburn
    c. constipation
    d. urinary retention

15. Which drug is a coating agent?
    a. Tums
    b. Zantac
    c. dexlansoprazole (Dexilant)
    d. sucralfate (Carafate)

16. Metoclopramide (Reglan) is given:
    a. 30 minutes before meals and at bedtime
    b. with food or milk
    c. on an empty stomach
    d. after meals

17. Which drug is prokinetic agent?
    a. metoclopramide (Reglan)
    b. esomeprazole (Nexium)
    c. misoprostol (Cytotec)
    d. ranitidine (Zantac)

18. Which drug class is a gastric stimulant?
    a. antacids
    b. coating agents
    c. prokinetic agents
    d. gastrointestinal prostaglandins

Answers to these questions can be found on the Evolve Resources site: http://evolve.elsevier.com/Anderson/medasst/

27

Drugs Used to Treat Nausea, Vomiting, Constipation, and Diarrhea

OBJECTIVES

- Define the key terms and key abbreviations used in this chapter.
- Describe nausea, vomiting, constipation, and diarrhea.
- Describe inflammatory bowel disease (IBD).
- Describe the drugs used to control nausea and vomiting.
- Explain how to assist with the nursing process when giving drugs to control nausea and vomiting.

- Describe the drugs used to control constipation.
- Explain how to assist with the nursing process when giving drugs to control constipation.
- Describe the drugs used to control diarrhea.
- Explain how to assist with the nursing process when giving drugs to control diarrhea.

KEY TERMS

Antidiarrheals Drugs that relieve the symptoms of diarrhea

Antiemetics Drugs used to treat nausea and vomiting

constipation The passage of a hard, dry stool

diarrhea The frequent passage of liquid stools

emesis Vomiting, vomitus

fecal impaction The prolonged retention and buildup of feces in the rectum

griping Severe and spasm-like pain in the abdomen caused by an intestinal disorder; gripping

laxatives Substances that cause evacuation of the bowel; *laxare* means *to loosen*

nausea The sensation of abdominal discomfort that may lead to the urge or need to vomit

retching The involuntary, labored, spasmodic contractions of the abdominal and respiratory muscles without vomitus; "dry heaves"

vomiting Expelling stomach contents through the mouth; emesis

vomitus The food and fluids expelled from the stomach through the mouth; emesis

KEY ABBREVIATIONS

GI   Gastrointestinal
h   Hour
IBD   Inflammatory bowel disease
MAR   Medication administration record
mg   Milligram

MI   Myocardial infarction
mL   Milliliter
PO   Per os (orally)
q   Every
VC   Vomiting center

Inflammatory bowel disease (IBD) is a group of disorders that involve chronic inflammation of the digestive tract. People with IBD may experience nausea, vomiting, diarrhea, or constipation. See Box 27-1.

Nausea is the sensation of abdominal discomfort that may lead to the urge or need to vomit. **Vomiting** (emesis) means expelling stomach contents through the mouth. It signals illness or injury. **Vomitus** (emesis) is the food and fluids expelled from the stomach through the mouth.

Nausea may occur without vomiting. Sudden vomiting may occur without prior nausea. However, nausea and vomiting often occur together.

Retching is the involuntary, labored, spasmodic contractions of the abdominal and respiratory muscles without vomitus. It is commonly called the "dry heaves."

BOX 27-1   Inflammatory Bowel Disease

Inflammatory bowel disease (IBD) is a group of disorders that involve chronic inflammation of the digestive tract. Two types of IBD are:

- Ulcerative colitis
- Crohn's disease

Ulcerative colitis. This involves inflammation and sores (ulcers) in the lining of the large intestine (colon) and rectum. The person may be constipated, but more often experiences severe diarrhea, abdominal pain, fatigue, and weight loss.

Crohn's disease. This involves inflammation of any part of the digestive tract. If the stomach and duodenum are involved, symptoms include nausea, vomiting, and epigastric pain. If the colon is inflamed, this typically causes abdominal pain, cramping, rectal bleeding, and diarrhea.

Treatment of IBD includes drug therapy, diet, and rest. The drugs in this chapter can be used to treat IBD symptoms.

Nausea and vomiting can occur with almost any illness. See Box 27-2 for the structures involved in vomiting. See Box 27-3 for the common causes of nausea and vomiting.

Constipation is the passage of a hard, dry stool. The person usually strains to have a bowel movement. Stools are large or marble-size. Large stools cause pain as they pass through the anus. Constipation occurs when feces move slowly through the bowel. This allows more time for water absorption.

See Box 27-4 for the common causes of constipation. Dietary changes, fluids, and activity prevent or relieve constipation. So do drugs and enemas.

Constipation can lead to fecal impaction if not relieved. Fecal impaction is the prolonged retention and buildup of feces in the rectum. Feces are hard or putty-like. The person cannot defecate. More water is absorbed from the already hard feces. Liquid feces pass around the hardened fecal mass in the rectum. The liquid feces seep from the anus.

Diarrhea is the frequent passage of liquid stools. Feces move through the intestines rapidly. This reduces the time for fluid absorption. The need to defecate is urgent. Some people may not get to a bathroom in time. Abdominal cramping, nausea,

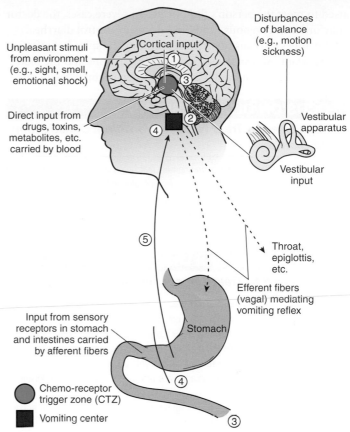

Fig. 27-1 Structures involved in vomiting. 1, Cerebral cortex. 2, Vestibular apparatus in the inner ear. 3, Chemoreceptor trigger zone and GI tract. 4, Serotonin receptors in the GI tract. 5, Neurokinin receptors in the vomiting center. (Adapted from Helms RA et al., eds: Textbook of therapeutics: drug and disease management, Philadelphia, 2006, Lippincott Williams & Wilkins.)

BOX 27-2   Structures Involved in Vomiting

The structures involved in vomiting are shown in Figure 27-1. The vomiting center (VC) is located in the medulla of the brain and coordinates the vomiting reflex. Nerves from sensory receptors in the pharynx, stomach, intestines, and other tissues connect directly with the VC through the vagus and splanchnic nerves. The nerves produce vomiting when stimulated.

The VC also responds to stimuli from other tissues—cerebral cortex, vestibular apparatus of the inner ear, and blood. These stimuli travel to the chemoreceptor trigger zone in the medulla. This activates the VC to induce vomiting.

When the VC is stimulated, nerve impulses are sent to the salivary, vasomotor, and respiratory centers. The vomiting reflex begins with a sudden deep inspiration that increases abdominal pressure. Abdominal muscles contract. The soft palate rises and the epiglottis closes. This prevents aspirating vomitus into the lungs. The pyloric sphincter contracts and the cardiac sphincter and esophagus relax. Stomach contents are expelled. Saliva increases to aid expulsion. Pallor, sweating, and tachycardia also occur with vomiting.

BOX 27-3   Common Causes of Nausea and Vomiting

- Chemotherapy
- Drug therapy
- Emotional disturbances
- GI disorders (Gastritis and liver, gallbladder, and pancreatic diseases are examples.)
- Infection
- Mental illness
- Motion sickness
- Overeating
- Pain
- Pregnancy
- Radiation therapy
- Stomach irritation by certain foods or liquids
- Surgical procedures
- Unpleasant sights and odors

BOX 27-4   Common Causes of Constipation and Diarrhea

Constipation
- A low-fiber diet
- Ignoring the urge to defecate
- Decreased fluid intake
- Inactivity
- Drugs
- Aging
- Certain diseases

- Spicy or fatty foods
- Lack of certain digestive enzymes
- Excessive use of laxatives
- Emotional stress
- Hyperthyroidism
- Inflammatory bowel disease
- Surgical bypass

Diarrhea
- Infections
- Some drugs

---

and vomiting may occur. See Box 27-4 for the common causes of diarrhea.

Fluid lost through diarrhea needs to be replaced. Otherwise, dehydration occurs and the person has pale or flushed skin, dry skin, and a coated tongue. The urine is dark and scant in amount (oliguria). Thirst, weakness, dizziness, and confusion may also occur. Falling blood pressure and increased pulse and respirations are serious signs. Death can occur. The nursing process is used to meet the person's fluid needs. In severe cases, the doctor may order intravenous fluids and drugs to control diarrhea.

Microbes can cause diarrhea. Preventing the spread of infection is important. Always follow Standard Precautions and the Bloodborne Pathogen Standard (Chapter 6) when in contact with stools.

FOCUS ON OLDER PERSONS

Drugs Used to Treat Nausea, Vomiting, Constipation, and Diarrhea

Older persons are at risk for dehydration from diarrhea. The amount of body water decreases with aging. Many diseases common in older persons affect body fluids. So do many drugs. Report signs of diarrhea at once. Ask the nurse to observe the stool. Death is a risk when dehydration is not recognized and treated.

DELEGATION GUIDELINES

Drugs Used to Treat Nausea, Vomiting, Constipation, and Diarrhea

Some drugs used to treat nausea, vomiting, constipation, and diarrhea are given parenterally—by intramuscular or intravenous injection. Because you do not give parenteral dose forms, they are not included in this chapter. Should a nurse delegate the administration of such to you, you must:

- Remember that parenteral dosages are often very different from dosages for other routes.
- Refuse the delegation but do not ignore the request. Make sure the nurse knows that you cannot give the drug and why.

See *Focus on Older Persons: Drugs Used to Treat Nausea, Vomiting, Constipation, and Diarrhea.*

See *Delegation Guidelines: Drugs Used to Treat Nausea, Vomiting, Constipation, and Diarrhea.*

DRUG THERAPY FOR NAUSEA AND VOMITING

Control of vomiting is important to:

- Relieve the distress caused by vomiting
- Prevent aspiration of stomach contents into the lungs
- Prevent dehydration
- Prevent electrolyte imbalance

Treatment is directed at the cause (see Box 27-2). Treatment measures may involve drug and non-drug measures. Antiemetics are drugs used to treat nausea and vomiting. They are generally more effective if given before the onset of nausea. Most antiemetics do one of the following:

- Suppress the action of the vomiting center (VC)
- Inhibit impulses going to or from the vomiting center (VC)

The goal of antiemetic therapy is relief of nausea and vomiting.

DRUG CLASS: Dopamine Antagonists

Dopamine antagonists inhibit dopamine receptors that are part of the pathway to the vomiting center. Dopamine receptors in other parts of the brain are blocked. See Chapters 15, 16, and 26.

Drugs in this class are the:

- Phenothiazines. They are used for mild to moderate nausea and vomiting associated with:
  - Anesthesia
  - Surgery
  - Radiation therapy
  - Chemotherapy
- Butyrophenones. These drugs are used as antiemetics in surgery and chemotherapy. Sedation is a side effect. Haldol is a butyrophenone that also works as an antipsychotic agent. See Chapter 16.
- Metoclopramide (Reglan). This drug also acts on receptors in the gastrointestinal (GI) tract. It is useful in treating nausea and vomiting associated with GI cancers, gastritis, peptic ulcer, radiation sickness, and migraine headache.

Assisting With the Nursing Process. When giving dopamine antagonists to relieve nausea and vomiting, you assist the nurse with the nursing process.

Assessment
- Observe the type, amount, and frequency of emesis.
- Observe the person's level of alertness.
Planning. See Table 27-1 for "Dose Forms."
Implementation. See Table 27-1 for "Adult Dosage Range."
Evaluation. Report and record:
- See Chapter 16 for phenothiazines.
- See Chapter 16 for haloperidol (Haldol).
- See Chapter 26 for metoclopramide (Reglan).

DRUG CLASS: Serotonin Antagonists

Serotonin antagonists block receptors in the medulla and GI tract that cause nausea and vomiting. They are used to treat emesis associated with:
- Chemotherapy
- Radiation therapy
- Postoperative nausea and vomiting

Assisting With the Nursing Process. When giving serotonin antagonists to relieve nausea and vomiting, you assist the nurse with the nursing process.

Assessment
- Observe the type, amount, and frequency of emesis.
- Observe the person's level of alertness.
Planning. See Table 27-1 for "Dose Forms."
Implementation. See Table 27-1 for "Adult Dosage Range."
Evaluation. Report and record:
- *Headache, diarrhea, constipation.* These are usually mild.
- *Sedation.* Provide for safety.

DRUG CLASS: Anticholinergic Agents

Motion sickness is thought to result from stimulation of structures in the inner ear. The stimuli are transmitted to areas near the VC. Excess acetylcholine is present. Anticholinergic agents are used to counterbalance the excessive amounts of acetylcholine present.

Assisting With the Nursing Process. When giving anticholinergic agents to relieve nausea and vomiting, you assist the nurse with the nursing process.

Assessment
- Observe the type, amount, and frequency of emesis.
- Observe the person's level of alertness.

TABLE 27-1 Antiemetic Agents

Generic Name	Brand Name	Dose Forms	Adult Dosage Range	Comments
Dopamine Antagonists				
Phenothiazines				Comments for All Phenothiazines
prochlorperazine	Compro	Tablets: 5, 10 mg Rectal suppositories: 25 mg	PO: 5-10 mg q6-8h Rectal: 25 mg twice daily	Phenothiazines may suppress the cough reflex. Ensure that the patient does not aspirate vomitus.
promethazine	Phenergan, Promethegan	Tablets: 12.5, 25, 50 mg Syrup: 6.25 mg/5 mL Oral solution: 6.25 mg/5 mL Suppositories: 12.5, 25, 50 mg	PO/PR: 12.5-25 mg q4-6h	Use with caution in patients (especially children) with undiagnosed vomiting. Phenothiazines can mask signs of toxicity of other drugs or mask symptoms of other diseases, such as brain tumor, Reye's syndrome, or intestinal obstruction. Use with extreme caution in patients with seizure disorders. Discontinue if rashes develop. May cause orthostatic hypotension.
Butyrophenones				
haloperidol (see Chapter 16)				
Metoclopramide				See Chapter 26, pgs. 251-252.
trimethobenzamide	Tigan	Capsules: 300 mg	PO: 300 mg three or four times daily	
Serotonin Antagonists				
dolasetron	Anzemet	Tablets: 50, 100 mg	100 mg within 1 hr before chemotherapy	Recommended for prevention of nausea and vomiting associated with chemotherapy.
granisetron	Sancuso (transdermal patch)	Tablets: 1 mg Liquid: 1 mg/5 mL Transdermal patch: 3.1 mg/24 hrs	1 mg up to 1 hr before chemotherapy, followed by a second dose 12 hrs later; or 2 mg once daily. Radiation therapy: 2 mg tablet once daily or 10 mL of oral solution within 1 hr of radiation therapy Apply one patch to the upper outer arm 24-48 hrs before chemotherapy. Patch may be worn for 7 days; do not remove for at least 24 hrs after chemotherapy.	Recommended for prevention of nausea and vomiting associated with cancer chemotherapy and radiation therapy.
ondansetron	Zofran, Zofran ODT	Tablets: 4, 8, 24 mg Tablets, orally disintegrating: 4, 8 mg Liquid: 4 mg/5 mL Oral film: 4, 8 mg	8 to 24 mg 30 minutes before chemotherapy, followed by 8 mg 8 hrs later 16 mg 1 hr before induction of anesthesia	Recommended for prevention of nausea and vomiting associated with cancer chemotherapy, radiation therapy, and post-operative nausea and vomiting.
Anticholinergic Agents Used For Motion Sickness				
dimenhydrinate	Dramamine	Tablets: 50 mg Chewable tablet: 50 mg	50-100 mg q4-6h; do not exceed 400 mg in 24 hrs	Will cause sedation. Beware of operating machinery.
diphenhydramine		Tablets: 12.5, 25, 50 mg Orally disintegrating strips: 12.5, 25 mg Capsules: 25, 50 mg Elixir: 12.5 mg/5 mL Liquid: 12.5, 25 mg/5 mL	PO: 12.5-25 mg three or four times a day; do not exceed 300 mg/24 hrs	
meclizine		Tablets: 12.5, 25 mg Chewable tablet: 25 mg	PO: 25-50 mg; may be repeated every 24 hrs	
scopolamine, transdermal	Transderm-Scop	Transdermal patch: 1.5 mg delivered over 72 hrs	Patch: Apply to skin behind ear at least 4 hrs before antiemetic effect is required; replace in 72 hrs if continued therapy required. Do not cut patches!	

TABLE 27-1   Antiemetic Agents—cont'd

Generic Name	Brand Name	Dose Forms	Adult Dosage Range	Comments
Corticosteroids dexamethasone		Tablets: 0.5, 0.75, 1, 1.5, 2, 4, 6 mg Elixir: 0.5 mg/5 mL Liquid: 1 mg/mL, 0.5 mg/5 mL	PO: 4-16 mg on day 1	Recommended for prevention of nausea and vomiting associated with chemotherapy. Used in combination with other antiemetics.
Benzodiazepines lorazepam	Ativan	Tablets: 0.5, 1, 2 mg Liquid: 2 mg/mL	0.5-2 mg q6h	Recommended for prevention of nausea and vomiting associated with chemotherapy.
Cannabinoids dronabinol (THC)	Marinol	Capsules: 2.5, 5, 10 mg	PO: Initial 5 mg/m2 1-3 hrs before chemotherapy, then q2-4h for a total of four to six doses/day Maximum: 15 mg/m2/dose	Schedule III controlled substance. Common adverse effects include drowsiness, dizziness, muddled thinking, and possible impairment of coordination, sensory, and perceptual functions. Use with caution in patients with hypertension or heart disease. Syndros is a Schedule II controlled substance requiring a new prescription.
nabilone	Cesamet	Capsules: 1 mg	PO: 1-2 mg two or three times daily Maximum: 6 mg daily in three doses	Schedule II controlled substance. Because of its potential for dysphoria, it should be used only when the patient can be supervised by a responsible individual.
Neurokinin-1 Receptor Inhibitor aprepitant	Emend	Capsules: 40, 80, 125 mg	125 mg 1 hr before chemotherapy on day 1; 80 mg daily in the morning of days 2 and 3 40 mg 3 hrs before anesthesia	Recommended for prevention of acute and delayed nausea and vomiting associated with initial and repeat courses of highly nauseating chemotherapy. Given to prevent post-operative nausea.
rolapitant	Varubi	Tablets: 90 mg	180 mg 1-2 hrs before chemotherapy in combination with dexamethasone and a serotonin antagonist	Use in combination with other antiemetics for the prevention of delayed nausea and vomiting in adults receiving highly emetogenic cancer chemotherapy
Fixed-dose combination: netupitant and palonosetron	Akynzeo	Capsule: netupitant 300 mg and palonosetron 0.5 mg	One capsule ~1 hr prior to initiation of chemotherapy on day 1 in combination with dexamethasone	Prevention of acute and delayed nausea and vomiting associated with initial and repeat courses of cancer chemotherapy, including, but not limited to, highly emetogenic chemotherapy.

Modified from Willihnganz M: Clayton's Basic Pharmacology for Nurses, ed 18, St Louis, 2020, Elsevier.

Planning. See Table 27-1 for "Dose Forms."
Implementation. See Table 27-1 for "Adult Dosage Range."
Evaluation. See Chapter 15.

DRUG CLASS: Corticosteroids

Corticosteroids used for nausea and vomiting are effective alone or when used with other antiemetics. They may help the person accept and control emesis because of these actions:
- Mood elevation
- Increased appetite
- A sense of well-being

Assisting With the Nursing Process. When giving corticosteroids to relieve nausea and vomiting, you assist the nurse with the nursing process.

Assessment
- Observe the type, amount, and frequency of emesis.
- Observe the person's level of alertness.

Planning. See Table 27-1 for "Dose Forms."
Implementation. See Table 27-1 for "Adult Dosage Range."
Evaluation. Report and record:
- Side effects do not occur often. Because only a few doses are given, the usual complications from long-term corticosteroid therapy do not occur (Chapter 28).

DRUG CLASS: Benzodiazepines

Benzodiazepines act as antiemetics through a combination of effects. They do the following:
- Cause sedation
- Reduce anxiety
- Depress the VC
- Have an amnesic effect (memory loss)

Benzodiazepines are effective in reducing the frequency of nausea and vomiting. They also reduce the anxiety associated with chemotherapy.

Assisting With the Nursing Process. When giving benzodiazepines to relieve nausea and vomiting, you assist the nurse with the nursing process.

> *Assessment*
- Observe the type, amount, and frequency of emesis.
- Observe the person's level of alertness.
> *Planning.* See Table 27-1 for "Dose Forms."
> *Implementation.* See Table 27-1 for "Adult Dosage Range."
> *Evaluation.* See Chapter 16.

DRUG CLASS: Cannabinoids

Smoking marijuana acts by inhibiting pathways to the VC. It is equally as effective as some phenothiazines, but less effective than metoclopramide. Because of the mind-altering effects and potential for abuse, they are mostly prescribed to people receiving chemotherapy.

Assisting With the Nursing Process
> *Assessment*
- Observe the type, amount, and frequency of emesis.
- Observe the person's level of alertness.
> *Planning.* See Table 27-1 for "Dose Forms."
> *Implementation.* See Table 27-1 for "Adult Dosage Range."
> *Evaluation.* Report and record:
- *Depressed mood, hallucinations, dreaming or fantasizing, distortion of perception, paranoid reactions, elation.* Frequently seen with higher doses. Provide for safety. The person must be warned not to drive, operate machinery, or perform duties that require alertness.

DRUG CLASS: Neurokinin-1 Receptor Inhibitor

Another antiemetic is used to prevent nausea and vomiting associated with chemotherapy and anesthesia:
- Aprepitant (a prep' eh tant); Emend (e mend')

The drug blocks the actions of substances that cause nausea and vomiting. It is used with a corticosteroid and a serotonin antagonist.

Assisting With the Nursing Process. When giving aprepitant (Emend) to relieve nausea and vomiting, you assist the nurse with the nursing process.
> *Assessment.* Observe the type, amount, and frequency of emesis.
> *Planning.* See Table 27-1 for "Dose Forms."
> *Implementation.* See Table 27-1 for "Adult Dosage Range."
> *Evaluation.* Report and record:
- *Tiredness, nausea, hiccups, constipation, diarrhea, loss of appetite, headache, hair loss.* The drug is taken for up to 3 days. Therefore, side effects are short-lived and rarely troublesome.

DRUG THERAPY FOR CONSTIPATION AND DIARRHEA

Laxatives are substances that cause evacuation of the bowel. (*Laxare* means *to loosen*). Antidiarrheals are drugs that relieve the symptoms of diarrhea.

DRUG CLASS: Laxatives

Types of laxatives are:
- Stimulant laxatives—act directly on the intestine. They cause an irritation that promotes peristalsis and evacuation.
  - Oral agents act within 6 to 10 hours.
  - Rectal agents act within 60 to 90 minutes.
- Saline laxatives—draw water into the intestine from surrounding tissues. The extra water affects stool consistency and distends the bowel. Peristalsis increases. These agents usually act within 1 to 3 hours.
- Osmotic laxatives—are similar to saline laxatives. They draw electrolytes and water into the intestine from surrounding tissues, resulting in diarrhea that cleanses the bowel so that the intestines can be seen during diagnostic procedures. These agents usually act within 15 to 30 minutes if takes as a suppository. If taken orally, they act within 24 to 96 hours.
- Lubricant laxatives—contain oils. They lubricate the intestinal wall and soften feces, allowing smooth passage of feces. Onset of action is often 6 to 8 hours but may be up to 48 hours. Peristalsis does not appear to increase. They are sometimes used to prevent constipation in persons who should not strain during defecation (e.g., persons recovering from myocardial infarction [MI] or abdominal surgery).
- Bulk-producing laxatives—are given with a full glass of water. The drug causes water to be retained in the feces. This increases bulk, which in turn stimulates peristalsis. Onset of action is usually 12 to 24 hours but may take as long as 72 hours.
- Stool softeners—draw water into the feces. This softens feces. These agents do not stimulate peristalsis. It may take 72 hours for a soft bowel movement to occur. These agents are often called *wetting agents*. Action from these agents depends on the person's hydration and their GI activity.
- Chloride channel activators—induce secretion of chloride-rich intestinal fluid without affecting sodium or potassium levels in the blood. This increases intestinal motility and helps with the passage of feces.
- Guanylate cyclase C agonists—are the newest class of drugs approved for the treatment of chronic constipation. They stimulate the secretion of chloride and bicarbonate into the intestine to increase fluid in the intestine and help with the passage of feces.

The goals of laxative therapy are:
- Relief from abdominal discomfort
- Passage of bowel contents within a few hours of administration

Assisting With the Nursing Process. When giving laxatives, you assist the nurse with the nursing process.
> *Assessment*
- Ask about the person's bowel elimination pattern.
- Ask the person to describe any abdominal pain.

TABLE 27-2 Laxatives

Generic Name	Brand Name	Laxative Type
bisacodyl	Dulcolax tablets	Stimulant
docusate sodium	Colace	Stool softener
glycerin	Glycerin suppositories	Osmotic
lactulose	Constulose	Osmotic
linaclotide	Linzess	Guanylate cyclase-C agonist
lubiprostone	Amitiza	Chloride channel activator
magnesium citrate	Citrate of Magnesia	Saline
magnesium hydroxide	Phillips' Milk of Magnesia	Saline
methylcellulose	Citrucel	Bulk-forming
methylnaltrexone	Relistor	Peripheral opioid antagonist
mineral oil	Mineral oil	Lubricant
naldemedine	Symproic	Peripheral opioid antagonist
naloxegol	Movantik	Peripheral opioid antagonist
plecanatide	Trulance	Guanylate cyclase-C agonist
polycarbophil	FiberCon	Bulk-forming
polyethylene glycol 3350	MiraLAX	Osmotic
polyethylene glycol–electrolyte solution	CoLyte GoLYTELY MoviPrep	Osmotic
psyllium hydrophilic mucilloid	Metamucil	Bulk-forming
sennosides	Ex-Lax Black Draught Senokot	Stimulant
sennosides and docusate sodium	Peri-Colace	Stool softener plus stimulant
sodium phosphates	Osmo-Prep	Saline

Modified from Willihnganz M: Clayton's Basic Pharmacology for Nurses, ed 18, St Louis, 2020, Elsevier.

Planning. See Table 27-2.
Implementation
- Follow directions on the MAR and container.
- Give adequate water with bulk-forming agents. Without enough water they can cause esophageal, gastric, intestinal, or rectal obstruction.

Evaluation. Report and record:
- *Griping (gripping), abdominal discomfort.* **Griping** (gripping) is a severe and spasm-like pain in the abdomen caused by an intestinal disorder. Griping and abdominal discomfort result from excessive bowel stimulation.
- *Abdominal tenderness, pain, bleeding, vomiting, diarrhea, abdominal distention.* No bowel movement or having only a small stool may signal an impaction. These are also symptoms of an acute abdominal condition. This is a serious problem that may require surgery.

DRUG CLASS: Antidiarrheal Agents

The two types of antidiarrheal agents are:
- Locally acting agents—absorb excess water to cause a formed stool. They absorb irritants or bacteria causing the diarrhea.
- Systemic agents—act through the nervous system to reduce peristalsis and GI motility. The intestinal lining can absorb nutrients, water, and electrolytes. This leaves formed feces in the colon. Reduced GI motility causes toxins to remain in the GI tract longer. This can cause further irritation.

Antidiarrheal agents are usually ordered:
- When diarrhea is of sudden onset, has lasted more than 2 or 3 days, and is causing significant fluid loss
- When persons with inflammatory bowel disease develop diarrhea
- Postoperatively for diarrhea after GI surgery
- When the cause of the diarrhea has been diagnosed and the healthcare provider determines that an antidiarrheal is appropriate for therapy

The goal of therapy is relief from diarrhea and its discomforts.

Assisting With the Nursing Process. When giving antidiarrheal agents, you assist the nurse with the nursing process.
Assessment
- Ask about the person's bowel elimination pattern.
- Ask the person to describe any abdominal pain.
Planning. See Table 27-3 for "Oral Dose Forms."
Implementation. See Table 27-3 for "Adult Dosage."
- Follow directions on the MAR and container.
- Give adequate water with bulk-forming agents. Without enough water they can cause esophageal, gastric, intestinal, or rectal obstruction.
Evaluation. Report and record:
- *Abdominal distention, nausea, constipation.* These may result from the excessive use of local agents.
- *Prolonged or worsening diarrhea.* Toxins may be present.

TABLE 27-3 Antidiarrheal Agents

Generic Name	Brand Name	Oral Dose Forms	Adult Dosage
Systemic Action			
difenoxin with atropine	Motofen	Tablets: 1 mg difenoxin with 0.025 mg atropine	Two tablets, then one tablet after each loose stool. Do not exceed eight tablets in 24 hrs
diphenoxylate with atropine	Lomotil	Tablets: 2.5 mg diphenoxylate with 0.025 mg atropine Liquid: 2.5 mg diphenoxylate, with 0.025 mg atropine per 5 mL	5 mg three to four times daily. Do not exceed 20 mg in 24 hrs

TABLE 27-3 Antidiarrheal Agents—cont'd

Generic Name	Brand Name	Oral Dose Forms	Adult Dosage
loperamide	Imodium A-D	Tablets: 2 mg Capsules: 2 mg Liquid: 1 mg/5 mL; 1 mg/7.5 mL	4 mg initially, followed by 2 mg after each un-formed movement. Do not exceed 16 mg/day.
Local Action Lactobacillus acidophilus	Lactinex	Capsules, granules	Two to four capsules, two to four times daily, with milk Granules: One packet added to cereal, fruit juice, or milk three or four times daily
bismuth subsalicylate	Pepto-Bismol	Tablets, chewable; 262 mg suspension; 262 mg/15 mL, 525 mg/15 mL	524 mg every 30 to 60 min or 1050 mg every 60 min as needed Maximum dosage: Approximately 4200 mg (eight doses of 262 mg; four doses of 525 mg) per 24 hrs

Modified from Willihnganz M: Clayton's Basic Pharmacology for Nurses, ed 18, St Louis, 2020, Elsevier.

REVIEW QUESTIONS

Circle the BEST answer.

1. Emesis means:
   a. diarrhea
   b. constipation
   c. retching or griping
   d. vomiting or vomitus
2. Drugs that cause bowel evacuation are called:
   a. antidiarrheals
   b. antiemetics
   c. laxatives
   d. enemas
3. Which is a phenothiazine used to control vomiting?
   a. prochlorperazine (Compro)
   b. haloperidol
   c. trimethobenzamide (Tigan)
   d. diphenhydramine
4. Which is often used to control motion sickness?
   a. ondansetron (Zofran)
   b. dexamethasone
   c. dronabinol (THC)
   d. dimenhydrinate (Dramamine)
5. Benzodiazepines are used to prevent nausea and vomiting from chemotherapy because they also:
   a. control diarrhea
   b. reduce anxiety
   c. improve alertness
   d. improve memory
6. Stimulant laxatives:
   a. cause an irritation that promotes peristalsis
   b. draw water into the intestine
   c. contain oils
   d. draw water into the feces
7. These statements are about lubricant laxatives. Which is *false*?
   a. They lubricate the intestinal wall.
   b. They soften feces.
   c. They may act within 6 to 8 hours.
   d. They increase the fecal mass in the bowel.

8. Which are often ordered to prevent straining during a bowel movement?
   a. stimulant laxatives
   b. saline laxatives
   c. fecal softeners
   d. bulk-forming laxatives
9. Which is *not* a laxative?
   a. Colace
   b. Metamucil
   c. Dulcolax
   d. Lomotil
10. A local-acting antidiarrheal agent:
    a. reduces peristalsis
    b. reduces GI motility
    c. absorbs excess water to cause a formed stool
    d. allows the toxin to remain in the intestine
11. Which is *not* an antidiarrheal agent?
    a. Imodium A-D
    b. Kaopectate
    c. Senokot
    d. Pepto-Bismol

Circle T if the statement is true. Circle F if the statement is false.

12. T F Some drugs used to control nausea and vomiting cause sedation.
13. T F Corticosteroids are sometimes used to treat constipation.
14. T F Phillips' Milk of Magnesia is a bulk-forming laxative.
15. T F Metamucil is a saline laxative.

Answers to these questions can be found on the Evolve Resources site: http://evolve.elsevier.com/Anderson/medasst/

28

Drugs Used to Treat Diabetes and Thyroid Diseases

OBJECTIVES

- Define the key terms and key abbreviations used in this chapter.
- Describe diabetes.
- Describe the drugs used to control diabetes.
- Explain how to assist with the nursing process when giving drugs to control diabetes.
- Describe hypothyroidism and hyperthyroidism.
- Describe the drugs used to treat thyroid diseases.
- Explain how to assist with the nursing process when giving drugs to treat thyroid diseases.

KEY TERMS

antidiabetic agents Drugs used to prevent or relieve the symptoms of diabetes

antithyroid agents Drugs used to suppress the production of thyroid hormones

cretinism Congenital hypothyroidism

diabetes A disorder in which the body cannot produce or use insulin properly

goiter An enlarged thyroid gland.

hyperglycemia High *(hyper)* sugar *(glyc)* in the blood *(emia)*

hyperthyroidism The disease that occurs from the excess *(hyper)* production of the thyroid hormones

hypoglycemia Low *(hypo)* sugar *(glyc)* in the blood *(emia)*

hypoglycemic agents Drugs that lower *(hypo)* the blood *(emic)* glucose *(glyc)* level

hypothyroidism The disease that results from inadequate *(hypo)* thyroid hormone production

insulin A hormone produced by the pancreas; it is needed for glucose to enter skeletal muscles, heart muscle, and fat

lactic acid A product of glucose metabolism

lactic acidosis A build-up of lactic acid in the blood

myxedema Hypothyroidism that occurs during adult life

thyroid replacement hormones Drugs that replace thyroid hormones in the treatment of hypothyroidism

KEY ABBREVIATIONS

F	Fahrenheit	mL	Milliliter
g	Gram	T_3	Tri-iodothyronine
GI	Gastrointestinal	T_4	Thyroxine
mcg	Microgram	TSH	Thyroid-stimulating hormone
mg	Milligram	TZD	Thiazolidinedione

The endocrine system is made up of glands (Fig. 28-1). The endocrine glands secrete hormones that affect other organs and glands. The pancreas and thyroid glands are part of the endocrine system. Diabetes is the most common endocrine disorder (Box 28-1). It involves the pancreas. Hyperthyroidism and hypothyroidism are thyroid disorders Box 28-2.

DRUG THERAPY FOR DIABETES

Insulin is required to control type 1 diabetes. If not controlled with diet and exercise, oral agents are used to treat type 2 diabetes. Many persons with type 2 diabetes need insulin:
- If it is not controlled with other measures Box 28-1
- During increased physical and psychological stress. Surgery, infection, and pregnancy are examples.

The goals of treatment for diabetes are:
- Normal blood glucose levels
- Fewer long-term complications from poorly controlled diabetes

DRUG CLASS: Insulin

Insulin is a hormone produced by the pancreas. Insulin is needed for glucose to enter skeletal muscles, heart muscle, and fat. It also is needed for protein and lipid metabolism.

The pancreas secretes insulin at a steady rate. It is released in greater amounts when the blood glucose rises, such as after a meal. Insulin deficiency reduces the rate of glucose transport into cells. This results in hyperglycemia.

See *Delegation Guidelines: Drug Class: Insulin.*
See *Promoting Safety and Comfort: Drug Class: Insulin.*

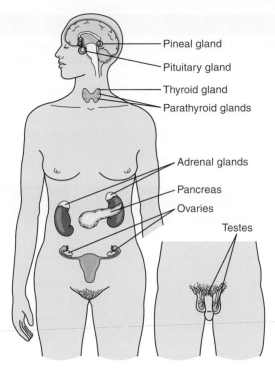

- Pineal gland
- Pituitary gland
- Thyroid gland
- Parathyroid glands
- Adrenal glands
- Pancreas
- Ovaries
- Testes

Fig. 28-1 Endocrine system.

DELEGATION GUIDELINES

Drug Class: Insulin

Insulin is given parenterally—by subcutaneous or intravenous injection. Because you do not give parenteral dose forms, you do not give insulin. Should a nurse delegate the administration of insulin to you, you must:

- Refuse the delegation but do not ignore the request. Make sure the nurse knows that you cannot give the drug and why.
- Some states allow MA-Cs to give insulin by the subcutaneous route. If you are allowed to give subcutaneous insulin, make sure that:
- You receive the necessary education about the drug and the dose form.
- You receive the necessary education and training to perform the skill correctly.
- A nurse is available to supervise you.
- A nurse is available to monitor how the drug affects the person.

PROMOTING SAFETY AND COMFORT

Drug Class: Insulin

Safety

Insulin should be stored in the refrigerator. It should not be allowed to freeze or be heated above 98° F. Once opened, an insulin bottle is discarded after 30 days, after which the contents may not be sterile. If not sterile, microbes can grow in the bottle. Prefilled insulin syringes are stored vertically with the needle up for up to 30 days.

Having cold insulin injected is uncomfortable. The agency may keep insulin at room temperature (68°F to 75° F). Insulin loses potency if kept above room temperature.

For most refrigerated insulins, the bottle or syringe is gently rolled between the hands (not shaken) to warm and remix the insulin. Label directions must be followed.

BOX 28-1 Diabetes

Diabetes is a disorder in which the body cannot produce or use insulin properly. Insulin is needed for glucose to move from the blood into the cells. The cells need glucose for energy. The pancreas secretes insulin. Without enough insulin, sugar builds up in the blood, resulting in high blood glucose (sugar). Cells do not have enough sugar for energy and cannot function. *Prediabetes* is when a person blood glucose is between normal and diabetes.

Three types of diabetes are:

- *Type 1*—occurs most often in children, teenagers, and young adults. The pancreas produces little or no insulin. Onset is over a few days to a few weeks.
- *Type 2*—can occur at any age, even during childhood. This is the most common form of diabetes. Persons over 40 years of age are at risk, but it can affect younger people also. Being overweight, lack of exercise, and hypertension are risk factors. The pancreas secretes insulin, but the body cannot use it well. Onset is slow. Infections are frequent. Wounds heal slowly. Gum disease is common.
- *Gestational diabetes*—develops during pregnancy. (*Gestare* means *to bear.*) It usually goes away after the baby is born but puts the mother at risk for type 2 diabetes later in life.
- There are some genetic defects, drugs, infections, surgeries, and diseases that can cause signs and symptoms that may appear similar to diabetes.

Risk Factors
- Family history
- Obesity
- Older than 45 years of age
- Lack of exercise
- Hypertension

These ethnic groups are at higher risk for diabetes:
- African Americans
- American Indians
- Alaskan Natives
- Hispanics

Signs and Symptoms
- Three P's.
  - *Polyuria*—urinating often
  - *Polyphagia*—feeling very hungry or tired
  - *Polydipsia*—feeling very thirsty
- Losing weight without trying
- Having sores that heal slowly
- Having dry, itchy skin
- Tingling or losing feeling in the feet
- Having blurred vision

Complications
- Blindness
- Dental diseases
- Renal failure
- Nerve damage
- Damage to the gums and teeth
- Sexual dysfunction and bladder incontinence
- Hypertension
- Stroke
- Heart attack

BOX 28-1   Diabetes—cont'd

- Slow healing (foot and leg wounds and ulcers can lead to infection and gangrene; amputation is sometimes necessary)

Treatment

Type 1 is treated with daily insulin therapy, healthy eating, and exercise. Type 2 is treated with healthy eating and exercise. Many persons with type 2 take oral drugs. Some need insulin. Overweight persons need to lose weight. Types 1 and 2 involve controlling blood pressure, cholesterol, and the risk factors for coronary artery disease.

The person's blood sugar level can fall too low or go too high. Blood glucose is monitored one to four times a day (Chapter 4). Observe the person for signs of:

- **Hypoglycemia** means low *(hypo)* sugar *(glyc)* in the blood *(emia)*.
- **Hyperglycemia** means high *(hyper)* sugar *(glyc)* in the blood *(emia)*.

See Table 28-1 for the causes, signs, and symptoms of hypoglycemia and hyperglycemia. Both can lead to death if not corrected. Alert the nurse at once.

Assisting With the Nursing Process. When a person receives insulin, you assist with the assessment and evaluation steps of the nursing process. If allowed to give insulin, you also assist with the planning and implementation steps. To assist the nurse, you need to understand the onset, peak, and duration for the type of insulin used (Table 28-2).

- *Onset*—the time required for the insulin to have an initial effect or action
- *Peak*—when the insulin will have the greatest effect
- *Duration*—the length of time that the insulin is active in the body

Knowing the onset, peak, and duration helps you know when a person is at risk for hypo- or hyperglycemia.

Assessment

- Measure blood glucose.
- Note the person's activity level.
- Note when and what the person eats.

Evaluation. Report and record:

- *Signs and symptoms of hypoglycemia.* See Table 28-1. These are more likely to occur when the insulin reaches its peak.
- *Signs and symptoms of hyperglycemia.* See Table 28-1.
- *Itching, swelling, redness at the injection site.* These signal an allergic reaction. Tell the nurse at once. If allowed to give insulin, do not give the next dose unless approved by the nurse.

DRUG CLASS: Biguanide Oral Antidiabetic Agents

Antidiabetic agents prevent or relieve the symptoms of diabetes. The following is a biguanide oral antidiabetic agent:

- Metformin (met for' mihn); Glucophage (glue' ko fagh)

Metformin (Glucophage) decreases the amount of glucose produced by the liver. It also decreases the amount of glucose absorbed by the small intestine. By improving insulin sensitivity, more glucose enters skeletal muscle cells and fat cells. Insulin must be present in the body for metformin to work. Therefore, this drug is not effective in treating type 1 diabetes.

The drug is used alone or with other oral antidiabetic agents.

Assisting With the Nursing Process. When giving metformin (Glucophage), you assist the nurse with the nursing process.

Assessment

- Measure blood glucose.
- Note the person's activity level.
- Note when and what the person eats.

Planning. The oral dose forms are:

- 500, 850, and 1000 mg tablets
- 500, 750, and 1000 mg 24-hr extended-release tablets
- 500 mg/5 mL oral solution

TABLE 28-1   Hypoglycemia and Hyperglycemia

	Causes	Signs and Symptoms
Hypoglycemia (low blood sugar)	Too much insulin or diabetic drugs Omitting or missing a meal Delayed meal Eating too little food Increased exercise Vomiting Drinking alcohol	Hunger Fatigue; weakness Trembling; shakiness Sweating Headache Dizziness Faintness Pulse: rapid Blood pressure: low Respirations: rapid and shallow Motions: clumsy and jerky Tingling around the mouth Confusion Vision: changes in Skin: cold and clammy Convulsions Unconsciousness
Hyperglycemia (high blood sugar)	Undiagnosed diabetes Not enough insulin or diabetic drugs Eating too much food Too little exercise Emotional stress Infection or sickness	Weakness Drowsiness Thirst Dry mouth (very) Hunger Urination: frequent Cramps: leg Face: flushed Breath odor: sweet Respirations: slow, deep, and labored Pulse: rapid, weak Blood pressure: low Skin: dry Vision: blurred Headache Nausea and vomiting Convulsions Coma

Modified from Willihnganz M: Clayton's Basic Pharmacology for Nurses, ed 18, St Louis, 2020, Elsevier.

Implementation. Adult dosages are:

- The initial dose is 500 mg twice daily or 850 mg once daily with the morning and evening meals.
- The dosage is increased by adding 500 mg to the daily dose each week or 850 mg every other week, up to 2000 or 2550 mg daily.

TABLE 28-2 Forms of Insulin

Type of Insulin	Strength (Units/MI)	Onset (Hours)	Peak (Hours)	Duration (Hours)*	Hyperglycemia†	Hypoglycemia†
Rapid-Acting Insulin **Insulin Analog Injection**						
Novolog (aspart)	100	0.2-0.33	1-3	3-5	After lunch (3)	Within 1-3 hours
Humalog (lispro)	100	0.2-0.33	0.5-2.5	3-5	After lunch (3)	Within 1-3 hours
Apidra (glulisine)	100	0.2-0.33	0.5-1.5	3-4	After lunch (3)	Within 1-3 hours
Short-Acting Insulin **Insulin Injection**						
Humulin R (human)	100, 500	0.5-1	2.5-5	5-10	Early AM (1)	Before lunch (3)
Novolin R (human)	100	0.5-1	2.5-5	8	Early AM	Before lunch
Intermediate-Acting Insulin **Isophane Insulin Suspension (NPH)**						
Humulin N (human)	100	1-2	4-12	16-28	Before lunch (2)	3 PM to supper (3)
Novolin N (human)	100	1-2	4-12	24	Before lunch	3 PM to supper
Isophane Insulin Suspension and Insulin Injection						
Humulin 70/30 (human)	100	0.5-1	4-12	24	Before lunch	3 PM to supper
Novolin 70/30 (human)	100	0.5-1	2-12	24	Before lunch	3 PM to supper
Lispro Protamine Suspension and Lispro Injection						
Humalog Mix 75/25	100	0.25-0.5	0.5-1.5	14-24	–	3 PM to supper
Novolog Mix 70/30	100	0.2-0.33	2.4	18-24	–	3 PM to supper
Long-Acting Insulin						
Lantus (glargine)	100	1.1	—‡	24	Mid-AM to mid-PM (1)	—‡
Levemir (detemir)	100	1	—‡	Up to 24	Mid-AM to mid-PM (1)	—‡
Toujeo (glargine)	300	1.1	—‡	24	Mid-AM to mid-PM	—‡
Basaglar (glargine)	100	1	—‡	Up to 24	Mid-PM	—‡
Tresiba (degludec)	100, 200	1	—‡	Up to 42	Mid-AM to mid-PM (1)	—‡
Long-Acting Insulin Plus Rapid-Acting Insulin						
Ryzodeg 70/30 (70% degludec/30% aspart)	100	0.2-0.33	1.15	Greater than 24	-	Mid-AM to mid-PM

*The times listed are averages based on a newly diagnosed diabetic patient or resident. Factors modifying these times include patient or resident variation, site and route of administration, and dosage.
†Most often occurs when insulin is administered: (1) at bedtime the previous night; (2) before breakfast the previous day; (3) before breakfast the same day.
‡No pronounced peak activity.
Modified from Willihnganz M: Clayton's Basic Pharmacology for Nurses, ed 18, St Louis, 2020, Elsevier.

- Most persons need at least 1500 mg daily for the desired effect.
- At dosages of 2000 mg and more, one of the following is ordered:
- The drug is given three times a day: 1000 mg with breakfast, 500 mg with lunch, 1000 mg with dinner.
- 850 mg is given three times a day with breakfast, lunch, and dinner.
  Evaluation. Report and record:
- *Nausea, vomiting, anorexia, abdominal cramps, flatulence.* These are usually mild and tend to resolve with continued therapy. Taking the drug with meals helps reduce these side effects.
- *Malaise, muscle pains, respiratory distress, hypotension.* These signal a buildup of lactic acid in the blood (**lactic acidosis**). **Lactic acid** is a product of glucose metabolism.

DRUG CLASS: Sulfonylurea Oral Hypoglycemic Agents

Hypoglycemic agents are drugs that lower *(hypo)* the blood *(emic)* glucose *(glyc)* level. Sulfonylureas lower blood glucose by stimulating the release of insulin from the pancreas. They also reduce the amount of sugar produced and metabolized by the liver. "First generation" sulfonylurea drugs were first produced over 30 years ago, The "second generation" of these drugs are used more often.

These drugs are used when the pancreas can still secrete insulin. Hypoglycemia may result if too much insulin is produced.

Assisting With the Nursing Process. When giving sulfonylureas, you assist the nurse with the nursing process.
   Assessment
- Measure blood glucose.

TABLE 28-3 Sulfonylurea Oral Hypoglycemic Agents

Generic Name	Brand Name	Oral Dose Forms	Initial Adult Dosage	Adult Dosage Range
First Generation				
chlorpropamide		Tablets: 100, 250 mg	100 mg daily	100-750 mg daily
tolazamide		Tablets: 250, 500 mg	100 mg daily	0.1-1 g daily
tolbutamide		Tablets: 500 mg	1 g twice daily	0.25-3 g daily
Second Generation				
glimepiride	Amaryl	Tablets: 1, 2, 4 mg	1-2 mg daily	1-8 mg daily
glipizide	Glucotrol	Tablets: 5, 10 mg	5 mg daily	15-40 mg daily
glipizide XL	Glucotrol XL	Extended-release 2.5, 5, 10 mg	2.5-10 mg daily	20 mg daily
glyburide	Glynase	Tablets: 1.25, 1.5, 2.5, 3, 5, 6 mg	2.5-5 mg daily	1.25-20 mg daily
		Tablets: 1.25, 2.5, 5 mg	2.5-5 mg daily	1.25-20 mg daily
		Tablets micronized: 1.5, 3, 6 mg	1.5-3 mg daily	0.75-12 mg daily

Modified from Willihnganz M: Clayton's Basic Pharmacology for Nurses, ed 18, St Louis, 2020, Elsevier.

- Note the person's activity level.
- Note when and what the person eats.
  Planning. See Table 28-3 for "Oral Dose Forms."
  Implementation
  See Table 28-3 for:
- "Initial Adult Dose"
- "Adult Dosage Range"
  Evaluation. Report and record:
- *Signs and symptoms of hypoglycemia.* See Table 28-1.
- *Anorexia, nausea, vomiting, jaundice.* These may signal liver toxicity.
- *Sore throat, fever, jaundice, weakness.* These may signal changes in red blood cells and white blood cells.
- *Rash, itching.* These may signal an allergic reaction. Tell the nurse at once. Do not give the next dose unless approved by the nurse.

DRUG CLASS: Meglitinide Oral Hypoglycemic Agents

Meglitinide oral hypoglycemic agents stimulate the pancreas to release insulin.

These drugs are used when the pancreas can still secrete insulin. They may cause hypoglycemia if too much insulin is produced. Insulin must be present in the body for meglitinide agents to work. Therefore, this drug is not effective in treating type 1 diabetes.

These drugs are used alone or with metformin (Glucophage). Meglitinides have a short duration of action. This reduces the risk of hypoglycemia.

Assisting With the Nursing Process. When giving meglitinides, you assist the nurse with the nursing process.
  Assessment
- Measure blood glucose.
- Note the person's activity level.
- Note when and what the person eats.

Planning. See Table 28-4 for "Oral Dose Forms."
Implementation. See Table 28-4 for "Daily Adult Dose."
- The dose is given 1 minute to 30 minutes before meals.
- Doses are taken two, three, or four times daily in response to changing mealtimes.
- The person should skip a dose if a meal is skipped to reduce the risk of hypoglycemia.
  Evaluation. Report and record:
- *Signs and symptoms of hypoglycemia.* See Table 28-1.

DRUG CLASS: Thiazolidinedione Oral Antidiabetic Agents

Thiazolidinedione (TZD) oral antidiabetic agents make muscle and fat cells more sensitive to insulin. This lowers blood glucose levels. TZDs also may decrease the amount of glucose produced and released by the liver.

These drugs are used when the pancreas can still secrete insulin. Insulin must be present for these agents to work.

Assisting With the Nursing Process. When giving TZDs, you assist the nurse with the nursing process.

TABLE 28-4 Meglitinide Oral Hypoglycemic Agents

Generic Name	Brand Name	Oral Dose Forms	Daily Adult Dose
repaglinide	Prandin	Tablets: 0.5, 1, 2 mg	Initial—0.5 mg before each meal Maximum dose—16 mg
nateglinide	Starlix	Tablets: 60, 120 mg	Initial—60-120 mg before each meal Maximum dose—360 mg

Modified from Willihnganz M: Clayton's Basic Pharmacology for Nurses, ed 18, St Louis, 2020, Elsevier.

TABLE 28-5 Thiazolidinedione Oral Hypoglycemic Agents			
Generic Name	Brand Name	Oral Dose Forms	Daily Adult Dose
pioglitazone	Actos	Tablets: 15, 30, 45 mg	Initial—15-30 mg once daily Maximum dose—45 mg
rosiglitazone	Avandia	Tablets: 2, 4 mg	Initial—2 mg twice daily or 4 mg once daily Maximum dose—8 mg

Modified from Willihnganz M: Clayton's Basic Pharmacology for Nurses, ed 18, St Louis, 2020, Elsevier.

Assessment
- Measure blood glucose.
- Note the person's activity level.
- Note when and what the person eats.
  Planning. See Table 28-5 for "Oral Dose Forms."
  Implementation. See Table 28-5 for "Daily Adult Dose."
  Evaluation. Report and record:
- *Nausea, vomiting, anorexia, abdominal cramps.* These are usually mild and tend to resolve with continued therapy.
- *Signs and symptoms of hypoglycemia.* See Table 28-1.
- *Anorexia, nausea, vomiting, jaundice.* These may signal liver toxicity.
- *Weight gain.* Weight gain of a few pounds is common. However, it may signal edema.

DRUG CLASS: Alpha-Glucosidase Inhibitor Agents

Alpha-glucosidase inhibitor agents block digestive enzymes that help the body digest sugars. This helps slow the absorption of glucose after meals. The advantage to using these agents is they will not cause hypoglycemia.

Assisting With the Nursing Process. When giving alpha-glucosidase inhibitor agents, you assist the nurse with the nursing process.
Assessment
- Measure blood glucose.
- Ask about GI symptoms.
- Note when and what the person eats.
  Planning. See Table 28-6 for "Oral Dose Forms."
  Implementation. See Table 28-6 for "Daily Adult Dose."
  Evaluation. Report and record:
- *Abdominal cramps, diarrhea, flatulence.* These are usually mild and tend to resolve with continued therapy.
- *Signs and symptoms of hypoglycemia.* See Table 28-1. Monitor for hypoglycemia if the drug is taken with other antidiabetic agents.
- *Anorexia, nausea, vomiting, jaundice.* These may signal liver toxicity.

DRUG CLASS: Sodium-Glucose Cotransporter 2 Inhibitors

Sodium-glucose cotransporter 2 inhibitors block the reabsorption of glucose from the kidneys into the blood. Glucose is excreted in the urine.

TABLE 28-6 Alpha-Glucosidase Inhibitor Agents			
Generic Name	Brand Name	Oral Dose Forms	Daily Adult Dose
acarbose	Precose	Tablets: 25, 50, 100 mg	PO: 25-100 mg three times a day. Take each dose with the first bite of each main meal. Maximum dose—≤132 lb (60 kg): 50 mg three times a day >132 lb (60 kg): 100 mg three times a day
miglitol	Glyset	Tablets: 25, 50, 100 mg	PO: 25-100 mg three times a day. Start at 25 mg once daily and gradually increase to 3 times a day to minimize GI adverse effects. Maximum dose—100 mg three times a day

Modified from Willihnganz M: Clayton's Basic Pharmacology for Nurses, ed 18, St Louis, 2020, Elsevier.

These drugs are used alone or in combination with other oral antidiabetic agents to treat type 2 diabetes.

Assisting With the Nursing Process. When giving sodium-glucose cotransporter 2 inhibitors, you assist the nurse with the nursing process.
Assessment
- Measure blood glucose.
- Monitor skin for sores or ulcers, especially on the feet and legs.
- Measure weight regularly.
  Planning. See Table 28-7 for "Oral Dose Forms."
  Implementation. See Table 28-7 for "Daily Adult Dose."
  Evaluation. Report and record:
- *Signs and symptoms of hypoglycemia.* See Table 28-1. Monitor for hypoglycemia if the drug is taken with other antidiabetic agents.
- *Urinary tract infection.* Notify nurse if urine appears cloudy or has a foul odor.
- *Hypotension, dehydration.* Provide for safety and maintain adequate hydration.
- *Pain, tenderness, or sores/ulcers to lower limbs.* Risk for limb amputation is higher when on this drug. Notify nurse immediately of these symptoms.

DRUG CLASS: Dipeptidyl Peptidase-4 Inhibitors

Dipeptidyl peptidase-4 inhibitors block the metabolism of the protein incretin. *Incretin* helps control blood glucose by:
- Helping with insulin secretion
- Decreasing the amount of glucose in the blood
- Slowing the absorption of sugars that come from food
- Maintain the cells that produce insulin

These drugs are used alone or in combination with other oral antidiabetic agents to treat type 2 diabetes.

Assisting With the Nursing Process. When giving dipeptidyl peptidase-4 inhibitors, you assist the nurse with the nursing process.

TABLE 28-7 Sodium-Glucose Cotransporter 2 Inhibitors

Generic Name	Brand Name	Oral Dose Forms	Daily Adult Dose
anagliflozin	Invokana	Tablets: 100, 300 mg	PO: 100 mg once daily Maximum dose—300 mg
dapagliflozin	Farxiga	Tablets: 5, 10 mg	PO: 5 mg once daily Maximum dose—10 mg
empagliflozin	Jardiance	Tablets: 10, 25 mg	PO: 10 mg once daily Maximum dose—25 mg
ertugliflozin	Steglatro	Tablets: 5, 15 mg	PO: 5 mg once daily Maximum dose—15 mg

Modified from Willihnganz M: Clayton's Basic Pharmacology for Nurses, ed 18, St Louis, 2020, Elsevier.

Assessment
- Measure blood glucose.
- Measure intake and output.
- Measure daily weight.
  Planning. See Table 28-8 for "Oral Dose Forms."
  Implementation. See Table 28-8 for "Daily Adult Dose."
  Evaluation. Report and record:
- *Signs and symptoms of hypoglycemia.* See Table 28-1. Monitor for hypoglycemia if the drug is taken with other antidiabetic agents.
- *Abdominal cramps, diarrhea, nausea, headache.* These are usually mild and tend to resolve with continued therapy.
- *Hives, rash, itching.* These may signal an allergic reaction. Tell the nurse at once. Do not give the next dose unless approved by the nurse.
- *Severe abdominal pain and vomiting.* These signal pancreatitis.
- *Nasal congestion, sore throat.* This could be a sign of an upper respiratory infection.
- *Edema, difficulty breathing, wheezing, frothy or blood-tinged sputum.* Check for swelling. See Chapter 22 for signs and symptoms of heart failure.

TABLE 28-8 Dipeptidyl Peptidase-4 Inhibitors

Generic Name	Brand Name	Oral Dose Forms	Daily Adult Dose
alogliptin	Nesina	Tablets: 6.25, 12.5, 25 mg	PO: 25 mg daily Maximum dose—25 mg
linagliptin	Tradjenta	Tablets: 5 mg	PO: 5 mg once daily Maximum dose—5 mg
saxagliptin	Onglyza	Tablets: 2.5, 5 mg	PO: 2.5-5 mg once daily Maximum dose—5 mg
sitagliptin	Januvia	Tablets: 25, 50, 100 mg	PO: 100 mg once daily Maximum dose—100 mg

Modified from Willihnganz M: Clayton's Basic Pharmacology for Nurses, ed 18, St Louis, 2020, Elsevier.

DRUG THERAPY FOR THYROID DISEASES

Hypothyroidism and hyperthyroidism are two thyroid disorders (see Box 28-1). There are two classes of drugs used to treat thyroid diseases:
- **Thyroid replacement hormones**—replace thyroid hormones. These are used in the treatment of hypothyroidism.
- **Antithyroid agents**—suppress the production of thyroid hormones. These are used in the treatment of hyperthyroidism. See *Delegation Guidelines: Drug Therapy for Thyroid Diseases.*

DRUG CLASS: Thyroid Replacement Hormones

Hypothyroidism is treated by replacing the thyroid hormones—T_3 and T_4. Thyroxine (T_4) is partially metabolized into T_3. Therapy with thyroxine (T_4) replaces both T_3 and T_4.

DELEGATION GUIDELINES
Drug Therapy for Thyroid Diseases

Some drugs used to treat thyroid diseases are given parenterally. Because you do not give parenteral dose forms, they are not included in this chapter. Should a nurse delegate the administration of such to you, you must:
- Remember that parenteral dosages are often very different from dosages for other routes.
- Refuse the delegation but do not ignore the request. Make sure the nurse knows that you cannot give the drug and why.

Assisting With the Nursing Process. When giving thyroid replacement hormones, you assist the nurse with the nursing process.
  Assessment
- Measure vital signs. Use the apical site to measure heart rate.
- Ask about bowel elimination.
- Measure weight.
- Observe for signs and symptoms of hyperthyroidism (see Box 28-2).
  Planning. See Table 28-9 for "Oral Dose Forms."
  Implementation. See Table 28-9 for "Adult Dosage Range."
- Levothyroxine should be taken on an empty stomach at least 45 minutes before eating.
- Most people take it immediately upon waking up, at least 45 minutes before breakfast.
  Evaluation. Report and record:
- *Signs and symptoms of hyperthyroidism.* See Box 28-2.

DRUG CLASS: Antithyroid Drugs

Antithyroid drugs block the formation of T_3 and T_4 in the thyroid gland. They do not destroy any T_3 and T_4 already produced. Once therapy is started, symptoms improve within a few days to 3 weeks.
  The following are antithyroid drugs:
- Propylthiouracil (pro' pil thy o you' rah sil); PTU, Propacil (pro' pa sil)
- Methimazole (meth im' ah zohl); Tapazole (tap' ah zoal)

Assisting With the Nursing Process. When giving antithyroid drugs, you assist the nurse with the nursing process.

TABLE 28-9 Thyroid Hormones

Generic Name	Brand Name	Oral Dose Forms	Composition	Adult Dosage Range
Levothyroxine	Synthroid Levoxyl	Tablets/capsules: 13, 25, 50, 75, 88, 100, 112, 125, 137, 150, 175, 200, 300 mcg	Thyroxine (T_4)	Initial: 12.5-50 mcg daily Maintenance: 100-200 mcg daily
Liothyronine	Cytomel	Tablets: 5, 25, 50 mcg	Liothyronine (T_3)	Initial—5-25 mcg daily Maintenance—25 to 75 mcg daily
Liotrix	Thyrola	Thyrolar-1/4: levothyroxine sodium 12.5 mcg/liothyronine sodium 3.1 mcg Thyrolar-1/2: levothyroxine sodium 25 mcg/liothyronine sodium 6.3 mcg Thyrolar-1: levothyroxine sodium 50 mcg/ liothyronine sodium 12.5 mcg Thyrolar-2: levothyroxine sodium 100 mcg/ liothyronine sodium 25 mcg Thyrolar-3: levothyroxine sodium 150 mcg/ liothyronine sodium 37.5 mcg	$T_4:T_3 = 4:1$	Initial: levothyroxine 25 mcg/liothyronine 6.25 mcg once daily Usual maintenance dose: levothyroxine 50-100 mcg/liothyronine 12.5 mcg
thyroid, USP	Armour Thyriod	Tablets: 15, 16.25, 30, 32.5, 48.75, 60, 65, 81.25, 90, 97.5, 113.75, 120, 130, 146.25, 162.5, 180, 195, 240, 260, 300, 325 mg	Unpredictable $T_4:T_3$ ratio	Maintenance—30-130 mg daily

Modified from Willihnganz M: Clayton's Basic Pharmacology for Nurses, ed 18, St Louis, 2020, Elsevier.

BOX 28-2 Thyroid Diseases

The anterior pituitary gland secretes thyroid-stimulating hormone (TSH). TSH stimulates the thyroid gland to release the hormones:

- Triiodothyronine (T_3)
- Thyroxine (T_4)

The thyroid hormones regulate metabolism. Imbalances in thyroid hormone production may interfere with:

- Growth and development
- Carbohydrate, protein, and fat metabolism
- Temperature regulation
- Cardiovascular function
- Lactation (producing and secreting breast milk)
- Reproduction

The goal of therapy for thyroid diseases is to return the person to a normal thyroid state.

Hypothyroidism

Hypothyroidism is the result of inadequate (hypo) thyroid hormone production. Severe hypothyroidism that is a life-threatening medical emergency with a high mortality rate is called Myxedema. It can lead to decreased level of consciousness, hypothermia, difficulty breathing, and myxedema coma. The onset of symptoms is usually mild and vague. They include:

- Slowness in motion, speech, and mental processes
- Lethargy—dullness, prolonged sleepiness, drowsiness, sluggishness
- Decreased physical activity
- Decreased appetite
- Weight gain
- Constipation
- Unable to tolerate cold temperatures
- Weakness
- Fatigue
- Low body temperature
- Dry, coarse, and thick skin
- Puffy face
- Low blood pressure
- Slow heart rate
- Anemia

- High cholesterol levels
- Increased susceptibility to infection

One cause of myxedema is the excessive use of antithyroid drugs. Such drugs are used to treat hyperthyroidism. Other causes include radiation exposure, thyroid surgery, and acute or chronic thyroiditis.

Congenital hypothyroidism is called **cretinism**. It occurs when a child is born without a thyroid gland or when the thyroid gland is hypoactive.

Fortunately, myxedema and cretinism are both rare occurrences.

Hypothyroidism is treated with thyroid hormones.

Hyperthyroidism

Hyperthyroidism occurs from the excess (hyper) production of the thyroid hormones. Signs and symptoms are:

- Rapid, bounding pulse (even during sleep)
- Palpitations
- Dysrhythmias
- Nervousness
- Agitation
- Tremors
- Low-grade fever
- Weight loss
- Increased appetite
- Insomnia
- Unable to tolerate heat
- Warm, flushed, and moist skin
- Increased sweating
- Edema around the eye
- Amenorrhea (no [a] menstruation [menorrhea])
- Dyspnea with minor exertion
- Hoarseness
- Rapid speech
- Increased susceptibility to infection

Causes of hyperthyroidism include thyroid cancer and tumors of the pituitary gland. Overdoses of thyroid hormones, thyroiditis, and goiter are also causes. **Goiter** is an enlarged thyroid gland.

Hyperthyroidism is treated with surgery, radioactive iodine, and antithyroid drugs.

Assessment
- Measure vital signs.
- Measure weight.
- Observe for signs and symptoms of hypothyroidism (see Box 28-2).
    Planning. The oral dose forms are:
- Propylthiouracil (PTU, Propacil): 50 mg tablets
- Methimazole (Tapazole): 5 and 10 mg tablets
    Implementation
- Propylthiouracil (PTU, Propacil):
    - The initial adult dose is 100 to 150 mg every 8 hours.
    - The dosage ranges up to 900 mg daily.
    - The maintenance dose is 50 mg two or three times a day.

- Methimazole (Tapazole):
    - The initial adult dose is 5 to 20 mg every 8 hours.
    - The maintenance dose is 5 to 15 mg daily.
    Evaluation. Report and record:
- *Rash, itching.* These often occur during the first 2 weeks of therapy. They usually resolve without treatment.
- *Headache, salivary gland and lymph node enlargement, loss of taste.* These are usually mild and tend to resolve with continued therapy.
- *Sore throat, fever, jaundice.* These may signal problems with blood cell production.
- *Anorexia, nausea, vomiting, jaundice.* These may signal liver toxicity.
- *Decreased urine output, bloody or smoky-colored urine.* These may signal kidney toxicity.

REVIEW QUESTIONS

Circle the BEST answer.

1. Insulin is a hormone produced by the:
    a. adrenal glands
    b. pancreas
    c. pituitary gland
    d. thyroid gland
2. Blood glucose is higher:
    a. before meals
    b. after meals
    c. at bedtime
    d. before breakfast
3. Once opened, an insulin bottle must be discarded in:
    a. 15 days
    b. 3 days
    c. 3 months
    d. 30 days
4. Insulin is usually stored:
    a. in the freezer
    b. in the refrigerator
    c. at room temperatures above 75° F
    d. for up to 45 days
5. To remix insulin, the nurse:
    a. shakes the bottle or syringe three times
    b. shakes the bottle or syringe six times
    c. turns the bottle or syringe upside down
    d. gently rolls the bottle or syringe between the hands
6. An insulin reaches its peak in 4 to 8 hours. This is when the insulin:
    a. has its initial action
    b. has its greatest effect
    c. remains active in the body
    d. must be discarded
7. A person received insulin. You assist the nurse by observing for:
    a. hypoglycemia
    b. hyperglycemia
    c. hypothyroidism
    d. hyperthyroidism

8. Metformin (Glucophage) is:
    a. a form of insulin
    b. an oral antidiabetic agent
    c. a hypoglycemic agent
    d. a first-generation sulfonylurea
9. The initial doses of metformin (Glucophage) are given:
    a. before each meal
    b. with the morning and evening meals
    c. after each meal
    d. on awakening and at bedtime
10. Sulfonylurea agents lower blood glucose by:
    a. decreasing the amount of glucose produced by the liver
    b. sensitizing muscle and fat cells to insulin
    c. stimulating the release of insulin
    d. inhibiting enzymes used to digest sugars
11. Which is *not* a sulfonylurea?
    a. glimepiride (Amaryl)
    b. glipizide (Glucotrol)
    c. glyburide (Glynase)
    d. repaglinide (Prandin)
12. Meglitinides are given:
    a. 1 hour before meals
    b. 1 hour after meals
    c. 1 to 30 minutes before meals
    d. 1 to 30 minutes after meals
13. Which is a thiazolidinedione?
    a. rosiglitazone (Avandia)
    b. chlorpropamide
    c. tolbutamide
    d. nateglinide (Starlix)
14. Sodium-glucose cotransporter 2 inhibitors block the reabsorption of glucose from the:
    a. liver
    b. stomach
    c. thyroid
    d. kidneys

15. A person is receiving a thyroid replacement hormone. You need to observe for:
    a. hypoglycemia
    b. hyperglycemia
    c. hypothyroidism
    d. hyperthyroidism
16. Which is a *not* a thyroid replacement hormone?
    a. liothyronine (Cytomel)
    b. levothyroxine (Synthroid)
    c. methimazole (Tapazole)
    d. liotrix (Thyrolar)
17. Levothyroxine (Synthroid, Levoxyl) is given:
    a. 30 minutes before eating
    b. 30 minutes after eating
    c. within 1 to 30 minutes of a meal
    d. 45 minutes before eating

Circle T if the statement is true. Circle F if the statement is false.
18. T   F   Insulin is always used to treat type 1 diabetes.
19. T   F   Incretin helps control blood glucose by slowing the absorption of sugar that comes from food.
20. T   F   Synthroid should be taken on an empty stomach.
21. T   F   Antithyroid drugs are used to treat myxedema.

Answers to these questions can be found on the Evolve Resources site: http://evolve.elsevier.com/Anderson/medasst/

29

Corticosteroids and Gonadal Hormones

OBJECTIVES

- Define the key terms and key abbreviations used in this chapter.
- Identify the purposes and uses of corticosteroids.
- Identify the corticosteroid preparations.
- Explain how to assist with the nursing process when giving corticosteroids.
- Identify the purposes and uses of gonadal hormones.
- Identify the estrogen preparations.
- Explain how to assist with the nursing process when giving estrogens.
- Identify the progestin preparations.
- Explain how to assist with the nursing process when giving progestins.
- Identify the androgen preparations.
- Explain how to assist with the nursing process when giving androgens.

KEY TERMS

androgens Steroid hormones that produce masculine effects

corticosteroids Hormones secreted by the adrenal cortex of the adrenal glands

endometriosis A condition (*osis*) in which the tissue that lines (*endo*) the inside of the uterus (*metri*) grows outside the uterus

estrogen The female hormone

eunuchism A condition in which the male lacks male hormones

glucocorticoids Hormones that regulate carbohydrate, protein, and fat metabolism; they have antiinflammatory, antiallergenic, and immunosuppressant activity

gonads The reproductive glands

hypogonadism A condition in which the body does not produce enough (*hypo*) testosterone

mineralocorticoids Hormones that maintain fluid and electrolyte balance

progesterone The hormone associated with body changes that favor pregnancy and lactation

testosterone The male hormone

KEY ABBREVIATIONS

g   Gram
mg Milligram

PO   Per os (orally)

CORTICOSTEROIDS

Corticosteroids are hormones secreted by the adrenal cortex of the adrenal glands (see Fig. 28-1 in Chapter 28). There are two categories:

- The **mineralocorticoids** maintain fluid and electrolyte balance. They are used to treat adrenal insufficiency caused by hypofunction of the pituitary or adrenal glands (Addison's disease).
- The **glucocorticoids** regulate carbohydrate, protein, and fat metabolism. They have antiinflammatory, antiallergenic, and immunosuppressant activity.

See *Delegation Guidelines: Corticosteroids and Gonadal Hormones.*

DRUG CLASS: Mineralocorticoids

The following is a mineralocorticoid:

- Fludrocortisone (flu droh kort' ih sown)

DELEGATION GUIDELINES
Corticosteroids and Gonadal Hormones

Some corticosteroids and gonadal hormones are given parenterally (by intramuscular or intravenous injection). Because you do not give parenteral dose forms, they are not included in this chapter. Should a nurse delegate the administration of such to you, you must:

- Remember that parenteral dosages are often very different from dosages for other routes.
- Refuse the delegation but do not ignore the request. Make sure the nurse knows that you cannot give the drug and why.

Fludrocortisone is a mineralocorticoid that affects fluid and electrolyte balance by causing:

- Sodium and water retention
- Potassium and hydrogen excretion

The drug is used with glucocorticoids. The goals of therapy are to:

- Control blood pressure
- Restore fluid and electrolyte balance

Assisting With the Nursing Process. When giving mineralo-corticoids, you assist the nurse with the nursing process.

Assessment
- Measure vital signs.
- Measure weight.
- Measure intake and output.
- Observe for signs and symptoms of infection. Corticosteroid therapy may mask signs and symptoms of infection.
- Observe level of alertness and orientation to person, time, and place.
- Test stools for occult blood.

Planning
- The oral dose form is 0.1 mg tablets.

Implementation. The adult dose is 0.1 mg daily.

Evaluation. Many side effects are related to dosage and duration of therapy. Report and record:

- *Changes in alertness and orientation to person, time, and place; confusion; muscle cramps; nausea.* These may signal electrolyte imbalance (potassium, sodium, and chloride).
- *Sore throat, fever, malaise, nausea, vomiting, other signs and symptoms of infection.* Corticosteroid therapy may mask signs and symptoms of infection.
- *Behavior changes.* Psychotic behaviors (Chapter 15) are more likely in persons with a history of mental health problems.
- *Signs and symptoms of hypoglycemia.* See Chapter 27.
- *Signs and symptoms of peptic ulcer.* See Chapter 25.
- *Vision problems.* These drugs may cause cataracts.
- *Delayed wound healing.* Observe surgical patients for signs of dehiscence (the separation of wound layers) (Fig. 29-1).

DRUG CLASS: Glucocorticoids

Glucocorticoids are given for their antiinflammatory, antiallergenic, and immunosuppressant effects. They relieve symptoms of inflammation, but do not cure disease. These drugs are used in the treatment of:
- Some cancers
- Organ transplants
- Autoimmune diseases
- Rheumatoid arthritis
- Allergy signs and symptoms
- Shock
- Nausea and vomiting from chemotherapy
  The goals of treatment are to:
- Reduce pain and inflammation
- Minimize shock and hasten recovery
- Reduce nausea and vomiting from chemotherapy

Assisting With the Nursing Process. When giving glucocorticoids, you assist the nurse with the nursing process.

Assessment
- Measure vital signs.
- Measure weight.
- Measure intake and output.
- Observe for signs and symptoms of infection. Corticosteroid therapy may mask signs and symptoms of infection.
- Observe level of alertness and orientation to person, time, and place.
- Test stools for occult blood.

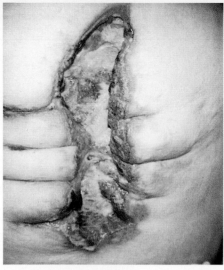

Fig. 29-1 Wound dehiscence. (Courtesy Kinetic Concepts, Inc. [KCI] Licensing, Inc., San Antonio, Tex.)

Planning. See Table 29-1 for "Dose Forms."

Implementation
- Persons taking these drugs for at least 1 week must not abruptly stop therapy. Abrupt stops in therapy may cause:
  - Fever
  - Malaise and fatigue
  - Weakness
  - Anorexia
  - Nausea
  - Dizziness
  - Hypotension
  - Fainting
  - Dyspnea
  - Hypoglycemia
  - Muscle and joint pain
  - Return of the disease process
- Follow the manufacturer's instructions to apply topical dose forms.
- Alternate-day therapy may be used for chronic conditions.
- Some corticosteroids are given between 0600 and 0900 on alternate days.
- Give oral dose forms with meals to lessen stomach irritation.

Evaluation. Many side effects are related to dosage and duration of therapy. Report and record:

- *Changes in alertness and orientation to person, time, and place; confusion; muscle cramps; nausea.* These may signal electrolyte imbalance (potassium, sodium, and chloride).
- *Sore throat, fever, malaise, nausea, vomiting, and other signs and symptoms of infection.* Corticosteroid therapy may mask signs and symptoms of infection.
- *Behavior changes.* Psychotic behaviors (Chapter 16) are more likely in persons with a history of mental health problems.
- *Signs and symptoms of hyperglycemia.* See Chapter 28.
- *Signs and symptoms of peptic ulcer.* See Chapter 26.
- *Vision problems.* These drugs may cause cataracts.
- *Delayed wound healing.* Observe surgical patients for signs of dehiscence (the separation of wound layers) (Fig. 29-1).

TABLE 29-1	Corticosteroid Preparations	
Generic Name	**Brand Name**	**Dose Forms**
alclometasone		Cream, ointment
amcinonide		Cream, ointment, lotion
betamethasone	Celestone Soluspan, Luxiq, Sernivo	Cream, ointment, lotion, emulsion, gel, foam, spray
budesonide	Entocort EC, Uceris	Oral extended-release capsule and tablet, rectal foam
clobetasol	Temovate, Clobex, Olux	Cream, ointment, solution, scalp shampoo, lotion, gel, foam
clocortolone	Cloderm	Cream
cortisone		Tablets
desonide	DesOwen, Verdeso	Cream, ointment, lotion, foam, gel
desoximetasone	Topicort	Cream, ointment, gel, liquid
dexamethasone	Decadron, Dexone, Hexadrol, Decaspray	Tablets, elixir, solution
diflorasone	ApexiCon E	Cream, ointment
fludrocortisone		Tablets
fluocinolone	Capex, Derma-Smoothe/FS, Synalar	Cream, ointment, solution, shampoo, oil
fluocinonide	Vanos	Cream, ointment, gel, solution
flurandrenolide	Cordran	Cream, ointment, tape, lotion
fluticasone	Cutivate	Cream, ointment, lotion
halcinonide	Halog	Cream, ointment
halobetasol	Ultravate	Cream, ointment, lotion
hydrocortisone	Cortef, Solu-Cortef, Hydrocortone	Cream, ointment, tablets, enema, gel, lotion, solution, suppositories, foam
methylprednisolone	Solu-Medrol, Depo-Medrol, Medrol	Tablets
mometasone	Elocon	Cream, ointment, lotion, solution
prednicarbate	Dermato	Cream, ointment
prednisolone	Veripred 20, Pediapred	Tablets, syrup, suspension, solution
prednisone	Deltasone, Rayos	Tablets, solution, liquid concentrate, delayed-release tablets
triamcinolone	Kenalog, Triderm	Cream, ointment, lotion, tablets, aerosol, paste

THE GONADS AND GONADAL HORMONES

The **gonads** are the reproductive glands: the testes of the male and the ovaries of the female (see Fig. 28-1 in Chapter 28). The testes produce sperm and **testosterone** (the male hormone). Testosterone controls the development of the male sex organs. It also controls the development of male secondary sex characteristics—voice, hair distribution, male body form. **Androgens** are other steroid hormones that produce masculine effects.

The ovaries produce estrogen and progesterone. These hormones stimulate development of the female sex organs. They influence breast development, voice quality, and the broader pelvis of the female body. **Estrogen** is the female hormone. It is responsible for most of the changes. **Progesterone** is the hormone needed for body changes favoring pregnancy and lactation.

DRUG CLASS: Estrogens

Estrogens are used:
- To relieve the hot flash symptoms of menopause
- For contraception
- For hormone replacement therapy after surgical removal of the ovaries
- As part of the treatment for osteoporosis
- To treat severe acne in females
- To slow the progress of advanced prostate cancers
- To slow the progress of some types of breast cancer

Assisting With the Nursing Process. When giving estrogen, you assist the nurse with the nursing process.

Assessment
- Measure vital signs.
- Measure weight.
  Planning. See Table 29-2 for "Dose Forms."
  Implementation. See Table 29-2 for "Adult Doses."
  Evaluation. Report and record:
- *Weight gain, edema, breast tenderness, nausea.* These tend to be mild and resolve with continued therapy.
- *Headache, migraine, dizziness, insomnia, anxiety, nervousness, emotional lability.* These tend to be mild and resolve with continued therapy.
- *Hypertension, signs and symptoms of hyperglycemia* (Chapter 28), *breakthrough uterine bleeding, signs and symptoms of thromboembolic diseases* (Chapter 24). These are complications of estrogen therapy.

DRUG CLASS: Progestins

Progesterone and the progestins inhibit ovulation. They are used to treat amenorrhea (no menstruation), breakthrough uterine bleeding, and endometriosis. **Endometriosis** is a condition (*osis*) in which the tissue that lines (*endo*) the inside of the uterus (*metri*) grows outside the uterus. The tissue usually grows on organs in the pelvic and abdominal areas. Symptoms include painful (often severe) menstrual cramps, lower back and pelvic pain, heavy menstrual periods, spotting between periods, and pain during or after sex.

The progestins may be used with estrogens as contraceptives (Chapter 30). The goals of progestin therapy are:
- Contraception
- Relief of endometriosis symptoms

TABLE 29-2 Estrogens

Generic Name	Brand Name	Dose Forms	Uses	Adult Doses
Conjugated estrogen	Premarin	Tablets: 0.3, 0.45, 0.625, 0.9, 1.25 mg Cream: 0.625 mg/g	Menopause Female hypogonadism Ovarian failure or postoophorectomy Osteoporosis prevention Breast carcinoma Prostatic carcinoma	PO: 0.3-1.25 mg daily cyclically* Intravaginal cream: 0.5-2 g intravaginally daily cyclically* PO: 0.3-0.625 mg daily cyclically* PO: 1.25 mg daily cyclically* PO: 0.3 mg initially daily cyclically*; dose may be titrated; use lowest effective dose PO: 10 mg three times daily for at least 3 months PO: 1.25-2.5 mg three times daily
conjugate estrogens and bazedoxifene	Duavee	Tablet: conjugated estrogens 0.45 mg, bazedoxifene 20 mg	Menopause; prevention of postmenopausal osteoporosis	PO: One tablet daily
Esterified estrogen	Menest	Tablets: 0.3, 0.625, 1.25, 2.5 mg	Menopause, atrophic vaginitis Female hypogonadism, postoophorectomy, ovarian failure Breast carcinoma Prostatic carcinoma	PO: 0.3-1.25 mg daily cyclically* PO: 1.25-7.5 mg daily cyclically* PO: 10 mg three times daily PO: 1.25-2.5 mg three times daily
estradiol	Estrace	Tablets: 0.5, 1, 2 mg	Menopause, atrophic vaginitis, hypogonadism, postoophorectomy, ovarian failure Prostatic carcinoma Breast carcinoma	PO: 1-2 mg daily cyclically* PO: 1-2 mg three times daily PO: 10 mg three times daily for at least 3 months
	Alora, Vivelle-Dot, Minivelle	Transdermal patch applied twice weekly: 0.025, 0.0375, 0.05, 0.075, 0.1 mg/24 hours	Menopause Female hypogonadism Primary ovarian failure Atrophic vaginitis Postoophorectomy Prevention of osteoporosis	Transdermal system: A patch should be placed on a clean, dry area of the skin on the trunk (usually abdomen or buttock) on a cyclic schedule. Rotate application site; interval of 1 week between uses of same site.
	Climara	Transdermal patch applied once weekly: 0.025, 0.037, 0.05, 0.6, 0.075, 0.1 mg/24 hours	Menopause Female hypogonadism Primary ovarian failure Atrophic vaginitis Postoophorectomy Prevention of osteoporosis	Transdermal system: A patch should be placed on a clean, dry area of the skin on the trunk (usually abdomen or buttock) on a cyclic schedule. Rotate application site; interval of 1 week between uses of same site.
	Menostar	Transdermal patch applied once weekly: 0.14 mg/24 hours	Prevention of postmenopausal osteoporosis	Transdermal system: A patch should be placed on a clean, dry area of the lower abdomen. Rotate site weekly. Remove old patch and discard appropriately.
	Divigel	Transdermal gel: 0.25 mg/0.25 g; 0.5 mg/0.5 g; 0.5 mg/0.5 g; 1mg/g	Menopause	0.25 g applied once daily; may apply 0.25 to 1 g daily based on symptoms
	Elestrin	Transdermal gel: 0.06%	Menopause	0.87 g applied once daily; may apply 0.87 to 1.7 g daily based on symptoms
	Estrogel	Topical gel: 0.06% in pump	Menopause; vaginal atrophy	Topical: Apply contents of one pump daily to one arm, spreading from wrist to upper arm on all sides. Allow to dry. Wash hands with soap and water. If uterus is intact, progestin should also be taken to prevent endometrial cancer. Alcohol gel is flammable until dry; avoid fire, flame, or smoking until dry.

Continued

TABLE 29-2   Estrogens—cont'd

Generic Name	Brand Name	Dose Forms	Uses	Adult Doses
	Evamist	Transdermal spray: 1.53 mg/spray	Menopause	Topical: One spray once every morning May apply one to three sprays daily based on symptoms
	Femring	Vaginal ring: 0.05/24 hours, 0.1 mg/24 hours	Menopause Vaginal atrophy	Intravaginally: 0.05 mg; adjust dose based on clinical response; ring should remain in place for 3 months
estropipate		Tablets: 0.75 mg	Menopause, atrophic vaginitis Female hypogonadism, postoophorectomy, ovarian failure Osteoporosis prevention	PO: 0.75-6 mg daily cyclically* PO: 1.25-9 mg daily cyclically* PO: 0.75 mg daily cyclically*

*Cyclically = 3 weeks of daily estrogen followed by 1 week off.

- Hormone balance to relieve amenorrhea or abnormal uterine bleeding

Assisting With the Nursing Process. When giving progestins, you assist the nurse with the nursing process.

Assessment
- Measure vital signs.
- Measure weight.
  Planning. See Table 29-3 for "Dose Forms."
  Implementation. See Table 29-3 for "Adult Doses."
  Evaluation. Report and record:
- *Weight gain, edema, nausea, vomiting, diarrhea, tiredness, oily scalp, acne.* These tend to be mild and resolve with continued therapy.
- *Breakthrough uterine bleeding, amenorrhea, breast enlargement, continuing headache, jaundice, depression.* These are complications of progestin therapy.
- *Pregnancy.* Birth defects are possible.

DRUG CLASS: Androgens

Androgens are used to treat:
- **Hypogonadism**—a condition in which the body does not produce enough *(hypo)* testosterone (the male hormone secreted from the male sex gland). This affects the development of the male sex organs and growth and development.
- **Eunuchism**—a condition in which the male lacks male hormones. The testicles were destroyed or removed. If this occurs before puberty, secondary sex characteristics do not develop.
- Androgen deficiency—lower than normal amounts of testosterone.
- Breast cancer in postmenopausal women. The goal is to suppress cancer growth and reduce discomfort.
- Wasting syndrome—a condition associated with acquired immunodeficiency (Chapter 35).

Assisting With the Nursing Process. When giving androgens, you assist the nurse with the nursing process.

TABLE 29-3   Progestins

Generic Name	Brand Name	Dose Forms	Uses	Adult Doses
medroxyprogesterone	Provera	Tablets: 2.5, 5, 10 mg	Secondary amenorrhea Abnormal uterine bleeding	PO: 5-10 mg daily for 5-10 days PO: 5-10 mg daily for 5-10 days, beginning on the 16th or 21st day of the menstrual cycle
norethindrone	Aygestin	Tablets: 5 mg	Amenorrhea, abnormal uterine bleeding Endometriosis	PO: 2.5-10 mg starting with the 20th and ending on the 25th day of the menstrual cycle PO: 5 mg for 2 weeks; increase in increments of 2.5 mg/day every 2 weeks until 15 mg/day is reached
progesterone	Progesterone, Prometrium	Tablets, capsules: 100, 200 mg; transdermal cream 10, 20% Vaginal gel: 4%, 8% Vaginal suppositories: 100, 200 mg	Amenorrhea, Endometrial Hyperplasia prevention	PO: 400 mg at bedtime for 10 days PO: 200 mg once daily at bedtime for 12 days sequentially per 28 day cycle

TABLE 29-4 Androgens

Generic Name	Brand Name	Dose Forms	Uses	Adult Doses
Short-Acting				
testosterone gel	AndroGel, Testim	Topical gel 1%, 1.62%	Male hypogonadism	Open one or more hormone packets (depending on dosage), squeeze entire contents onto palm of hand, and apply to clean, dry, intact skin of shoulders, upper arms, and abdomen. Allow to dry prior to dressing. Wash hands with soap and water. Do not apply to genitals.
testosterone USP in gel base	Androderm	Transdermal patch: 2, 4 mg	Male hypogonadism	One to three patches applied on hips, abdomen, thighs, or buttocks nightly for 24 hours; replace every 24 hours; do not apply to scrotum.
Oral Products				
testosterone	Striant	Buccal system: 30 mg	Hypogonadism	One buccal system applied to the gum above the incisor tooth every 12 hours. Alternate with opposite side for each new dose. When applying, hold the rounded surface against the gum for 30 seconds to ensure adhesion. Do not chew or swallow.
methyltestosterone	Methitest, Testred	Tablets: 10, 25 mg Capsules: 10 mg	Eunuchism Male hypogonadism Breast carcinoma	PO: 10-50 mg daily PO: 10-50 mg daily 50-200 mg daily, in one to four divided doses

Assessment

- Measure vital signs.
- Measure weight.
- Measure blood glucose. Androgens may cause hypoglycemia in persons with diabetes.

  Planning. See Table 29-4 for "Dose Forms."

  Implementation. See Table 29-4 for "Adult Doses."

  Evaluation. Report and record:

- *Stomach irritation.* Give the drug with food or milk.
- *Changes in alertness and orientation to person, time, and place; confusion; muscle cramps; nausea; edema.* These may signal electrolyte imbalance (potassium, sodium, chloride).
- *Women: masculine characteristics such as deepening voice, hoarseness, growth of facial hair, menstrual irregularities.* These may not reverse when therapy is discontinued.
- *Men: excessive sexual stimulation, priapism (prolonged or constant penis erection), breast enlargement. These signal androgen overdose.*
- *Nausea, vomiting, constipation, poor muscle tone, lethargy.* These signal hypercalcemia—high *(hyper)* blood *(emia)* calcium *(calc)* levels.
- *Anorexia, nausea, vomiting, jaundice.* These may signal liver toxicity.

REVIEW QUESTIONS

Circle the BEST answer.

1. Which maintain fluid and electrolyte balance?
   a. androgens
   b. estrogens
   c. glucocorticoids
   d. mineralocorticoids

2. Which have antiinflammatory, antiallergenic, and immunosuppressant activity?
   a. androgens
   b. estrogens
   c. testosterone
   d. mineralocorticoids

3. Testosterone is produced by the:
   a. adrenal glands
   b. gonads
   c. ovaries
   d. testes

4. Fludrocortisone is:
   a. an androgen
   b. an estrogen
   c. a glucocorticoid
   d. a mineralocorticoid

5. Fludrocortisone is used to:
   a. control blood pressure
   b. relieve inflammation
   c. treat nausea and vomiting from chemotherapy
   d. prevent conception

6. Oral glucocorticoids are given:
   a. before meals
   b. with meals
   c. after meals
   d. at bedtime

7. Which is *not* a corticosteroid?
   a. triamcinolone (Kenalog)
   b. dexamethasone (Decadron)
   c. conjugated estrogen (Premarin)
   d. methylprednisolone (Solu-Medrol)
8. Corticosteroids may cause signs and symptoms of:
   a. electrolyte imbalance
   b. masculine characteristics
   c. infection and inflammation
   d. allergies
9. A person has a history of mental health problems. Behavior changes may occur when taking:
   a. corticosteroids
   b. estrogens
   c. progestins
   d. androgens
10. Estrogens may be used in the treatment of the following, *except:*
    a. endometriosis
    b. menopause
    c. advanced prostate cancers
    d. some types of breast cancer
11. Which is a progestin?
    a. estradiol (Estrace)
    b. esterified estrogen (Menest)
    c. estropipate
    d. medroxyprogesterone (Provera)

12. Progestins are used for the following, *except:*
    a. breast cancer in postmenopausal women
    b. contraception
    c. endometriosis
    d. abnormal uterine bleeding
13. Male hormones are lacking because the testes were removed. This is called:
    a. androgen deficiency
    b. eunuchism
    c. hypogonadism
    d. priapism
14. Which is an androgen?
    a. medroxyprogesterone (Provera)
    b. fluocinonide (Vanos)
    c. methyltestosterone (Methitest)
    d. estradiol (Alora)

Circle T if the statement is true. Circle F if the statement is false.

15. T   F   Corticosteroids are secreted by the cerebral cortex.
16. T   F   Estrogen and progesterone are female hormones.
17. T   F   Many corticosteroids are applied topically.
18. T   F   Thromboembolic disease is a complication of estrogen therapy.

Answers to these questions can be found on the Evolve Resources site: http://evolve.elsevier.com/Anderson/medasst/

30

Drugs Used in Men's and Women's Health

OBJECTIVES

- Define the key terms and key abbreviations used in this chapter.
- Describe the sexually transmitted infections.
- Identify the drugs used to treat sexually transmitted infections.
- Describe the various types of contraceptives.
- Explain how to assist with the nursing process when contraceptives are taken.
- Identify the purposes for using drugs in obstetrics.
- Explain osteoporosis.
- Identify the drugs used to treat osteoporosis.

- Explain how to assist with the nursing process when giving drugs to treat osteoporosis.
- Explain benign prostatic hyperplasia.
- Identify the drugs used to treat benign prostatic hyperplasia.
- Explain how to assist with the nursing process when giving drugs to treat benign prostatic hyperplasia.
- Explain erectile dysfunction.
- Explain how to assist with the nursing process when drugs to treat erectile dysfunction are taken.

KEY TERMS

contraception The processes or methods used to prevent (contra) pregnancy

erectile dysfunction (ED) The inability of the male to have an erection; impotence

impotence See "erectile dysfunction"

leukorrhea An abnormal whitish (leuko) vaginal discharge (rrhea)

oral contraceptives Birth control pills

osteoporosis A bone disease that causes bones to become fragile and fracture easily

priapism A prolonged or constant erection

KEY ABBREVIATIONS

BPH Benign prostatic hyperplasia
ED Erectile dysfunction
GERD Gastroesophogeal reflux disease
MAR Medication administration record

mg Milligram
STI Sexually transmitted infection
TURP Transurethral resection of the prostate

Drug therapy for men's and women's health involves treating genital infections and sexually transmitted infections (STIs). Many women use contraceptives for birth control. Drugs also are used in obstetrics. Some men require treatment of prostatic hyperplasia or erectile dysfunction. Both men and women can be affected by osteoporosis.

DRUG THERAPY FOR LEUKORRHEA AND GENITAL INFECTIONS

Having vaginal secretions is normal. Excessive discharge is abnormal. **Leukorrhea** is an abnormal whitish (leuko) vaginal discharge (rrhea). A symptom of an underlying disorder, it can occur at any age. The most common cause is an infection.

STIs are described in Table 30-1. See Table 30-2 for drugs used to treat genital infections. Also see Chapter 35.

DRUGS USED FOR CONTRACEPTION

Contraception means the process or methods used to prevent (contra) pregnancy. **Oral contraceptives** (birth control

pills) are the most common form of birth control in the United States. The goal of contraceptive therapy is to prevent pregnancy.

See Box 30-1 for a review of menstruation and fertilization.

DRUG CLASS: Oral Contraceptives

Oral contraceptives prevent ovulation. The two types of oral contraceptives are:

- The combination pill. It contains both estrogen and progestin. These pills are packaged with 28 tablets. The last 7 tablets contain iron but no hormones. The package has 28 tablets so there is no break in the daily routine of taking a pill. The four types of combination pills are:
  - Monophasic. They contain a fixed amount of estrogen and progestin given daily for 21 days. The first dose is taken on day 5 of the menstrual cycle.
  - Biphasic. They contain a fixed amount of estrogen and progestin on days 1 through 10 that is lower than the dose given on days 11 through 21 of the menstrual cycle.

TABLE 30-1   Sexually Transmitted Infections

Disease	Signs and Symptoms	Treatment
Herpes	Painful, blister-like sores on or near the genitals, mouth, or anus The sores may have a watery discharge Pain, itching, burning, and tingling in the affected area Vaginal discharge Pain during urination or intercourse Fever Swollen glands	No known cure Antiviral drugs
Genital warts	*Male*—Warts in or on the penis, anus, genitalia, mouth, or throat *Female*—Warts in or on the vagina, cervix, labia, anus, mouth, or throat	Application of special ointment that causes the warts to dry up and fall off
HIV/AIDS	Loss of appetite Cough Depression Diarrhea lasting more than 1 week Lack of energy Fever Headache Memory loss, confusion, and forgetfulness Mouth or tongue: • Brown, red, pink, or purple spots or blotches • Sores or white patches Night sweats Pneumonia Shortness of breath Skin: • Rashes or flaky skin • Brown, red, pink, or purple spots or blotches on the skin, eyelids, or nose Painful or difficult swallowing Swollen glands in the neck, underarms, and groin Tiredness: may be extreme Vision loss Weight loss	Antiviral and antifungal drugs
Gonorrhea	Burning and pain during urination Urinary frequency and urgency Genital discharge (vagina, urethra, rectum)	Antibiotic drugs
Chlamydia	May not show symptoms Discharge from the penis or vagina Burning or pain during urination Testicular pain or swelling Vaginal bleeding Rectal inflammation and/or discharge Pain during intercourse Diarrhea Nausea Abdominal pain Fever	Antibiotic drugs
Pubic lice	Intense itching	Over-the-counter or prescription lice treatment; washing or dry-cleaning all exposed clothing, bedding, and towels
Trichomoniasis (occurs in women; men are carriers)	No symptoms in men Frothy, thick, foul-smelling, yellow vaginal discharge Genital itching and irritation Burning and pain during urination Genital swelling	Metronidazole
Syphilis	*Stage 1:* Ten to 90 days after exposure • Painless sores (chancres) on the penis, in the vagina, or on the genitalia; the chancre may also be on the lips, inside of the mouth, or anywhere on the body	Penicillin and other antibiotic drugs

TABLE 30-1	Sexually Transmitted Infections—cont'd	
Disease	Signs and Symptoms	Treatment
Syphilis—cont'd	*Stage 2:* About 3 to 6 weeks after the sores • General fatigue, loss of appetite, nausea, fever, headache, rash, swollen glands, sore throat, bone and joint pain, hair loss, lesions on the lips and genitalia • Symptoms may come and go for many years • *Stage 3:* Three to 15 years after infection • Central nervous system damage (including paralysis), heart damage, blindness, liver damage, mental health problems, death	

Modified from Willihnganz M: Clayton's Basic Pharmacology for Nurses, ed 18, St Louis, 2020, Elsevier.

TABLE 30-2 Causative Organisms and Products Used to Treat Genital Infections

Causative Organism	Generic Name	Brand Name
Vaginitis		
Candida albicans (fungus)	butoconazole vaginal cream	Gynazolel 1;
	clotrimazole vaginal cream, vaginal tablets	Gyne-Lotrimin,
	fluconazole oral tablets	Diflucan
	itraconazole oral capsules	Sporanox
	miconazole vaginal cream, suppositories	Monistat 3, Monistat 7
	terconazole vaginal cream, suppositories	
Trichomonas vaginalis (protozoa)	metronidazole oral tablets	Flagyl
	tinidazole oral tablets	Tindamax
Bacterial vaginosis	metronidazole oral tablets, vaginal gel	Flagyl; MetroGel-Vaginal
	clindamycin vaginal cream	Cleocin
	tinidazole oral tablets	Tindamax
Gonorrhea		
Neisseria gonorrhea (bacteria)	ceftriaxone	
	cefixime	Suprax
	azithromycin	Zithromax
	doxycycline	Vibramycin
Syphilis		
Treponema pallidum (spirochete)	penicillin G benzathine	Bicillin L-A
	tetracycline	Tetracycline
	doxycycline	Vibramycin
	azithromycin	Zithromax
Genital Herpes		
Herpes simplex genitalis (virus)	acyclovir oral capsules	Zovirax
	famciclovir oral tablets	
	valacyclovir oral tablets	Valtrex
Chlamydia		
Chlamydia trachomatis (chlamydia)	azithromycin	Zithromax
	doxycycline	Vibramycin
	erythromycin	Erythromycin
	levofloxacin	
	ofloxacin	

Data from Workowski KA, Bolan GA; Centers for Disease Control and Prevention. Sexually transmitted diseases treatment guidelines, 2015. MMWR Recomm Rep. 2015;64(No. RR-3):1-137; Gilbert DN, Chambers HF, Eliopoulos GM, et al. The Sanford Guide to Antimicrobial Therapy 2014, 44th ed. Sperryville, VA: Antimicrobial Therapy, Inc.; 2014.

BOX 30-1 Menstruation and Fertilization

Menstruation. The endometrium is rich in blood to nourish the cell that grows into a fetus. If pregnancy does not occur, the endometrium breaks up and is discharged from the body through the vagina. This process is called *menstruation*. Menstruation occurs about every 28 days. Therefore, it is called the *menstrual cycle (period).*

The first day of the menstrual cycle begins with menstruation. Blood flows from the uterus through the vaginal opening. Menstrual flow usually lasts 3 to 7 days. Ovulation occurs during the next phase. An ovum matures in an ovary and is released. Ovulation usually occurs on or around day 14 of the cycle.

Meanwhile, estrogen and progesterone (the female hormones) are secreted by the ovaries. These hormones cause the endometrium to thicken for pregnancy. If pregnancy does not occur, the hormones decrease in amount. This causes the blood supply to the endometrium to decrease. The endometrium breaks up. It is discharged through the vagina. Another menstrual cycle begins.

Fertilization. To reproduce, a male sex cell (sperm) must unite with a female sex cell (ovum). The uniting of the sperm and ovum into one cell is called *fertilization.* A sperm has 23 chromosomes. An ovum has 23 chromosomes. The fertilized cell has 46 chromosomes.

During intercourse, millions of sperm are deposited into the vagina. Sperm travel up the cervix, through the uterus, and into the fallopian tubes (Fig. 30-1). If a sperm and an ovum unite in a fallopian tube, fertilization results, and pregnancy occurs. The fertilized cell travels down the fallopian tube to the uterus. After a short time, the fertilized cell implants in the thick endometrium and grows during pregnancy.

• Triphasic. They contain three concentrations of estrogen and progestin to provide the lowest doses necessary to prevent conception.
• Quadriphasic. They contain four concentrations of estrogen and progestin to provide the lowest doses necessary to prevent conception.
• The minipill. It contains only progestin. All 28 tablets contain an active hormone.

Extended-cycle and continuous-cycle oral contraceptives are new combination oral contraceptives. The woman has only four menstrual periods each year. The drug shortens the duration of the menstrual cycle and for some may eliminate menses altogether. The drug contains estrogen and progestin in lower doses than other combination oral contraceptives. The package has 24 active tablets and 4 that contain no hormones (24/4), or 84 active tablets and 7 that contain no hormones (84/7). One tablet is taken daily.

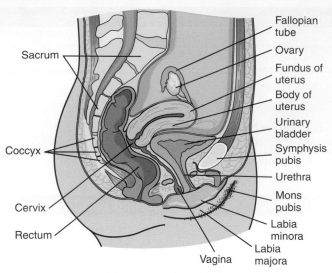

Fig. 30-1 Female reproductive system.

Assisting With the Nursing Process. When giving oral contraceptives, you assist the nurse with the nursing process.

Assessment
- Measure weight.
- Measure blood pressure in the supine and sitting positions.

Planning. See Box 30-2.

Implementation
- Combination pills: The first pill is taken on the first Sunday after the period begins. One pill is taken daily at the same time until the pack is gone.
- 21-day pack—wait 1 week and start a new pack on Sunday.
- 28-day pack—start a new pack the day after finishing a pack.
- Minipills: The first pill is taken on the first day of the period.

BOX 30-2   Oral Contraceptives

Monophasic Oral Contraceptives	Enpresse-28
Altavera	Estrostep Fe
Apri	Ortho Tri-Cyclen Lo
Aviane	
Brevicon	**Quadriphasic Oral Contraceptives**
Cryselle	Natazia
Junel 1/20	
Kelnor 1/35	**Progestin-only Contraceptives**
Ortho-Cyclen	Camila
Quasense	Errin
Yaz	Heather
	Jolivette
Biphasic Oral Contraceptives	Ortho-Micronor
Amenthia	Nora-BE
Lo Loestrin FE	Norlyda
Mircette	Sharobel
Necon 10/11	Tulana
Triphasic Oral Contraceptives	
Aranelle	
Caziant	

- Another form of birth control is needed the first month.
- One pill is taken daily at the same time of day until the pack is gone.
- Follow the nurse's directions for missed doses.

Evaluation. Report and record:
- *Nausea, weight gain, spotting, changed menstrual flow, missed periods, depression, mood changes, headaches, and brown pigmentation on the forehead, cheeks, and nose. These are common side effects. A prescription change is needed if they do not resolve after 3 months.*
- *Vaginal discharge, breakthrough bleeding, yeast infection. A prescription change and additional drugs may be needed.*
- *Blurred vision, severe headaches, dizziness, leg pain, chest pain, shortness of breath, acute abdominal pain. These may signal serious complications.*

DRUG CLASS: Transdermal Contraceptive

The following is a transdermal contraceptive:
- Norelgestromin-ethinyl estradiol transdermal system (nor ehl ges' troh min); Xulane (zoo' lane)

The drug contains estrogen and progestin to inhibit ovulation. Cervical mucus becomes thick and inhibits sperm from traveling up the cervix to the uterus and fallopian tubes. The hormones also change the endometrial wall. This impairs implantation of a fertilized ovum.

One of the following methods is used:
- First day start. Apply the first patch during the first 24 hours of the menstrual period. Note the day of the week. This becomes "patch change day."
- Sunday start. Apply the first patch on the first Sunday after menstruation begins. This becomes "patch change day."

Assisting With the Nursing Process. When applying a transdermal contraceptive, you assist the nurse with the nursing process.

Assessment
- Measure blood pressure in the supine and sitting positions.

Planning
- The dose form is a transdermal patch with 4.86 mg norelgestromin and 0.53 mg ethinyl estradiol.

Implementation
- Apply a new patch on the same day of the week. This day is called "patch change day."
- Apply a patch to clean, dry, intact, healthy skin. Do not apply the patch to an irritated area.
- The patch sites are the buttock, abdomen, upper outer arm, or upper torso. Do not apply a patch on a breast. Avoid areas where tight clothing can rub the patch.
- Do not apply makeup, powder, lotion, or cream to the skin or patch area. The patch may not adhere properly. Hormone absorption may be impaired.
- Follow the nurse's directions if a patch is loose or comes off.
- Another form of birth control is needed the first 7 days of the first menstrual cycle.

Evaluation. Report and record:
- *Nausea, weight gain, spotting, changed menstrual flow, missed periods, depression, mood changes, headaches, and brown pigmentation*

on the forehead, cheeks, and nose. These are common side effects. A prescription change is needed if they do not resolve after 3 months.

- *Vaginal discharge, breakthrough bleeding, yeast infection.* A prescription change and additional drugs may be needed.
- *Blurred vision, severe headaches, dizziness, leg pain, chest pain, shortness of breath, acute abdominal pain.* These may signal serious complications.

DRUGS USED IN OBSTETRICS

Obstetrics is the field of healthcare practice associated with pregnancy, labor, childbirth, and the first 6 to 8 weeks after birth. Drugs are used in obstetrics to:

- Induce labor
- Control bleeding after delivery
- Maintain uterine firmness after delivery
- Induce therapeutic abortion
- Prevent premature labor
- Control seizure activity
- Promote ovulation
- Prevent mother-child blood incompatibilities in future pregnancies

Some of the drugs used in obstetrics are listed in Table 30-3. See *Delegation Guidelines: Drugs Used in Obstetrics.*

DELEGATION GUIDELINES

Drugs Used in Obstetrics

Drugs used in obstetrics must be given carefully to protect the health of the mother and fetus. If allowed to give such drugs, you need to learn more about them. Ask for the necessary education and supervision.

Some drugs are given parenterally—by intramuscular or intravenous injection. Because you do not give parenteral dose forms, they are not included in this chapter. Should a nurse delegate the administration of such to you, you must:

- Remember that parenteral dosages are often very different from dosages for other routes.
- Refuse the delegation but do not ignore the request. Make sure the nurse knows that you cannot give the drug and why.

DRUG THERAPY FOR OSTEOPOROSIS

As men and women age, they may be affected by osteoporosis (Box 30-3). Biphosphonates and denosumab are used to treat osteoporosis. Dietary and supplemental calcium and vitamin D are also used for treatment.

DRUG CLASS: Biphosphonates

Biphosphonates inhibit bone resorption. This prevents low bone mass. The goal of therapy is to reduce fractures in persons with osteoporosis.

BOX 30-3 Osteoporosis

- Osteoporosis is the most common bone disease. The bones become fragile, which increases the risk of fracture.

Risk factors include:

- Increased age
- Female sex
- Postmenopausal women
- Hypogonadism
- Low body weight
- History of parental hip fracture
- White persons are at higher risk than black persons
- Rheumatoid arthritis
- Smoking
- Drinking alcohol (more than 3 drinks a day)
- Vitamin D deficiency
- Low calcium intake
- Long term use of some drugs

Some ways to prevent osteoporosis and fractures include:

- Adequate intake of calcium
- Adequate intake of vitamin D
- Lifelong participation in regular weight-bearing exercises
- Regular muscle-strengthening exercises
- No smoking
- Identification and treatment of alcoholism
- Prevent falls

TABLE 30-3 Drugs Used in Obstetrics

Generic Name	Brand Name	Dose Forms	Adult Dosage Range	Uses
dinoprostone	Prostin E2 Prepidil Cervidil	Vaginal suppository: 20 mg Cervical gel: 0.5 mg/3 g Vaginal insert: 10 mg		Expel uterine contents Start and continue cervical ripening at term
mifepristone	Mifeprex	Tablets: 200 mg	200 mg as a single dose	Termination of intrauterine pregnancy
misoprostol	Cytotec	Tablets: 100, 200 mcg	800 mcg buccally 24 to 48 hours after Mifeprex. Place two 200 mg tablets in each cheek pouch for 30 minutes.	Termination of intrauterine pregnancy
methylergonovine maleate		Tablets: 0.2 mg	0.2 mg every 6 to 8 hours after delivery for up to 1 week	Stimulate post-partum uterine contractions to control bleeding and maintain uterine firmness
clomiphene citrate	Clomid	Tablets: 50 mg	50 mg daily for 5 days (first course; follow the MAR for second and third courses)	Induce ovulation in women who are not ovulating

Modified from Willihnganz M: Clayton's Basic Pharmacology for Nurses, ed 18, St Louis, 2020, Elsevier.

TABLE 30-4   Biphosphonates

Generic Name	Brand Name	Oral Dose Forms	Daily Adult Dose
alendronate	Fosamax Binosto	Solution: 70 mg/75 mL Tablets: 5, 10, 35, 70 mg Effervescent tablet: 70 mg	Glucocorticoid-induced osteoporosis: PO: 5 mg once daily; Postmenopausal women not receiving estrogen PO: 10 mg once daily Osteoporosis in men: PO: 70 mg once weekly or 10 mg once daily Osteoporosis in postmenopausal women: Prevention: PO: 35 mg once weekly or 5 mg once daily Treatment: PO: 70 mg once weekly or 10 mg once daily
risedronate	Actonel	Tablets: 5, 35, 150 mg	Glucocorticoid-induced osteoporosis: PO: 5 mg daily Osteoporosis in men: PO: 35 mg once weekly Osteoporosis in postmenopausal women: PO: 5 mg daily or 35 mg once weekly or 150 mg once a month

Modified from Willihnganz M: Clayton's Basic Pharmacology for Nurses, ed 18, St Louis, 2020, Elsevier.

Assisting With the Nursing Process. When giving biphosphonates to treat osteoporosis, you assist the nurse with the nursing process.

Assessment
- Measure vital signs.
  Planning. See Table 30-4 for "Oral Dose Forms."
  Implementation. See Table 30-4 for "Daily Adult Dose."
  Evaluation. Report and record:
- *Abdominal pain, GERD (Chapter 26), heartburn, constipation, diarrhea, muscle pain.* These tent to be mild and resolve with continued use.
- *Difficulty swallowing, heartburn, severe muscle, or joint pain.* Stop therapy and alert the healthcare provider.
- *Thigh or groin pain.* This could be a sign of a femoral fracture that may occur with minimal or no trauma to the area.
- *Decreasing urinary output, bloody or smoky-colored urine.* These signal kidney toxicity.

DRUG THERAPY FOR BENIGN PROSTATIC HYPERPLASIA

The prostate is a gland in men. It lies in front of the rectum and just below the bladder (Fig. 30-2). The prostate also surrounds the urethra. In young men, the prostate is about the size of a walnut. The prostate grows larger (enlarges) as the man grows older. This is called benign prostatic hyperplasia (BPH). (*Benign* means *non-malignant. Hyper* means *excessive. Plasia* means *formation* or *development.*) Benign prostatic hypertrophy is another name for enlarged prostate. (*Trophy* means *growth.*)

Usually, BPH does not cause problems until after age 50. Most men in their 60s, 70s, and 80s display some symptoms of BPH.

BPH causes urinary problems. The enlarged prostate presses against the urethra. This obstructs urine flow through the urethra. Bladder function is gradually lost. These problems are common:
- A weak urine stream
- Frequent voiding of small amounts of urine
- Urgency and leaking or dribbling of urine
- Frequent urination at night
- Urinary retention

Treatment depends on the extent of the problem. For mild BPH, the doctor may order drugs. Drugs can shrink the prostate or stop its growth. Some microwave and laser treatments destroy the excess prostate tissue.

Transurethral resection of the prostate (TURP) is a common surgical procedure. A lighted scope is inserted through the penis. The scope has a wire loop. The doctor uses the loop to cut tissue and seal blood vessels. The removed tissue is flushed out of the bladder at the end of the surgery. A special catheter is inserted and left in place for a few days. Flushing fluid enters the bladder through the catheter. Urine and the flushing fluid flow out of the bladder through the same catheter. Some bleeding and blood clots are normal.

DRUG CLASS: Alpha-1 Adrenergic Blocking Agents

Alpha-1 adrenergic blocking agents are used to treat BPH. They block alpha-1 receptors on the prostate gland and certain areas of the bladder neck. Muscles relax, allowing greater urine flow.

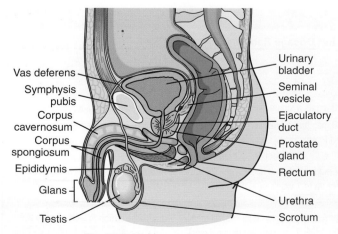

Vas deferens
Symphysis pubis
Corpus cavernosum
Corpus spongiosum
Epididymis
Glans
Testis

Urinary bladder
Seminal vesicle
Ejaculatory duct
Prostate gland
Rectum
Urethra
Scrotum

Fig. 30-2 Male reproductive system.

TABLE 30-5 Alpha-1 Adrenergic Blocking Agents Used for BPH

Generic Name	Brand Name	Oral Dose Forms	Adult Dosage Range
alfuzosin	Uroxatral	Tablets, extended-release (24 hr): 10 mg	PO: 10 mg daily to be taken immediately after the same meal each day Tablets should not be crushed or chewed
doxazosin	Cardura	Tablets: 1, 2, 4, 8 mg	PO: 1-8 mg once daily
	Cardura XL	Tablets, extended-release (24 hr): 4, 8 mg	
silodosin	Rapaflo	Capsules: 4, 8 mg	PO: 8 mg daily; 4 mg daily for patients with renal impairment
tamsulosin	Flomax	Capsules: 0.4 mg	PO: 0.4 mg daily, taken approximately 30 min following the same meal each day If symptoms are not adequately controlled after 2-4 wks of therapy, the dose may be increased to 0.8 mg once daily If administration is discontinued or interrupted for several days, at either the 0.4- or 0.8-mg dose, start therapy again with the 0.4-mg once-daily dose
terazosin	—	Capsules: 1, 2, 5, 10 mg	PO: Initial: 1 mg daily at bedtime Increase stepwise to 2 mg, 5 mg, or 10 mg daily to achieve desired response of symptoms and flow rate Maximum dose is 20 mg divided twice daily

Modified from Willihnganz M: Clayton's Basic Pharmacology for Nurses, ed 18, St Louis, 2020, Elsevier.

The drugs are used to treat mild to moderate urinary obstruction in men with BPH. The goals of therapy are to:
- Reduce symptoms of BPH
- Improve urine flow

Assisting With the Nursing Process. When giving alpha-1 adrenergic blocking agents to treat BPH, you assist the nurse with the nursing process.
  Assessment
- Measure blood pressure in the supine and standing positions.
  Planning. See Table 30-5 for "Oral Dose Forms."
  Implementation. See Table 30-6 for "Adult Dose Range."
  Evaluation. Report and record:
- *Drowsiness, headache, dizziness, weakness, lethargy.* These tend to be self-limiting. Provide for safety.
- *Dizziness, tachycardia, fainting.* These may develop 15 to 90 minutes after the first dose. Give the drug with food to avoid these symptoms. Have the person lie down if they occur. Provide for safety.

DRUG CLASS: Antiandrogen Agents
The following antiandrogen agents are used to treat BPH:
- Dutasteride (du tas' ter ide); Avodart (av'oh dart)
- Finasteride (fin as' ter ide); Proscar (pro' scar)
  These drugs reduce the cell growth associated with BPH. The goals of therapy are to:
- Reduce BPH symptoms
- Improve urine flow
- Reduce the need for surgery

Assisting With the Nursing Process. When giving antiandrogen drugs to treat BPH, you assist the nurse with the nursing process.

  Assessment. Ask the nurse what to observe and report.
  Planning
- Dutasteride (Avodart): the dose form is 0.5 mg capsules.
- Finasteride (Proscar): the dose form is 5 mg tablets.
  Implementation
- Dutasteride (Avodart): a 0.5 mg capsule is given once a day with or without food.
- Finasteride (Proscar): a 5 mg tablet is given once a day with or without food.
  Evaluation. Report and record:
- *Complaints of impotence, decreased sexual drive, decreased volume of ejaculate.* These tend to be self-limiting.

DRUG THERAPY FOR ERECTILE DYSFUNCTION

Erectile dysfunction (ED) or impotence is the inability of the male to have an erection sufficient for satisfactory sexual activity. Causes include diabetes, spinal cord injuries, multiple sclerosis, prostate problems, alcoholism, heart and circulatory disorders, drug abuse, and psychological factors. Some drugs for high blood pressure can cause impotence, as can some drugs not used to treat high blood pressure. Some drugs treat impotence.

DRUG CLASS: Phosphodiesterase Inhibitors
Drugs in this class result in smooth muscle relaxation. This allows blood to fill the erectile tissue in the penis during sexual stimulation. The resulting erection can last an hour or so.
  The goals of therapy are:
- Improved erectile function
- Sexual satisfaction in men with ED

TABLE 30-6   Drugs Used for Erectile Dysfunction

Generic Name	Brand Name	Oral Dose Forms	Adult Dosage Range
avanafil	Stendra	Tablets: 50, 100, 200 mg	Initial: 100 mg Maximum: 200 mg/24 hours
sildenafil	Viagra	Tablets: 25, 50, 100 mg	Initial: 50 mg Maximum: 100 mg/24 hours
tadalafil	Cialis	Tablets: 5, 10, 20 mg	Initial: 10 mg Maximum: 20 mg/24 hours
vardenafil	Levitra Staxyn	Tablets: 2.5, 5, 10, 20 mg Tablets, dispersible: 10 mg	Initial: 10 mg Maximum: 20 mg/24 hours Initial: 10 mg Maximum: 10 mg; if dosage adjustment is needed, switch to Levitra

Modified from Willihnganz M: Clayton's Basic Pharmacology for Nurses, ed 18, St Louis, 2020, Elsevier.

Assisting With the Nursing Process. When drugs are used to treat ED, you assist the nurse with the nursing process.

Assessment
- Measure vital signs.
  Planning. See Table 30-6 for "Oral Dose Forms."
  Implementation. See Table 30-6 for "Adult Dosage Range."
- A dose is taken 30 minutes to 4 hours before sexual activity.
- Do not take nitroglycerin for angina when taking these drugs.
  Evaluation. Report and record:
- *Headache, flushing of the face and neck.* These tend to be self-limiting.
- *Color (blue or green) vision impairment.* The dosage may need to be reduced.
- *Hypotension, dizziness, angina.* The person should lie down and stop sexual activity. The person should not take nitroglycerin for angina.
- *Loss of vision, loss of hearing.* These are rare.
- *Priapism.* **Priapism** is a prolonged or constant erection. Medical attention is needed if this lasts longer than 4 hours.

REVIEW QUESTIONS

Circle the BEST answer.

1. Contraceptives are used to:
   a. prevent pregnancy
   b. treat benign prostatic hyperplasia
   c. treat erectile dysfunction
   d. prevent leukorrhea
2. Combination oral contraceptives contain:
   a. estrogen only
   b. progestin only
   c. estrogen and progestin
   d. progestin and testosterone
3. Combination oral contraceptives are packaged with 28 tablets. The last 7 contain:
   a. estrogen
   b. progestin
   c. testosterone
   d. no hormones
4. Minipill oral contraceptives are packaged with 28 tablets. All tablets contain only:
   a. estrogen
   b. progestin
   c. testosterone
   d. no hormones
5. Which oral contraceptive results in four periods in one year?
   a. monophasic
   b. biphasic
   c. triphasic
   d. extended-cycle
6. The following are side effects from contraceptives. Which may signal a serious complication?
   a. weight gain
   b. leg pain
   c. vaginal discharge
   d. breakthrough bleeding
7. A transdermal contraceptive patch can be applied to the following areas, *except:*
   a. the breast
   b. a buttock
   c. the abdomen
   d. the upper outer arm
8. Drugs are used in obstetrics for the following reasons, *except:*
   a. to induce labor
   b. to control bleeding after delivery
   c. to prevent premature labor
   d. to change the mother's blood type
9. Which is not used to treat osteoporosis?
   a. biphosphonates
   b. mosoprostol (Cytotec)
   c. calcium
   d. vitamin D
10. When giving alfuzosin (Uroxatral) and tamsulosin (Flomax), the dose form:
    a. can be chewed or crushed
    b. is given after the same meal each day
    c. is given at bedtime
    d. is changed on "change day"

11. Which drug is *not* used to treat erectile dysfunction?
    a. tadalafil (Cialis)
    b. vardenafil (Levitra)
    c. finasteride (Proscar)
    d. sildenafil (Viagra)

Circle T if the statement is true. Circle F if the statement is false.

12. T F Angina is experienced after taking a drug for erectile dysfunction. Nitroglycerin tablets should be taken.

13. T F Priapism is another term for erectile dysfunction.
14. T F Drugs for impotence are taken 30 minutes to 4 hours before sexual activity.

Answers to these questions can be found on the Evolve Resources site: http://evolve.elsevier.com/Anderson/medasst/

31

Drugs Used to Treat Urinary System Disorders

OBJECTIVES

- Define the key terms and key abbreviations used in this chapter.
- Describe urinary tract infections.
- Describe overactive bladder syndrome.
- Describe the drugs used to treat urinary tract infections.
- Explain how to assist with the nursing process when giving drugs to treat urinary tract infections.
- Describe the drugs used to treat overactive bladder syndrome.
- Explain how to assist with the nursing process when giving drugs to treat overactive bladder syndrome.

KEY TERMS

cystitis Inflammation *(itis)* of the bladder *(cyst)*

healthcare-associated infection (HAI) An infection that develops in a person cared for in any setting where health care is given; the infection is related to receiving health care

overactive bladder (OAB) A syndrome characterized by urinary frequency, urgency, and incontinence; urge syndrome or urgency/frequency syndrome

prostatitis Inflammation *(itis)* of the prostate *(prostat)*

pyelonephritis Inflammation *(itis)* of the kidney *(nephr)* pelvis *(pyelo)*

urethritis Inflammation *(itis)* of the urethra *(urethr)*

urinary antimicrobial agents Substances that have an antiseptic effect on urine and the urinary tract

KEY ABBREVIATIONS

g Gram

GI Gastrointestinal

HAI Healthcare-associated infection

mg Milligram

mL Milliliter

OAB Overactive bladder

UTI Urinary tract infection

Urinary tract infections (UTIs) are common. Infection in one area can involve the entire system. Microbes can enter the system through the urethra. Common causes include catheterization, urological exams, intercourse, poor perineal hygiene, immobility, and poor fluid intake. UTI is a common healthcare-associated infection. A **healthcare-associated infection (HAI)** is an infection that develops in a person cared for in any setting where health care is given (Chapter 6). The infection is related to receiving health care.

Women are at high risk for UTIs because microbes can easily enter the short female urethra. Prostate gland secretions help protect men from UTIs. However, an enlarged prostate increases the risk of UTI in older men (Chapter 30).

Older persons are at high risk for UTIs. Incomplete bladder emptying, perineal soiling from fecal incontinence, poor fluid intake, and poor nutrition increase the risk of UTI in older men and women.

UTIs include:

- **Cystitis**—inflammation *(itis)* of the bladder *(cyst)*
- **Pyelonephritis**—inflammation *(itis)* of the kidney *(nephr)* pelvis *(pyelo)*
- **Prostatitis**—inflammation *(itis)* of the prostate *(prostat)*
- **Urethritis**—inflammation *(itis)* of the urethra *(urethr)*

Overactive bladder (OAB) is another urinary disorder. It is characterized by urinary frequency, urgency, and incontinence (p. 289).

For a review of the urinary system, see Box 31-1.

DRUG THERAPY FOR URINARY TRACT INFECTIONS

Urinary antimicrobial agents are substances that have an antiseptic effect on urine and the urinary tract. The drug ordered depends on the pathogen causing the infection. Other antibiotics used to treat UTIs are described in Chapter 35.

The person should have a fluid intake of 2000 mL daily. The length of treatment depends on:

- If the infection is acute, chronic, or recurrent
- The pathogen
- The drug ordered

DRUG CLASS: Fosfomycin Antibiotics

The following is a fosfomycin antibiotic:

- Fosfomycin (fos foh my' sin); Monurol (mohn' urh ol)

The drug affects the cell walls of bacteria. It also reduces the ability of bacteria to adhere to the urinary tract.

The digestive system rids the body of solid wastes. The lungs rid the body of carbon dioxide. Water and other substances leave the body through sweat. There are other waste products in the blood from cells burning food for energy. These wastes are removed through the urinary system (Fig. 31-1). The urinary system also maintains water balance within the body.

The bladder is a hollow, muscular sac that lies toward the front of the lower part of the abdominal cavity. A tube, called the *ureter*, is attached to the renal pelvis of the kidney. Each ureter is about 10 to 12 inches long. The ureters carry urine from the kidneys to the *bladder*.

Urine is stored in the bladder until the need to urinate is felt. This usually occurs when there is about a half pint (250 mL) of urine in the bladder. Urine passes from the bladder through the *urethra*. The opening at the end of the urethra is the *meatus*. Urine passes from the body through the meatus. Urine is a clear, yellowish fluid.

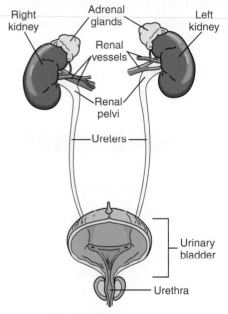

Fig. 31-1 Urinary system.

The drug is used as a single dose to treat uncomplicated acute cystitis in women. The goal of therapy is to resolve the UTI.

Assisting With the Nursing Process. When giving fosfomycin (Monurol), you assist the nurse with the nursing process.
Assessment
- Note the amount, color, clarity, and odor of urine.
- Ask about urgency, burning, pain, or other problems.
- Measure vital signs.
- Ask about gastrointestinal (GI) complaints.
Planning
- The dose form is 3 g packets of granules.
Implementation
- Pour the entire contents of a single-dose packet of granules into 90 to 120 mL (3 to 4 ounces) of water. Stir to dissolve. Do not use hot water.

- Have the person take the drug at once after the granules dissolve in water.
- The drug may be taken with or without food.
- The drug must be mixed with water. It is not taken in its dry form.
Evaluation. Report and record:
- *Nausea, diarrhea, abdominal cramps, flatulence.* These are mild and tend to resolve without the need for therapy.
- *Perineal burning, dysuria.* Burning with voiding may be due to the infection. Symptoms should improve in 2 to 3 days after taking the drug.

DRUG CLASS: Urinary Antibacterial Agents

The following antibacterial agents are used to treat UTIs:
- Nitrofurantoin (ny tro fuhr' an toe in); Macrodantin (mak ro dan' tin), Furadantin (fuhr ah dan' tin), and Macrobid (mak' ro bid)

These drugs interfere with several bacterial enzyme ystems. They are not effective against microbes in blood or tissues outside the urinary tract.

Assisting With the Nursing Process. When giving nitrofurantoin (Macrodantin, Furadantin, and Macrobid), you assist the nurse with the nursing process.
Assessment
- Note the amount, color, clarity, and odor of urine.
- Ask about urgency, burning, pain, or other problems.
- Measure vital signs.
- Ask about GI complaints.
- Ask about numbness or tingling in the extremities.
Planning. The oral dose forms are:
- 25, 50, and 100 mg capsules
- 25 mg/5 mL suspension
Implementation
- The adult oral dosage for Macrodantin and Furadantin is 50 to 100 mg four times a day for 10 to 14 days. The drug is given every 6 hours to maintain adequate urine concentrations.
- The adult oral dosage for Macrobid is 100 mg two times a day for 7 days.
- Give the drug with food or milk to reduce GI side effects.
Evaluation. Report and record:
- *Nausea, vomiting, anorexia.* Give the drug with food or milk to reduce GI irritation.
- *Rust brown to yellow-colored urine.* This is harmless.
- *Dyspnea, chills, rash, itching.* These signal an allergic reaction. Alert the nurse at once. Do not give the next dose unless approved by the nurse.
- *Numbness and tingling in the extremities.* The drug needs to be discontinued.
- *Dysuria, foul-smelling urine, fever.* These signal a second infection.

DRUG THERAPY FOR OVERACTIVE BLADDER

The major symptoms of OAB are urinary:
- *Frequency*—the need to void 8 or more times a day. Nocturia is common (the need to void at night).

- *Urgency*—a sudden, compelling desire to pass urine that is hard to ignore.
- *Incontinence*—the inability to control urine from passing from the bladder.

DRUG CLASS: Anticholinergic Drugs

Anticholinergic drugs are the treatment of choice for OAB. They also are known as urinary antispasmodic agents. They relax the outer muscle layer of the bladder. Involuntary bladder contractions decrease and the bladder can hold more urine. Urinary frequency and urgency are reduced and the desire to void is delayed.

The goals of therapy are to:

- Decrease frequency by increasing the amount voided
- Decrease urgency
- Reduce incidents of incontinence

Cholinergic receptors are located throughout the body (Chapter 15). Therefore, anticholinergic agents can lead to dry mouth, blurred vision, constipation, confusion, and sedation.

Assisting With the Nursing Process. When giving anticholinergic agents to control OAB, you assist the nurse with the nursing process.

Assessment

- Note the amount, color, clarity, and odor of urine.
- Ask about urgency, burning, pain, or other problems.
- Measure vital signs.
  Planning. See Table 31-1 for "Dose Forms."
  Implementation. See Table 31-1 for "Adult Dosage Range."
  Evaluation. Report and record:
- *Dry mouth, urinary hesitancy, urinary retention, sedation.* These are usually dose related. They may respond to a lower dosage. The nurse may allow the person to chew gum or suck on ice chips or hard candy. Sedation resolves with continued use.
- *Constipation, bloating.* Follow the care plan for diet and fluid intake.
- *Blurred vision.* The person should not drive or operate machinery. Provide for safety.

DRUG CLASS: Beta-3 Adrenergic Agonists

The following Beta-3 adrenergic agonist is used to treat OAB:

- Mirabegron (mir a beg' ron); Myrbetriq (mer beh' trik)

This drug relaxes the outer muscle layer of the bladder when the bladder is filling. The bladder can hold more urine. Urinary

TABLE 31-1   Urinary Anticholinergic Agents

Generic Name	Brand Name	Dose Forms	Adult Dosage Range
darifenacin	Enablex	Tablets: 7.5 and 15 mg	Initial dose: 7.5 mg once daily. Based on individual response, the dose may be increased to 15 mg once daily as early as 2 weeks after starting therapy. May be taken with or without food.
oxybutynin	Ditropan Ditropan XL Gelnique Oxytrol	Tablets: 5 mg Syrup: 5 mg/5 mL Extended-release tablets: 5, 10, and 15 mg Topical gel: 10% Transdermal patch: 36 mg (3.9 mg/day release)	Initial dose: 5 mg (tablets or syrup) two or three times daily. Maximum dose: 20 mg daily. Initial dose: 5 mg once daily. Dosage may be adjusted at weekly intervals in 5 mg increments. Maximum dose: 30 mg daily. May be administered with or without food and must be swallowed whole with the aid of liquids. Do not crush or chew. Apply the contents of one sachet once daily to clean, dry interact skin on abdomen, thighs, or upper arms/shoulder. Rotate site; do not apply to same site on consecutive days. Wash hands after use. Cover treated area with clothing after gel has dried to prevent transfer to others. Do not bathe, shower, or swim until 1 hour after gel is applied. Initial dose: Apply one patch every 3 to 4 days to dry, intact skin on the abdomen, hip, or buttock. Select a new application site with each new patch to avoid reapplication to the same site within 7 days.
fesoterodine	Toviaz	24-hr extended-release tablets: 4, 8 mg	4-8 mg daily; 4 mg daily for people with renal impairment
solifenacin	VESIcare	Tablets: 5 and 10 mg	Initial dose: 5 mg once daily. If well tolerated, the dose may be increased to 10 mg once daily. May be taken with or without food.
tolterodine	Detrol Detrol LA	Tablets: 1 and 2 mg 24-hr extended-release capsules: 2 and 4 mg	Initial dose: 1-2 mg twice daily based on individual response and tolerance. Initial dose: 2-4 mg once daily taken with liquids and swallowed whole.
trospium		Tablets: 20 mg 24-hr extended-release capsules: 60 mg	Initial dose: 20 mg twice daily at least 1 hour before meals on an empty stomach. For persons with reduced kidney function, the recommended dose is 20 mg once daily at bedtime.

frequency and urgency are reduced. The desire to void is delayed.

Assisting With the Nursing Process. When giving mirabegron (Myrbetriq) for OAB, you assist the nurse with the nursing process.
   Assessment
- Note the amount, color, clarity, and odor of urine.
- Ask about urgency, burning, pain, or other problems.
- Measure vital signs.
   Planning
- The oral dose forms are 25 and 50 mg 24-hour extended-release tablets.
   Implementation
- The adult oral dosage is 25 to 50 mg once daily.
   Evaluation. Report and record:
- *Constipation, diarrhea, dry mouth.* Adding bulk to the diet will help alleviate constipation and diarrhea. Encourage fluid intake. The nurse may allow the person to chew gum or suck on ice chips or hard candy.
- *Urinary retention.* Start with a lower dose.
- *Dysuria, foul-smelling urine, fever.* These signal a UTI. Do not stop mirabegron. Notify nurse so the infection can be treated.
- *Hypertension.* Notify nurse if this occurs.

MISCELLANEOUS URINARY AGENTS

The following agents are also used to treat urinary symptoms:
- Bethanechol chloride (be than' e kol); Urecholine (yur e kol' een)
- Phenazopyridine hydrochloride (fen a zo peer' a deen); Pyridium (pie rid' ee um)

Bethanechol Chloride (Urecholine)

This drug helps stimulate urination. It is commonly used in postoperative and postpartum patients.

Assisting With the Nursing Process
- When giving bethanechol chloride (Urecholine), you assist the nurse with the nursing process.
   Assessment
- Note the amount, color, clarity, and odor of urine.
- Ask about urgency, burning, pain, or other problems.
- Measure vital signs.
- Ask about GI symptoms.
   Planning
- The oral dose forms are 5, 10, 25, and 50 mg tablets.
   Implementation
- The adult oral dosage is 10-50 mg two to four times daily.
- Maximum dosage is 120 mg.
   Evaluation. Report and record:
- *Nausea, vomiting, sweating, abdominal pain and cramps, belching, flushing of skin, headache.* Start with a lower dose.

Phenazopyridine Hydrochloride (Pyridium)

Pyridium relieves burning, pain, urgency, and frequency associated with UTIs.

Assisting With the Nursing Process
- When giving phenazopyridine hydrochloride (Pyridium), you assist the nurse with the nursing process.
   Assessment
- Note the amount, color, clarity, and odor of urine.
- Ask about urgency, burning, pain, or other problems.
- Note skin color.
   Planning
- The oral dose forms are 95, 100, and 200 mg tablets.
   Implementation
- The adult oral dosage is 200 mg three times daily.
   Evaluation. Report and record:
- *Reddish-orange urine discoloration.* This is harmless.
- *Yellow sclera or skin.* Report this to the nurse. Do not stop treatment.

■ REVIEW QUESTIONS

Circle the BEST answer.

1. Cystitis is an inflammation of the:
   a. bladder
   b. kidney pelvis
   c. prostate
   d. urethra
2. Which does *not* occur in overactive bladder syndrome?
   a. urgency
   b. frequency
   c. incontinence
   d. diuresis
3. Which is inflammation of the kidney pelvis?
   a. urethritis
   b. prostatitis
   c. cystitis
   d. pyelonephritis
4. Which is given as a single dose to treat cystitis?
   a. oxybutynin (Oxytrol)
   b. nitrofurantoin (Furadantin)
   c. fosfomycin (Monurol)
   d. mirabegron (Myrbetriq)
5. The dose form of fosfomycin (Monurol) is 3 g packets of granules. To give the drug, you:
   a. dissolve the granules in 90 to 120 mL of cool water
   b. give the drug right before the granules fully dissolve
   c. give the drug in its dry form
   d. mix the granules with hot food
6. Nitrofurantoin (Macrodantin or Furadantin) is given:
   a. to treat overactive bladder
   b. before meals
   c. every 6 hours
   d. dissolved in water

7. Nitrofurantoin (Macrodantin, Furadantin, and Macrobid) is used to treat:
   a. urinary frequency
   b. overactive bladder
   c. incontinence
   d. urinary tract infections
8. The following are given to control overactive bladder, *except:*
   a. tolterodine (Detrol XL)
   b. darifenacin (Enablex)
   c. bethanechol chloride (Urecholine)
   d. solifenacin (VESIcare)
9. Which drug relieves burning, pain, urgency and frequency associated with UTIs?
   a. mirabegron (Myrbetriq)
   b. trospium
   c. phenazopyridine hydrochloride (Pyridium)
   d. nitrofurantoin (Macrobid)

Circle T if the statement is true. Circle F if the statement is false.

10. T F Women are at high risk for urinary tract infections.
11. T F Overactive bladder syndrome is treated with urinary antimicrobial agents.
12. T F Urecholine is used to treat OAB in postpartum patients.

Answers to these questions can be found on the Evolve Resources site: http://evolve.elsevier.com/Anderson/medasst/

Drugs Used to Treat Eye Disorders

OBJECTIVES

- Define the key terms and key abbreviations used in this chapter.
- Describe the common eye disorders.
- Describe the drugs used to treat eye disorders.
- Explain how to assist with the nursing process when giving drugs to treat eye disorders.

KEY TERMS

miosis Narrowing of the pupil
mydriasis Dilation of the pupil

osmotic agents Drugs that cause fluid to be drawn from outside of the vascular system into the blood

KEY ABBREVIATIONS

g Gram
GI Gastrointestinal
IOP Intraocular pressure
kg Kilogram

mg Milligram
mL Milliliter
PO Per os (orally)

The structures and functions of the eye are reviewed in Box 32-1. For common eye disorders, see Box 32-2. To safely give topical ophthalmic agents, see Chapter 13. Also follow these rules:
- Do not use more than one drop (unless otherwise ordered). The eye can only hold a small amount of fluid.
- Wait at least 5 minutes if more than one drug is ordered. This prevents:
  - The second drug from washing away the first drug
  - The second drug from diluting the first drug
- Apply drops before ointments.
- Wait a few hours to apply drops after applying an ointment.
- Provide for safety after applying ointments. They may cause blurred vision.
- Know the standard colors for ophthalmic labels and bottle caps:
  - Antiinfectives—tan
  - Beta-adrenergic blocking agents—yellow or dark blue
  - Miotics—dark green
  - Mydriatics and cycloplegics—red (*Cycloplegics* paralyze the ciliary muscle of the eye and are used for eye exams)
  - Nonsteroidal antiinflammatory agents—gray
  See *Delegation Guidelines: Drugs Used to Treat Eye Disorders.*

DELEGATION GUIDELINES
Drugs Used to Treat Eye Disorders

Some drugs used to treat eye disorders are given parenterally—by intramuscular or intravenous injection. Because you do not give parenteral dose forms, they are not included in this chapter. Should a nurse delegate the administration of such to you, you must:
- Remember that parenteral dosages are often very different from dosages for other routes.
- Refuse the delegation but do not ignore the request. Make sure the nurse knows that you cannot give the drug and why.

DRUG THERAPY FOR GLAUCOMA

Several drug classes are used to treat glaucoma. The goals of therapy are to:
- Reduce intraocular pressure (IOP)
- Prevent further blindness

DRUG CLASS: Carbonic Anhydrase Inhibitors

These agents inhibit carbonic anhydrase (an enzyme). Inhibiting the enzyme causes decreased production of aqueous humor. This lowers IOP.

Assisting With the Nursing Process. When giving carbonic anhydrase inhibitors, you assist the nurse with the nursing process.
Assessment
- Measure vital signs.
- Measure weight.
- Measure intake and output.
- Observe for alertness and orientation to person, time, and place.
- Ask about gastrointestinal (GI) signs and symptoms.
Planning. See Table 32-1 for "Dose Forms."
Implementation. See Table 32-1 for "Adult Dosage Range."
- Remove contact lenses for topical dose forms.
- Do not give the drug if the person is allergic to sulfonamide antibiotics (Chapter 35).
- Give oral dose forms with food or milk to lessen stomach irritation.
Evaluation. Report and record:
- *Thirst; changes in alertness and orientation to person, time, and place; confusion; muscle cramps; nausea.* These may signal dehydration or electrolyte imbalance (potassium, sodium, chloride).

BOX 32-1   The Eye: Structures and Functions

Receptors for vision are in the *eyes* (Fig. 32-1). The eye is easily injured. Bones of the skull, eyelids and eyelashes, and tears protect the eyes from injury. The eye has three layers:

- The *sclera*, the white of the eye, is the outer layer. It is made of tough connective tissue. The *cornea* is the clear, outer layer over the eyeball.
- The *choroid* is the second layer. Blood vessels, the *ciliary muscle,* and the *iris* make up the choroid. The iris gives the eye its color. The opening in the middle of the iris is the *pupil.* Pupil size varies with the amount of light entering the eye (Fig. 32-2). The pupil constricts (narrows) in bright light. Narrowing of the pupil is called **miosis** *(to become less).* The pupil dilates (widens) in dim or dark places. Dilation of the pupil is called **mydriasis** *(hot mass).*
- The *retina* is the inner layer. It has receptors for vision and the nerve fibers of the *optic nerve.*

Light enters the eye through the cornea. Light rays pass to the *lens,* which lies behind the pupil. The light is then reflected to the retina. Light is carried to the brain by the optic nerve.

The *aqueous chamber* separates the cornea from the lens. The chamber is filled with a fluid called *aqueous humor.* The fluid helps the cornea keep its shape and position. The *vitreous humor* is behind the lens. It is a gelatin-like substance that supports the retina and maintains the eye's shape.

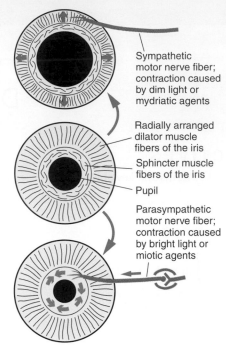

Fig. 32-2 Effect of light or ophthalmic agents on the iris of the eye.

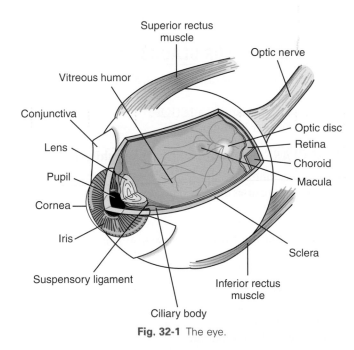

Fig. 32-1 The eye.

- *Signs and symptoms of allergic reaction to sulfonamide antibiotics.* See Chapter 35. Tell the nurse at once. Do not give the next dose unless approved by the nurse.
- *Confusion.* Provide for safety.
- *Drowsiness.* This is usually mild and tends to resolve with continued therapy. Provide for safety.

DRUG CLASS: Cholinergic Agents

Cholinergic agents produce strong contractions of the iris (miosis). They also produce muscle contractions that allow the eye to adjust to distances.

The following is a cholinergic agent used to glaucoma:
- Pilocarpine (pye" loe kar' peen); Isopto Carpine

This drugs lowers IOP in persons with glaucoma by permitting the outflow of aqueous humor. It also reduceds pupil dilation after eye surgery or eye exams.

Assisting With the Nursing Process. When giving pilocarpine (Isopto Carpine), you assist the nurse with the nursing process.

> ***Assessment***
- Measure vital signs.
> ***Planning***
- The topical dose forms are 1%, 2%, and 4% suspensions.
> ***Implementation***
- One drop, up to four times daily.
> ***Evaluation.*** Report and record:
- *Problems adjusting to changes in light, problems seeing at night, blurred vision.* Provide for safety. The person should not drive or perform dangerous tasks in poor light.
- *Eye irritation, eye redness, headache.* These are usually mild and tend to resolve with continued therapy.
- *Pain, discomfort.* These may occur in bright light.
- *Sweating, increased saliva, abdominal discomfort, diarrhea, bronchospasm, tremors, hypotension, dysrhythmias, bradycardia.* These signal that the person is receiving too much of a cholinergic agent.

DRUG CLASS: Alpha-Adrenergic Agents

Alpha-adrenergic agents are used for eye disorders because they cause:
- Pupil dilation
- Increased outflow of aqueous humor
- Vasoconstriction

BOX 32-2   Eye Disorders

Glaucoma

Glaucoma results in damage to the optic nerve. The eye produces a fluid that nourishes certain structures in the eye. The fluid normally drains from the eye (Fig. 32-3, A). Fluid builds up in the eye when it cannot drain properly (Fig. 32-3, B). This causes pressure on the optic nerve—intraocular pressure (IOP). The optic nerve is damaged. Vision loss with eventual blindness occurs.

Glaucoma can develop in one or both eyes. Onset may be sudden or gradual. Peripheral vision (side vision) is lost. The person sees through a tunnel (Fig. 32-4). Other signs and symptoms vary and include blurred vision and halos around lights. With sudden onset, the person has severe eye pain, nausea, and vomiting.

Risk Factors. Glaucoma is a leading cause of vision loss in the United States. Persons at risk include:

- African Americans over 40 years of age
- Everyone over 60 years of age
- Those with a family history of the disease
- Those who have diabetes, high blood pressure, or heart disease
- Those who have eye diseases or eye injuries
- Those who have had eye surgery

Treatment. Glaucoma has no cure. Prior damage cannot be reversed. Drugs and surgery can control glaucoma and prevent further damage to the optic nerve.

Cataracts

Cataract is a clouding of the lens in the eye (Fig. 32-5). Normally the lens is clear. *Cataract* comes from the Greek word that means *waterfall.* Trying to see is like looking through a waterfall. A cataract can occur in one or both eyes. Signs and symptoms include:

- Cloudy, blurry, or dimmed vision (Fig. 32-6).
- Colors seem faded. Blues and purples are hard to see.
- Sensitivity to light and glares.
- Poor vision at night.
- Halos around lights.
- Double vision in one eye.

Risk Factors. Most cataracts are caused by aging. By age 80, more than 50% of all Americans have a cataract or have had cataract surgery. Risk factors include diabetes, smoking, alcohol use, prolonged exposure to sunlight, and a family history of cataracts.

Treatment. Surgery is the only treatment. Surgery is done when the cataract starts to interfere with daily activities. Driving, reading, and watching TV are examples.

Surgery involves removing the lens. Then a plastic lens is implanted. Vision improves after surgery. Postoperative care includes the following:

- Keep the eye shield or patch in place as directed. Some doctors allow the shield or patch off during the day if eyeglasses are worn. The shield or patch is worn for sleep, including naps.
- Follow measures for persons who are visually impaired or blind when an eye shield or patch is worn. The person may have vision loss in the other eye.
- Remind the person not to rub or press the affected eye.
- Do not bump the eye.
- Place the overbed table and the bedside stand on the inoperative side.
- Place the signal light within reach.
- Report eye drainage or complaints of pain to the nurse immediately.

TABLE 32-1   Carbonic Anhydrase Inhibitors

Generic Name	Brand Name	Dose Forms	Adult Dosage Range
acetazolamide	Diamox	Tablets: 125, 250 mg 12-hr extended-release capsules: 500 mg	PO: 250 mg one to four times daily or 500 mg extended-release twice daily
brinzolamide	Azopt	Ophthalmic solution: 1% in 10 and 15 mL dropper bottles	Intraocular: One drop in affected eye(s) three times daily; if more than one ophthalmic agent is to be administered in the same eye, separate the administration by at least 10 minutes
dorzolamide	Trusopt	Ophthalmic solution: 2% in 10 mL dropper bottles	Intraocular: One drop in affected eye(s) three times daily; if more than one ophthalmic agent is to be administered in the same eye, separate the administration by at least 10 minutes
Methazolamide	Neptazane	Tablets: 25, 50 mg	50 to 100 mg, two or three times daily

Modified from Willihnganz M: Clayton's Basic Pharmacology for Nurses, ed 18, St Louis, 2020, Elsevier.

- Relaxation of the ciliary muscle
- A decrease in the formation of aqueous humor
  The goals of therapy are to:
- Dilate the pupils (mydriasis) for eye exams
- Reduce IOP
- Reduce redness of the eyes from irritation

Assisting With the Nursing Process. When giving alpha-adrenergic agents in the treatment of eye disorders, you assist the nurse with the nursing process.

Assessment
- Measure vital signs.

Planning. See Table 32-2 for "Topical Dose Forms."
Implementation. See Table 32-2 for "Adult Dosage."
Evaluation. Report and record:

- *Sensitivity to bright light.* When pupils are dilated, excess amounts of light enter the eyes. This causes squinting. Sunglasses help reduce brightness. Provide for safety. The person should not drive or perform dangerous tasks in poor light.
- *Eye irritation, tearing.* These tend to be mild and resolve with continued therapy.
- *Palpitations, tachycardia, dysrhythmias, hypertension, faintness, trembling, sweating.* These signal overdose or excessive amounts of an adrenergic agent.

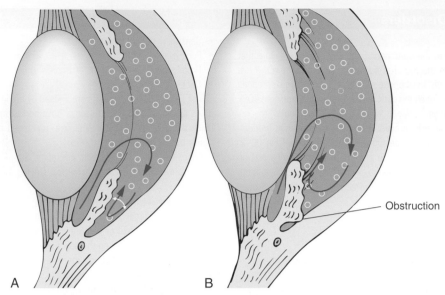

Fig. 32-3 A, Fluid drains normally from the eye. **B,** Flow of fluid from the eye is obstructed.

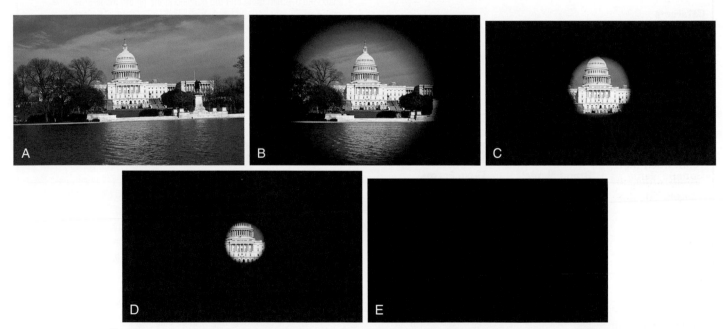

Fig. 32-4 Vision loss from glaucoma. **A,** Normal vision. **B,** Loss of peripheral vision begins. **C, D,** and **E,** Vision loss continues, with eventual blindness.

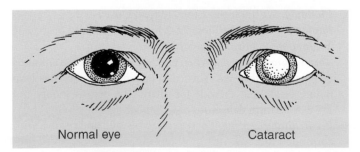

Fig. 32-5 One eye is normal. The other has a cataract. (From Phipps WJ and others: *Medical-surgical nursing: concepts and clinical practice,* ed 5, St Louis, 1995, Mosby.)

DRUG CLASS: Beta-Adrenergic Blocking Agents

Beta-adrenergic blocking agents are used to reduce elevated IOP. These agents are thought to reduce the production of aqueous humor.

Assisting With the Nursing Process. When giving beta-adrenergic blocking agents in the treatment of IOP, you assist the nurse with the nursing process.

Assessment
- Measure vital signs.

Planning. See Table 32-3 for "Topical Dose Forms."

Implementation. See Table 32-3 for "Initial Adult Dosage."

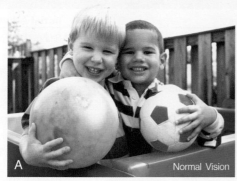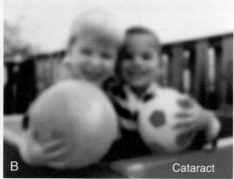

Fig. 32-6 Vision loss from a cataract. **A,** Normal vision. **B,** Scene viewed with a cataract. (From National Eye Institute: *Cataract: what you should know,* National Institutes of Health, Bethesda, Md.)

TABLE 32-2 Alpha-Adrenergic Agents

Generic Name	Brand Name	Topical Dose Forms	Adult Dosage
apraclonidine	Iopidine	Ophthalmic solution: 0.5%, 1%	One drop 1 hour before surgery and immediately after surgery
brimonidine	Alphagan P	Ophthalmic solution: 0.1%, 0.15%, 0.2%	One drop every 8 hours in affected eye(s)
naphazoline hydrochloride	Clear Eyes	Ophthalmic solution: 0.0125%	One to two drops every 3-4 hours
phenylephrine	Altafrin	Ophthalmic solution: 2.5%, 10%	One to two drops two or three times daily
tetrahydrozoline hydrochloride	Opti-Clear; Good Sense Eye Drops	Ophthalmic solution: 0.05%	One to two drops two or three times daily

Modified from Willihnganz M: *Clayton's Basic Pharmacology for Nurses,* ed 18, St Louis, 2020, Elsevier.

Evaluation. Report and record:
- *Eye irritation, tearing.* These tend to be mild and resolve with continued therapy.
- *Bradycardia, dysrhythmias, hypotension, faintness, bronchospasm.* The dosage may need adjustment.

DRUG CLASS: Prostaglandin Agonists

Prostaglandin agonists reduce IOP by increasing the outflow of aqueous humor. They are used to reduce IOP in persons with glaucoma who have not responded well to other IOP-lowering agents.

Assisting With the Nursing Process. When giving prostaglandin agonists in the treatment of IOP, you assist the nurse with the nursing process.

   Assessment. Measure vital signs.

   Planning. See Table 32-4 for "Topical Dose Form."

   Implementation. See Table 32-4 for "Adult Dosage Range."

   Evaluation. Report and record:
- *Eye irritation, burning and stinging, tearing.* These tend to be mild and resolve with continued therapy.
- *Changes in eye color.* Eye color may gradually change. The amount of brown pigment in the eye may increase. This may take several months to years and is likely permanent. Eyelids may develop color changes. Eyelashes may increase in growth.

OTHER OPHTHALMIC AGENTS

Other drug classes used to treat eye disorders are:
- Anticholinergic agents
- Antifungal agents
- Antiviral agents
- Antibacterial agents
- Corticosteroids
- Ophthalmic antiinflammatory agents
- Antihistamines
- Antiallergenic agents
- Artificial tear solutions

DRUG CLASS: Anticholinergic Agents

Anticholinergic agents cause relaxation of certain eye muscles. As a result, the pupils dilate, allowing:
- Examination of the interior of the eye
- Resting of the eye during uveitis—inflammation of the uveal tract (middle coat of the eye)
- Measurement of lens strength for eyeglasses (refraction)

Assisting With the Nursing Process. When giving anticholinergic agents in the treatment of IOP, you assist the nurse with the nursing process.

   Assessment
- Measure vital signs.

   Planning. See Table 32-5 for "Topical Dose Forms."

   Implementation. See Table 32-5 for "Adult Dosage."

   Evaluation. Report and record:
- *Sensitivity to bright light.* When pupils are dilated, excess amounts of light enter the eyes. This causes squinting. Sunglasses help reduce brightness. Provide for safety. The person should not drive or perform dangerous tasks in poor light.

TABLE 32-3 Beta-Adrenergic Blocking Agents

Generic Name	Brand Name	Topical Dose Forms	Initial Adult Dosage
betaxolol hydrochloride	Betoptic S	Ophthalmic solution: 0.25%, 0.5% solutions in 5, 10, and 15 mL dropper bottles	One to two drops twice daily
carteolol		Ophthalmic solution: 1% solution in 5, 10, 15 mL dropper bottles	One drop twice daily
levobunolol hydrochloride	Betagan	Ophthalmic solution: 0.5% solutions in 5, 10, and 15 mL dropper bottles	One drop once or twice daily
metipranolol		Ophthalmic solution: 0.3% solution in 5 and 10 mL dropper bottles	One drop twice daily in affected eye(s)
timolol maleate	Timoptic	Ophthalmic solution: 0.25%, 0.5% solutions in 5, 10, and 15 mL dropper bottles Gel-forming ophthalmic solution: 0.25%, 0.5% solutions	One drop of 0.25% solution twice daily; One drop of gel solution once daily

Modified from Willihnganz M: Clayton's Basic Pharmacology for Nurses, ed 18, St Louis, 2020, Elsevier.

TABLE 32-4 Prostaglandin Agonists

Generic Name	Brand Name	Topical Dose Forms	Adult Dosage Range
bimatoprost	Lumigan	Ophthalmic solution: 0.01%, 0.03% solution in 2.5, 5, and 7.5 mL dropper bottles	One drop in each affected eye in the evening
latanoprost	Xalatan	Ophthalmic solution: 0.005% solution in 2.5, 7.5 mL dropper bottle	One drop in each affected eye in the evening
afluprost	Zioptan	Ophthalmic solution: 0.0015% solution in 0.3 mL pouch	One drop in each affected eye in the evening
travoprost	Travatan Z	Ophthalmic solution: 0.004% solution in 2.5, 5 mL dropper bottle	One drop in each affected eye in the evening

TABLE 32-5 Anticholinergic Agents

Generic Name	Brand Name	Topical Dose Forms	Adult Dosage
atropine sulfate		Ointment: 1%; Ophthalmic solution: 0.5%, 1%, 2%	Uveitis: One to two drops up to three times daily
cyclopentolate hydrochloride	Cyclogyl	Ophthalmic solution: 0.5%, 1%, 2%	Refraction: One drop followed by another drop in 5-10 minutes
homatropine hydrobromide		Ophthalmic solution: 5%	Uveitis: One to two drops every 3-4 hours
tropicamide	Mydriacyl	Ophthalmic solution: 0.5%, 1%	Refraction: One to two drops, repeated in 5 minutes

Modified from Willihnganz M: Clayton's Basic Pharmacology for Nurses, ed 18, St Louis, 2020, Elsevier.

* *Eye irritation, tearing.* These tend to be mild and resolve with continued therapy.
* *Flushing, dry skin, dry mouth, blurred vision, tachycardia, dysrhythmias, urinary hesitancy and retention, vasodilation, constipation.* These signal overdose or excessive administration of an anticholinergic agent.

DRUG CLASS: Antifungal Agents

The following is an antifungal agent used to treat fungal infections of the eye:

* Natamycin (na tah my' sin); Natacyn (na' tah sin)

Assisting With the Nursing Process. When giving natamycin (Natacyn), you assist the nurse with the nursing process.

Assessment
* Ask about eye symptoms.
* Ask about the amount and type of visual impairment.

Planning
* The topical dose form is a 5% suspension.

Implementation
* One drop in the eye at 1- or 2-hour intervals for the first 3 to 4 days.
* The dosage may then be reduced to one drop every 3 to 4 hours.
* Therapy is continued for 14 to 21 days.

Evaluation. Report and record:
* *Sensitivity to bright light.* When pupils are dilated, excess amounts of light enter the eyes. This causes squinting. Sunglasses help reduce brightness. Provide for safety. The person should not drive or perform dangerous tasks in poor light.
* *Blurred vision, tearing, redness.* These are usually mild and tend to resolve with continued therapy. Provide for safety. Remind the person not to forcefully rub their eyes when tearing.
* *Eye pain.* The person needs medical attention.
* *Worsening of symptoms.* The person needs medical attention if symptoms worsen or do not improve after several days.

TABLE 32-6 Antiviral Agents

Generic Name	Brand Name	Topical Dose Forms	Adult Dosage
ganciclovir	Zirgan	Ophthalmic Gel: 0.15%	Initial dosage: One drop in affected eye five times daily (about q3h while awake) until the corneal ulcer heals Maintenance dosage: 1 drop three times daily for 7 days
trifluridine	Viroptic	Ophthalmic solution: 1% in 7.5 mL dropper bottle	Intraocular: Place one drop onto the cornea of the affected eye q2h during waking hours; do not exceed nine drops daily Continue for 7 more days to prevent recurrence, using one drop q4h (five drops daily)

Modified from Willihnganz M: Clayton's Basic Pharmacology for Nurses, ed 18, St Louis, 2020, Elsevier.

TABLE 32-7 Ophthalmic Antibiotics

Antibiotic	Brand Name	Dose Forms
azithromycin	AzaSite	Drops
bacitracin	Bacitracin ophthalmic	Ointment
besifloxacin	Besivance	Drops
ciprofloxacin	Ciloxan	Drops, ointment
erythromycin		Ointment
gatifloxacin	Zymaxid	Drops
gentamicin	Gentak	Drops, ointment
levofloxacin	—	Drops
moxifloxacin	Moxeza, Vigamox	Drops
ofloxacin	Ocuflox	Drops
sulfacetamide	Bleph-10	Drops
tobramycin	Tobrex ophthalmic	Drops, ointment
Combinations		
trimethoprim-polymyxin B	Polytrim ophthalmic	Drops
polymyxin B-bacitracin	Polycin	Ointment
neomycin-polymyxin B-bacitracin	Neo-Polycin ophthalmic	Ointment
neomycin-polymyxin B-gramicidin	Neosporin ophthalmic	Solution

Modified from Willihnganz M: Clayton's Basic Pharmacology for Nurses, ed 18, St Louis, 2020, Elsevier.

DRUG CLASS: Antiviral Agents

Ophthalmic antiviral agents inhibit the virus from reproducing. They are used to treat herpes infections of the eye.

Assisting With the Nursing Process. When giving antiviral agents for eye conditions, you assist the nurse with the nursing process.

  Assessment
- Ask about eye symptoms.
- Ask about the amount and type of visual impairment.
  Planning. See Table 32-6 for "Topical Dose Forms."
  Implementation. See Table 32-6 for "Adult Dosage."
  Evaluation. Report and record:
- *Visual haze, tearing, redness, burning.* These are usually mild and tend to resolve with continued therapy. Provide for safety. Remind the person not to forcefully rub their eyes when tearing.
- *Sensitivity to bright light.* When pupils are dilated, excess amounts of light enter the eyes. This causes squinting. Sunglasses help reduce brightness. Provide for safety. The person should not drive or perform dangerous tasks in poor light.
- *Allergic reactions.* The person needs medical attention.

DRUG CLASS: Ophthalmic Antibiotics

Ophthalmic antibiotics are used to treat superficial eye infections. Prolonged or frequent use of topical antibiotics should be avoided because of these risks:
- Hypersensitivity reactions
- The development of resistant organisms, including fungi
  See Table 32-7.

DRUG CLASS: Corticosteroids

Corticosteroids are used for allergic reactions of the eye. They also are used for other acute noninfectious inflammatory conditions of the eye. Prolonged therapy may cause glaucoma and cataracts. See Table 32-8.

DRUG CLASS: Ophthalmic Antiinflammatory Agents

The following ophthalmic antiinflammatory agents stop the production of prostaglandins. Prostaglandins increase intraocular inflammation and pressure. Some agents are used before and after cataract surgery.

The following are ophthalmic antiinflammatory agents are used to treat conditions of the eye:
- Flurbiprofen sodium—inhibits miosis (constriction of the pupil) during cataract surgery.
- Bromfenac—used to treat postoperative inflammation after cataract removal surgery.

TABLE 32-8 Corticosteroids

Generic Name	Brand Name	Dose Forms
dexamethasone	Maxidex	Suspension
difluprednate	Durezol	Suspension
fluorometholone	FML FML Liqiuifilm	Ointment Suspension
loteprednol	Lotemax	Suspension; ointment; gel
prednisolone	Omnipred	Suspension

Modified from Willihnganz M: Clayton's Basic Pharmacology for Nurses, ed 18, St Louis, 2020, Elsevier.

TABLE 32-9   Ophthalmic Antihistamines

Generic Name	Brand Name	Topical Dose Forms	Adult Dosage
alcaftadine	Lastacaft	Solution: 0.25% in 3 mL dropper bottle	Instill one drop in each eye once daily
azelastine		Solution: 0.5 mg/mL in 6 mL dropper bottle	Instill one drop in each affected eye twice daily
Bepotastine	Bepreve	Solution: 1.5% in 5 and 10 mL dropper bottle	Instill one drop in each affected eye twice daily
cetirizine	Zerviate	Solution: 0.24% in 7.5 and 10mL dropper bottle	Instill one drop in affected eye twice daily (~8 hr apart)
emedastine	Emadine	Solution: 0.05% in 5 mL dropper bottle	Instill one drop in each eye up to four times daily
epinastine	Elestat	Solution: 0.05% in 5 mL dropper bottles	Instill one drop in each eye two times daily
ketotifen	Zaditor	Solution: 0.025% in 5 and 10 mL dropper bottles	Instill one drop in each eye every 8-12 hours
olopatadine	Patanol	Solution: 0.1% in 5 mL dropper bottle	Instill one or two drops in each affected eye two times daily at an interval of 6 to 8 hours
	Pataday	Solution: 0.2% in 2.5 mL dropper bottle	Instill one drop in each affected eye once daily
	Pazeo	Solution: 0.7% in 2.5 mL dropper bottle	Instill one drop in each affected eye once daily

Modified from Willihnganz M: Clayton's Basic Pharmacology for Nurses, ed 18, St Louis, 2020, Elsevier.

- Diclofenac sodium—used to treat postoperative inflammation after cataract removal surgery.
- Nepafenac—used to treat postoperative inflammation after cataract removal surgery.
- Ketorolac tromethamine—used to relieve itchy eyes from seasonal allergies.

DRUG CLASS: Antihistamines

Antihistamines are used to relieve the signs and symptoms associated with allergic conjunctivitis. They also prevent itching. For best results, they should be instilled before exposure to allergens. See Table 32-9.

DRUG CLASS: Antiallergenic Agents

Antiallergenic agents inhibit the release of histamine. These agents are used to treat allergic eye disorders:
- Cromolyn sodium 4% solution—one or two drops in each eye four to six times a day at regular intervals.

- Lodoxamide 0.1% solution (Alomide) —one or two drops in each affected eye four times a day.
- Nedocromil 2% solution (Alocril)—one or two drops in each eye twice a day at regular intervals.

DRUG CLASS: Artificial Tear Solutions

Artificial tear solutions are like natural eye secretions. They lubricate dry eyes. They may be used as lubricants for artificial eyes.

The dosage is one to three drops in each eye three or four times a day as needed. Product names include:
- Systane Ultra
- Refresh
- Tears Naturale Free
- Artificial Tears
- HypoTears

▮ REVIEW QUESTIONS

Circle the BEST answer.

1. Two types of eye drops are ordered. You apply the first type. How long should you wait before applying the second type?
   a. at least 5 minutes
   b. 30 minutes
   c. 1 hour
   d. a few hours
2. A person has glaucoma. The goal of drug therapy is to:
   a. prevent infection
   b. reduce intraocular pressure
   c. reverse blindness
   d. restore normal vision
3. After cataract surgery, postoperative care includes all of the following, *except:*
   a. keeping the eye shield in place as directed, including during naps
   b. placing the bedside table on the same side as the affected eye
   c. reminding the person not to rub or press the affected eye
   d. reporting eye drainage to the nurse immediately

4. When giving carbonic anhydrase inhibitors:
   a. do not give the drug if the person is allergic to sulfonamide antibiotics
   b. do not give the drug if the person is taking sulfonamide antibiotics
   c. it is not necessary to measure vital signs
   d. always give it on an empty stomach
5. Acetazolamide (Diamox Sequels) is used to treat glaucoma because it:
   a. prevents infection
   b. reduces intraocular pressure
   c. reverses blindness
   d. restores normal vision
6. Cholinergic agents are used to treat glaucoma because they:
   a. prevent infection
   b. reduce intraocular pressure
   c. reverse blindness
   d. restore normal vision

7. Which is a cholinergic agent used to treat glaucoma?
   a. brinzolamide (Azopt)
   b. tetrahydrozoline hydrochloride (Opti-Clear)
   c. pilocarpine (Pilocar)
   d. naphazoline hydrochloride (Clear Eyes)
8. Cholinergic agents and cholinesterase inhibitors may cause:
   a. increased intraocular pressure
   b. infection
   c. problems seeing at night
   d. kidney failure
9. Adrenergic agents:
   a. dilate the pupils
   b. increase intraocular pressure
   c. cause problems seeing at night
   d. cause heart failure
10. Beta-adrenergic blocking agents:
    a. decrease intraocular pressure
    b. increase intraocular pressure
    c. dilate the pupils
    d. constrict the pupils
11. Which is a beta-adrenergic blocking agent?
    a. bimatoprost (Lumigan)
    b. tropicamide (Mydracyl)
    c. carteolol
    d. ganciclovir (Zirgan)
12. Prostaglandin agonists:
    a. decrease intraocular pressure
    b. increase intraocular pressure
    c. dilate the pupils
    d. constrict the pupils
13. Anticholinergic agents:
    a. decrease intraocular pressure
    b. increase intraocular pressure
    c. dilate the pupils
    d. constrict the pupils
14. Anticholinergic agents:
    a. lubricate the eyes
    b. prevent infection
    c. cause problems seeing at night
    d. cause sensitivity to bright light
15. Corticosteroids are used:
    a. to increase intraocular pressure
    b. to decrease intraocular pressure
    c. before and after cataract surgery
    d. to treat allergic reactions of the eye
16. Which is an antiinflammatory agent used in the treatment of eye disorders?
    a. bacitracin (Bacitracin Ophthalmic)
    b. dexamethasone (Maxidex)
    c. emedastine (Emadine)
    d. flurbiprofen sodium
17. Which is *not* an antiallergenic agent?
    a. ketorolac tromethamine
    b. cromolyn sodium
    c. nedocromil (Alocril)
    d. lodoxamide (Alomide)
18. Artificial tears are used to:
    a. treat allergies
    b. dilate the pupils
    c. constrict the pupils
    d. lubricate the eyes

Circle T if the statement is true. Circle F if the statement is false.

19. T F Ointments are applied before eye drops.
20. T F Eye ointments may blur vision.
21. T F Ophthalmic labels and bottle caps are color coded.
22. T F HypoTears is an artificial tear solution.

Answers to these questions can be found on the Evolve Resources site: http://evolve.elsevier.com/Anderson/medasst/

33

Drugs Used in the Treatment of Cancer

OBJECTIVES

- Define the key terms used in this chapter.
- Explain the difference between benign tumors and cancer.
- Identify cancer risk factors.
- Identify the signs and symptoms of cancer.
- Explain the common cancer treatments.
- Identify the agents used for chemotherapy.
- Identify the common side effects of chemotherapy.

KEY TERMS

alopecia Hair loss

benign tumor A tumor that does not spread to other body parts but can grow to a large size

cancer Malignant tumor

malignant tumor A tumor that invades and destroys nearby tissue and can spread to other body parts; cancer

metastasis The spread of cancer to other body parts

stomatitis Inflammation *(itis)* of the mouth *(stomat)*

tumor A new growth of abnormal cells; tumors are either benign or malignant

---

Cells reproduce for tissue growth and repair. Cells divide in an orderly way. Sometimes cell division and growth are out of control. A mass or clump of cells develops. This new growth of abnormal cells is called a **tumor.** Tumors are benign or malignant (Fig. 33-1):

- **Malignant tumors (cancer)** invade and destroy nearby tissue (Fig. 33-2). They can spread to other body parts. They may be life-threatening. They sometimes grow back after removal.
- **Benign tumors** do not spread to other body parts. They can grow to a large size, but are rarely life-threatening. They usually do not grow back when removed.

Metastasis is the spread of cancer to other body parts (Fig. 33-3). Cancer cells break off the tumor and travel to other body parts. New tumors grow in other body parts. This occurs if cancer is not treated and controlled.

Cancer can occur almost anywhere. Common sites are the skin, lung and bronchus, colon and rectum, breast, prostate, uterus, ovary, urinary bladder, kidney, mouth and pharynx, pancreas, and thyroid gland (Fig. 33-4). Cancer is the second leading cause of death in the United States.

Certain factors increase the risk of cancer. The National Cancer Institute describes these risk factors:

- *Growing older.* Cancer occurs in all age groups. However, most cancers occur in persons over 65 years of age.
- *Tobacco.* This includes using tobacco (smoking, snuff, and chewing tobacco) and being around tobacco (secondhand smoke). This risk can be avoided.
- *Sunlight.* Sun, sunlamps, and tanning booths cause early aging of the skin and skin damage. These can lead to skin cancer. Time in the sun should be limited. Sunlamps and tanning booths should be avoided.

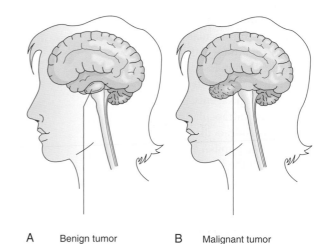

A   Benign tumor   B   Malignant tumor

Fig. 33-1 Tumors. **A,** A benign tumor grows within a local area. **B,** A malignant tumor invades other tissues.

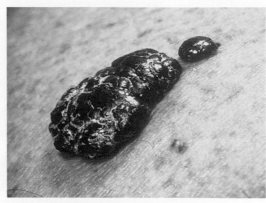

Fig. 33-2 Malignant tumor on the skin. (From Belcher AE: *Cancer nursing,* St Louis, 1992, Mosby.)

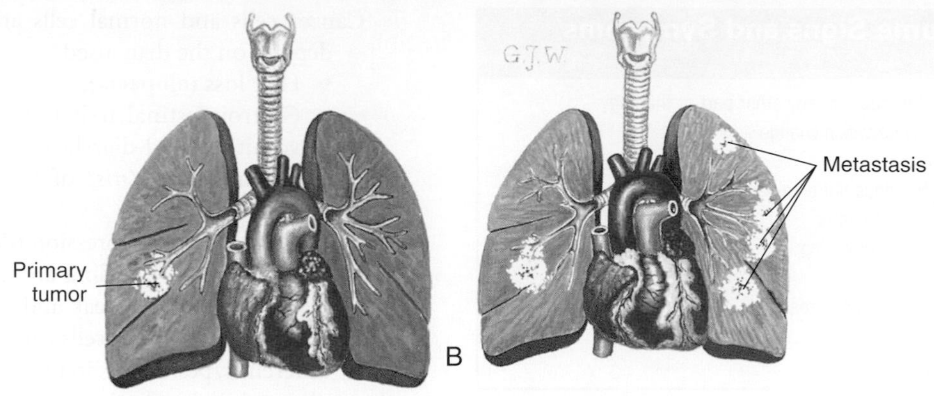

Fig. 33-3 A, Tumor in the lung. **B,** Tumor has metastasized to the other lung. (Modified from Belcher AE: *Cancer nursing,* St Louis, 1992, Mosby.)

Estimated new cases

Male			Female		
Pancreas	29,940	3%	Leukemia	25,860	3%
Leukemia	35,920	4%	Pancreas	26,830	3%
Oral cavity & pharynx	38,140	4%	Kidney & renal pelvis	29,700	3%
Non-Hodgkin lymphoma	41,090	5%	Non-Hodgkin lymphoma	33,110	4%
Kidney & renal pelvis	44,120	5%	Thyroid	37,810	4%
Melanoma of the skin	57,200	7%	Melanoma of the skin	39,260	5%
Urinary bladder	61,700	7%	Uterine corpus	61,880	7%
Colon & rectum	78,500	9%	Colon & rectum	67,100	7%
Lung & bronchus	116,440	13%	Lung & bronchus	111,710	13%
Prostate	174,650	20%	Breast	268,600	30%
All sites	**870,970**		**All sites**	**891,480**	

Estimated deaths

Male			Female		
Brain & other nervous system	9,910	3%	Brain & other nervous system	7,850	3%
Non-Hodgkin lymphoma	11,510	4%	Non-Hodgkin lymphoma	8,460	3%
Urinary bladder	12,870	4%	Leukemia	9,690	3%
Esophagus	13,020	4%	Liver & intrahepatic bile duct	10,180	4%
Leukemia	13,150	4%	Uterine corpus	12,160	4%
Liver & intraphepatic bile duct	21,600	7%	Ovary	13,980	5%
Pancreas	23,800	7%	Pancreas	21,950	8%
Colon & rectum	27,640	9%	Colon & rectum	23,380	8%
Prostate	31,620	10%	Breast	41,760	15%
Lung & bronchus	76,650	24%	Lung & bronchus	66,020	23%
All sites	**321,670**		**All sites**	**285,210**	

Estimate are rounded to the nearest 10, and cases exclude basal cell and squamous cell skin cancers and in situ carcinoma except urinary bladder. Estimates do not include Puerto Rico or other US territories. Ranking is based on modeled projections and may differ from the most recent observed data.

Fig. 33-4 Leading sites of new cancer cases and deaths—2019 estimates. (Data from American Cancer Society. Cancer Facts & Figures 2019. Atlanta, American Cancer Society, Inc.)

- *Ionizing radiation.* This can cause cell damage that leads to cancer. X-rays are one source, as is radon gas formed in the soil and certain rocks. People who work in mines are at risk for radon exposure. Radon can be found in homes in some parts of the country. Radioactive fallout, which can come from nuclear power plant accidents, is another source. Radon may also come from the production, testing, or use of atomic weapons.
- *Certain chemicals and other substances.* Painters, construction workers, and those in the chemical industry are at risk. Household substances also carry risks—paint, pesticides, used engine oil, and other chemicals.
- *Some viruses and bacteria.* Being infected with certain viruses increases the risk of the following cancers—cervical, liver, lymphoma, leukemia, stomach, Kaposi's sarcoma (a cancer associated with acquired immunodeficiency syndrome—AIDS).
- *Certain hormones.* Hormone replacement therapy for menopause may increase the risk of breast cancer. Diethylstilbestrol (DES), a form of estrogen, was given to some pregnant women between the early 1940s and 1971. Women who took the drug are at risk for breast cancer. Their daughters are at risk for a certain type of cervical cancer.
- *Family history of cancer.* Certain cancers tend to occur in families. They include melanoma and cancers of the breast, ovary, prostate, and colon.
- *Alcohol.* The risk of certain cancers increases with more than two drinks a day. Such cancers are of the mouth, throat, esophagus, larynx, liver, and breast. Women should have no more than one drink a day. Men should have no more than two drinks a day.
- *Poor diet, lack of physical activity, being overweight.* A high-fat diet increases the risk of cancers of the colon, uterus, and

prostate. Lack of physical activity and being overweight increase the risk for cancers of the breast, colon, esophagus, kidney, and uterus.

If detected early, cancer can be treated and controlled (Box 33-1). Treatment depends on the type of tumor, its site and size, and whether or not it has spread. The goal of cancer treatment may be one of the following:

- Cure the cancer
- Control the disease
- Reduce symptoms for as long as possible

Some cancers respond to one type of treatment. Others respond best to two or more types. Cancer treatments also damage healthy cells and tissues. Side effects depend on the type and extent of the treatment.

- *Surgery.* Surgery removes tumors and may be carried out to cure or control cancer. Surgery also relieves pain from advanced cancer. The person has some pain after surgery, which is controlled with pain relieving drugs. The person may feel weak or tired for a while. Some surgeries are very disfiguring and may affect self-esteem and body image.
- *Radiation therapy.* Radiation therapy also is called radiotherapy. It kills cells. X-ray beams are aimed at the tumor. Sometimes radioactive material is implanted in or near the tumor. Cancer cells and normal cells receive radiation. Both are destroyed. Radiation therapy:
  - Destroys certain tumors
  - Shrinks a tumor before surgery
  - Destroys cancer cells that remain in an area after surgery
  - Controls tumor growth to prevent or relieve pain

Side effects depend on the body part being treated. Burns, skin breakdown, and hair loss can occur at the treatment site. The doctor may order special skin care measures. Fatigue is common. Extra rest is needed. Discomfort, nausea and vomiting, diarrhea, and loss of appetite are other side effects.

- *Chemotherapy.* Chemotherapy involves drugs that kill cells. It is used to:
  - Shrink a tumor before surgery.
  - Kill cells that break off the tumor. The goal is to prevent metastasis.
  - Relieve symptoms caused by the cancer.

Cancer cells and normal cells are affected. Side effects depend on the drug used:

- Hair loss (**alopecia**).
- Gastrointestinal irritation. Poor appetite, nausea, vomiting, and diarrhea can occur. **Stomatitis,** an inflammation (*itis*) of the mouth (*stomat*), may occur.
- Bone marrow depression (decreased production of blood cells). Bleeding and infection are risks. The person may feel weak and tired.

- *Stem cell transplants.* Stem cells can potentially develop into many different types of cells in the body. When high doses of chemotherapy and radiation destroy blood cells, stem cell transplants help the body develop more blood-forming stem cells. Stem cells can come from the person or a donor. They may come from the bloodstream, bone marrow, or umbilical cord. There can be side effects to stem cell transplants. The person must be protected from infections and abnormal bleeding. Rejection can also be a complication. It can be a long process and the person's immune system needs time to recover.
- *Hormone therapy.* Hormone therapy prevents cancer cells from using hormones needed for their growth. Drugs are given that prevent the production of certain hormones. Organs or glands that produce a certain hormone are removed. For example, a breast cancer might need estrogen for growth. Then the ovaries are removed. A prostate cancer may need testosterone for growth. Then the testicles may be removed. Side effects of hormone therapy include fatigue, fluid retention, weight gain, hot flashes, nausea and vomiting, appetite changes, and blood clots. Fertility is affected in men and women. Men also may experience impotence and loss of sexual desire.
- *Biological therapy.* Biological therapy (*immunotherapy*) helps the immune system fight the cancer. It also protects the body from the side effects of cancer treatments. Side effects include flu-like symptoms—chills, fever, muscle aches, weakness, loss of appetite, nausea, vomiting, and diarrhea. Bleeding, bruising, swelling, and skin rashes may occur.

DRUG THERAPY FOR CANCER

Chemotherapy is most effective when the tumor is small and when cells divide rapidly. The agent used depends on the type of tumor cells, rate of growth, and tumor size.

Because approaches to cancer treatment are changing rapidly, specific agents and dosages are not discussed. See Table 33-1.

Chemotherapy can be very toxic to the normal cells. Chemoprotective agents (Table 33.2) help reduce the toxicity of chemotherapy.

Some drugs kill healthy bone marrow cells while also killing cancer cells. Bone marrow stimulants (Table 33.3) are used to help stimulate bone marrow cells to recover quicker. This helps the person's immune system respond to and fight infections.

See *Delegation Guidelines: Drugs Used in the Treatment of Cancer.*

TABLE 33-1 Cancer Chemotherapeutic Agents

Generic Name	Brand Name	Major Indications
busulfan	Myleran	Chronic myelogenous leukemia
cisplatin	Platinol-AQ	Testicular and ovarian cancers, bladder cancer
cyclophosphamide	Cytoxan	Hodgkin's disease and other lymphomas, multiple myeloma, lymphocytic leukemia, many solid cancers
capecitabine	Xeloda	Breast cancer, colorectal cancer
fluorouracil	5-FU, FU	Breast, large bowel, ovarian, pancreatic, stomach carcinoma
mercaptopurine	6-MP, Purinethol	Acute lymphocytic and granulocytic leukemia
methotrexate	MTX	Acute lymphocytic leukemia, choriocarcinoma, carcinoma of cervix and head and neck area, mycosis fungoides, solid cancers
etoposide	VePesid, Toposar	Testicular tumors, small cell carcinoma of the lung, Hodgkin's disease and non-Hodgkin's lymphoma, acute non-lymphocytic leukemia, ovarian carcinoma, Kaposi's sarcoma
docetaxel	Taxotere	Breast cancer, prostate cancer
paclitaxel	Taxol	Ovarian carcinoma, breast carcinoma, AIDS-related Kaposi's sarcoma, lung cancer
vinblastine sulfate	Velban	Hodgkin's disease and other lymphomas, solid cancers
vincristine sulfate	Oncovin	Acute lymphocytic leukemia, Hodgkin's disease and other lymphomas, solid cancers
Antibiotics		
dactinomycin	Actinomycin D; Cosmegen	Testicular carcinoma, Wilms' tumor, rhabdomyosarcoma, Ewing's and osteogenic sarcoma, and other solid tumors
daunorubicin	Cerubidine	Acute non-lymphocytic leukemia in adults, acute lymphocytic leukemia in children and adults
doxorubicin	Adriamycin	Soft tissue, osteogenic and miscellaneous sarcomas, Hodgkin's disease, non-Hodgkin's lymphoma, bronchogenic and breast carcinoma, thyroid cancer, leukemias
aldesleukin	Proleukin	Melanoma, renal cell carcinoma, T-cell lymphoma
dacarbazine	DTIC-Dome; DIC	Metastatic malignant melanoma, Hodgkin's disease
hydroxyurea	Hydrea	Chronic granulocytic leukemia, ovarian cancer, melanoma
interferon alfa-2a	Roferon-a	Hairy cell leukemia, Kaposi's sarcoma
interferon alfa-2b	Intron a	Hairy cell leukemia, Kaposi's sarcoma, malignant melanoma
leuprolide acetate	Lupron	Prostatic carcinoma, breast carcinoma
mitotane	Lysodren	Adrenal cortical carcinoma
procarbazine hydrochloride	Matulane	Hodgkin's disease, non-Hodgkin's lymphoma, lung cancer, melanoma
Hormones		
anastrozole	Arimidex	Breast cancer in postmenopausal women with disease progression following tamoxifen therapy
bicalutamide	Casodex	Prostate cancer
estramustine	Emcyt	Prostate cancer
Ethinyl estradiol		Breast and prostate carcinomas
exemestane	Aromasin	Breast cancer in postmenopausal women with disease progression following tamoxifen therapy
fluoxymesterone		Breast carcinoma
flutamide	Eulexin	Metastatic prostatic carcinoma
fulvestrant	Faslodex	Breast cancer
goserelin	Zoladex	Prostate and breast cancer
histrelin	Vantas	Prostate cancer
letrozole	Femara	Breast cancer in postmenopausal women with disease progression following antiestrogen therapy
medroxyprogesterone acetate	Provera	Endometrial carcinoma, renal cell, breast cancer
nilutamide	Nilandron	Prostate cancer
tamoxifen	Nolvadex	Breast cancer (estrogen sensitive)
toremifene	Fareston	Metastatic breast cancer in postmenopausal women with estrogen positive tumors
triptorelin	Trelstar	Prostate cancer
irinotecan	Camptosar	Carcinoma of the colon and rectum

Modified from Willihnganz M: Clayton's Basic Pharmacology for Nurses, ed 18, St Louis, 2020, Elsevier.

TABLE 33-2   Chemoprotective Agents

Generic Name	Brand Name
amifostine	Ethyol
dexrazoxane	Zinecard
glucarpidase	Voraxaze
leucovorin	
Mesna	Mesnex

Modified from Willihnganz M: Clayton's Basic Pharmacology for Nurses, ed 18, St Louis, 2020, Elsevier.

TABLE 33-3   Bone Marrow Stimulants

Generic Name	Brand Name
darbepoetin	Aranesp
epoetin alfa	Procrit, Epogen
filgrastim	Neupogen
pegfilgrastim	Neulasta
sargramostim	Leukine

Modified from Willihnganz M: Clayton's Basic Pharmacology for Nurses, ed 18, St Louis, 2020, Elsevier.

DELEGATION GUIDELINES
Drugs Used in the Treatment of Cancer

Some drugs used to treat cancer are given parenterally—by subcutaneous, intramuscular, or intravenous injection. You do not give parenteral dose forms. Should a nurse delegate the administration of such to you, you must:
- Remember that parenteral dosages are often very different from dosages for other routes.
- Refuse the delegation but do not ignore the request. Make sure the nurse knows that you cannot give the drug and why.

Your state and agency may allow you to give some oral dose forms. Make sure you receive the necessary education about any chemotherapy agents that you will give.

■ REVIEW QUESTIONS

Circle the BEST answer.

1. A person has cancer. You know that:
   a. the tumor will not threaten life
   b. the tumor can spread to other body parts
   c. the tumor is benign
   d. the person's mouth is inflamed
2. Which is *not* a warning sign of cancer?
   a. painful, swollen joints
   b. a sore that does not heal
   c. unusual bleeding or discharge
   d. discomfort after eating
3. A person had surgery for cancer. The person's care will likely include:
   a. pain-relieving measures
   b. mouth care for stomatitis
   c. skin care for burns at the treatment site
   d. measures to prevent hair loss

4. Chemotherapy is most effective:
   a. when the tumor is first diagnosed
   b. after surgery
   c. after radiation therapy
   d. when the tumor is small
5. A person receiving chemotherapy will likely experience:
   a. diarrhea
   b. burns
   c. skin breakdown
   d. weight gain

Circle T if the statement is true. Circle F if the statement is false.
6. T F   Nausea and vomiting are common side effects from chemotherapy.
7. T F   Hormones are used to treat some cancers.
8. T F   Some antibiotics are used in the treatment of cancer.

Answers to these questions can be found on the Evolve Resources site: http://evolve.elsevier.com/Anderson/medasst/

34

Drugs Affecting Muscles and Joints

OBJECTIVES

- Define the key terms and key abbreviations used in this chapter.
- Describe the goals of therapy when muscle relaxants are given.
- Describe the different types of muscle relaxants.
- Explain how to assist with the nursing process when giving muscle relaxants.
- Describe gout.
- Describe the drugs used to treat gout.
- Explain how to assist with the nursing process when giving drugs to treat gout.

KEY TERMS

clonus Rapidly alternating involuntary contraction and relaxation of skeletal muscles

hyperreflexia Increased reflex actions

spasm An involuntary muscle contraction of sudden onset

KEY ABBREVIATIONS

CNS Central nervous system
g Gram
GI Gastrointestinal

mg Milligram
PO Per os (orally)

Musculoskeletal disorders may produce varying degrees of pain and immobility. Nervous system disorders often affect the muscles. The person's ability to perform activities of daily living is affected. The person may need drug therapy to relax the muscles. See Box 34-1 for structure and function of the muscles.

Arthritis is a common joint disease. It is treated with nonsteroidal antiinflammatory agents (Chapter 18) and corticosteroids (Chapter 29). Gout is a very painful form of arthritis (p. 309).

See *Delegation Guidelines: Drugs Affecting Muscles and Joints.*

DELEGATION GUIDELINES
Drugs Affecting Muscles and Joints

Some drugs affecting muscles and joints are given parenterally—by intramuscular or intravenous injection. Some are injected into the spinal column. Because you do not give such dose forms, they are not included in this chapter. Should a nurse delegate the administration of such to you, you must:
- Remember that parenteral dosages are often very different from dosages for other routes.
- Refuse the delegation but do not ignore the request. Make sure the nurse knows that you cannot give the drug and why.

DRUG THERAPY FOR MUSCLE SPASMS

A spasm is an involuntary muscle contraction of sudden onset. Muscle spasms are often painful. Drugs in this class depress the central nervous system (CNS). They do not have a direct effect on muscles or nerve conduction. All drugs in this class cause some degree of sedation.

BOX 34-1   Muscles: Structure and Function

The human body has more than 500 *muscles* (Fig. 34-1 and Fig. 34-2). Some are voluntary and others are involuntary.
- *Voluntary muscles* can be consciously controlled. Muscles attached to bones *(skeletal muscles)* are voluntary. Arm muscles do not work unless you move your arm, and leg muscles do not work unless you move your arm. Skeletal muscles are *striated*, meaning they look striped or streaked.
- *Involuntary muscles* work automatically. You cannot control them. They control the action of the stomach, intestines, blood vessels, and other body organs. Involuntary muscles are also called *smooth muscles*. They look smooth; not streaked or striped.
- *Cardiac muscle* is in the heart. It is an involuntary muscle. However, it appears striated like skeletal muscle.

Muscles have three functions:
- Movement of body parts
- Maintenance of posture
- Production of body heat

Strong, tough connective tissues called *tendons* connect muscles to bones. When muscles contract (shorten), tendons at each end of the muscle cause the bone to move. The body has many tendons. See the Achilles tendon in Figure 34-2. Some muscles constantly contract to maintain the body's posture. When muscles contract, they burn food for energy. Heat is produced. The more muscle activity, the greater the amount of heat produced. Shivering is how the body produces heat when exposed to cold. Shivering is from rapid, general muscle contractions.

DRUG CLASS: Centrally Acting Skeletal Muscle Relaxants

Centrally acting skeletal muscle relaxants are used to relieve acute muscle spasms.

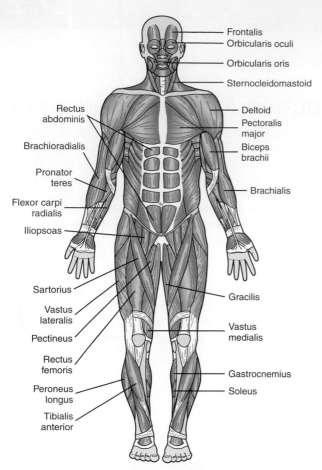

Fig. 34-1 Anterior view of the muscles of the body.

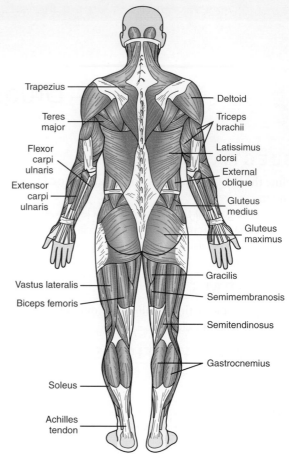

Fig. 34-2 Posterior view of the muscles of the body.

The drugs listed in Table 34-1 are used with physical therapy, rest, and analgesics. The goal of therapy is relief of muscle spasm.

Assisting With the Nursing Process. When giving centrally acting skeletal muscle relaxants, you assist the nurse with the nursing process.

   Assessment
* Measure vital signs.
* Observe level of alertness.
   Planning. See Table 34-1 for "Oral Dose Forms."
   Implementation. See Table 34-1 for "Adult Dosage."
   Evaluation. Report and record:
* *Sedation, weakness, lethargy, gastrointestinal (GI) complaints.* These are usually mild and tend to resolve with continued therapy. Provide for safety. Remind the person to avoid driving or using machines.
* *Dizziness.* Provide for safety.
* *Sore throat, fever, jaundice, weakness.* These may signal changes in red blood cells and white blood cells.
* *Anorexia, nausea, vomiting, jaundice.* These may signal liver toxicity.

DRUG CLASS: Direct-Acting Skeletal Muscle Relaxant

The following is a direct-acting skeletal muscle relaxant:
* Dantrolene (dan' tro leen); Dantrium (dan' tree um)

This drug acts directly on skeletal muscle. It produces mild weakness of skeletal muscles. It decreases the force of reflex muscle contractions, muscle stiffness, involuntary muscle movements, and spasticity. It also decreases:
* Clonus—rapidly alternating involuntary contraction and relaxation of skeletal muscles
* Hyperreflexia—increased reflex actions
   The drug is used to control spasticity of chronic disorders such as cerebral palsy, multiple sclerosis, spinal cord injury, and stroke. The goal of therapy is relief from muscle spasm.

Assisting With the Nursing Process. When giving dantrolene (Dantrium), you assist the nurse with the nursing process.
   Assessment
* Measure vital signs.
* Observe muscle spasms that may be present.
   Planning. The oral dose forms are 25, 50, and 100 mg capsules.
   Implementation
* The initial adult dose is 25 mg daily for 7 days.
* The dose is then increased to 25 mg three times daily for 7 days.
* The dose is then increased to 50 mg three times daily for 7 days.
* The final dosage is gradually increased up to 100 mg three times a day.
* Some persons may require 100 mg four times daily.

TABLE 34-1	Centrally Acting Muscle Relaxants		
Generic Name	**Brand Name**	**Oral Dose Forms**	**Adult Dosage**
carisoprodol	Soma	Tablets: 250, 350 mg	PO: 250-350 mg four times daily for a maximum of two to three weeks.
chlorzoxazone	Lorsone	Tablets: 250, 375, 500, 750 mg	PO: 250-750 mg three or four times daily
cyclobenzaprine	Amrix	Tablets: 5, 7.5, 10 mg Capsules, extended-release (24-hr): 15, 30 mg	PO: 10-20 mg three times daily; do not exceed 60 mg PO: extended-release: 15-30 mg once daily; do not exceed 30 mg daily
metaxalone	Skelaxin	Tablets: 400, 800 mg	PO: 800 mg three or four times daily
methocarbamol	Robaxin	Tablets: 500, 750 mg	PO: 1-1.5 g four times daily
orphenadrine citrate		Tablets, 12-hr extended-release: 100 mg	PO: 100 mg two times daily
tizanidine	Zanaflex	Tablets: 2, 4 mg Capsules: 2, 4, 6 mg	PO: 4-8 mg every 6 to 8 hours; do not exceed 36 mg daily

Modified from Willihnganz M: Clayton's Basic Pharmacology for Nurses, ed 18, St Louis, 2020, Elsevier.

Evaluation. Report and record:
- *Weakness, diarrhea, drowsiness.* These are usually mild and tend to resolve with continued therapy.
- *Dizziness, lightheadedness.* Provide for safety.
- *Photosensitivity.* This is sensitivity to sunlight and ultraviolet light (sunlamps, tanning beds). The person should avoid exposure to sunlight, sunlamps, and tanning beds. They should apply sunscreen and wear long-sleeved garments, a hat, and sunglasses when outdoors. Sunburn needs medical attention.
- *Anorexia, nausea, vomiting, jaundice.* These may signal liver toxicity.

OTHER MUSCLE RELAXANTS

The following drug relaxes muscles by partially inhibiting reflex activity at the spinal cord:
- Baclofen (bak' lo fen); Lioresal (ly or' e sahl)

Baclofen (Lioresal)

The drug is used to manage muscle spasticity from multiple sclerosis, spinal cord injury, and other spinal cord diseases. The goal of therapy is relief of muscle spasm.

Assisting With the Nursing Process. When giving baclofen (Lioresal), you assist the nurse with the nursing process.
Assessment
- Observe level of alertness.
Planning
- The oral dose forms are:
  - 5, 10, and 20 mg tablets
  - 1 mg/mL and 5 mg/mL oral suspension
Implementation
- The oral adult dose is 5 mg three times a day.
- The dosage may be increased by 5 mg every 3 to 7 days based on the person's response.
- The best effects usually occur with dosages of 40 to 80 mg daily.
- Do not abruptly discontinue baclofen therapy.
Evaluation. Report and record:
- *Nausea, fatigue, headache, drowsiness.* These are usually mild and tend to resolve with continued therapy.
- *Dizziness.* Provide for safety.

DRUGS USED TO TREAT GOUT

Gout occurs when uric acid builds up in the body. The buildup can lead to kidney stones and sharp uric acid crystal deposits in the joints. Uric acid comes from the breakdown of substances called *purines.* Purines are in all body tissues and in some foods. Liver, dried beans, peas, and anchovies are examples.

Uric acid is normally excreted from the body through urine. It can build up in the blood when:
- The body makes too much uric acid
- The kidneys do not excrete enough uric acid
- A person eats too many foods high in purine

The first gout attack often occurs in the big toe. The toe is very sore, red, warm, and swollen. Gout can also affect the insteps, ankles, heels, knees, wrists, fingers, and elbows (Fig. 34-3). Signs and symptoms include:
- Pain
- Swelling
- Redness
- Heat
- Stiff joints

Stress, alcohol, drugs, and other illnesses can lead to gout. The next attack may not occur for months or years.

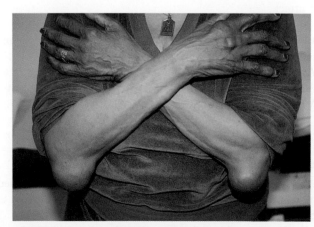

Fig. 34-3 Gout. (From Swartz MH: *Textbook of physical diagnosis, history, and examination,* ed 4, Philadelphia, 2002, Saunders.)

Drugs used to treat gout are:
- Nonsteroidal antiinflammatory agents (Chapter 18)
- Corticosteroids (Chapter 29)
- Other agents:
  - Allopurinol (al oh pur' in ol); Zyloprim (zy' lo prim)
  - Colchicine (kol' chi seen)
  - Probenecid (pro ben' eh sid)

Allopurinol (Zyloprim)

Allopurinol (Zyloprim) prevents uric acid from forming. The goals of therapy are to:
- Reduce uric acid blood levels
- Reduce the frequency of acute gout attacks

Assisting With the Nursing Process. When giving allopurinol (Zyloprim), you assist the nurse with the nursing process.
Assessment
- Ask about GI complaints.
Planning
- The oral dose forms are 100 and 300 mg tablets.
Implementation
- The initial adult dose is 100 mg daily.
- The daily dosage is 300 mg.
- The maximum daily dosage is 800 mg.
- Give the drug with food or milk if gastric irritation occurs.
Evaluation. Report and record:
- *Anorexia, nausea, vomiting, jaundice.* These may signal liver toxicity.
- *Sore throat, fever, jaundice, weakness.* These may signal changes in red blood cells and white blood cells.
- *Fever, itching, rash.* These may signal an allergic reaction. Tell the nurse at once. Do not give the next dose unless approved by the nurse.
- *Nausea, vomiting, diarrhea, dizziness, headache.* These are usually mild and tend to resolve with continued therapy.

Colchicine

Colchicine is used to prevent or relieve acute gout attacks. Joint pain and swelling begin to subside within 48 to 72 hours after therapy is started.

The goal of therapy is to relieve joint pain caused by an acute gout attack.

Assisting With the Nursing Process. When giving colchicine, you assist the nurse with the nursing process.
Assessment
- Ask about GI complaints.
- Measure intake and output.

Planning. The oral dose forms are 0.6 mg tablets and capsules.
Implementation
- 1.2 mg at first sign of gout flare, followed by 0.6 mg 1 hour later; do not exceed 1.8 mg over 1 hour.
- After the acute attack, 0.6 mg should be administered one to two times daily to prevent relapse.
- Do not repeat high-dose therapy for at least 3 days.
- The person should drink 8 to 12 eight-ounce glasses of fluid daily.

Evaluation. Report and record:
- *Nausea, vomiting, diarrhea.* Drug therapy is discontinued when these develop.
- *Red blood in vomitus, "coffee ground" vomitus, dark tarry stools.* These signal GI bleeding.
- *Sore throat, fever, jaundice, weakness.* These may signal changes in red blood cells and white blood cells.

Probenecid

Probenecid promotes the excretion of uric acid through the urine. It prevents the kidneys from reabsorbing urate. This results in reduced uric acid in the blood.

The goal of therapy is to treat chronic gouty arthritis. It is not effective for acute attacks of gout and is not used to treat pain.

Assisting With the Nursing Process. When giving probenecid, you assist the nurse with the nursing process.
Assessment
- Ask about GI complaints.
Planning
- The oral dose form is 500 mg tablets.
Implementation
- The initial adult dose is 250 mg twice a day for 1 week. It is then increased to 500 mg twice a day.
- The dosage may be increased by 500 mg every few weeks.
- The maximum daily dosage is 2 to 3 g.
- Give the drug with food or milk to prevent gastric irritation.
- The person should drink 8 to 12 eight-ounce glasses of fluid daily.

Evaluation. Report and record:
- *Sign and symptoms of acute gout attacks* (p. 309). These may increase for the first few months of therapy.
- *Nausea, anorexia, vomiting.* These may signal peptic ulcer disease.
- *Red blood in vomitus, "coffee ground" vomitus, dark tarry stools.* These signal GI bleeding.
- *Hives, itching, rash.* These may signal an allergic reaction. Tell the nurse at once. Do not give the next dose unless approved by the nurse.

REVIEW QUESTIONS

Circle the BEST answer.

1. An involuntary muscle contraction of sudden onset is called:
   a. clonus
   b. hyperreflexia
   c. a spasm
   d. a jerk

2. The rapidly alternating involuntary contraction and relaxation of skeletal muscles is called:
   a. clonus
   b. hyperreflexia
   c. a spasm
   d. jerking

3. Centrally acting skeletal muscle relaxants act:
   a. directly on the muscle
   b. by depressing the CNS
   c. by inhibiting reflex activity at the spinal cord
   d. by blocking nerve impulses

4. All centrally acting skeletal muscle relaxants cause some degree of:
   a. confusion
   b. orthostatic hypotension
   c. sedation
   d. spasticity

5. The goal of therapy for centrally acting muscle relaxants is relief of:
   a. clonus
   b. hyperreflexia
   c. muscle spasm
   d. jerking

6. Which has a dose form of oral suspension?
   a. dantrolene (Dantrium)
   b. baclofen (Lioresal)
   c. carisoprodol (Soma)
   d. tizanidine (Zanaflex)

7. Which is *not* a centrally acting muscle relaxant?
   a. dantrolene (Dantrium)
   b. cyclobenzaprine (Amrix)
   c. methocarbamol (Robaxin)
   d. carisoprodol (Soma)

8. Direct-acting skeletal muscle relaxants decrease:
   a. clonus, hyperreflexia, and muscle spasm
   b. cerebral palsy and multiple sclerosis
   c. spinal cord injury and stroke
   d. photosensitivity, sedation, and drowsiness

9. Which is a direct-acting skeletal muscle relaxant?
   a. dantrolene (Dantrium)
   b. baclofen (Lioresal)
   c. metaxalone (Skelaxin)
   d. orphenadrine citrate

10. Baclofen (Lioresal) is used in the management of:
    a. clonus, hyperreflexia, and muscle spasm
    b. cerebral palsy and stroke
    c. spinal cord injury and multiple sclerosis
    d. photosensitivity, sedation, and drowsiness

11. Allopurinol (Zyloprim) is given for gout. The initial adult dose is:
    a. 100 mg daily
    b. 200 mg daily
    c. 300 mg daily
    d. 400 mg daily

12. Allopurinol (Zyloprim) is given:
    a. before meals
    b. on an empty stomach
    c. with food or milk
    d. at bedtime

13. After therapy is started, a person receiving colchicine should begin to see symptom relief within:
    a. 12 to 24 hours
    b. 1 to 2 days
    c. 2 to 3 days
    d. 1 week

14. Persons receiving colchicine or probenecid should drink:
    a. 4 to 8 eight-ounce glasses of fluid daily
    b. 8 to 12 eight-ounce glasses of fluid daily
    c. milk with every meal
    d. milk at bedtime

15. Persons receiving drug therapy for gout should be observed for:
    a. dysrhythmias
    b. tremors
    c. GI symptoms
    d. confusion

Answers to these questions can be found on the Evolve Resources site: http://evolve.elsevier.com/Anderson/medasst/

35

Drugs Used to Treat Infections

OBJECTIVES

- Define the key terms and key abbreviations used in this chapter.
- Identify the signs and symptoms of an infection.
- Describe healthcare-associated infections and how to prevent them.
- Identify the pathogens destroyed by antimicrobial agents.
- Identify the safety measures needed when giving antimicrobial agents.
- Identify the signs of an allergic reaction to antimicrobial agents.

KEY TERMS

aerobe A microbe that lives and grows in the presence of oxygen *(aer)*

anaerobe A microbe that lives and grows in the absence *(an)* of oxygen *(aer)*

antibiotics Antimicrobials derived from living microorganisms

antimicrobial agents Chemicals that eliminate pathogens

bacteria One-celled plant life that multiply rapidly and can cause an infection in any body system; germs

carrier A human or animal that is a reservoir for microbes but does not have the signs and symptoms of infection

fungi Plants that live on other plants or animals

germs See "bacteria"

microbe See "microorganism"

microorganism A small *(micro)* living plant or animal *(organism)* seen only with a microscope; a microbe

non-pathogen A microbe that does not usually cause an infection

opportunistic infection An infection caused by non-pathogens in a person with a weakened immune system

pathogen A microbe that is harmful and can cause an infection

protozoa One-celled animals that can infect the blood, brain, intestines, and other body areas

secondary infection An infection caused by a microbe that follows the first infection caused by a different microbe

viruses Microbes that grow in living cells

KEY ABBREVIATIONS

AIDS Acquired immunodeficiency syndrome
CDC Centers for Disease Control and Prevention
g Gram
GI Gastrointestinal
HAI Healthcare-associated infection
HBV Hepatitis B virus
HIV Human immunodeficiency virus
IM Intramuscular

IV Intravenous
kg Kilogram
mg Milligram
mL Milliliter
STI Sexually transmitted infection
TB Tuberculosis
UTI Urinary tract infection

A **microorganism (microbe)** is a small *(micro)* living plant or animal *(organism)*. It is seen only with a microscope. **Microbes** are everywhere—in the mouth, nose, respiratory tract, stomach, and intestines. They are on the skin and in the air, soil, water, and food. They are also found on animals, clothing, and furniture. See Chapter 6.

Some microbes are harmful and can cause infections. These are called **pathogens. Non-pathogens** are microbes that do not usually cause an infection.

Normal flora are microbes that live and grow in a certain area (Chapter 6). Certain microbes are in the respiratory tract, in the intestines, and on the skin. They are non-pathogens when in or on a natural reservoir. A non-pathogen becomes a pathogen

when it is transmitted from its natural site to another site or host. When a non-pathogen causes an infection in a person with a weakened immune system, this is called an **opportunistic infection.** *Escherichia coli (E. coli)* is found in the colon. If it enters the urinary system, it can cause an infection.

INFECTION

The immune system protects the body from disease and infection (Box 35-1). As discussed in Chapter 6, an infection is a disease state resulting from the invasion and growth of microbes in the body. A *local infection* is in a body part. A *systemic infection* involves the whole body. *(Systemic means entire.)* The person has

BOX 35-1 The Immune System: Structure and Function

The immune system protects the body from disease and infection. Abnormal body cells can grow into tumors. Sometimes the body produces substances that cause the body to attack itself. Microbes (bacteria, viruses, and other germs) can cause an infection. The immune system defends against threats inside and outside the body.

The immune system gives the body *immunity*, meaning a person has protection against a disease or condition. The person will not get or be affected by the disease. There are two types of immunity:

- *Specific immunity* is the body's reaction to a certain threat.
- *Non-specific immunity* is the body's reaction to anything it does not recognize as a normal body substance.

some or all the signs and symptoms listed in Chapter 6, Box 6-1. Common infections are discussed in Box 35-2.

Infection prevention and healthcare-associated infections are discussed in Chapter 6.

See *Focus on Older Persons: Infection.*

ANTIMICROBIAL AGENTS

Antimicrobial agents are chemicals that eliminate pathogens. **Antibiotics** are antimicrobials derived from living microorganisms. For example, penicillin was first derived from a mold. Most antibiotics are harvested from large colonies of microbes. The microbes are purified and chemically modified into semi-synthetic antimicrobial agents.

BOX 35-2 Common Infections

Acquired Immunodeficiency Syndrome

Acquired immunodeficiency syndrome (AIDS) is caused by a virus. The virus is called the *human immunodeficiency virus (HIV)*. It attacks the immune system.

The virus is spread through body fluids—blood, semen, vaginal secretions, and breast milk. HIV is not spread by saliva, tears, sweat, sneezing, coughing, insects, or casual contact. The virus is mainly transmitted by:

- Unprotected anal, vaginal, or oral sex with an infected person ("Unprotected" meaning engaging in these sexual activities without a new latex or polyurethane condom.)
- Needle and syringe sharing among IV drug users
- HIV-infected mothers before or during childbirth
- HIV-infected mothers through breast-feeding

Box 35-3 lists the signs and symptoms of AIDS. Some persons infected with HIV have symptoms within a few months. Others may be symptom-free for more than 10 years. Although asymptomatic, they still carry the virus and can spread it to others.

Healthcare-Associated Infection

A **healthcare-associated infection (HAI)** is an infection that develops in a person cared for in any setting where health care is given. The infection is related to receiving health care. Hospitals, nursing centers, clinics, and home care settings are examples. HAIs also are called *nosocomial infections*. (*Nosocomial* comes from the Greek word for hospital.) HAIs are caused by normal flora. Or they are caused by microbes transmitted to the person from other sources.

For example, *E. coli* is normally in the colon. Feces contain *E. coli*. Poor wiping after bowel movements can cause *E. coli* to enter the urinary system. The hands can transmit *E. coli* to other body areas. If hand washing is poor, *E. coli* may spread to any body part or anything the hands touch. It also can be transmitted to other people.

Microbes can enter the body through equipment used in treatments, therapies, and tests. Such items must be free of microbes. Staff can transfer microbes from one person to another and from themselves to others. Common sites for HAIs are:

- The urinary system
- The respiratory system
- Wounds
- The bloodstream

Patients and residents are weak from disease or injury. Some have wounds or open skin areas. Infants and older persons have a hard time fighting infections. The health team must prevent the spread of infection. HAIs are prevented by:

- Medical asepsis (This includes hand hygiene.)
- Surgical asepsis
- Standard Precautions

- Transmission-Based Precautions
- The Bloodborne Pathogen Standard (Appendix C)

Hepatitis B

Hepatitis B is caused by the hepatitis B virus (HBV). It is present in the blood and body fluids (saliva, semen, vaginal secretions) of infected persons. It is spread by:

- IV drug use and sharing needles
- Accidental needle sticks
- Sex without a condom, especially anal sex
- Contaminated tools used for tattoos or body piercings
- Sharing a toothbrush, razor, or nail clippers with an infected person

Hepatitis C

Hepatitis C is spread by blood contaminated with the virus. A person may have the virus but no symptoms. Serious liver disease and damage may show up years later. Even without symptoms, the person can transmit the disease. Hepatitis C is treated with drugs. The virus is spread by:

- Blood contaminated with the virus
- IV drug use and sharing needles
- Inhaling cocaine through contaminated straws
- Contaminated tools used for tattoos or body piercings
- High-risk sexual activity—sex with an infected person, multiple sex partners
- Sharing a toothbrush, razor, or nail clippers with an infected person

Herpes Zoster (Shingles)

This is caused by the same virus that causes chickenpox. The virus lies dormant in nerve tissue. (*Dormant* means to be *inactive.*) The virus can become active years later. The person has a rash or blisters on the skin. At first, the person has a burning or tingling pain, numbness, or itching. This occurs in an area on one side of the body or one side of the face. After a few days or a week, a rash with fluid-filled blisters appears (Fig. 35-1). The person has mild to intense pain. Itching is a common complaint. The doctor orders antiviral drugs and drugs for pain relief.

Tuberculosis

Tuberculosis (TB) is a bacterial infection in the lungs. It also can occur in the kidneys, bones, joints, nervous system (including the spine), muscles, and other parts of the body. If TB is not treated, the person can die.

TB is spread by airborne droplets with coughing, sneezing, speaking, singing, or laughing. Nearby persons can inhale the bacteria. Those who have close, frequent contact with an infected person are at risk.

TB can be present in the body but not cause signs and symptoms. An active infection may not occur for many years. Only persons with an active infection can spread the disease to others.

BOX 35-3   Signs and Symptoms of AIDS

- Appetite: loss of
- Cough
- Depression
- Diarrhea lasting more than a week
- Energy: lack of
- Fever
- Headache
- Memory loss, confusion, and forgetfulness
- Mouth or tongue:
  - Brown, red, pink, or purple spots or blotches
  - Sores or white patches
- Night sweats
- Pneumonia
- Shortness of breath
- Skin:
  - Rashes or flaky skin
  - Brown, red, pink, or purple spots or blotches on the skin, eyelids, or nose
- Swallowing: painful or difficult
- Swollen glands: neck, underarms, and groin
- Tiredness: may be extreme
- Vision loss
- Weight loss

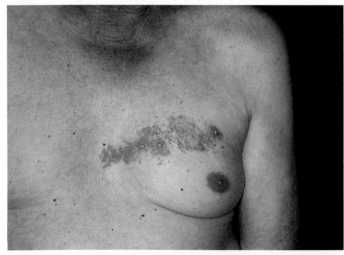

Fig. 35-1 Shingles. (Courtesy Department of Dermatology, School of Medicine, University of Utah. In McCance KL, Huether SE: *Pathophysiology: the biologic basis for disease in adults and children,* ed 5, 2006, St Louis.)

FOCUS ON OLDER PERSONS

Infection

Like other body systems, changes occur in the immune system with aging. When an older person has an infection, he or she may not show the signs and symptoms listed in Chapter 6, Box 6-1. The person may have only a slight fever or no fever at all. Redness and swelling may be very slight. The person may not complain of pain. Confusion and delirium may occur.

An infection can become life-threatening before the older person has obvious signs and symptoms. You must be alert to even the most minor changes in the person's behavior or condition. Report any concerns to the nurse at once.

Older persons are at risk for infection. Healing takes longer than in younger persons. Therefore, rehabilitation can take longer. The person's independence and quality of life are affected.

Antimicrobials are first classified according to the type of pathogen to be destroyed (see Chapter 6):

- Bacteria are treated with antibacterial agents. **Bacteria** are one-celled plant life that multiply rapidly. They are often called **germs.** They can cause an infection in any body system. A staining method is used to classify bacteria. (This method is named after Hans Gram. He was the Danish doctor who developed the staining method.)
  - Gram-negative bacteria—have a pink color when stained.
  - Gram-positive bacteria—have a violet color when stained.
- Fungi are treated with antifungal agents. **Fungi** are plants that live on other plants or animals. Mushrooms, yeasts, and molds are common fungi. Fungi can infect the mouth, vagina, skin, feet, and other body areas.
- Viruses are treated with antiviral agents. **Viruses** are microbes that grow in living cells. They cause many diseases including the common cold, herpes, acquired immunodeficiency syndrome (AIDS), hepatitis, and COVID-19.

Antibacterials are further classified into drug classes. Penicillins and tetracyclines are examples. The antibacterial ordered depends on the pathogen present.

The goal of antimicrobial therapy is to eliminate the infection. Secondary infections may develop. A **secondary infection** is an infection caused by a microbe that follows the first infection. The first infection was caused by a different microbe.

See *Delegation Guidelines: Antimicrobial Agents.*

See *Promoting Safety and Comfort: Antimicrobial Agents.*

DELEGATION GUIDELINES

Antimicrobial Agents

Some drugs used to treat infections are given parenterally—by intramuscular (IM) or intravenous (IV) injection. Because you do not give parenteral dose forms, they are not included in this chapter. Should a nurse delegate the administration of such to you, you must:

- Remember that parenteral dosages are often very different from dosages for other routes.

- Refuse the delegation but do not ignore the request. Make sure the nurse knows that you cannot give the drug and why.

PROMOTING SAFETY AND COMFORT
Antimicrobial Agents

Safety
Always check for allergies any time you give any drugs, including antimicrobials. Closely observe all persons for allergic reactions to antimicrobials. Persons with histories of allergies, asthma, or rhinitis are at risk, as are persons taking many other drugs.

Everyone should be observed carefully for at least the first 20 to 30 minutes after the drug is given. However, some drug reactions may not occur for several days. Alert the nurse at once should a reaction occur. Do not give the next dose until the nurse directs you to do so.

A serious allergic reaction may occur with the first dose. Repeated exposures can be life-threatening. Tell the nurse at once if the person shows any sign of an allergic reaction:

- Swelling, redness, or pain at an injection site
- Hives
- Rash
- Itching
- Nasal congestion and discharge
- Wheezing
- Dyspnea
- Severe respiratory distress
- Nausea
- Vomiting
- Diarrhea
- Fever
- Malaise

Follow the nurse's directions. You may be asked to:

- Activate the agency's rapid response team.
- Bring the emergency cart (crash cart) to the person's bedside.
- Provide cardiopulmonary resuscitation.

Comfort
Antimicrobials are usually given at regular intervals to maintain blood levels of the drug. For example, an antibiotic is given every 6 hours. You may need to wake the person.

DRUG CLASS: Aminoglycosides

Aminoglycosides are antibiotics that kill bacteria by inhibiting protein synthesis. They are used against gram-negative microbes that cause gram-negative infections including:

- Urinary tract infections (UTIs)—Chapter 31
- Meningitis—an infection or inflammation of the membranes covering the brain and spinal cord
- Wound infections
- Septicemia—a systemic infection in which pathogens are present in the blood; it can be caused by the spread of an infection from any body part

Most drugs in this class are given IM or IV. The following is an aminoglycoside that is given orally:

- Neomycin (nee oh my e sin)

Neomycin is commonly used to treat infections involving the liver. It is sometimes given to people before gastrointestinal surgery.

Assisting With the Nursing Process. When giving neomycin, you assist the nurse with the nursing process.

Assessment

- Ask about the person's signs and symptoms.
- Measure vital signs.
- Measure intake and output.
- Observe for hearing loss.
Planning. The oral dose form is:
- 500 mg tablets
Implementation
- The usual adult oral dose is 4 to 12 g daily in four divided doses.
Evaluation. Report and record:
- *Dizziness, tinnitus (ringing in the ears), signs of hearing loss.* The drug can cause hearing damage.
- *Decreasing urinary output, bloody or smoky-colored urine.* These signal kidney toxicity.
- See *Promoting Safety and Comfort: Antimicrobial Agents.*

DRUG CLASS: Cephalosporins

Cephalosporins inhibit cell wall synthesis in bacteria. These drugs are related to the penicillins. They may be used for persons allergic to penicillins.

Cephalosporins are used for:

- UTIs
- Respiratory tract infections
- Abdominal infections
- Bacteremia (the presence of bacteria in the blood)
- Meningitis
- Osteomyelitis (an infection of the bone and bone marrow)

Assisting With the Nursing Process. When giving cephalosporins, you assist the nurse with the nursing process.

Assessment

- Ask about the person's signs and symptoms.
- Measure vital signs.
- Measure intake and output.
Planning. See Table 35-1 for "Oral Dose Forms."
Implementation. See Table 35-1 for "Adult Dosage Range."
Evaluation. Report and record:
- *Diarrhea.* The normal flora of the GI tract is altered. Observe for signs and symptoms of dehydration if diarrhea is severe or does not resolve.
- *Decreasing urinary output, bloody or smoky-colored urine.* These signal kidney toxicity.
- *Genital and anal itching, vaginal discharge, thrush (a fungal infection of the mouth).* These signal secondary infections. Remind the person of the need for good oral and perineal hygiene.
- *Bleeding, easy bruising, bleeding gums, nosebleeds.* These signal changes in platelets.
- *Changes in alertness and orientation to person, time, and place; confusion; muscle cramps; nausea.* These may signal electrolyte imbalance (potassium, sodium, and chloride).
- See *Promoting Safety and Comfort: Antimicrobial Agents.*

DRUG CLASS: Macrolides

Macrolides inhibit protein synthesis in susceptible bacteria. They kill bacteria or prevent bacteria from multiplying.

Drugs in this class are often used when other classes of drugs cannot be used. They may be used for:

- Respiratory infections
- GI infections

TABLE 35-1   Cephalosporins

Generic Name	Brand Name	Oral Dose Forms	Adult Dosage Range
cefaclor		250, 500 mg capsules 500 mg 12-hr extended-release tablets 125, 250, 375 mg/5 mL suspension	250-500 mg every 8 hours; do not exceed 4 g/day
cefadroxil		500 mg capsules 1000 mg tablets 250, 500 mg/5 mL suspension	1-2 g daily in one to two daily doses. Treatment generally lasts at least 10 days.
cefdinir		300 mg capsules 125, 250 mg/5 mL suspension	300 mg every 12 hours or 600 mg once daily
cefixime	Suprax	100, 200 mg chewable tablets 400 mg capsules 100, 200, 500 mg/5 mL suspension	200 mg every 12 hours or 400 mg once daily. Treatment generally lasts at least 10 days.
cefpodoxime		100, 200 mg tablets 50, 100 mg/5 mL suspension	200 mg every 12 hours for 7-14 days
cefprozil		250, 500 mg tablets 125, 250 mg/5 mL suspension	250-500 mg every 12 hours for 10 days
ceftibuten	Cedax	400 mg capsules 180 mg/5 mL suspension	400 mg once daily 2 hours before or 1 hour after meals for 10 days
cefuroxime		250, 500 mg tablets 125, 250 mg/5 mL suspension	250-500 mg every 12 hours
cephalexin	Keflex Daxbia	250, 500 mg tablets 250, 333, 500, 750 mg capsules 125, 250 mg/5 mL suspension	250-1000 mg every 6 hours or 500 mg every 12 hours

Modified from Willihnganz M: Clayton's Basic Pharmacology for Nurses, ed 18, St Louis, 2020, Elsevier.

- Skin infections
- Soft tissue infections
- Sexually transmitted infections (STIs)

Assisting With the Nursing Process. When giving macrolides, you assist the nurse with the nursing process.

Assessment
- Ask about the person's signs and symptoms.
- Measure vital signs.
- Measure intake and output.
- Ask about GI symptoms.
    Planning. See Table 35-2 for "Oral Dose Forms."
    Implementation. See Table 35-2 for "Adult Dosage Range."
    Evaluation. Report and record:
- *Diarrhea, nausea, vomiting, abnormal taste.* These are the most common side effects from this drug. They are usually mild and tend to resolve with continued therapy.
- See *Promoting Safety and Comfort: Antimicrobial Agents.*

DRUG CLASS: Penicillins

Penicillins were the first true antibiotics. They remain one of the most widely used classes of antibiotics.

Penicillins interfere with bacterial cell wall synthesis. The resulting cell wall is weak because of a defective structure. Bacteria are destroyed.

Penicillins are most effective against bacteria that multiply rapidly. Many bacteria that are sensitive to penicillin develop a protective mechanism against the drug, meaning they can resist

penicillin therapy. Some penicillin drugs have been modified to prevent this problem.

Penicillins are used to treat:
- Middle ear infections (otitis media)
- Pneumonia
- Meningitis
- UTIs
- Syphilis

Penicillins may also be ordered for some persons before surgery and before dental procedures. The goal is to prevent infection in persons with a history of rheumatic fever. *Rheumatic fever* is a systemic inflammatory disease that may develop as a delayed reaction to a poorly treated upper respiratory infection. It usually occurs in young school-age children. Rheumatic fever may affect the brain, heart, joints, skin, or subcutaneous tissues.

Assisting With the Nursing Process. When giving penicillins, you assist the nurse with the nursing process.

Assessment
- Ask about the person's signs and symptoms.
- Measure vital signs.
- Measure intake and output.
    Planning. See Table 35-3 for "Oral Dose Forms."
    Implementation. See Table 35-3 for "Adult Dosage Range."
    Evaluation. Report and record:
- *Diarrhea.* Penicillins alter the normal flora of the GI tract. Observe for signs and symptoms of dehydration if diarrhea is severe or does not resolve.

TABLE 35-2 Macrolides

Generic Name	Brand Name	Oral Dose Forms	Adult Dosage Range
azithromycin	Zithromax	250, 500, 600 mg tablets 100, 200 mg/5 mL suspension 1 g packet	500 mg for 5 days for hospitalized pneumonia patients. 500 mg daily for 3 days for sinus infection.
clarithromycin		250, 500 mg tablets 125, 250 mg/5 mL suspension 500 mg 24-hr extended-release tablets	250-500 mg every 12 hours for 7-14 days
erythromycin	Erythrocin; many others	3250, 400, 500 mg tablets 250, 333, 500 mg delayed-release tablets 250, 333 mg delayed-release particles 200, 400 mg/5 mL suspension	250 mg four times daily for 10-14 days
fidaxomicin	Dificid	200 mg tablets	200 mg two times daily for 10 days

Modified from Willihnganz M: Clayton's Basic Pharmacology for Nurses, ed 18, St Louis, 2020, Elsevier.

TABLE 35-3 Penicillins

Generic Name	Brand Name	Oral Dose Forms	Adult Dosage Range
amoxicillin	-	500, 875 mg tablets 775 mg 24-hr extended-release tablets 125, 200, 250, 400 mg chewable tablets 250, 500 mg capsules 125, 200, 250, 400 mg/5 mL suspension	250-875 mg every 8-12 hours
ampicillin	-	250, 500 mg capsules 125, 250 mg/5 mL	250-500 mg every 6 hours
dicloxacillin	-	250, 500 mg capsules	250-500 mg every 6 hours
penicillin V potassium	-	250, 500 mg tablets 125, 250 mg/5 mL suspension	125-500 mg every 6 hours
Combination Products amoxicillin and potassium clavulanate (co-amoxiclav)	Augmentin	200, 400 mg chewable tablets 250, 500, 875 mg tablets 1000 mg 12-hr extended-release tablets 125, 250, 400, 600 mg/5 mL suspension	250 mg every 8 hours or 500-875 mg every 12 hours 2000 mg extended-release tablets every 12 hours 600 mg suspension every 12 hours

Modified from Willihnganz M: Clayton's Basic Pharmacology for Nurses, ed 18, St Louis, 2020, Elsevier.

- *Changes in alertness and orientation to person, time, and place; confusion; muscle cramps; nausea.* These may signal electrolyte imbalance (potassium, sodium, and chloride).
- *Decreasing urinary output, bloody or smoky-colored urine.* These signal kidney toxicity.
- *Anorexia, nausea, vomiting, jaundice.* These may signal liver toxicity.
- See *Promoting Safety and Comfort: Antimicrobial Agents.*

DRUG CLASS: Quinolones

Quinolone antibiotics prevent bacteria from reproducing. They are effective in treating initial and recurrent UTIs.

A subclass known as the fluoroquinolones inhibit the activity of an enzyme needed for bacteria to multiply. Drugs in this subclass are effective against many gram-positive and gram-negative bacteria. This includes some anaerobes—microbes that live and grow in the absence *(an)* of oxygen *(aer)*. Aerobes are microbes that live and grow in the presence of oxygen *(aer)*.

Assisting With the Nursing Process. When giving quinolones, you assist the nurse with the nursing process.
 Assessment
- Ask about the person's signs and symptoms.
- Measure vital signs.
- Measure intake and output.
- Ask about GI symptoms.
 Planning. See Table 35-4 for "Oral Dose Forms."
 Implementation. See Table 35-4 for "Adult Dosage Range."
 Evaluation. Report and record:
- *Nausea, vomiting, diarrhea, GI discomfort.* These are usually mild and tend to resolve with continued therapy.
- *Dizziness, light-headedness.* These tend to be self-limiting. Remind the person not to drive or do dangerous tasks. Provide for safety.
- *Photosensitivity.* This is sensitivity to sunlight and ultraviolet light (sunlamps, tanning beds). The person should avoid exposure to sunlight, sunlamps, and tanning beds. The person

TABLE 35-4   Quinolones

Generic Name	Brand Name	Oral Dose Forms	Adult Dosage Range
ciprofloxacin	Cipro	Tablets: 100, 250, 500, 750 mg Tablets, 24-hr extended-release: 500, 1000 mg Suspension: 250, 500 mg/5 mL	0.2-1.5 g daily in two divided doses 2 hours after meals
delafloxacin	Baxdela	Tablets: 450 mg	450 mg every 12 hours
gemifloxacin	Factive	Tablets: 320 mg	320 mg once daily. It may be taken without regard to meals.
levofloxacin		Tablets: 250, 500, 750 mg Suspension: 25 mg/mL	250-750 mg once daily
moxifloxacin	Avelox	Tablets: 400 mg	400 mg once daily. It may be taken without regard to meals.
ofloxacin		Tablets: 300, 400 mg	400-800 mg daily in two divided doses every 12 hours, 1 hour before or 2 hours after meals, with a large glass of fluid

Modified from Willihnganz M: Clayton's Basic Pharmacology for Nurses, ed 18, St Louis, 2020, Elsevier.

should apply a sunscreen and wear long-sleeved garments, a hat, and sunglasses when outdoors. Sunburn needs medical attention.
- *Tinnitus (ringing in the ears), headache, dizziness, depression, drowsiness, confusion.* These are nervous system effects. Provide for safety.
- *Anorexia, nausea, vomiting, jaundice.* These may signal liver toxicity.
- *Decreasing urinary output, bloody or smoky-colored urine.* These signal kidney toxicity.
- See *Promoting Safety and Comfort: Antimicrobial Agents.*

DRUG CLASS: Sulfonamides

Sulfonamides are highly effective antibacterial agents. They inhibit bacteria from making folic acid, causing bacterial death. Folic acid is needed for cell growth and reproduction.

Drugs in this class are used to treat UTIs and otitis media. They may be used to treat other infections in persons allergic to penicillin.

Assisting With the Nursing Process. When giving sulfonamides, you assist the nurse with the nursing process.
Assessment
- Ask about the person's signs and symptoms.
- Measure vital signs.
- Measure intake and output.
- Ask about GI symptoms.
Planning. See Table 35-5 for "Oral Dose Forms."
Implementation. See Table 35-5 for "Adult Dosage Range."
- The person should drink water several times a day.
Evaluation. Report and record:
- *Nausea, vomiting, diarrhea, GI discomfort.* These are usually mild and tend to resolve with continued therapy.
- *Photosensitivity.* This is sensitivity to sunlight and ultraviolet light (sunlamps, tanning beds). The person should avoid exposure to sunlight, sunlamps, and tanning beds. The person should apply a sunscreen and wear long-sleeved garments, a

hat, and sunglasses when outdoors. Sunburn needs medical attention.
- *Sore throat, fever, jaundice, weakness.* These may signal changes in red blood cells and white blood cells.
- *Tinnitus (ringing in the ears), headache, dizziness, depression, drowsiness, confusion.* These are nervous system effects. Provide for safety.
- See *Promoting Safety and Comfort: Antimicrobial Agents.*

DRUG CLASS: Tetracyclines

Tetracyclines are effective against gram-negative and gram-positive bacteria. They inhibit bacteria cells from making protein.

These drugs are often used in persons allergic to penicillin to treat:
- Certain STDs
- UTIs
- Upper respiratory infections
- Pneumonia
- Meningitis
- Acne

Tetracyclines may stain the teeth if taken during tooth development—last half of pregnancy through 8 years of age. These drugs are secreted in breast milk. Nursing mothers should feed infants formula or cow's milk.

Assisting With the Nursing Process. When giving tetracyclines, you assist the nurse with the nursing process.
Assessment
- Ask about the person's signs and symptoms.
- Measure vital signs.
- Measure intake and output.
- Ask about GI symptoms.
Planning. See Table 35-6 for "Oral Dose Forms."
Implementation. See Table 35-6 for "Adult Dosage Range."
- Give the drug 1 hour before or 2 hours after the person ingests antacids, milk or other dairy products, or products containing

TABLE 35-5 Sulfonamides

Generic Name	Brand Name	Oral Dose Forms	Adult Dosage Range
sulfadiazine	Sulfadiazine	500 mg tablets	Initial dose: 2-4 g, then 2-4 g daily in three to six divided doses
sulfasalazine	Azulfidine	500 mg tablets 500 mg delayed-release tablets	Initial therapy: 3-4 g daily in divided doses; maintenance dosage is 2 g daily
co-trimoxazole	Bactrim, Bactrim DS	Tablets: 400/80, 800/160 mg sulfamethoxazole/trimethoprim Suspension: 200/40, 400/80 mg sulfamethoxazole/trimethoprim	Two to four tablets daily, depending on strength and the disease being treated

Modified from Willihnganz M: Clayton's Basic Pharmacology for Nurses, ed 18, St Louis, 2020, Elsevier.

TABLE 35-6 Tetracyclines

Generic Name	Brand Name	Oral Dose Forms	Adult Dosage Range
doxycycline	Vibramycin	20, 50, 75, 100, 150 mg tablets 50, 75, 100, 120, 150, 200 mg delayed-release tablets 50, 75, 100, 150 mg capsules 40 mg delayed-release capsules 25, 50 mg/5 mL syrup	100 mg two times a day
minocycline	Minocin	50, 75, 100 mg capsules 50, 75, 100 mg tablets 45, 55, 65, 80, 90, 105, 115, 135 mg 24-hr extended-release tablets 90, 135 mg 24-hr extended-release capsules	200 mg, followed by 100 mg every 12 hours
tetracycline		250, 500 mg capsules	250-500 mg four times daily

Modified from Willihnganz M: Clayton's Basic Pharmacology for Nurses, ed 18, St Louis, 2020, Elsevier.

calcium, aluminum, magnesium, or iron. (Note: Food and milk interfere with the absorption of demeclocycline.)

Evaluation. Report and record:

- *Nausea, vomiting, diarrhea, GI discomfort.* These are usually mild and tend to resolve with continued therapy.
- *Photosensitivity.* This is sensitivity to sunlight and ultraviolet light (sunlamps, tanning beds). The person should avoid exposure to sunlight, sunlamps, and tanning beds. The person should apply a sunscreen and wear long-sleeved garments, a hat, and sunglasses when outdoors. Sunburn needs medical attention.
- See *Promoting Safety and Comfort: Antimicrobial Agents.*

ANTITUBERCULAR AGENTS

Tuberculosis (TB) is described in Box 35-2. These drugs are used in the treatment of TB:
- Ethambutol (e tham' bu tol)
- Isoniazid (i so ny' ah zid); INH
- Pyrazinamide (pie rah zin' a mide); Tebrazid (teb rah' zid)
- Rifampin (rif am' pin); Rifadin (rif' ah din)

Ethambutol

This drug inhibits bacterial growth. It is used with other antitubercular agents to prevent the development of resistant organisms. The goal of therapy is to eliminate the TB.

Assisting With the Nursing Process. When giving ethambutol, you assist the nurse with the nursing process.

Assessment
- Ask about the person's signs and symptoms.
- Measure vital signs.
- Measure intake and output.
- Ask about GI symptoms.
- Observe level of alertness and orientation to person, time, and place.

Planning. The oral dose forms are 100 and 400 mg tablets.

Implementation
- The dosage is based on the person's body weight.
- The drug is given once a day with food or milk.

Evaluation. Report and record:
- *Nausea, vomiting, diarrhea, abdominal cramps.* These are usually mild and tend to resolve with continued therapy. Give the drug with food to lessen nausea and vomiting.
- *Confusion, hallucinations.* Provide for safety.
- *Blurred vision, red-green vision changes.* Provide for safety during blurred vision.
- See *Promoting Safety and Comfort: Antimicrobial Agents.*

Isoniazid (INH)

This drug appears to disrupt the bacteria's cell wall and inhibits the cell from multiplying.

The drug is used to prevent and treat TB. If TB is active, it is used with other antitubercular agents. The goals of therapy are to:
- Prevent TB in persons who test positive for the disease
- Eliminate TB in persons with active TB

Assisting With the Nursing Process. When giving isoniazid (INH), you assist the nurse with the nursing process.

Assessment
- Ask about the person's signs and symptoms.
- Measure vital signs.
- Measure intake and output.
- Ask about GI symptoms.

Planning. The oral dose forms are:
- 100 and 300 mg tablets
- 50 mg/5 mL syrup

Implementation
- The dosage is based on the person's body weight.
- The dosage is usually a single daily dose. It may be given in divided doses.
- Give the drug on an empty stomach.

Evaluation. Report and record:
- *Tingling and numbness of the hands and feet.* These are common and are dose related. Observe for signs of skin breakdown. Test water temperature to prevent burns.
- *Nausea, vomiting.* These are common and are dose related.
- *Dizziness, ataxia (staggering gait, imbalance, poor coordination).* Provide for safety during ambulation.
- *Anorexia, nausea, vomiting, jaundice.* These may signal liver toxicity.
- See *Promoting Safety and Comfort: Antimicrobial Agents.*

Pyrazinamide (Tebrazid)

This drug must be used in combination with other antitubercular agents. It may inhibit uric acid excretion. This may cause a gouty attack (Chapter 34).

The goal of therapy is to eliminate TB in persons with active TB.

Assisting With the Nursing Process. When giving pyrazinamide (Tebrazid), you assist the nurse with the nursing process.

Assessment
- Ask about the person's signs and symptoms.
- Measure vital signs.
- Measure intake and output.
- Ask about GI symptoms.
- Observe level of alertness and orientation to person, time, and place.

Planning. The oral dose form is 500 mg tablets.

Implementation
- The dosage is based on the person's body weight.
- The dosage is usually a single daily dose. It may be given in divided doses.

Evaluation. Report and record:
- *Anorexia, nausea, vomiting, jaundice.* These may signal liver toxicity.
- *Nausea, vomiting, anorexia, joint pain, muscle pain.* These are usually mild and tend to resolve with continued therapy.
- See *Promoting Safety and Comfort: Antimicrobial Agents.*

Rifampin (Rifadin)

This drug blocks key pathways needed for cells to grow and multiply. It is used with other drugs to treat TB.

Rifampin (Rifadin) also is used to eliminate certain bacteria in the nasopharynx of carriers showing no symptoms. A carrier is a human or animal that is a reservoir for microbes but does not have the signs and symptoms of infection.

Assisting With the Nursing Process. When giving rifampin (Rifadin), you assist the nurse with the nursing process.

Assessment
- Ask about the person's signs and symptoms.
- Measure vital signs.
- Measure intake and output.
- Ask about GI symptoms.

Planning
- The oral dose forms are:
  - 150 and 300 mg capsules
  - 25 mg/mL per 120 mL bottle suspension

Implementation
- The dosage is based on the person's body weight.
- The drug is given 1 hour before or 2 hours after a meal.

Evaluation. Report and record:
- *Reddish-orange secretions.* Urine, feces, saliva, sputum, sweat, and tears may be tinged reddish-orange. This is harmless and resolves with continued therapy.
- *Nausea, vomiting, anorexia, abdominal cramps.* These are usually mild and tend to resolve with continued therapy.
- *Nausea, vomiting, fever, chills, muscle or bone pain, bruising, yellowish color of the skin or eyes.* The person needs further medical attention.
- See *Promoting Safety and Comfort: Antimicrobial Agents.*

OTHER ANTIBIOTICS

Other antibiotics used to treat infections are:
- Clindamycin (klin dah my; sin); Cleocin (klee o' sin)
- Metronidazole (met row nyd' a zol); Flagyl (fla' jil)
- Tinidazole (tin id' a zol); Tindamax (tin' dah max)
- Vancomycin (van ko my' sin); Vancocin (van ko' sin)

Clindamycin (Cleocin)

This drug inhibits the bacteria from making protein. It is used against:
- Gram-negative aerobes
- Gram-positive anaerobes
- Gram-negative anaerobes

Assisting With the Nursing Process. When giving clindamycin (Cleocin), you assist the nurse with the nursing process.

Assessment
- Ask about the person's signs and symptoms.
- Measure vital signs.
- Measure intake and output.
- Ask about bowel elimination patterns.

Planning. The oral dose forms are:
- 75, 150, and 300 mg capsules
- 75 mg/5 mL suspension

Implementation
- The usual adult oral dose is 150 to 450 mg every 6 hours.
- Do not refrigerate the suspension. It is stable at room temperature for 14 days.

Evaluation. Report and record:
- *Diarrhea.* This is usually mild and tends to resolve with continued therapy.
- *Severe diarrhea.* This is signaled by five or more stools per day.
- *Blood or mucus in the stool.* The person needs further medical attention.
- See *Promoting Safety and Comfort: Antimicrobial Agents.*

Metronidazole (Flagyl)

This drug kills bacteria and some protozoa. **Protozoa** are one-celled animals. They can infect the blood, brain, intestines, and other body areas.

Assisting With the Nursing Process. When giving metronidazole (Flagyl), you assist the nurse with the nursing process.
   Assessment
- Ask about the person's signs and symptoms.
- Measure vital signs.
- Measure intake and output.
- Ask about GI symptoms.
- Observe level of alertness and orientation to person, time, and place.
   Planning. The oral dose forms are:
- 250 and 500 mg tablets
- 375 mg capsules
- 750 mg 24-hour extended-release tablets
   Implementation
- The dosage depends on the infection needing treatment.
- The person should avoid alcoholic beverages and drugs containing alcohol (cough medications, mouthwashes).
   Evaluation. Report and record:
- *Nausea, vomiting, diarrhea, metallic taste.* These are usually mild and tend to resolve with continued therapy.
- *Dizziness.* Provide for safety.
- *Confusion, seizures.* Provide for safety. Follow the care plan for seizure precautions.
- See *Promoting Safety and Comfort: Antimicrobial Agents.*

Tinidazole (Tindamax)

This drug is similar to metronidazole (Flagyl). The goal of therapy is to eliminate the infection.

Assisting With the Nursing Process. When giving tinidazole (Tindamax), you assist the nurse with the nursing process.
   Assessment
- Ask about the person's signs and symptoms.
- Measure vital signs.
- Measure intake and output.
- Ask about GI symptoms.
- Observe level of alertness and orientation to person, time, and place.
   Planning. The oral dose forms are 250 and 500 mg tablets.
   Implementation
- The dosage depends on the infection needing treatment.
- The person should avoid alcoholic beverages and drugs containing alcohol (cough medications, mouthwashes).

Evaluation. Report and record:
- *Nausea, vomiting, diarrhea.* These are usually mild and tend to resolve with continued therapy.
- *Dizziness.* Provide for safety.
- *Confusion, seizures.* Provide for safety. Follow the care plan for seizure precautions.
- See *Promoting Safety and Comfort: Antimicrobial Agents.*

Vancomycin (Vancocin)

This drug prevents cell walls from forming. It is effective against gram-positive bacteria. The drug has severe adverse effects. Therefore, it is reserved for persons with potentially life-threatening infections who cannot be treated with penicillins or cephalosporins.

Assisting With the Nursing Process. When giving vancomycin (Vancocin), you assist the nurse with the nursing process.
   Assessment
- Ask about the person's signs and symptoms.
- Measure vital signs.
- Measure intake and output.
- Observe for hearing loss.
   Planning. The oral dose forms are 125 and 250 mg capsules and 50 mg/mL oral solution.
   Implementation. The usual adult dose is 500-2000 mg every 6 hours in divided doses.
   Evaluation. Report and record:
- *Dizziness, tinnitus (ringing in the ears), signs of hearing loss.* The drug can cause hearing damage.
- *Decreasing urinary output, bloody or smoky-colored urine.* These signal kidney toxicity.
- *Genital and anal itching, vaginal discharge, thrush (a fungal infection of the mouth).* These signal secondary infections. Remind the person that they need to practice good oral and perineal hygiene.
- See *Promoting Safety and Comfort: Antimicrobial Agents.*

TOPICAL ANTIFUNGAL AGENTS

Antifungal agents change cell membranes. Proteins and electrolytes can leak from cells. Cells cannot take in the nutrients needed for their growth.
   Topical agents are used to treat:
- Athlete's foot
- Jock itch
- Ringworm
- Thrush
- Diaper rash
- Vaginal yeast infection
- The goal of therapy is to eliminate the fungal infection.

Assisting With the Nursing Process. When applying topical antifungal agents, you assist the nurse with the nursing process.
   Assessment. Ask about the person's signs and symptoms.
   Planning. See Table 35-7 for "Topical Dose Forms."
   Implementation. See Table 35-7 for "Adult Dosage Range."
- See Chapter 12 for applying topical agents. Wear gloves.
- For athlete's foot: the person should wear cotton socks. They should be changed two or three times a day.

TABLE 35-7 Topical Antifungal Agents

Generic Name	Brand Name	Topical Dose Forms	Adult Dosage Range
butenafine	Lotrimin Ultra, Mentax	Cream: 1%	For ringworm, jock itch, athlete's foot: Apply topically to affected area one or two times daily for 1-4 weeks
butoconazole	Gynazole-1	Vaginal cream: 2%	For vaginal candidiasis: Insert one applicatorful intravaginally at bedtime once
ciclopirox	Loprox	Cream: 0.77% Gel: 0.77% Shampoo: 1% Solution for nails: 8% Topical suspension: 0.77%	For ringworm, jock itch, athlete's foot, cutaneous candidiasis, and tinea versicolor: Massage product into affected skin twice daily for at least 4 weeks; shampoo: twice weekly for 4 weeks
clotrimazole	Gyne-Lotrimin 3 Desenex, Alevazol Lotrimin AF	Vaginal cream: 2% Cream and ointment: 1% Solution: 1% Oral lozenges: 10 mg (troches)*	For vaginal candidiasis: Cream: One full applicator at bedtime for 3-7 nights For ringworm, jock itch, athlete's foot: Apply topically to affected skin morning and evening; gently rub in For oral candidiasis: Allow one lozenge to dissolve slowly in mouth five times daily for 14 consecutive days
econazole	Ecoza	Cream: 1% Foam: 1%	For ringworm, jock itch, athlete's foot, tinea versicolor: Apply over affected area once daily For cutaneous candidiasis: Apply twice daily, morning and evening
efinaconazole	Jublia	Solution: 10%	For fungal infections of the toes: Apply to affected toenails once daily for 48 weeks
ketoconazole	Nizoral	Cream: 2% Foam: 2% Gel: 2% Shampoo: 1%, 2%	For ringworm, jock itch, athlete's foot, cutaneous candidiasis, tinea versicolor: Massage cream into affected and surrounding tissue once daily; may require 2-4 weeks of treatment For seborrheic dermatitis: Cream and foam: Massage into affected area twice daily for 4 weeks Gel: Massage into affected area once daily for 2 weeks For dandruff: Moisten hair and scalp with water; apply shampoo and lather gently for 1 min; rinse and reapply, leaving lather on scalp for 3 min; rinse thoroughly and dry hair; apply shampoo twice weekly for 4 weeks with at least 3 days between shampooing
luliconazole	Luzu	Cream, external 1%	For jock itch, truncal lesions: Apply once daily for 1 week For athlete's foot: Apply once daily for 2 weeks
miconazole	Monistat 3 Monistat 7 Micatin	Vaginal suppositories: 200 mg Vaginal cream: 2% Vaginal suppositories: 100 mg Vaginal cream: 2% Cream: 2% Powder: 2% Solution: 2% Spray: 2% Ointment: 2%	For vaginal candidiasis: Monistat 3: Insert one suppository intravaginally at bedtime for 3 days Monistat 7: Insert one full applicator or one suppository intravaginally at bedtime for 3-7 days For ringworm, jock itch, athlete's foot, cutaneous candidiasis, and tinea versicolor: Cover affected areas twice daily, morning and evening; treatment may require 2-4 weeks
naftifine	Naftin	Cream: 1%, 2% Gel: 1%, 2%	For ringworm, jock itch, athlete's foot: Cream: Massage into affected area once daily Gel: Massage into affected area twice daily
nystatin		Vaginal tablets: 100,000 units Oral suspension: 100,000 units/mL* Oral tablets: 500,000 units Cream, ointment, powder	For vaginal candidiasis: One tablet intravaginally daily for 2 weeks For oral candidiasis: Sip 4-6 mL four times daily; retain in mouth as long as possible before swallowing One or two tablets three times daily For cutaneous candidiasis: Apply to affected area two to three times daily
oxiconazole nitrate	Oxistat	Cream: 1% Lotion: 1%	For ringworm, jock itch, athlete's foot: Massage into affected areas once daily at bedtime
sertaconazole	Ertaczo	Cream: 2%	For athlete's foot: Apply twice daily for 4 weeks
sulconazole	Exelderm	Cream: 1% Solution: 1%	For ringworm, jock itch, athlete's foot: Massage into affected area twice daily
tavaborole	Kerydin	Solution: 5%	For onychomycosis of the toenail: Apply to affected toenail(s) once daily for 48 weeks

TABLE 35-7 Topical Antifungal Agents—cont'd

Generic Name	Brand Name	Topical Dose Forms	Adult Dosage Range
terbinafine	Lamisil AT	Cream: 1% Spray: 1% Gel: 1%	Massage into affected area twice daily; treatment may require 2-4 weeks
terconazole	Terazol 7 Terazol 3 Zazole	Vaginal cream: 0.4% Vaginal cream: 0.8% Vaginal suppository: 80 mg	For vaginal candidiasis: Insert one full applicator intra-vaginally daily at bedtime for 3 (Terazol 3) or 7 (Terazol 7) consecutive days Insert one suppository intravaginally once daily at bedtime for 3 consecutive days
tioconazole	Vagistat-1	Vaginal ointment: 6.5%	For vaginal candidiasis: Insert one full applicator intravaginally at bedtime once
tolnaftate	Tinactin	Cream: 1% Solution: 1% Spray: 1% Powder: 1%	For ringworm, jock itch, athlete's foot, cutaneous candidiasis, and tinea versicolor: Cover affected areas twice daily, morning and evening; treatment may require 2-4 weeks

*This is an oral dose form.
Modified from Willihnganz M: Clayton's Basic Pharmacology for Nurses, ed 18, St Louis, 2020, Elsevier.

- For jock itch or ringworm: the person should wear clothing that fits well, is not constrictive, and is well-ventilated.
- Eye contact: eye contact with the drug should be avoided. Wash eyes at once if contact occurs.
  Evaluation. Report and record:
- *Vaginal applications: vaginal or perineal burning, itching, discharge, soreness, swelling.* These are usually mild and tend to resolve with continued therapy.
- *Redness, swelling, blistering, oozing.* These may signal an allergic reaction.
- See *Promoting Safety and Comfort: Antimicrobial Agents.*

SYSTEMIC ANTIFUNGAL AGENTS

The following systemic antifungal agents are given orally:
- Fluconazole (flu kon' a zol); Diflucan (dye' flu can)
- Griseofulvin (griz ee o ful' vin)
- Itraconazole (it rah kon'a zol); Sporanox (spor' ahn ox)
- Terbinafine (ter bin' ah feen)

Fluconazole (Diflucan)

This drug interferes with cell wall formation. The drug is used:
- For fungal infections affecting:
  - The meninges
  - Mouth and pharynx
  - Esophagus
  - Vagina
- To prevent fungal infections in:
  - Bone marrow transplant patients who are receiving radiation or chemotherapy
  - Persons with HIV
  - Persons with weakened immune systems

Assisting With the Nursing Process. When giving fluconazole (Diflucan), you assist the nurse with the nursing process.
  Assessment
- Ask about the person's signs and symptoms.
- Measure vital signs.
- Measure intake and output.
- Ask about GI symptoms.
  Planning. The oral dose forms are:
- 50, 100, 150, and 200 mg tablets
- 10 and 40 mg/mL
  Implementation
- The usual adult dose is 100 to 400 mg daily.
- The dosage depends on the infection being treated.
  Evaluation. Report and record:
- *Nausea, vomiting, and diarrhea.* These are usually mild and tend to resolve with continued therapy.
- *Anorexia, nausea, vomiting, jaundice.* These may signal liver toxicity.
- *Rash.* Report to nurse for further evaluation.
- See *Promoting Safety and Comfort: Antimicrobial Agents.*

Griseofulvin

This drug stops cell division and new cell growth. They are used to treat ringworm of the scalp, body, nails, and feet.

Assisting With the Nursing Process. When giving griseofulvin, you assist the nurse with the nursing process.
  Assessment
- Ask about the person's signs and symptoms.
- Measure vital signs.
- Measure intake and output.
- Ask about GI symptoms.
  Planning. The oral dose forms are:
- 125, 250, and 500 mg tablets
- 125 mg/5 mL oral suspension
  Implementation
- Dosage depends on the microbe and location of the infection—usually 500 mg to 1 g in one dose or in divided doses daily.
- A high-fat meal may increase drug absorption.
  Evaluation. Report and record:
- *Nausea, vomiting, anorexia, abdominal cramps.* These are usually mild and tend to resolve with continued therapy.

- *Rash, itching.* These are relatively common and may be relieved by adding baking soda to the bath water.
- *Confusion, dizziness.* Provide for safety.
- *Genital and anal itching, vaginal discharge, thrush (a fungal infection of the mouth).* These signal secondary infections. Remind the person that they need to practice good oral and perineal hygiene.
- *Photosensitivity.* This is sensitivity to sunlight and ultraviolet light (sunlamps, tanning beds). The person should avoid exposure to sunlight, sunlamps, and tanning beds. The person should apply a sunscreen and wear long-sleeved garments, a hat, and sunglasses when outdoors. Sunburn needs medical attention.
- *Sore throat, fever, jaundice, weakness.* These may signal changes in red blood cells and white blood cells.
- *Decreasing urinary output, bloody or smoky-colored urine.* These signal kidney toxicity.
- *Anorexia, nausea, vomiting, jaundice.* These may signal liver toxicity.
- See *Promoting Safety and Comfort: Antimicrobial Agents.*

Itraconazole (Sporanox)

This drug interferes with the cell wall. Cell contents leak out of the cell. It is used to treat a variety of fungal infections.

Assisting With the Nursing Process. When giving itraconazole (Sporanox), you assist the nurse with the nursing process.

Assessment
- Ask about the person's signs and symptoms.
- Measure vital signs.
- Measure intake and output.
- Ask about GI symptoms.
- Observe for signs and symptoms of heart failure (Chapter 22).
Planning. The oral dose forms are:
- 100 mg capsules
- 200 mg tablets
- 10 mg/mL oral solution in 150 mL containers
Implementation
- The usual adult dose is 100 to 400 mg daily.
- Doses greater than 200 mg are given in two divided doses.
- Give the drug with a full meal.
Evaluation. Report and record:
- *Nausea, vomiting.* These are usually mild and tend to resolve with continued therapy.
- *Anorexia, nausea, vomiting, jaundice.* These may signal liver toxicity.
- *Dyspnea, chest pain, fatigue, edema, syncope (fainting), palpitations.* These are signs of heart failure.
- *Rash, itching.* These are relatively common and may be relieved by adding baking soda to the bath water.
- See *Promoting Safety and Comfort: Antimicrobial Agents.*

Terbinafine

Terbinafine affects enzymes that cells need to live. The drug is used to treat fungal infections affecting toenails and fingernails.

Assisting With the Nursing Process. When giving terbinafine, you assist the nurse with the nursing process.
Assessment
- Ask about the person's signs and symptoms.
- Measure vital signs.
- Measure intake and output.
- Ask about GI symptoms.
Planning. The oral dose form is 250 mg tablets.
Implementation
- Fingernail infections: 250 mg daily for 6 weeks
- Toenail infections: 250 mg daily for 12 weeks
Evaluation. Report and record:
- *Decreasing urinary output, bloody or smoky-colored urine.* These signal kidney toxicity.
- *Anorexia, nausea, vomiting, jaundice.* These may signal liver toxicity.
- *Rash, itching.* These are relatively common. This may be relieved by adding baking soda to the bath water.
- See *Promoting Safety and Comfort: Antimicrobial Agents.*

ANTIVIRAL AGENTS

The following are antiviral agents:
- Acyclovir (a sy' klo veer); Zovirax (zoh' ve rahx)
- Famciclovir (pham sik' lo veer)
- Valacyclovir (vahl ah syk' lo veer); Valtrex (vahl'trex)
- Oseltamivir (oh sel tahm' ah veer); Tamiflu (tahm' ih fluh)
- Zanamivir (zahn am' ah veer); Relenza (rehl en'zah)
- Ribavirin (ribe ah vi' rihn); Rebetol (rehb et' ohl) and Ribasphere (rye' ba sfeer)

Acyclovir (Zovirax)

This drug prevents viral cells from multiplying. It is used to treat genital and oral herpes infections (Chapter 30).

Assisting With the Nursing Process. When giving acyclovir (Zovirax), you assist the nurse with the nursing process.
Assessment
- Ask about the person's signs and symptoms.
- Measure vital signs.
- Measure intake and output.
- Observe level of alertness and orientation to person, time, and place.
Planning. The dose forms are:
- Topical: 5% ointment and cream
- Oral:
  - 200 mg capsules
  - 400 and 800 mg tablets
  - 200 mg/5 mL suspension
Implementation
- Topical: apply to each lesion every 3 hours six times a day for 7 days. Wear gloves and practice hand hygiene.
- Oral:
  - Initial treatment: The usual adult dosage is 200 mg every 4 hours while awake. The total daily dosage is 1000 mg for 10 days.
  - Suppressive therapy: 400 mg two to five times a day for up to 12 months.

- Intermittent therapy: 200 mg every 4 hours while awake. The total daily dosage is 1000 mg for 5 days. The drug is started at the earliest sign of symptoms.
  Evaluation. Report and record:
- *Sweating.* Follow the care plan for fluid intake.
- *Rash, itching.* These are relatively common. This may be relieved by adding baking soda to the bath water.
- *Decreasing urinary output, bloody or smoky-colored urine.* These signal kidney toxicity.
- *Hypotension.* Blood pressure is measured in the supine and standing positions. Provide for safety. Remind the person to rise slowly from a supine or sitting position. Have the person sit or lie down if feeling faint.
- *Confusion.* Provide for safety.
- See *Promoting Safety and Comfort: Antimicrobial Agents.*

Famciclovir

This drug prevents the virus cell from multiplying. It is used to treat:
- Recurrent genital herpes
- Herpes zoster (shingles)

Assisting With the Nursing Process. When giving famciclovir, you assist the nurse with the nursing process.
Assessment
- Ask about the person's signs and symptoms.
- Measure vital signs.
- Measure intake and output.
- Ask about GI symptoms.
- Observe level of alertness and orientation to person, time, and place.
  Planning. The oral dose forms are 125, 250, and 500 mg tablets.
  ### Implementation
- For genital herpes: 1000 mg two times a day for 1 day. Therapy should be started within 6 hours of the first sign or symptom.
- For herpes zoster (shingles): 500 mg every 8 hours for 7 days. Therapy should be started within 72 hours of symptom onset.
  Evaluation. Report and record:
- *Nausea, vomiting, headache.* These are usually mild and resolve with continued therapy.
- *Confusion.* Provide for safety.
- See *Promoting Safety and Comfort: Antimicrobial Agents.*

Valacyclovir (Valtrex)

This drug inhibits the viral cell from multiplying. It is used to treat herpes zoster (shingles). The drug also is used to treat or suppress genital herpes.

Assisting With the Nursing Process. When giving valacyclovir (Valtrex), you assist the nurse with the nursing process.
Assessment
- Ask about the person's signs and symptoms.
- Measure vital signs.
- Measure intake and output.
- Observe level of alertness and orientation to person, time, and place.
  Planning. The oral dose forms are 500 mg and 1 g tablets.

Implementation
- For herpes zoster: 1 g three times a day for 7 days. Therapy should be started within 48 hours of the first sign or symptom.
- For genital herpes: 1 g two times a day for 10 days. Therapy should be started within 48 hours of the first sign or symptom.
- For recurrent episodes: 500 mg two times a day for 3 days.
  Evaluation. Report and record:
- *Sweating.* Follow the care plan for fluid intake.
- *Rash, itching.* These are relatively common and may be relieved by adding baking soda to the bath water.
- *Decreasing urinary output, bloody or smoky-colored urine.* These signal kidney toxicity.
- *Hypotension.* Blood pressure is measured in the supine and standing positions. Provide for safety. Remind the person to rise slowly from a supine or sitting position. Have the person sit or lie down if feeling faint.
- *Confusion.* Provide for safety.
- See *Promoting Safety and Comfort: Antimicrobial Agents.*

Oseltamivir (Tamiflu)

This drug inhibits an enzyme on the viral cell coat. The enzyme is needed for cell reproduction and the spread of viral cell particles. The drug is used to reduce flu symptoms—nasal congestion, sore throat, cough, muscle aches, fatigue, headache, chills, sweats.

Assisting With the Nursing Process. When giving oseltamivir (Tamiflu), you assist the nurse with the nursing process.
Assessment
- Ask about the person's signs and symptoms.
- Measure vital signs.
- Measure intake and output.
- Ask about GI symptoms.
  Planning. The oral dose forms are:
- 30, 45, and 75 mg capsules
- 6 mg/mL oral suspension
  ### Implementation
- The usual adult dosage is 75 mg two times a day for 5 days.
- Treatment should begin within 2 days of flu symptom onset.
- Give the drug with food or milk.
  Evaluation. Report and record:
- *Nausea, vomiting.* Give the drug with food or milk to lessen nausea and vomiting.
- *Cough, yellow or green sputum, sore throat, fever, continuing symptoms.* The person needs further medical attention.
- See *Promoting Safety and Comfort: Antimicrobial Agents.*

Zanamivir (Relenza)

This drug inhibits an enzyme on the viral cell coat. The enzyme is needed for cell reproduction and the spread of viral cell particles. The drug is used to reduce flu symptoms—nasal congestion, sore throat, cough, muscle aches, fatigue, headache, chills, sweats. The drug may prevent the secondary infection of pneumonia.

Assisting With the Nursing Process. When giving zanamivir (Relenza), you assist the nurse with the nursing process.
Assessment
- Ask about the person's signs and symptoms.

- Measure vital signs.
- Measure intake and output.
  Planning. The dose form is 5 mg blisters of powder for inhalation.
  Implementation. The usual adult dosage is:
- Two inhalations (one 5 mg blister per inhalation for a total of 10 mg) every 12 hours for 5 days.
- Treatment should begin within 2 days of flu symptom onset.
- Inhaled bronchodilators should be taken before this drug.
  Evaluation. Report and record:
- *Asthma, bronchospasm, shortness of breath, chest soreness.* The person must stop taking the drug and seek medical attention.
- *Cough, yellow or green sputum, sore throat, fever, continuing symptoms.* The person needs further medical attention.
- See *Promoting Safety and Comfort: Antimicrobial Agents.*

Ribavirin (Rebetol and Ribasphere)

This drug inhibits viral activity. It is used with other drugs in the treatment of hepatitis C in adults. See Box 35-2.

Assisting With the Nursing Process. When giving ribavirin (Rebetol and Ribasphere), you assist the nurse with the nursing process.

Assessment
- Ask about the person's signs and symptoms.
- Measure vital signs.
- Measure intake and output.
- Ask about GI symptoms.
  Planning. The oral dose forms are:
- 200, 400, 600 mg tablets
- 200 mg capsules
- 40 mg/mL oral solution
  Implementation
- For persons weighing less than 165 pounds (75 kg):
  - 400 mg capsule in the morning
  - 600 mg capsule in the evening
- For persons weighing more than 165 pounds (75 kg):
  - 600 mg capsule in the morning
  - 600 mg capsule in the evening
  - Tablets: 800-1200 mg in two divided doses. Give with food.
  Evaluation. Report and record:
- *Fatigue, dizziness, headache, pallor, dyspnea on exertion.* These may signal changes in red blood cell production.
- *Shortness of breath, chest soreness.* The person must stop taking the drug and seek medical attention.
- See *Promoting Safety and Comfort: Antimicrobial Agents.*

▌ REVIEW QUESTIONS

Circle the BEST answer.

1. Microbes that are harmful and cause infection are called:
   a. bacteria
   b. fungi
   c. normal flora
   d. pathogens
2. Plants that live on other plants or animals are called:
   a. bacteria
   b. fungi
   c. germs
   d. viruses
3. Chemicals that eliminate pathogens are called:
   a. antibiotics
   b. antimicrobials
   c. antivirals
   d. non-pathogens
4. An older person with an infection:
   a. always shows signs and symptoms
   b. does not typically become confused
   c. takes longer to heal than a younger person
   d. always experiences pain
5. A person is being treated for an infection. Another infection develops. This is called:
   a. a bacterial infection
   b. a healthcare-associated infection
   c. a viral infection
   d. a secondary infection

6. Before giving any antimicrobial, you must first:
   a. check for allergies
   b. observe for an allergic reaction
   c. put on gloves
   d. observe the person for 20 to 30 minutes
7. The following signal an allergic reaction, *except:*
   a. bleeding
   b. dyspnea
   c. hives
   d. nasal congestion
8. To maintain blood levels of the drug, antimicrobials are usually given:
   a. at regular intervals
   b. at the same time every day
   c. every 6 hours
   d. every 12 hours
9. Neomycin is an aminoglycoside. It can cause:
   a. diabetes
   b. hearing loss
   c. meningitis
   d. septicemia
10. Which drug class can cause staining of the teeth?
    a. cephalosporins
    b. penicillins
    c. sulfonamides
    d. tetracyclines

11. Cephalosporins and macrolides are given to treat infections caused by:
    a. bacteria
    b. fungi
    c. penicillins
    d. viruses
12. Which is *not* a cephalosporin?
    a. co-amoxiclav (Augmentin)
    b. cefaclor
    c. cephalexin (Keflex)
    d. cefixime (Suprax)
13. Which is *not* an antitubercular agent?
    a. metronidazole (Flagyl)
    b. isoniazid (INH)
    c. ethambutol
    d. rifampin (Rifadin)
14. Which is *not* a penicillin?
    a. amoxicillin
    b. ciprofloxacin (Cipro)
    c. ampicillin
    d. dicloxacillin
15. A common side effect from penicillin is:
    a. diarrhea
    b. hearing loss
    c. phototoxicity
    d. tingling
16. Doxycycline (Vibramycin) is a:
    a. cephalosporin
    b. penicillin
    c. sulfonamide
    d tetracycline
17. Fluoroquinolones are effective against many of the following, *except:*
    a. gram-positive bacteria
    b. anaerobic bacteria
    c. gram-negative bacteria
    d. fungi and viruses
18. Isoniazid (INH) is given:
    a. on an empty stomach
    b. with food or milk
    c. 30 minutes before a meal
    d. 30 minutes after a meal
19. Antitubercular agents are usually given:
    a. in a single daily dose
    b. in divided doses
    c. every 4 hours
    d. every 6 hours
20. Which antibiotic has the most severe adverse effects?
    a. clindamycin (Cleocin)
    b. metronidazole (Flagyl)
    c. tinidazole (Tindamax)
    d. vancomycin (Vancocin)
21. Which is similar to metronidazole (Flagyl)?
    a. clindamycin (Cleocin)
    b. tinidazole (Tindamax)
    c. terbinafine (Lamisil)
    d. vancomycin (Vancocin)

22. Which is a systemic antifungal agent?
    a. fluconazole (Diflucan)
    b. butenafine (Lotrimin)
    c. tioconazole (Vagistat-1)
    d. nystatin
23. Which antifungal agent is used to treat fungal infections affecting the scalp, body, nails, and feet?
    a. itraconazole (Sporanox)
    b. fluconazole (Diflucan)
    c. griseofulvin
    d. terbinafine
24. The following are used to treat genital herpes, *except:*
    a. famciclovir
    b. oseltamivir (Tamiflu)
    c. valacyclovir (Valtrex)
    d. acyclovir (Zovirax)
25. Which antiviral agent is used to reduce symptoms of the flu?
    a. ribavirin (Ribasphere)
    b. zanamivir (Relenza)
    c. oseltamivir (Tamiflu)
    d. acyclovir (Zovirax)
26. Which drug comes in an ointment and a cream?
    a. valacyclovir (Valtrex)
    b. famciclovir
    c. oseltamivir (Tamiflu)
    d. acyclovir (Zovirax)
27. Which drug is inhaled?
    a. acyclovir (Zovirax)
    b. zanamivir (Relenza)
    c. ribavirin (Ribasphere)
    d. oseltamivir (Tamiflu)
28. Which is used to treat hepatitis C?
    a. ribavirin (Rebetol)
    b. zanamivir (Relenza)
    c. acyclovir (Zovirax)
    d. oseltamivir (Tamiflu)

Circle T if the statement is true. Circle F if the statement is false.

29. T F Aerobic microbes live and grow in the presence of oxygen.
30. T F Sulfonamides are used to treat HIV and opportunistic infections.
31. T F Tetracyclines are given with dairy products to promote drug absorption.
32. T F Clindamycin (Cleocin) suspension should be refrigerated.
33. T F Metronidazole (Flagyl) is applied topically.
35. T F Famciclovir and valacyclovir (Valtrex) are used to treat shingles.

Answers to these questions can be found on the Evolve Resources site: http://evolve.elsevier.com/Anderson/medasst/

36

Nutrition and Herbal and Dietary Supplement Therapy

KEY TERMS

aspiration Breathing fluid, food, vomitus, or an object into the lungs

calorie The amount of energy produced when the body burns food

enteral nutrition Giving nutrients into the gastrointestinal (GI) tract (*enteral*) through a feeding tube

gastrostomy tube A tube inserted through a surgically created opening (*stomy*) in the stomach (*gastro*); stomach tube

jejunostomy tube A feeding tube inserted into a surgically created opening (*stomy*) in the *jejunum* of the small intestine

macronutrients The energy sources needed for balanced metabolism

malnutrition Any disorder of nutrition; *mal* means *bad*

nasoduodenal tube A feeding tube inserted through the nose (*naso*) into the *duodenum* of the small intestine

nasogastric (NG) tube A feeding tube inserted through the nose (*naso*) into the stomach (*gastro*)

nasointestinal tube A feeding tube inserted through the nose (*naso*) into the small intestine (*intestinal*)

nasojejunal tube A feeding tube inserted through the nose (*naso*) into the *jejunum* of the small intestine

nutrient A substance that is ingested, digested, absorbed, and used by the body

nutrition The processes involved in the ingestion, digestion, absorption, and use of foods and fluids by the body

parenteral nutrition Giving nutrients through a catheter inserted into a vein; *para* means *beyond*; *enteral* relates to the *bowel*

percutaneous endoscopic gastrostomy (PEG) tube A feeding tube inserted into the stomach (*gastro*) through a small incision (*stomy*) made through (*per*) the skin (*cutaneous*); a lighted instrument (*scope*) allows the doctor to see inside a body cavity or organ (*endo*)

regurgitation The backward flow of stomach contents into the mouth

KEY ABBREVIATIONS

AIDS Acquired immunodeficiency syndrome
BPH Benign prostatic hyperplasia
CNS Central nervous system
GI Gastrointestinal
IV Intravenous
MAR Medication administration record

Mg Milligram
mL Milliliter
NG Nasogastric
PEG Percutaneous endoscopic gastrostomy
TPN Total parenteral nutrition

The body needs a regular source of energy to support and maintain its functions. Bodily functions include respiration, nerve transmission, circulation, physical work, and maintaining body temperature. For some people, the daily diet provides needed energy sources. Others may use herbs and dietary supplements to enhance the daily diet.

NUTRITION

Nutrition is the processes involved in the ingestion, digestion, absorption, and use of foods and fluids by the body. Good nutrition is needed for growth, healing, and supporting body functions. A well-balanced diet and correct calorie intake are needed. A high-fat and high-calorie diet causes weight gain and obesity. Weight loss occurs with a low-calorie diet.

Foods and fluids contain nutrients. A **nutrient** is a substance that is ingested, digested, absorbed, and used by the body. Nutrients are grouped into fats, proteins, carbohydrates, vitamins, minerals, and water.

Fats, proteins, and carbohydrates give the body fuel for energy. The amount of energy provided by a nutrient is measured in calories. A **calorie** is the amount of energy produced when the body burns food:

- 1 gram of fat—9 calories
- 1 gram of protein—4 calories
- 1 gram of carbohydrate—4 calories

Dietary Guidelines

The *2015-2020 Dietary Guidelines for Americans* are for persons 2 years of age and older (Box 36-1). Through diet and physical activity, the guidelines serve to:
- Promote health
- Reduce the risk of chronic diseases

Certain diseases are linked to poor diet and the lack of physical activity. They include cardiovascular diseases, hypertension (high blood pressure), diabetes, being overweight, obesity, osteoporosis, and some cancers.

MyPlate

The *MyPlate Food Guide* (Fig. 36-1) is based on the *2015-2020 Dietary Guidelines for Americans*. Smart and healthy food choices are encouraged. It is a reminder to find your healthy eating style and build it throughout your lifetime. This means:
- Focus on variety, amount, and nutrition.
- Choose foods and beverages with less saturated fat, sodium, and added sugars.
- Start with small changes to build healthier eating styles.
- Support healthy eating for everyone.

A healthy eating pattern includes:
- A variety of dark-green vegetables, starchy vegetables, red and orange vegetables, beans and peas, and other vegetables
- Fruits, especially whole fruits
- Grains, at least half of which are whole grains
- Fat-free or low-fat dairy, including milk, yogurt, cheese, and/or fortified soy beverages
- A variety of protein foods, including seafood, lean meats and poultry, eggs, legumes (beans and peas), and nuts, seeds, and soy products
- Oils

The guidelines also make recommendations for healthy eating pattern limits, which include:
- Limiting saturated fats and *trans* fats, added sugars, and sodium
- Consuming less than 10% of calories per day from added sugars
- Consuming less than 10% of calories per day from saturated fats
- Consuming less than 2300 mg per day of sodium
- If alcohol is consumed, it should be consumed in moderation and only by adults of legal drinking age

Nutrients and Macronutrients

No food or food group has every essential nutrient. A well-balanced diet ensures an adequate intake of essential nutrients and macronutrients. Macronutrients are the energy sources needed for balanced metabolism. They include proteins, carbohydrates, fats, and fiber. Essential nutrients include vitamins, minerals, and water.

BOX 36-1 Recommendations of Dietary Guidelines for Americans, 2015–2020

Five Dietary Guidelines:
1. Follow a healthy eating pattern across the life span.
   - All food and beverage choices matter.
   - Choose a healthy eating pattern at an appropriate calorie level to help achieve and maintain a healthy body weight, support nutrient adequacy, and reduce the risk of chronic disease.
2. Focus on variety, nutrient density, and amount.
   - To meet nutrient needs within calorie limits, choose a variety of nutrient-dense foods across and within all food groups in recommended amounts.
   - Shifts are needed within the protein foods group to increase seafood intake, but the foods to be replaced depend on the individual's current intake from the other protein subgroups.
   - Strategies to increase the variety of protein foods include incorporating seafood as the protein foods choice in meals twice per week in place of meat, poultry, or eggs, and using legumes or nuts and seeds in mixed dishes instead of some meat or poultry.
   - For example, choosing a salmon steak, a tuna sandwich, bean chili, or almonds on a main-dish salad could all increase protein variety.
3. Limit calories from added sugars and saturated fats and reduce sodium intake.
   - Consume an eating pattern low in added sugars, saturated fats, and sodium.
   - Cut back on foods and beverages higher in these components to amounts that fit within healthy eating patterns.
   - The most commonly used oil in the United States is soybean oil. Other commonly used oils include canola, corn, olive, cottonseed, sunflower, and peanut oil. Oils also are found in nuts, avocados, and seafood.
4. Coconut, palm, and palm kernel oils (tropical oils) are solid at room temperature because they have high amounts of saturated fatty acids and are therefore classified as a solid fat rather than as an oil. Shift to healthier food and beverage choices.
   - Choose nutrient-dense foods and beverages across and within all food groups in place of less healthy choices.
- Consider cultural and personal preferences to make these shifts easier to accomplish and maintain.
- Shift to eating more vegetables.
- One strategy to do that would mean choosing a green salad or a vegetable as a side dish and incorporating vegetables into most meals and snacks.
- Shift to eating more fruits by choosing more fruits as snacks, in salads, as side dishes, and as desserts in place of foods with added sugars, such as cakes, pies, cookies, doughnuts, ice cream, and candies.
- Shift to make half of all grains consumed be whole grains.
- Strategies to increase dairy intake include drinking fat-free or low-fat milk (or a fortified soy beverage) with meals, choosing yogurt as a snack, or using yogurt as an ingredient in prepared dishes such as salad dressings or spreads.
- Strategies for choosing dairy products in nutrient-dense forms include choosing lower-fat versions of milk, yogurt, and cheese in place of whole milk products and regular cheese.
5. Support healthy eating patterns for all.
   - Everyone has a role in helping to create and support healthy eating patterns in multiple settings nationwide, including home, school, work, and other communities.
   - In order to improve individual and population lifestyle choices, strategies need to be implemented such as expanding access to healthy, safe, and affordable food choices that align with the Dietary Guidelines.
   - Adopt organizational changes and practices, including those that increase the availability, accessibility, and consumption of foods that align with the Dietary Guidelines.
   - Provide nutrition assistance programs that support education and promotional activities tailored to the needs of the community.

Adapted from U.S. Department of Agriculture and U.S. Department of Health and Human Services. *Dietary Guidelines for Americans, 2015-2020.* 8th ed. Washington, DC: U.S. Government Printing Office; 2015.

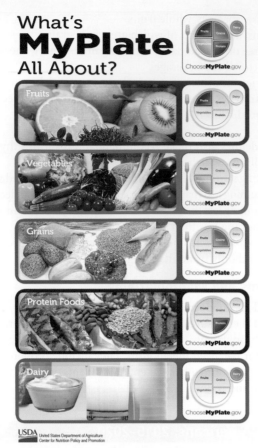

Fig. 36-1 MyPlate Food Guide. (Courtesy of US Department of Health and Human Services/US Department of Agriculture, 2011.)

- *Protein*—is needed for tissue growth and repair. Sources include meat, fish, poultry, cheese, eggs, milk and milk products, cereals, beans, peas, and nuts.
- *Carbohydrates*—provide energy for activities and metabolism. They are often referred to as sugars because many of them taste sweet. They are found in fruits, vegetables, breads, cereals, and sugar. Carbohydrates break down into sugars during digestion. The sugars are absorbed into the bloodstream.
- *Fats*—provide energy. They are also known as lipids (Chapter 19). They add flavor to food and help the body use certain vitamins. Sources include meats, lard, butter, shortening, oils, milk, cheese, egg yolks, and nuts. Dietary fat not needed by the body is stored as body fat *(adipose tissue)*.
- *Fiber*—comes from undigestible carbohydrates. It makes people feel full from eating and can help with weight control. It helps with blood glucose control and can reduce the absorption of dietary fat and cholesterol. Fiber also adds bulk to fecal content, which helps prevent constipation.
- *Vitamins*—are needed for certain body functions. They do not provide calories. The body stores vitamins A, D, E, and K. Vitamin C and the B complex vitamins are not stored and therefore must be ingested daily. The lack of a certain vitamin results in signs and symptoms of an illness. Table 36-1 lists the sources and major functions of common vitamins.
- *Minerals*—are used for many body processes. They are needed for bone and tooth formation, nerve and muscle function, fluid balance, blood clotting, and other body

processes. Table 36-2 lists the major functions and dietary sources of common minerals.
- *Water*—is needed for all body processes. Death can result from too much or too little water. Water is ingested through fluids and foods. Water is lost through urine, feces, and vomit. It is also lost through the skin (perspiration) and the lungs (expiration). An adult needs 1500 mL of water daily to survive. About 2000 to 2500 mL of fluid per day are needed for normal fluid balance. The water requirement increases with hot weather, exercise, fever, illness, and excess fluid losses.

It is recommended that to meet the body's energy and nutritional needs and to decrease the risk for chronic disease, adults should get:

- 45% to 65% of their calories from carbohydrates
- 20% to 35% of their calories from fats
- 10% to 35% of their calories from protein

Malnutrition

Nutrition plays a vital role in the recovery from illness, surgery, and injury. Adequate nutrient intake is needed to restore normal body processes and to rebuild and repair tissue. If nutritional needs are not met, malnutrition results. **Malnutrition** is any disorder of nutrition. *(Mal* means *bad.)*

Persons who are malnourished are at risk for infections and organ failure. Complications, other diseases, and death may occur. Malnutrition usually results from:

- Inadequate intake of protein and calories
- A deficiency of one or more vitamins and minerals

Therapy for Malnutrition. Therapy for malnutrition involves partial or full supplementation. To *supplement* means to complete or add to. The diet can be supplemented by:

- *Oral supplements.* The person drinks one of the oral formulas listed in Table 36-3.
- *Enteral nutrition.* **Enteral nutrition** is giving nutrients into the gastrointestinal (GI) tract *(enteral)* through a feeding tube. The doctor orders the type of formula, the amount to give, and when to give tube feedings. Most formulas contain proteins, carbohydrates, fats, vitamins, and minerals. Tube feedings are given at certain times (scheduled feedings) or over a 24-hour period (continuous feedings). Common feeding tubes are:
  - **Nasogastric (NG) tube.** A feeding tube is inserted through the nose *(naso)* into the stomach *(gastro).* See Fig. 36-2.
  - **Nasointestinal tube.** A feeding tube is inserted through the nose *(naso)* into the small intestine *(intestinal).* A **nasoduodenal tube** is inserted into the *duodenum.* A **nasojejunal tube** is inserted into *the jejunum.* See Fig. 36-3.
  - **Gastrostomy tube.** Also called a *stomach tube,* it is inserted into the stomach. A doctor surgically creates an opening *(stomy)* in the stomach *(gastro).* See Fig. 36-4.
  - **Jejunostomy tube.** A feeding tube inserted into a surgically created opening *(stomy)* in the *jejunum* of the small intestine. See Fig. 36-5.
  - **Percutaneous endoscopic gastrostomy (PEG) tube.** The doctor inserts the feeding tube with an endoscope. An endoscope is a lighted instrument *(scope)* used to see inside a body cavity or organ *(endo).* The tube is inserted through the mouth and esophagus and into the stomach. The doctor

TABLE 36-1 Functions and Sources of Common Vitamins

Vitamin	Major Functions	Sources
Vitamin A (retinol)	Growth; vision; healthy hair, skin, and mucous membranes; resistance to infection; reproduction	Liver, fish liver oils, eggs, whole milk, sweet potatoes, cantaloupe, carrots, spinach, broccoli, raw apricots
Vitamin B_1 (thiamin)	Muscle tone, nerve function, digestion, appetite, normal elimination, carbohydrate use	Pork products, whole grains, wheat germ, meats, peas, cereal, dry beans, peanuts
Vitamin B_2 (riboflavin)	Growth and development, healthy eyes, protein and carbohydrate metabolism, healthy skin and mucous membranes	Green leafy vegetables, fruit, eggs and dairy products, enriched cereal products, organ meats, peanuts and peanut butter
Vitamin B_3 (niacin)	Protein, fat, and carbohydrate metabolism; nervous system function; appetite; digestive system function; decreases cholesterol levels	Meat, pork, liver, fish, peanuts, breads and cereals, green vegetables, dairy products
Vitamin B_{12} (cyanocobalamin)	Formation of red blood cells, protein metabolism, nervous system function	Liver, meats, poultry, fish, eggs, milk, cheese
Folate (folic acid)	Formation of red blood cells, intestinal function, protein metabolism	Liver, beans, green vegetables, yeast, nuts, fruit
Vitamin C (ascorbic acid)	Formation of substances that hold tissues together; healthy blood vessels, skin, gums, bones, and teeth; wound healing; prevention of bleeding; resistance to infection	Citrus fruits, tomatoes, potatoes, broccoli, cabbage, strawberries, green vegetables, melons
Vitamin D	Absorption and metabolism of calcium and phosphorus, healthy bones	Fish liver oils, milk, butter, egg yolks, liver, exposure to sunlight
Vitamin E	Normal reproduction, formation of red blood cells, muscle function	Vegetable oils, milk, eggs, meats, cereals, green leafy vegetables, almonds, peanuts
Vitamin K	Blood clotting	Liver, green leafy vegetables, egg yolks, cheese, broccoli, asparagus, pickles, pine nuts, blueberries

TABLE 36-2 Functions and Sources of Common Minerals

Mineral	Major Functions	Sources
Calcium	Formation of teeth and bones, blood clotting, muscle contraction, heart function, nerve function	Milk, cheese, vegetables
Phosphorus	Formation of bones and teeth; use of proteins, fats, and carbohydrates; nerve and muscle function	Milk, cheese, grains, meats, green leafy vegetables, fish
Iron	Allows red blood cells to carry oxygen	Liver, meat, clams, eggs, green leafy vegetables, breads and cereals, dried peas and beans, nuts, prunes, raisins
Iodine	Thyroid gland function, growth, metabolism	Iodized salt, seafood, shellfish, vegetables, dairy products
Sodium	Fluid balance, nerve and muscle function	Almost all foods
Potassium	Nerve function, muscle contraction, heart function	Fruits, vegetables, cereals, meats, dried peas and beans
Magnesium	Formation of bones and enzymes; protein synthesis, nerve function	Grains, green leafy vegetables, nuts, legumes, oysters, crab, cornmeal

TABLE 36-3 Oral Nutritional Supplements

Formula Type	Brand Names	Comments
Oral supplements	Ensure Liquid Ensure HN Ensure Plus Boost	These products are dietary supplements available in a variety of flavors for oral use. Requires full digestive capability by gut. At recommended dosages, these formulas provide 100% of the recommended dietary allowance for vitamins and minerals.

makes a small incision (*stomy*) through (*per*) the skin (*cutaneous*) and into the stomach (*gastro*). A tube is inserted into the stomach through the incision (Fig. 36-6). The endoscope allows the doctor to see correct tube placement in the stomach.

- *Parenteral nutrition.* **Parenteral nutrition** is giving nutrients through a catheter inserted into a vein (Fig. 36-7). (*Para* means *beyond*; *enteral* relates to the *bowel*). A nutrient solution is given directly into the bloodstream. Nutrients do not enter the GI tract for absorption. Parenteral nutrition is often called *total parenteral nutrition (TPN)* or *hyperalimentation.* (*Hyper* means *high* or *excessive. Alimentation* means *nourishment.*) The nutrient solution contains water, proteins, carbohydrates, vitamins, and minerals. The solution drips through a catheter inserted into a large vein. This method is used when the person cannot receive oral feedings or enteral feedings, or when oral or enteral feedings are not enough to meet the person's needs.

See *Delegation Guidelines: Therapy for Malnutrition.*
See *Promoting Safety and Comfort: Therapy for Malnutrition.*

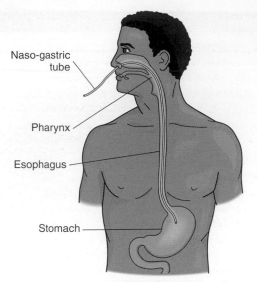

Fig. 36-2 A nasogastric tube inserted through the nose and esophagus and into the stomach.

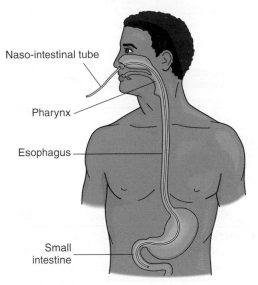

Fig. 36-3 A nasointestinal tube is inserted through the nose and into the duodenum or jejunum of the small intestine.

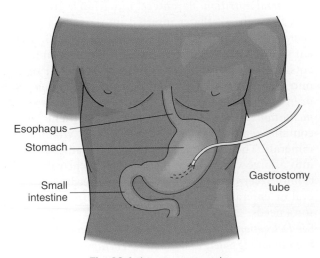

Fig. 36-4 A gastrostomy tube.

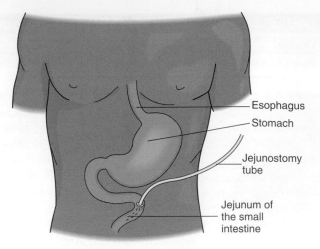

Fig. 36-5 A jejunostomy tube.

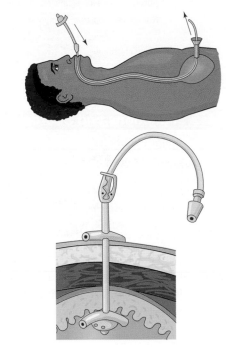

Fig. 36-6 A percutaneous endoscopic gastrostomy (PEG) tube.

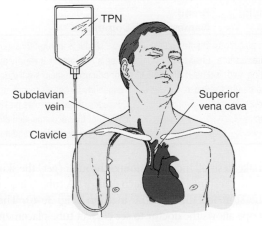

Fig. 36-7 Parenteral nutrition. (*Mosby's dictionary of medicine, nursing, and health professions,* ed 8, St Louis, 2009, Mosby.)

DELEGATION GUIDELINES

Therapy for Malnutrition

The nurse is responsible for all aspects of TPN. You assist the nurse by carefully observing the person.

You assist the nurse with tube feedings. In some states and agencies, you are allowed to give tube feedings. *Remember, you are never responsible for inserting feeding tubes or checking their placement.* This is the RN's responsibility.

Before giving tube feedings, make sure that:

- Your state allows you to perform the procedure
- The procedure is in your job description
- You have had the necessary education and training
- You know how to use the agency's equipment and supplies
- You review the procedure in the agency's procedure manual
- You review the procedure with the nurse
- A nurse is available to answer questions and to supervise you
- An RN has identified and labeled all other tubes, catheters, and needles
- An RN checks tube placement

If the above conditions are met, you need this information from the nurse, the MAR, and the care plan:

- The type of tube—NG, nasointestinal, PEG, or jejunostomy
- What feeding method to use—syringe, feeding bag, or feeding pump
- What size syringe to use—usually 30 or 60 mL for an adult
- How to position the person for the feeding—Fowler's or semi-Fowler's
- How to position the person after the feeding and for how long—Fowler's or semi-Fowler's
- What formula to use
- How much formula to give
- How high to raise the syringe or hang the feeding bag—usually 18 inches above the stomach or intestines
- The amount of flushing solution to use—usually 30 to 60 mL (1 to 2 ounces) of water for an adult
- How fast to give the feeding if using a syringe—usually over 30 minutes
- The flow rate if a feeding bag is used (Flow rate is the number of drops per minute.)
- The flow rate if a feeding pump is used
- If ice is kept around the bag for a continuous feeding
- What observations to report and record:
  - Nausea
  - Discomfort during the feeding
  - Vomiting
  - Distended (enlarged and swollen) abdomen
  - Coughing
  - Complaints of indigestion or heartburn
  - Redness, swelling, drainage, odor, or pain at the ostomy site
  - Fever
  - Signs and symptoms of respiratory distress
  - Increased pulse rate
  - Complaints of flatulence
  - Diarrhea
  - When to report observations
  - What specific patient or resident concerns to report immediately

PROMOTING SAFETY AND COMFORT

Therapy for Malnutrition

Safety

The person may have an intravenous (IV) line, a breathing tube (tracheostomy or endotracheal tube), and drainage tubes. You must know the purpose of each tube. Ask the nurse to label each tube to identify its purpose. Formula must enter only the feeding tube. Otherwise, the person can die.

Before giving a tube feeding always:

- Turn on the light if the room is dark. Do so even if the person is sleeping.
- Check and inspect the feeding tube and label with the nurse.
- Make sure an RN checks for tube placement.
- Make sure every tube, catheter, and needle is labeled.
- Trace the feeding tube back to the insertion site. Start at the end of the tube into which you will give the feeding. Trace the tube backward. For example, if the person has an NG tube, you will end at the nose. If the person has a gastrostomy tube, you will end at the abdomen. If you do not end at the correct place, do not give the tube feeding. Call for the nurse.

Aspiration is a major risk that can occur from tube feedings. **Aspiration** is breathing fluid, food, vomitus, or an object into the lungs. It can cause pneumonia and death. Aspiration can occur:

- *During* insertion. NG tubes and nasointestinal tubes are passed through the esophagus and then into the stomach or small intestine. The tube can slip into the airway. An x-ray is taken after insertion to check tube placement.
- From *tube movement out of place.* Coughing, sneezing, vomiting, suctioning, and poor positioning are common causes. A tube can move from the stomach or intestines into the esophagus and then into the airway. The RN checks tube placement before every scheduled tube feeding. With continuous feedings, the RN checks tube placement every 4 hours. To do so, the RN attaches a syringe to the tube. Gastrointestinal secretions are withdrawn through the syringe. Then the pH of the secretions is measured. *You are never responsible for checking feeding tube placement.*
- *From* regurgitation. **Regurgitation** is the backward flow of stomach contents into the mouth. Delayed stomach emptying and overfeeding are common causes.

To assist the nurse in preventing regurgitation and aspiration:

- Position the person in Fowler's or semi-Fowler's position before the feeding. Follow the care plan and the nurse's directions.
- Maintain Fowler's or semi-Fowler's position after the feeding. The person may be required to maintain the position for 1 to 2 hours after the feeding or at all times. The position allows formula to move through the GI tract. Follow the care plan and the nurse's directions.
- Avoid the left side-lying position. When the person lies on the left side, the stomach cannot empty into the small intestine.

Persons with NG or gastrostomy tubes are at great risk for regurgitation. The risk is less with intestinal tubes. Formula passes directly into the small intestine. Also, formula is given at a slow rate. During digestion, food slowly passes from the stomach into the small intestine. The stomach handles larger amounts of food at one time than does the small intestine.

Nasal secretions may contain blood or microbes. So can drainage at an ostomy site. Wear gloves. Follow Standard Precautions and the Bloodborne Pathogen Standard (Chapter 6).

Remind visitors to call for a nurse if any tube becomes disconnected or needs to be reconnected. They could connect the wrong tubes together.

HERBAL AND DIETARY SUPPLEMENTS

Many people use herbs and dietary supplements to promote and maintain health. Hundreds of herbal medicines and dietary supplements are marketed in the United States. The vast majority of health benefit claims made for herbal and dietary supplements are not proven. See Table 36-4 for some commonly used herbs. See Table 36-5 for some common dietary supplements.

TABLE 36-4   Herbal Therapy

Common Name	Other Names	Uses	Dose Forms	Side Effects

aloe	aloe vera
	salvia
	burn plant
		Arthritis
		Colitis
		Common cold
		Ulcers
		Hemorrhoids
		Seizures
		Glaucoma
		Pain
		Inflammation
		Itching
		Sunburn
		Skin ulcers
		Psoriasis
		Frostbite
			Aloe gel:
			Moisturizing lotion
			Shampoo
			Hair conditioner
			Gels
			Toothpaste
			Aloe juice for topical
			    application
			Capsules and tinctures
			    for oral use
			Aloe latex:
			    Juice drinks
			    Juice
				Oral forms may cause diarrhea

black cohosh	squawroot black snakeroot bugbane bugwort	Premenstrual syndrome Menstrual cramps Menopause	Elixirs Tablets Capsules	Upset stomach is a rare side effect

chamomile	German or Hungarian chamomile
	pinhead
	chamomilla
	genuine chamomile
	ground apple
	whig plant
	common chamomile
		Bloating
		Antiinflammatory in the gastrointestinal
		    (GI) tract
		Menstrual cramps
		Skin irritation
		Mouthwash for minor mouth irritation or
		    gum infections
			Ointment
			Gel
			Tea
			Bath additive
				Allergic reactions can occur but are
				    rare

echinacea	purple coneflower coneflower black Sampson	Common cold Flu Urinary tract infection Wounds	Dried roots Teas Tinctures Powder	Allergic reactions can occur but are rare
feverfew	featherfoil flirtwort bachelor's buttons	Migraine headache Rheumatoid arthritis	Leaf powder for tea Tablets	Mouth ulcers Lip swelling Allergic reactions

garlic		Reduce cholesterol and triglycerides
		Lower blood pressure
		Antiplatelet activity
			Cloves
			Oil
			Enteric-coated tablets
			Capsules
			Elixirs
				Taste
				Odor
				Commercial preparations may cause
				    nausea, vomiting, and burning of
				    the mouth and stomach

ginger	African ginger Jamaica ginger race ginger	Nausea and vomiting Rheumatoid arthritis Osteoarthritis Muscle discomfort	Powdered ginger-root Tea from ginger-root	Heartburn Diarrhea Mouth and throat irritation
ginkgo	maidenhair tree	Short-term memory loss Headache Dizziness Tinnitus Emotional instability Anxiety Alzheimer's disease Improve walking distance Erectile dysfunction Improve peripheral blood flow in diabetes Hearing	Liquid Tablets Capsules	Restlessness Diarrhea Nausea Vomiting Dizziness

Continued

TABLE 36-4 Herbal Therapy—cont'd

Common Name	Other Names	Uses	Dose Forms	Side Effects
ginseng	aralia cinquefoil five fingers tartar root red berry	Health maintenance Stress Vitality	Teas Powders Capsules Tablets Liquids	Insomnia Diarrhea Skin eruptions
goldenseal	yellow root Indian dye Indian paint jaundice root	Canker sores Sore mouth Cracked and bleeding lips	Powder for tea Tincture Fluid extract Freeze-dried root	High doses may cause: Nausea Vomiting Diarrhea CNS stimulation
green tea	Chinese tea Teagreen	CNS stimulation Increased blood pressure and heart rate Diuretic Diarrhea Lower cholesterol and triglycerides Reduce the risk of bladder, esophageal, and pancreatic cancers	Tea bags	Anxiety Nervousness Headache Diuresis Insomnia Tremors Irritability Palpitations Dysrhythmias Dependence
St. John's wort	klamath weed hardhay amber	Depression Heal wounds	Powder Tablets Capsules Liquid Semi-solids for topical use	Photosensitivity Serotonin syndrome (from taking two or more drugs that affect serotonin levels): Confusion Agitation Shivering Fever Sweating Nausea Diarrhea Muscle spasms Tremors Coma
valerian	amantilla setwall heliotrope vandal root	Restlessness Sleep	Tea Tincture Extract Tablets Capsules	Excitability Uneasiness Headache

TABLE 36-5 Other Dietary Supplements

Common Name	Other Names	Uses	Dose Forms	Side Effects
coenzyme Q_{10}	CoQ_{10} Ubiquinone	Heart failure Angina Hypertension Dysrhythmias Heart valve replacement Cancers of the breast, lung, prostate, pancreas, colon Muscular dystrophy Periodontal disease AIDS	Powder-filled capsules Tablets Liquid-filled gel capsules Chewable wafers Intraoral spray	Insomnia

TABLE 36-5 Other Dietary Supplements—cont'd

Common Name	Other Names	Uses	Dose Forms	Side Effects
creatine	creatine monohydrate	Muscle performance	Powder Candy Gum Liquid	Weight gain from water retention
lycopene		May reduce the risk of prostate cancer and possibly lung, colon, and breast cancer Lower cholesterol Protect against heart attack and stroke Cataracts Macular degeneration	Tomato powder Tomato extract	None reported
melatonin	sleep hormone MEL MLT	Insomnia Jet lag Antiaging	Tablets Chewable tablets Oral disintegrating tablets Extended-release tablets Capsules Liquid	Drowsiness Sedation Lethargy Agitation Insomnia
policosanol	policosanol N-octacosanol wheat germ oil octacosanol	Lower cholesterol Inhibit platelets	Tablets	Nervousness Headache Diarrhea Insomnia Weight loss Excess urination Insomnia
omega-3 fatty acids	fish oil	Reduce the risk of heart failure and myocardial infarction	Liquid Capsules Enteric-coated tablets	
s-adenosylmethionine (SAM-e)	Sammy SAM	Depression Osteoarthritis Fibromyalgia	Tablets Capsules	Mild stomach distress

REVIEW QUESTIONS

Circle the BEST answer.

1. Nutrition is:
   a. fats, proteins, carbohydrates, vitamins, and minerals
   b. the many processes involved in the ingestion, digestion, absorption, and use of foods and fluids by the body
   c. the MyPlate Food Guide
   d. the balance between calories taken in and used by the body

2. The MyPlate Food Guide encourages the following, *except*:
   a. the same diet for everyone
   b. focusing on variety, amount, and nutrition
   c. choosing foods and beverages with less saturated fat, sodium, and added sugars
   d. taking small steps to improve diet and lifestyle

3. A healthy eating pattern includes the following, *except*:
   a. fried foods
   b. fruits, especially whole fruits
   c. oils
   d. a variety of protein foods

4. Which is *not* a macronutrient?
   a. garlic
   b. protein
   c. fiber
   d. fats

5. Fats are also known as:
   a. lipids
   b. iodine
   c. glucose
   d. nutrients

6. Fiber in the diet helps with the following, *except*:
   a. prevents constipation
   b. blood glucose control
   c. weight control
   d. bloating

7. Which is needed for nerve and heart function?
   a. phosphorus
   b. iron
   c. iodine
   d. potassium

8. Enteral nutrition:
   a. requires an NG tube
   b. is given into a central venous site
   c. is given into the GI tract
   d. requires an IV

9. For a tube feeding, the person is positioned in:
   a. Fowler's or semi-Fowler's position
   b. the left side-lying position
   c. the right side-lying position
   d. the supine position
10. The nurse checks feeding tube placement to prevent:
    a. aspiration
    b. regurgitation
    c. over-feeding
    d. cramping
11. Which position is used to prevent regurgitation after a tube feeding?
    a. Fowler's or semi-Fowler's position
    b. the supine position
    c. the left or right side-lying position
    d. the prone position
12. A nurse asks you to give a tube feeding. The procedure is not in your job description. What should you do?
    a. refuse to perform the task
    b. give the tube feeding
    c. tell the director of nursing
    d. ask another nurse what you should do

13. Which is an oral nutritional supplement?
    a. Ensure
    b. aloe
    c. green tea
    d. St. John's wort
14. Herbs and dietary supplements have proven nutritional value.
    a. True
    b. False
15. Which is an herb?
    a. folic acid
    b. ginger
    c. iodine
    d. thiamin

Answers to these questions can be found on the Evolve Resources site: http://evolve.elsevier.com/Anderson/medasst/

A Review of Arithmetic

FRACTIONS

OBJECTIVE

- Demonstrate proficiency in mathematical problems using addition, subtraction, multiplication, and division of fractions. Fractions are one or more of the separate parts of a whole number or amount.

  EXAMPLE:

$$1 - \frac{1}{2} = \frac{1}{2}$$

Common Fractions

A common fraction is part of a whole number. The numerator (dividend) is the number above the line. The denominator (divisor) is the number below the line.

The line separating the numerator and denominator tells us to divide.

<u>Numerator (names how many parts are used)</u>
Denominator (tells how many pieces
into which the whole is divided)

EXAMPLES:

The denominator represents the number of parts or pieces into which the whole is divided.

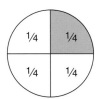

Graphically, $\frac{1}{4}$ means that the whole circle is divided into four (4) parts; one (1) of the parts is being used.

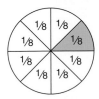

Graphically, $\frac{1}{8}$ means that the whole circle is divided into eight (8) parts; one (1) of the parts is being used.

From these two examples ($\frac{1}{4}$ and $\frac{1}{8}$), you can see that the *larger* the *denominator* number, the *smaller* the *portion*. In the example above, each section in the $\frac{1}{8}$ circle is smaller than each section in the $\frac{1}{4}$ circle.

Common fractions are an important concept to understand when calculating drug doses. For example, the medicine ordered may be $\frac{1}{4}$ g and the drug source available is $\frac{1}{2}$ g tablet. Before proceeding to do any formal calculations, you should first decide if the dose you need to give is smaller or larger than the drug source available.

EXAMPLES:
Visualize:

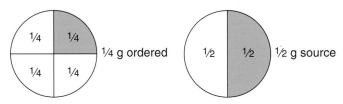

Decision: "Is the needed dosage a larger or smaller portion than the drug available?"

Answer: $\frac{1}{4}$ g is smaller. Therefore, it would be less than one tablet.

Try a second example: $\frac{1}{8}$ g is ordered. The drug source is $\frac{1}{2}$ g.

Visualize:

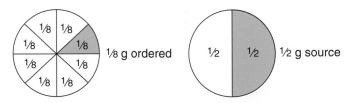

Decision: "Is the needed dosage a larger or smaller portion than the drug available?"

Answer: $\frac{1}{8}$ g is smaller than the drug source. Therefore, it would be less than one tablet.

Types of Common Fractions

Common fractions are expressed in various formats:
1. *Simple:* Contains *one* numerator and *one* denominator: $\frac{1}{4}$, $\frac{1}{20}$, $\frac{1}{60}$, $\frac{1}{100}$

2. *Complex:* May have a simple fraction in the numerator or denominator:

$$\frac{1}{2} \text{ over } 4 = \frac{\frac{1}{2}}{4}$$

or

$$\frac{1}{2} \div 4 =$$

$$\frac{1}{2} \div \frac{4}{1} =$$

$$\frac{1}{2} \times \frac{1}{4} = \frac{1}{8}$$

3. *Proper:* Numerator is smaller than denominator: $\frac{1}{8}, \frac{2}{5}, \frac{1}{100}$
4. *Improper:* Numerator is larger than denominator: $\frac{4}{3}, \frac{6}{4}, \frac{100}{10}$
5. *Mixed number:* A whole number and a fraction: $4\frac{5}{8}, 6\frac{2}{3}, 1\frac{5}{100}$
6. *Decimal:* Fractions written on the basis of a multiple of 10: $0.5 = \frac{5}{10}, 0.05 = \frac{5}{100}, 0.005 = \frac{5}{1000}$
7. *Equivalent:* Fractions that have the same value: $\frac{1}{3}$ and $\frac{2}{6}$

Working With Fractions

Reducing to Lowest Terms

Divide the numerator and the denominator by a number that will divide into both evenly (a common denominator).

EXAMPLE:

$$\frac{25}{125} \div \frac{25}{25} = \frac{1}{5}$$

Finding the lowest common denominator of a series of fractions is not always easy. Remember:

- If the numerator and denominator are even numbers, 2 will work as a common denominator but it may not be the smallest one.
- If the numerator and denominator end with 0 or 5, 5 will work as a common denominator but it may not be the smallest one.
- Check to see if the numerator divides evenly into the denominator; this will be the smallest term. When all else fails, use the prime number method to find the lowest common denominator. A prime number is a whole number, greater than 1, that can be divided only by itself and 1 (2, 3, 5, 7, 11, 19, 23, etc.).

Addition

Adding common fractions. When denominators are the same figure, add the numerators.

EXAMPLE:

$$\frac{1}{4} + \frac{2}{4} + \frac{3}{4} = \frac{6}{4} = 1\frac{1}{2}$$

Add the following:

$$\frac{2}{6} + \frac{3}{6} + \frac{4}{6} = \frac{9}{6} = 1\frac{1}{2}$$

$$\frac{1}{100} + \frac{3}{100} + \frac{5}{100} = \frac{9}{100}$$

When the denominators are unlike, change the fractions to equivalent fractions. Do so by finding the lowest common denominator.

EXAMPLE:

$$\frac{2}{5} + \frac{3}{10} + \frac{1}{2} = \underline{\quad\quad}$$

1. Determine the lowest common denominator. In this example, 10 is the lowest common denominator.
2. Divide the denominator of the fraction being changed into the common denominator. Then, multiply the product (answer) by the numerator.

$$\frac{2}{5} = \frac{4}{10}$$ Divide 5 into 10. Multiply the answer [2] by 2.

$$\frac{3}{10} = \frac{3}{10}$$ Divide 10 into 10. Multiply the answer [1] by 3.

$$\frac{1}{2} = \frac{5}{10}$$ Divide 2 into 10. Multiply the answer [5] by 1.

$$\frac{12}{10} = 1\frac{1}{5}$$ Add the numerators and place the total over the denominator [10]. Convert the improper fraction to a mixed number and reduce to lowest terms.

Add the following:

a.
$$\frac{2}{8} = \frac{}{64}$$

$$+\frac{4}{64} = \frac{}{64}$$

$$+\frac{5}{16} = \frac{}{64}$$

$$\overline{\frac{}{64}} \quad Answer: \frac{5}{8}$$

b.
$$\frac{3}{7} = \frac{}{28}$$

$$+\frac{9}{14} = \frac{}{28}$$

$$+\frac{1}{28} = \frac{}{28}$$

$$\overline{\frac{}{28}} \quad Answer: 1\frac{3}{28}$$

Adding mixed numbers. Add the fractions first, then add whole numbers.

EXAMPLE:

$$2\frac{3}{4} + 2\frac{1}{2} + 3\frac{3}{8} = \underline{\quad\quad}$$

1. Determine the lowest common denominator. In this example, 8 is the common denominator.

2. Divide the denominator of the fraction being changed into the common denominator. Multiply the product (answer) by the numerator.

$$2\frac{3}{4}=2\frac{6}{8}$$ Divide 4 into 8. Multiply the answer [2] by 3.

$$2\frac{1}{2}=2\frac{4}{8}$$ Divide 2 into 8. Multiply the answer [4] by 1.

$$+3\frac{3}{8}=3\frac{3}{8}$$ Divide 8 into 8. Multiply the answer [1] by 3.

$$\frac{13}{8}$$ Add the numerators. Place the total over the denominator [8].

Convert the improper fraction $3\frac{13}{84}$ to a mixed number $3\frac{5}{84}$. Add it to the whole numbers.

$$7+\frac{13}{8}=7+1\frac{5}{8}=8\frac{5}{8}$$

Add the following:

a.
$$\frac{1}{4}$$
$$+\frac{3}{4}$$
$$\frac{-}{4}\quad Answer:\frac{4}{4}=1$$

b.
$$\frac{1}{2}=\frac{}{6}$$
$$+\frac{1}{3}=\frac{}{6}$$
$$+\frac{1}{6}=\frac{}{6}$$
$$=\frac{}{6}\quad Answer:\frac{6}{6}=1$$

c.
$$\frac{3}{5}=\frac{}{50}$$
$$+\frac{4}{50}=\frac{}{50}\quad Answer:\frac{34}{50}=\frac{17}{25}$$
$$=\frac{}{50}\quad (Reduced\ to\ lowest\ term)$$

Subtraction

Subtracting fractions. When the denominators are not alike, change the fractions to an equivalent fraction by finding the lowest common denominator.

EXAMPLE:

$$\frac{1}{4}-\frac{3}{16}=\underline{\quad}$$

1. Determine the lowest common denominator. In this example, 16 is the lowest common denominator.
2. Divide the denominator of the fraction being changed into the common denominator. Multiply the product (answer) by the numerator.

$$\frac{1}{4}=\frac{4}{16}$$ Divide 4 into 16. Multiply the answer [4] by 1.

$$-\frac{3}{16}=\frac{3}{16}$$

$$\frac{1}{16}$$ Subtract the numerators. Place the total [1] over the denominator [16].

Subtract the following:

a.
$$\frac{3}{8}$$
$$-\frac{2}{8}$$
$$\frac{-}{8}\quad Answer:\frac{1}{8}$$

b.
$$\frac{1}{100}=\frac{}{300}$$
$$-\frac{1}{150}=\frac{}{300}$$
$$\frac{}{300}\quad Answer:\frac{1}{300}$$

Subtracting mixed numbers. Subtract the fractions first. Then subtract the whole numbers.

EXAMPLE:

$$4\frac{1}{4}-1\frac{3}{4}=\underline{\quad}$$

$$4\frac{1}{4}=3\frac{5}{4}$$ You cannot subtract $\frac{3}{4}$ from $\frac{1}{4}$.
$$-1\frac{3}{4}=1\frac{3}{4}$$ Therefore borrow 1 (which equals $\frac{4}{4}$) from the whole numbers. Then add
$$3\frac{5}{4}-1\frac{3}{4}=2\frac{2}{4}$$ $\frac{4}{4}+\frac{1}{4}=\frac{5}{4}$.

$$2\frac{2}{4}=2\frac{1}{2}$$ Subtract the numerators. Place answer over the denominator (4). Reduce to lowest terms. Subtract the whole numbers.

When the denominators are not alike, change the fractions to equivalent fractions by finding the lowest common denominator.

EXAMPLE:

$$2\frac{5}{8}-1\frac{1}{4}=\underline{\quad}$$

1. Determine the lowest common denominator. In this example, 8 is the common denominator.

2. Divide the denominator of the fraction being changed into the common denominator. Multiply the product (answer) by the numerator.

$$2\frac{5}{8} = 2\frac{5}{8}$$ Divide 8 into 8. Multiply the answer (1) by 5.

$$-1\frac{1}{4} = 1\frac{2}{8}$$ Divide 4 into 8. Multiply the answer (2) by 1.

$$2\frac{5}{8} - 1\frac{2}{8} = 1\frac{3}{8}$$ Subtract the numerators. Place the total (3) over the denominator (8) and reduce to lowest terms. Subtract the whole numbers.

Subtract the following:

a. $$\frac{7}{8} = \frac{}{24}$$

   $$-\frac{3}{6} = \frac{}{24}$$

   $$\frac{}{24}$$ Answer: $\frac{9}{24} = \frac{3}{8}$

b. $$6\frac{7}{8} = \frac{}{16}$$

   $$-3\frac{1}{16} = \frac{}{16}$$

   $$\frac{}{16}$$ Answer: $3\frac{13}{16}$

Multiplication
Multiplying a whole number by a fraction

EXAMPLE:

$$3 \times \frac{5}{8} = \underline{\quad}$$

1. Place the whole number over $1\left(\frac{3}{1}\right)$.
2. Multiply the numerators (top numbers) and denominators (bottom numbers).

$$\frac{3}{1} \times \frac{5}{8} = \frac{15}{8}$$

3. Change the improper fraction to a mixed number.

$$\frac{15}{8} = 1\frac{7}{8}$$

Multiply the following:

a. $2 \times \frac{3}{4} = \underline{\quad}$ Answer: $\frac{3}{2} = 1\frac{1}{2}$

b. $15 \times \frac{3}{5} = \underline{\quad}$ Answer: $\frac{9}{1} = 9$

Multiplying two fractions

EXAMPLE:

$$\frac{1}{4} \times \frac{2}{3} = \underline{\quad}$$

1. Use cancellation to speed the process.

$$\frac{1}{2\cancel{4}} \times \frac{\cancel{2}^{1}}{3} = \frac{1}{6}$$

2. Multiply the numerators and denominators.

$$\frac{1}{2} \times \frac{1}{3} = \frac{1}{6}$$

Multiplying mixed numbers

EXAMPLE:

$$3\frac{1}{2} \times 2\frac{1}{5} = \underline{\quad}$$

1. Change the mixed numbers (a whole number and a fraction) to an improper fraction (wherein the numerator is larger than the denominator).

$$3\frac{1}{2} \times 2\frac{1}{5} = \underline{\quad}$$ Multiply the denominator times the whole number and add the numerator.

$$\frac{7}{2} \times \frac{11}{5} = \underline{\quad}$$

2. Multiply the numerators and denominators.

$$\frac{7}{2} \times \frac{11}{5} = \frac{77}{10}$$

3. Change the product (answer), an improper fraction, to a mixed number. Divide the denominator into the numerator and reduce to lowest terms.

$$\frac{7}{2} \times \frac{11}{5} = \frac{77}{10} = 7\frac{7}{10}$$

Multiply the following:

a. $1\frac{2}{3} \times \frac{3}{6} = \underline{\quad}$ Answer: $\frac{5}{6}$

b. $1\frac{7}{8} \times 1\frac{1}{4} = \underline{\quad}$ Answer: $\frac{75}{32} = 2\frac{11}{32}$

Division
Dividing fractions

EXAMPLE:

$$4 \div \frac{1}{2} = \underline{\quad}$$

1. Change the division sign to a multiplication sign.
2. Invert the divisor (the number after the division sign).
3. Reduce the fractions using cancellation.

4. Multiply the numerators and denominators.

$$4 \div \frac{1}{2} = \frac{4}{1} \times \frac{2}{1} = \frac{8}{1} = 8$$

Dividing with a mixed number

1. Change the mixed number to an improper fraction.
2. Change the division sign to a multiplication sign.
3. Invert the divisor.
4. Reduce whenever possible.

EXAMPLES:

$$4\frac{1}{2} \div \frac{3}{4} = \frac{9}{2} \div \frac{3}{4} = \frac{\cancel{9}^3}{\cancel{2}_1} \times \frac{\cancel{4}^2}{\cancel{3}_1} = \frac{6}{1} \text{ or } 6$$

$$6\frac{1}{4} \div 1\frac{1}{4} = \frac{25}{4} \div \frac{5}{4} = \frac{\cancel{25}^5}{\cancel{4}_1} \times \frac{\cancel{4}^1}{\cancel{5}_1} = \frac{5}{1} \text{ or } 5$$

Fractions as Decimals

Fractions can be changed to a decimal form by dividing the numerator by the denominator.

EXAMPLE:

$$\frac{1}{2} = 2\overline{)1.0}^{\,0.5}$$

Change the following fractions to decimals:

$\dfrac{1}{100} = \underline{\hspace{1cm}}$ *Answer:* 0.01

$\dfrac{5}{8} = \underline{\hspace{1cm}}$ *Answer:* 0.625

$\dfrac{1}{2} = \underline{\hspace{1cm}}$ *Answer:* 0.5

Using Cancellation to Speed Your Work

1. Determine a number that will divide evenly into both the numerator and denominator.
2. Continue the process of dividing both the numerator and denominator by the same number until all numbers are reduced to the lowest terms.
3. Complete the multiplication of the problem.

EXAMPLE:

$$\frac{\cancel{5}^1}{\cancel{6}_2} \times \frac{\cancel{9}^3}{\cancel{10}_2} = \underline{\hspace{1cm}}$$

$$\frac{1}{2} \times \frac{3}{2} = \frac{3}{4}$$

4. Complete the division of the problem.

EXAMPLE:

$$\frac{6}{9} \div \frac{5}{8} = \underline{\hspace{1cm}}$$

Change the division sign to a multiplication sign and invert the number after the division sign. Reduce and complete the multiplication of the problem.

$$\frac{2}{3} \times \frac{8}{5} = \frac{16}{15} = 1\frac{1}{15}$$

DECIMAL FRACTIONS

OBJECTIVES

- Calculate problems using addition, subtraction, multiplication, and division of decimals.
- Convert decimals to fractions and fractions to decimals.
- When fractions are written in decimal form, the denominators are not included. Decimal means "10."

When reading decimals, the numbers to the left of the decimal point are whole numbers. It helps to think of them as whole dollars. Numbers to the right of the decimal are fractions of the whole number. Think of them as "cents."

EXAMPLES:
   1.0 = one
   11.0 = eleven
   111.0 = one hundred eleven
   1111.0 = one thousand one hundred eleven

Numbers to the right of the decimal point are read as follows:

EXAMPLES:

Decimal(s):	Fraction(s):
0.1 = one tenth	1/10
0.01 = one hundredth	1/100
0.465 = four hundred sixty-five thousandths	465/1000
0.0007 = seven ten thousandths	7/10,000

Here is another way to view reading decimals:

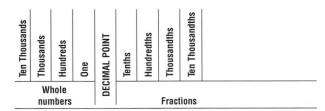

Ten Thousands	Thousands	Hundreds	One	DECIMAL POINT	Tenths	Hundredths	Thousandths	Ten Thousandths
Whole numbers					Fractions			

. 1 equals one-tenth (1/10)

. 2 2 equals twenty-two hundredths (22/100)

. 1 1 2 equals one hundred twelve thousandths (112/1000)

. 0 1 1 2 equals one hundred twelve ten thousandths (112/10,000)

1 . equals number one

1 0 . equals number ten

1 0 0 . equals number one hundred

1 0 0 0 . equals number one thousand

On prescriptions another way of expressing the decimal is by using a slanted line.

EXAMPLES:

   1 mg = 0.001 g = 0/001 g
   0.1 mg = 0.0001 g = 0/0001 g
   30 mg = 0.030 g = 0/030 g
   100 mg = 0.100 g = 0/100 g
   1000 mg = 1.000 g = 1   g

Note: Often the decimal point is not recognized, and very large doses have been accidentally administered. *The rule is: Do not use trailing 0s to the right of decimal points.*

$$250 \text{ mg} = 0.250 \text{ g} = 0/250 \text{ g}$$

Multiplying Decimals

Multiplying whole numbers and decimals

1. The multiplicand is the top number.
2. The multiplier is the bottom number with the x (multiplication sign) before it.
3. Count as many places in the answer, starting from the right, as there are places in the decimal involved in the multiplication.

EXAMPLES:

500	1000	1000
×0.02	×0.04	×0.009
10.00 (10)	40.00 (40)	9.000 (9)

	7.25	500
	× 4	×0.009
	29.00 (29)	4.500 (or 4.5)

Multiplying a Decimal by a Decimal

1. Multiply the problem as if the numbers were both whole numbers.
2. Count decimal places in the answer, starting from the right, as many decimal places as there are in both of the numbers that were multiplied.

EXAMPLE:

```
   3.75
×  0.5
  1.875
```

There are two decimal places in 3.75 and one decimal place in 0.5, making three decimal places. Count three decimal places from the right.

Multiplying Numbers With Zero

EXAMPLES:

1. Multiply 223 by 40.
   a. Multiply 223 by 0. Write the answer, 0, in the unit column of the answer.
   b. Then multiply 223 by 4. Write this answer in front of the 0 in the product.

```
   223
×   40
   000
   892
  8920
```

2. Multiply 124 by 304.
   a. First, multiply 124 by 4. The answer is 496.
   b. Now, multiply 124 by 0. Write the answer, 0, under the 9 in 496.

c. Multiply 124 by 3. Write this answer in front of the 0 in the product.

```
    124
×   304
    496
    000
    372
 37,696
```

Dividing Decimals

1. If the divisor (number by which you divide) is a decimal, make it a whole number. Do so by moving the decimal point to the right of the last number.
2. Move the decimal point in the dividend (the number inside the bracket) as many places to the right as you move the decimal point in the divisor.
3. Place the decimal point for the quotient (answer) directly above the new decimal point of the dividend and divide dividend by the divisor.

EXAMPLES:

$$0.25\overline{)10} = 25\overline{)1000.}\;\;^{40.} \qquad 0.3\overline{)99.3} = 3\overline{)993.}\;\;^{331.}$$

$$0.4\overline{)1.68} = 4\overline{)16.8}\;\;^{4.2}$$

Changing Decimals to Common Fractions

1. Remove the decimal point.
2. Place the appropriate denominator under the number.
3. Reduce to lowest terms.

EXAMPLES:

$$0.2 = \frac{2}{10} = \frac{1}{5} \qquad 0.2 = \frac{20}{100} = \frac{1}{5}$$

Changing Common Fractions to Decimal Fractions

Divide the numerator of the fraction by the denominator.

EXAMPLE:

$$\frac{1}{4} \text{ means } 1 \div 4 \text{ or } 4\overline{)1.00}\;\;^{0.25}$$

▮ PERCENTS

OBJECTIVES

- Calculate problems using percentages.
- Convert percentages to fractions, percentages to decimals, decimal fractions to percentages, and common fractions to percentages.

Determining the Percent of One Number Relative to Another

1. Divide the smaller number by the larger number.
2. Multiply the quotient by 100. Add the percent sign.

EXAMPLE:

A certain 1000-part solution is 10 parts drug. What percent of the solution contains the drug?

$$1000 \overline{)10.00} \quad \text{(0.01)}$$

$0.01 \times 100 = 1.$ or 1%

Changing Percents to Fractions

1. Omit the percent sign to form the numerator.
2. Use 100 for the denominator.
3. Reduce the fraction.

EXAMPLES:

$5\% \dfrac{5}{100} = \dfrac{1}{20}$ $75\% \dfrac{75}{100} = \dfrac{3}{4}$

Changing Percents to Decimal Fractions

1. Omit the percent signs.
2. Insert a decimal point *two places to the left* of the last number; or express decimally as hundredths.

EXAMPLES:

$5\% = 0.05$ $15\% = 0.15$

Numbers that are already expressed in hundredths, such as 10%, 15%, 25%, 50%, merely need to have the decimal point placed in front of the first digits. That is because they are already expressed in hundredths, whereas 1%, 2%, 4%, 5% needed to have a zero placed in front of the number to express them as hundredths.

If the percent is a mixed number, it should have the fraction expressed as a decimal. Then change the percent to a decimal. Do so by moving the decimal point two places to the left.

EXAMPLES:

$12\dfrac{1}{2}\% = 12.5\%$ or 0.125 $\dfrac{1}{4}\% = 0.25\%$ or 0.0025

Changing Common Fractions to Percents

1. Divide the numerator by the denominator.
2. Multiply the quotient by 100. Then add the percent sign.

EXAMPLE:

$\dfrac{1}{50} = 50 \overline{)1.00} \;\; {}^{0.02} = 0.02 \times 100 = 2\%$

Change the following:

$\dfrac{1}{400} = \underline{\qquad}$ Answer $= 0.25\%$

$\dfrac{1}{8} = \underline{\qquad}$ Answer $= 12.5\%$

Changing Decimal Fractions to Percents

1. Move the decimal point two places to the right.
2. Omit the decimal point if a whole number results.
3. Add the percent sign. This is the same as multiplying the decimal fraction by 100 and adding the percent sign.

EXAMPLE:

$0.01 = 1.00 = 1\%$ (or $\dfrac{1}{100}$)

Points to Remember in Reading Decimals

1. One (1) is the whole number 1. When it is written 1.0, it is still one or 1.
2. The whole number is usually written like this: 1 or 2 or 3 or 4, and so on. Remember, do not use trailing 0s.
3. Can you read 0.1? This is one tenth. There is one number after the decimal point.
4. Can you read .1? This is also one tenth. The zero in front of the decimal point is a leading zero. It does not change its value. One tenth can be written in two ways: 0.1 and .1. The leading 0 to the left of the decimal should be used to help prevent errors.
5. One can also be written 1.0. The zero after the decimal is called a trailing zero. It does not change the value of the number. The trailing zero should be left off to prevent errors. 1.0 g can be misread as 10 g if the decimal point is not clearly written.

SYSTEMS OF WEIGHTS AND MEASURES

OBJECTIVES

- Know the basic equivalents of the household and metric systems.
- Convert drug problems using the household and metric systems.

Two systems of measurement are used during the calculation, preparation, and administration of medicines: household and metric.

Household Measurements

Household measurements are often the way drugs are given at home. However, they are the least accurate. Household measurements include drops, teaspoons, tablespoons, teacups, cups, glasses, pints, quarts, and gallons. The first three measurements—drops, teaspoons, and tablespoons—are used for drugs, depending on the amount prescribed.

COMMON HOUSEHOLD EQUIVALENTS

1 quart	=	4 cups
1 pint	=	2 cups
1 cup	=	8 ounces
1 teacup	=	6 ounces
1 tablespoon	=	3 teaspoons
1 teaspoon	=	approximately 5 mL

The metric system uses the **meter** as the standard unit of length. The **liter** is the standard unit of volume and the **gram** is the standard unit of weight.

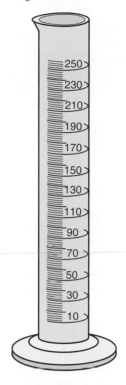

UNITS OF LENGTH (METER)

1 millimeter = 0.001   meaning 1/1000
1 centimeter = 0.01   meaning 1/100
1 decimeter −0.1   meaning 1/10
1 meter = 1   meter

UNITS OF VOLUME (LITER)

1 milliliter = 0.001   meaning 1/1000
1 centiliter = 0.01   meaning 1/100
1 deciliter = 0.1   meaning 1/10
1 liter = 1   liter

UNITS OF WEIGHT (GRAM)

1 microgram = 0.000001   meaning 1/1,000,000
1 milligram = 0.001   meaning 1/1000
1 centigram = 0.01   meaning 1/100
1 decigram = 0.1   meaning 1/10
1 gram = 1   gram

Other Prefixes

Deca means ten or 10 times as much. *Hecto* means one hundred or 100 times as much. *Kilo* means one thousand or 1000 times as much. These three prefixes can be combined with the words *meter, gram, or liter.*

EXAMPLES:

1 decaliter   =   10 liters
1 hectometer =   100 meters
1 kilogram   =   1000 grams

Arabic numbers are used to write metric doses.

EXAMPLES:

500 milligrams, 5 grams, 15 milliliters

Prefixes added to the units (meter, liter, or gram) indicate smaller or larger units. All units are derived by dividing or multiplying by 10, 100, or 1000.

COMMON METRIC EQUIVALENTS

1000 milliliters (mL) = 1 liter (L)
1000 milligrams (mg) = 1 gram (g)
1000 micrograms (mcg) = 1 milligram (mg)
1,000,000 micrograms (mcg) = 1 gram (g)
1000 grams (g) = 1 kilogram (kg)

Differentiate among metric weight and metric volume. Mark each of the following MW for metric weight or MV for metric volume.

1. microgram =_____   Answer: MW
2. liter =   _____   Answer: MV
3. gram =   _____   Answer: MW

Conversion of Metric Units

The first step in calculating the drug dosage is to ensure that the drug ordered and the drug source on hand are *both* using the same *system of measurement* (preferably in the metric system) and are expressed in the *same unit of weight* (for example, both **milligrams** or **grams**).

Converting Milligrams to Grams (1000 mg = 1 g)

Divide the number of milligrams by 1000 or move the decimal point of the milligrams three places to the left.

EXAMPLES:

200 mg = 0.2 g
0.6 mg = 0.0006 g

In the following example, both the doctor's order and the drug available use the metric system. However, they are *not* both in the *same unit of weight* within the metric system.

EXAMPLE:

The doctor orders 0.25 g of a drug. The label on the drug bottle says 250 mg. This means that each capsule contains 250 mg of the drug.

To change the gram dose into milligrams, multiply 0.25 by 1000. Move the decimal point three places to the right (a milligram is one thousandth of a gram). 0.250 g = 250 mg. You would give one tablet of this drug.

TRY THIS ONE: The doctor orders 0.1 g of a drug. The bottle label states that the strength of the drug is 100 mg/capsule.

To change the gram dose into milligrams, move the decimal point three places to the right: 0.1 g = 100 mg. That is exactly what the bottle label strength states.

Converting Kilograms (kg) to Pounds (lb)

(1 kg = 2.2 lb)
Multiply the number of kilograms by 2.2.
Example: 40 kg x 2.2 = 88 lb

Converting Pounds to Kilograms

Divide the number of pounds by 2.2.
Example: 143 lb ÷ 2.2 = 65 kg

Solid Dosage for Oral Administration

If the dosage on hand and dosage ordered are both expressed using the same system of measurement and use the same unit of weight, calculate the dosage using one of these methods.

EXAMPLE:

The doctor orders 1 g of ampicillin. The ampicillin bottle states that each tablet in the bottle contains 0.5 g.

PROBLEM:

You do not have the 1 g as ordered. How many tablets will you give? Notice that the amount ordered and the amount available use the same system of measurement (metric) and the same unit of weight (grams).

SOLUTION:

$$\frac{\text{Dose desired}}{\text{Dose on hand}} = \frac{1\,g}{0.5\,g} = 2$$

You will give two 0.5 g capsules for the 1 g ordered.

The dosage on hand and dosage ordered are both expressed in the same system of measurement, but they are *not* in the same unit of weight within the system. The units of weight must first be converted.

EXAMPLE:

The doctor orders 1000 milligrams (metric) of ampicillin. On hand: 0.25 gram (metric) per tablet.

Rule: Converting grams (metric) to milligrams (metric) (1 g = 1000 mg)

Multiply the number of grams by 1000. Move the decimal point of the grams three places to the right. 0.25 g = 250 mg

SOLUTION:

$$\frac{\text{Dose desired}}{\text{Dose on hand}} = \frac{1000\,mg}{250\,mg} = 4$$

Give four 0.25 g tablets.

Conversion Problems

Some students may better understand problems in tablet or capsule dosage for oral administration if presented with their fractional equivalents as follows:

1. The doctor orders 2 g of a drug in oral tablet form. The medicine bottle label states that the strength on hand is 0.5 g. This means each tablet in the bottle contains 0.5 g of the drug.
   How many tablets should you give? 1, 2, 3, 4, or 5? *Answer:* 4
   What strength is ordered? 2 g
   What strength is on the bottle label? 0.5 g
   What is the fractional equivalent of 0.5 g? $\frac{1}{2}$ g
   How many $\frac{1}{2}$ g (0.5 g) tablets would equal 2 g? 4

   $$2 \div \frac{1}{2} = \frac{2}{1} \times \frac{2}{1} = 4 \text{ tablets}$$

2. The doctor orders 0.2 mg of a drug in oral tablet form. The medicine bottle label states that the strength on hand is

0.1 mg. This means each tablet in the bottle contains 0.1 mg of the drug.
How many tablets should you give? 1, 2, 3, or 4? *Answer:* 2 tablets
What strength is ordered? 0.2 mg
What is the fractional equivalent of 0.2 mg? $\frac{2}{10}$
What strength is on the bottle label? 0.1 mg
What is the fractional equivalent of 0.1 mg? $\frac{1}{10}$
How many $\frac{1}{10}$ mg (0.1 mg) tablets would equal $\frac{2}{10}$ mg (0.2 mg)? 2

$$\begin{array}{l} 0.1\ mg = \frac{1}{10}\ mg\ or\ 1\ tablet \\ + 0.1\ mg = \frac{1}{10}\ mg\ or\ 1\ tablet \\ \hline 0.2\ mg = \frac{2}{10}\ mg\ or\ 2\ tablets \end{array}$$

Dosage desired ÷ dosage on hand =

$$or\ \ \frac{2}{10} \div \frac{1}{10} = \frac{2}{\cancel{10}} \times \frac{\cancel{10}^{1}}{1} = 2 \text{ tablets}$$

3. The doctor orders 0.5 mg of a drug in oral capsule form. The medicine bottle label states that the strength on hand is 0.25 mg. This means each capsule in the bottle contains 0.25 mg of the drug.
   How many tablets should you give? 1, 2, 3, 4, or 5? *Answer:* 2 tablets
   What strength is ordered? 0.5 mg
   What fractional equivalent equals 0.5 mg? $\frac{1}{2}$ mg
   What strength is on the bottle label? 0.25 mg
   What fractional equivalent equals the strength on hand? $\frac{1}{4}$ mg
   How many $\frac{1}{4}$ mg (0.25 mg) tablets would equal $\frac{1}{2}$ mg (0.5 mg)? 2

   $$\begin{array}{l} 0.25\ mg = \frac{1}{4}\ mg\ or\ 1\ tablet \\ + 0.25\ mg = \frac{1}{4}\ mg\ or\ 1\ tablet \\ \hline 0.50\ mg = \frac{1}{2}\ mg\ or\ 2\ tablets \end{array}$$

   Dosage desired ÷ dosage on hand =

   $$or\ \ \frac{1}{2} \div \frac{1}{4} = \frac{1}{2} \times \frac{4}{1} = 2 \text{ tablets}$$

4. The doctor orders 0.25 mg of a drug in oral capsule form. The medicine bottle label states that the strength on hand is 0.5 mg. This means that every capsule in the bottle contains 0.5 mg of the drug.
   How many tablets should you give? $\frac{1}{2}$, 1, $1\frac{1}{2}$, 2, $2\frac{1}{2}$, 3, 4, or 5? *Answer:* $\frac{1}{2}$ tablet
   What strength did the doctor order? 0.25 mg
   What is the fractional equivalent of the strength ordered? $\frac{1}{4}$ mg
   What strength is on the bottle label? 0.5 mg
   What is the fractional equivalent of the strength on the bottle label? $\frac{1}{2}$ mg
   Which is less: 0.5 mg ($\frac{1}{2}$ mg) or 0.25 mg ($\frac{1}{4}$ mg)? *Answer:* 0.25 mg ($\frac{1}{4}$ mg)
   Was the amount ordered less than the strength on hand or more? *Answer:* Less

   $$0.5\ mg = \frac{1}{2}\ mg\ or\ 1\ tablet$$

$0.25 \text{ mg} = \dfrac{1}{4} \text{ mg or half as much or } \dfrac{1}{2} \text{ tablet}$

$or \ \dfrac{1}{4} \div \dfrac{1}{2} = \dfrac{1}{4} \times \dfrac{2}{1} = \dfrac{1}{2} \text{ tablet}$

Note: If the drug is available in 0.25 mg tablets, request this size from the pharmacy. A tablet should be divided only when scored. Even then, the practice is not advised because the tablet often fragments into unequal pieces.

ARITHMETIC EXERCISES—ON YOUR OWN

WORKING WITH FRACTIONS

Reduce the following fractions to lowest terms.
1. 5/100 = _____
2. 3/21 = _____
3. 6/36 = _____
4. 12/44 = _____
5. 2/4 = _____

Changing Decimals to Common Fractions

Convert the following decimals to common fractions.
6. 0.3 = _____
7. 0.25 = _____
8. 0.4 = _____
9. 0.50 = _____
10. 0.5 = _____
11. 0.75 = _____
12. 0.05 = _____
13. 0.002 = _____

Changing Common Fractions to Decimal Fractions

Convert the following common fractions to decimal fractions.
14. ½ = _____
15. ¾ = _____
16. 1/6 = _____
17. 1/50 = _____
18. 2/3 = _____

Changing Percentages to Fractions

Convert the following percentages to fractions.
19. 25% = 25/100 = _____
20. 2% = 2/100 = _____
21. 15% = 15/100 = _____
22. 12 1/2% = 12.5/100 = _____
23. 10% = 10/100 = _____
24. ¼% = 1/4/100 = _____
25. 20% = 20/100 = _____
26. 150% = 150/100 = _____

27. 50% = 50/100 = _____
28. 4% = 4/100 = _____

Changing Percentages to Decimal Fractions

Convert the following percentages to decimal fractions.
29. 4% = _____
30. 25% = _____
31. 1% = _____
32. 50% = _____
33. 2% = _____
34. 10% = _____

Changing Decimal Fractions to Percentages

Convert the following decimal fractions to percentages.
35. 0.05 = _____
36. 0.25 = _____
37. 0.15 = _____
38. 0.125 = _____
39. 0.0025 = _____

Converting Milligrams to Grams

Convert the following milligrams (mg) to grams (g).
40. 0.4 mg = _____g
41. 0.12 mg = _____g
42. 0.2 mg = _____g
43. 0.1 mg = _____g
44. 500 mg = _____g
45. 125 mg = _____g
46. 100 mg = _____g
47. 200 mg = _____g
48. 50 mg = _____g
49. 400 mg = _____g

Convert the following grams (g) to milligrams (mg).
50. 0.2 g = _____mg
51. 0.250 g = _____mg
52. 0.125 g = _____mg
53. 0.006 g = _____mg
54. 0.004 g = _____mg
55. 2.5 g = _____mg

Converting Between Kilograms and Pounds

Convert the following kilograms (kg) to pounds (lb).
56. 92 kg = _____lb
57. 75.5 kg = _____lb

Convert the following pounds (lb) to kilograms (kg).
58. 154 lb = _____kg
59. 211.2 lb = _____kg

Answers:

1. 1/20   2. 1/7   3. 1/6   4. 3/11   5. ½   6. 3/10
7. ¼   8. 2/5   9. ½   10. ½   11. ¾   12. 1/20
13. 1/500   14. 0.5   15. 0.75   16. 0.1666   17. 0.02
18. 0.66   19. ¼   20. 1/5   21. 3/20   22. 1/8
23. 1/10   24. 1/400   25. 1/5   26. 3/2 or 1 1/2
27. ½   28. 1/25   29. 0.04   30. 0.25   31. 0.01
32. 0.5   33. 0.02   34. 0.1   35. 5%   36. 25%
37. 15%   38. 12.5%   39. 0.25%   40. 0.0004 g

41. 0.00012 g   42. 0.0002 g   43. 0.0001 g   44. 0.5 g
45. 0.125 g   46. 0.1 g   47. 0.2 g   48. 0.05 g
49. 0.4 g   50. 200 mg   51. 250 mg   52. 125 mg
53. 0.6 g   54. 4 mg   55. 2500 mg   56. 202.4 lb
57. 166.1 lb   58. 70 kg   59. 96 kg

Adapted from Willihnganz MJ, Gurevitz SM, Clayton BD: Clayton's Basic pharmacology for nurses, ed 18, St. Louis, 2020, Mosby.

absorption   The process by which a drug is transferred from its site of body entry to circulating body fluids (blood, lymph) for distribution

abuse   The intentional mistreatment or harm of another person

accountable   Being responsible for one's actions and the actions of others who performed the delegated tasks; answering questions about and explaining one's actions and the actions of others

adrenergic blocking agent   A drug that inhibits adrenergic effects

adrenergic fibers   Nerve endings that release norepinephrine (a neurotransmitter)

advance directive   A document stating a person's wishes about health care when that person cannot make his or her own decisions

adverse drug reaction (ADR)   An unintended effect on the body from using a legal drug, illegal drug, or two or more drugs; adverse effect

aerobe   A microbe that lives and grows in the presence of oxygen (aer)

agonist   A drug that acts on a certain type of cell to produce a predictable response

aldosterone   A substance that causes the kidneys to retain sodium

allergic reaction   An unfavorable response to a substance that causes a hypersensitivity reaction

alopecia   Hair loss

anaerobe   A microbe that lives and grows in the absence (an) of oxygen (aer)

analgesic   A drug that relieves pain; an means without, algesic means pain

anaphylactic reaction   See "anaphylaxis"

anaphylaxis   A severe, life-threatening sensitivity to an antigen; anaphylactic reaction

androgens   Steroid hormones that produce masculine effects

angiotensin   A substance that causes vasoconstriction, increased blood pressure, and the release of aldosterone

antacids   Drugs that buffer, neutralize, or absorb hydrochloric acid in the stomach; ant means against, acid means sour

antagonist   A drug that exerts an opposite action to that of another; or it competes for the same receptor sites

antianxiety drugs   Drugs used to treat anxiety

antibiotics   Antimicrobials derived from living microorganisms; drugs that kill microbes that cause infections

anticholinergic agent   A drug that blocks or inhibits cholinergic activity

anticoagulants   Drugs that prevent arterial and venous thrombi; "blood thinners"

anticonvulsants   Drugs used to prevent or reduce seizures; antiepileptic drugs

antidepressants   Several classes of drugs used to treat mood disorders

antidiabetic agents   Drugs used to prevent or relieve symptoms of diabetes

antidiarrheals   Drugs that relieve symptoms of diarrhea

antidysrhythmic agents   Drugs used to prevent or correct abnormal heart rhythms

antiemetics   Drugs used to treat nausea and vomiting

antiepileptic drugs   Drugs used to prevent or reduce seizures; anticonvulsants

antihistamines   Drugs that compete with released histamine for receptor sites in the arterioles, capillaries, and glands in mucous membranes

antihypertensive agents   Drugs that reduce blood pressure

antimicrobial agents   Chemicals that eliminate pathogens

antithyroid agents   Drugs used to suppress the production of thyroid hormones

antitussives   Drugs that suppress the cough center in the brain; cough suppressants

anxiety   A vague, uneasy feeling in response to stress

anxiolytics   Antianxiety drugs; tranquilizers

arrhythmia   Without (a) a rhythm (rhythmia); dysrhythmia

artery   A blood vessel that carries blood away from the heart

asepsis   Being free of disease-producing microbes

aspiration   Breathing fluid, food, vomitus, or an object into the lungs

assault   Intentionally attempting or threatening to touch a person's body without the person's consent

assessment   Collecting information about the person; a step in the nursing process

bacteria   One-celled plant life that multiply rapidly and can cause an infection in any body system; germs

barbiturate   A drug that depresses the central nervous system, respirations, blood pressure, and temperature

battery   Touching a person's body without the person's consent

benign tumor   A tumor that does not spread to other body parts; it can grow to a large size

blood pressure   The amount of force exerted against the walls of an artery by the blood

boundary crossing   A brief act or behavior outside of the helpful zone

boundary signs   Acts, behaviors, or thoughts that warn of a boundary crossing or violation

boundary violation   An act or behavior that meets your needs, but not the person's

brand name   The name the manufacturer gives to a specific drug; trademark, trade name

bronchodilators   Drugs that relax the smooth muscles of the tracheobronchial tree

buccal   Inside the cheek (bucco)

calorie   The amount of energy produced when the body burns food

cancer   Malignant tumor

capillary   A tiny blood vessel; food, oxygen, and other substances pass from the capillaries to the cells

capsule   A gelatin container that holds a drug in a dry powder or liquid form

carrier   A human or animal that is a reservoir for microbes but does not have the signs or symptoms of infection

cell   The basic unit of body structure

cerumen   Ear wax

chart   See "medical record"

cholesterol   A waxy, fat-like substance found in all body cells

cholinergic fibers   Nerve endings that release acetylcholine (a neurotransmitter)

civil law   Laws concerned with relationships between people

clinical record   See "medical record"

clonus   Rapidly alternating involuntary contraction and relaxation of skeletal muscles

coating agents   Drugs that form a substance that adheres to the crater of an ulcer

constipation   The passage of a hard, dry stool

contamination   The process of becoming unclean

contraception   The processes or methods used to prevent (contra) pregnancy

corticosteroids   Hormones secreted by the adrenal cortex of the adrenal glands

cough suppressants   See "antitussives"

cream   A semi-solid emulsion containing a drug

cretinism   Congenital hypothyroidism

crime   An act that violates a criminal law

criminal law   Laws concerned with offenses against the public and society in general

cross-contamination   Passing microbes from one person to another by way of contaminated hands, equipment, or supplies

cystitis   Inflammation (itis) of the bladder (cyst)

debride   To remove

decongestants   Drugs that cause vasoconstriction of the nasal mucosa

defamation   Injuring a person's name and reputation by making false statements to a third party

delegate   To authorize another person to perform a nursing task in a certain situation

desired action   Expected response

diabetes   A disorder in which the body cannot properly produce or use insulin

diarrhea   The frequent passage of liquid stools

diastole   The resting phase of the heartbeat; heart chambers fill with blood

digestion   The process of physically and chemically breaking down food so that it can be absorbed for use by the cells

digitalization   Giving a larger dose of digoxin for the first 24 hours, then giving the person a daily dose

dilute   To add the correct amount of water or other liquid

distribution   The ways drugs are transported by circulating body fluids to the sites of action (receptors) and to the sites of metabolism and excretion

diuresis   The increased formation and excretion of urine; *dia* means *through*, *ur* means *urine*

diuretic   A drug that promotes the formation and excretion of urine; *dia* means *through*, *ur* means *urine*

dose   The amount of drug to give

drug   A chemical substance that influences a living organism

drug blood level   The amount of a drug present in the blood

drug diversion   Taking a person's drugs for your own use

drug interaction   When the action of one drug is altered by the action of another drug

drug order   An order for a drug written on the agency's (hospital, nursing center) physician's order form or entered electronically into the agency's computer system for a patient or resident; medication order

drug reaction   See "adverse drug reaction"

drug tolerance   When a person needs increasingly higher doses of a drug to treat their pain

dyslipidemia   An abnormality of one or more of the blood fats (lipids)

dysrhythmia   An abnormal *(dys)* rhythm *(rhythmia)*; arrhythmia

electronic health record (EHR)   An electronic version of a person's medical record; electronic medical record

electronic medical record (EMR)   See "electronic health record"

elixir   A clear liquid made up of a drug dissolved in alcohol and water

embolus   A small part of a thrombus that breaks off and travels through the vascular system until it lodges in a blood vessel

emesis   Vomiting, vomitus

emulsion   An oral dose form containing small droplets of water-in-oil or oil-in-water

end-of-shift report   A report that the nurse gives at the end of the shift to the on-coming shift

endometriosis   A condition *(osis)* in which the tissue that lines *(endo)* the inside of the uterus *(metri)* grows outside the uterus

enteral nutrition   Giving nutrients into the gastrointestinal (GI) tract *(enteral)* through a feeding tube

enteral route   Drugs are given directly into the gastrointestinal (GI) tract; *enteral* means *bowel*

enzymes   Substances produced by body cells; using oxygen, enzymes break down glucose and other nutrients to release energy for cellular work

epidemic   A disease that affects many people within a community, population, or region

epilepsy   A brain disorder in which clusters of nerve cells sometimes signal abnormally

erectile dysfunction (ED)   The inability of the male to have an erection; impotence

estrogen   The female hormone

ethics   Knowledge of what is right conduct and wrong conduct

eunuchism   A condition in which the male lacks male hormones

euphoria   An exaggerated feeling or state of physical or mental well-being

evaluation   To measure if goals in the planning step were met; a step in the nursing process

excretion   The elimination of a drug from the body

expectorants   Drugs that liquify mucus to promote the ejection of mucus from the lungs and tracheobronchial tree

false imprisonment   Unlawful restraint or restriction of a person's freedom of movement

fecal impaction   The prolonged retention and build-up of feces in the rectum

fraud   Saying or doing something to trick, fool, or deceive a person

fungi   Plants that live on other plants or animals

gastrointestinal prostaglandins   Drugs that inhibit gastric acid secretion

gastrostomy tube   A tube inserted through a surgically created opening *(stomy)* in the stomach *(gastro)*; stomach tube

generic name   The drug's common name

germs   See "bacteria"

glucocorticoids   Hormones that regulate carbohydrate, protein, and fat metabolism; they have antiinflammatory, antiallergenic, and immunosuppressant activity

goiter   An enlarged thyroid gland

gonads   The reproductive glands

griping   Severe and spasm-like pain in the abdomen caused by an intestinal disorder; gripping

gynecologic   Pertains to diseases of the female reproductive organs and breasts

healthcare-associated infection (HAI)   An infection that develops in a person cared for in any setting where health care is given; the infection is related to receiving health care

Health Insurance Portability and Accountability Act (HIPAA)   An act created in 1996 that protects people's privacy and health information. A HIPAA violation may result in severe fines.

hemoglobin   The substance in red blood cells that carries oxygen and gives blood its color

hemorrheologic agent   A drug that prevents the clumping of red blood cells and platelets; hemorrheologic relates to the science *(logic)* of blood *(hemo)* flow *(rrheo)*

histamine   A substance released in response to allergic reactions and tissue damage from trauma or infection

histamine (H2)-receptor antagonists   Drugs that block the action of histamine; histamine blockers

hives   See "urticaria"

homeostasis   A constant internal environment

hormone   A chemical substance secreted by the endocrine glands into the bloodstream

hyperglycemia   High *(hyper)* sugar *(glyc)* in the blood *(emia)*

hyperlipidemia   Excess *(hyper)* lipids *(fats)* in the blood *(emia)*

hyperreflexia   Increased reflex actions

hypertension   The systolic pressure is 140 mm Hg or higher *(hyper)* or the diastolic pressure is 90 mm Hg or higher; high blood pressure

hyperthyroidism   The disease that occurs from the excess *(hyper)* production of the thyroid hormones

hypnotic   A drug that produces sleep

hypoglycemia   Low *(hypo)* sugar *(glyc)* in the blood *(emia)*

hypoglycemic agents   Drugs that lower *(hypo)* the blood *(emic)* glucose *(glyc)* level

hypogonadism   A condition in which the body does not produce enough *(hypo)* testosterone

hypothyroidism   The disease that results from inadequate *(hypo)* thyroid hormone production

idiosyncratic reaction   Something unusual or abnormal that happens when a drug is first given

immunity   Protection against a disease or condition; the person will not get or be affected by the disease

implementation   To perform or carry out nursing measures in the care plan; a step in the nursing process

impotence   See "erectile dysfunction"

infarction   A local area of tissue death

infection   A disease state resulting from the invasion and growth of microbes in the body

inhibitor   A drug that prevents or restricts a certain action

inotropic agents   Drugs that stimulate the heart to increase the force of contractions

insomnia   A chronic condition in which the person cannot sleep or stay asleep all night

instill   To enter drop by drop

insulin   A hormone produced by the pancreas; it is needed for glucose to enter skeletal muscles, heart muscle, and fat

intermittent claudication A pain pattern usually described as aching, cramping, tightness, or weakness in the calves usually during walking; it is relieved with rest

intramuscular (IM) Within (*intra*) a muscle (*muscular*)

intranasal Within (*intra*) the nose (*nasal*)

intravenous (IV) Within (*intra*) a vein (*venous*)

invasion of privacy Violating a person's right not to have his or her name, photo, or private affairs exposed or made public without the person's consent

ischemia A decreased supply of oxygenated blood to a body part

jejunostomy tube A feeding tube inserted into a surgically created opening (*stomy*) in the jejunum of the small intestine

lactic acid A product of glucose metabolism

lactic acidosis A buildup of lactic acid in the blood

lavage Washing out the stomach

law A rule of conduct made by a government body

laxatives Substances that cause evacuation of the bowel; *laxare* means *to loosen*

leukorrhea An abnormal whitish (*leuko*) vaginal discharge (*rrhea*)

libel Making false statements in print, writing, or through pictures or drawings

lipids Fats

lotion A watery preparation containing suspended particles

lozenge A flat disk containing a medicinal agent with a flavored base; troche

macronutrients The energy sources needed for balanced metabolism

malignant tumor A tumor that invades and destroys nearby tissue and can spread to other body parts; cancer

malnutrition Any disorder of nutrition; *mal* means *bad*

malpractice Negligence by a professional person

medical asepsis Practices used to remove or destroy pathogens and to prevent their spread from one person or place to another person or place; clean technique

medical diagnosis The identification of a disease or condition by a doctor

medical record The written or electronic account of a person's condition and response to treatment and care; chart or clinical record

medication A drug used to prevent and treat disease; medicine

medication assistant-certified (MA-C) Nursing assistants who are allowed by state law to give drugs

medication order See "drug order"

medication reminder Reminding the person to take drugs, observing the person taking the drugs as prescribed, and charting that they were taken

medicine See "medication"

medicine cup A plastic container with measurement scales

medicine dropper A small glass or plastic tube with a hollow rubber ball at one end

meniscus The lowest point of liquid in a medicine cup

menstruation The process in which the lining of the uterus breaks up and is discharged from the body through the vagina

metabolism The burning of food for heat and energy by the cells; the process by which the body in-activates drugs

metabolite A product of drug metabolism

metastasis The spread of cancer to other body parts

microbe See "microorganism"

microorganism A small (*micro*) living plant or animal (*organism*) seen only with a microscope; a microbe

mineralocorticoids Hormones that maintain fluid and electrolyte balance

miosis Narrowing of the pupil

misappropriation To dishonestly, unfairly, or wrongly take for one's own use

mucolytic agents Drugs that reduce the stickiness and thickness of pulmonary secretions

mydriasis Dilation of the pupil

myxedema Hypothyroidism that occurs during adult life

nasal Pertains to the nose

nasoduodenal tube A feeding tube inserted through the nose (*naso*) into the duodenum of the small intestine

nasogastric (NG) tube A feeding tube inserted through the nose (*naso*) into the stomach (*gastro*)

nasointestinal tube A feeding tube inserted through the nose (*naso*) into the small intestine (*intestinal*)

nasojejunal tube A feeding tube inserted through the nose (*naso*) into the *jejunum* of the small intestine

nausea The sensation of abdominal discomfort that may lead to the urge or need to vomit

neglect Failure to provide the person with the goods or services needed to avoid physical harm, mental anguish, or mental illness

negligence An unintentional wrong in which a person did not act in a reasonable and careful manner and a person or the person's property was harmed

neuron The basic nerve cell of the nervous system

neurotransmitter A chemical substance that transmits nerve impulses

non-pathogen A microbe that does not usually cause an infection

normal flora Microbes that live and grow in a certain area

nurse practice act The law that regulates nursing practice in a state

nursing assistants Individuals employed to give direct hands-on care and perform delegated nursing care tasks under the supervision of a licensed nurse

nursing care plan A written guide about the person's care; care plan

nursing diagnosis Describes a health problem that can be treated by nursing measures; a step in the nursing process

nursing intervention An action or measure taken by the nursing team to help the person reach a goal

nursing process The method nurses use to plan and deliver nursing care; its five steps are assessment, nursing diagnosis, planning, implementation, and evaluation

nursing task Nursing care or a nursing function, procedure, activity, or work that does not require an RN's or LPN's/LVN's professional knowledge or judgment

nutrient A substance that is ingested, digested, absorbed, and used by the body

nutrition The processes involved in the ingestion, digestion, absorption, and use of foods and fluids by the body

objective data Information that is seen, heard, felt, or smelled by an observer; signs

observation Using the senses of sight, hearing, touch, and smell to collect information

ocular Pertains to the eye

ointment A semi-solid preparation containing a drug in an oily base

ophthalmic Pertains to the eye

opiate A drug that contains opium, is derived from opium, or has opium-like activity

opioids Drugs that provide pain relief. They come from opium or are man-made.

opportunistic infection An infection caused by non-pathogens in a person with a weakened immune system

oral contraceptives Birth control pills

organ Groups of tissues with the same function

osmotic agents Drugs that cause fluid to be drawn from outside of the vascular system into the blood

osteoporosis A bone disease that causes bones to become fragile and fracture easily

otic Pertains to the ear

overactive bladder (OAB) A syndrome characterized by urinary frequency, urgency, and incontinence; urge syndrome or urgency/frequency syndrome

pain To ache, hurt, or be sore; discomfort

pandemic An epidemic that has spread to multiple countries or continents

parenteral nutrition Giving nutrients through a catheter inserted into a vein; *para* means *beyond*; *enteral* relates to the bowel

parenteral route Drugs bypass the GI tract; *para* means *beyond*; *enteral* means *bowel*

pathogen A microbe that is harmful and can cause an infection

peptic Pertains to digestion or the enzymes and secretions needed for digestion

peptic ulcer   An ulcer in the stomach, duodenum, or other part of the GI system exposed to gastric juices

percutaneous endoscopic gastrostomy (PEG) tube   A feeding tube inserted into the stomach *(gastro)* through a small incision *(stomy)* made through *(per)* the skin *(cutaneous)*; a lighted instrument *(scope)* allows the doctor to see inside a body cavity or organ *(endo)*

percutaneous route   Drugs are given through *(per)* the skin *(cutaneous)* or a mucous membrane

peristalsis   Involuntary muscle contractions in the digestive system that move food down the esophagus through the alimentary canal

pharmacology   The study of drugs and their actions on living organisms

placebo   A drug dosage form that has no active ingredients

planning   Setting priorities and goals; a step in the nursing process

platelet aggregation inhibitor   A drug that prevents platelets from clumping together and causes vasodilation

platelet inhibitors   Drugs that prevent platelet aggregation (clumping)

powder   A finely ground drug in a talc base

prescription   A drug or drugs ordered for a person leaving the hospital or nursing center or for a person seen in a clinic or doctor's office; it is written on a prescription pad or called in, faxed, or emailed to the pharmacy by the prescriber

priapism   A prolonged or constant erection

PRN order   The nurse decides when to give the drug based on the person's needs

professional boundaries   That which separates helpful behaviors from behaviors that are not helpful

professional sexual misconduct   An act, behavior, or comment that is sexual in nature and occurs within the scope of employment

progesterone   The hormone associated with body changes that favor pregnancy and lactation

prokinetic agents   Drugs that stimulate movement or motility

prostatitis   Inflammation *(itis)* of the prostate *(prostat)*

protected health information   Identifying information about the person's health care that is maintained or sent in any form (paper, electronic, oral)

proton pump inhibitors   Drugs that inhibit the gastric acid pump of the parietal cells

protozoa   One-celled animals that can infect the blood, brain, intestines, and other body areas

psychosis   A state of severe mental impairment; the person does not view the real or unreal correctly

pyelonephritis   Inflammation *(itis)* of the kidney *(nephr)* pelvis *(pyelo)*

reconstitute   To add water or other liquid to a powder or solid form of a drug

regurgitation   The backward flow of stomach contents into the mouth

renin   An enzyme that affects blood pressure

respiration   The process of supplying the cells with oxygen and removing carbon dioxide from them

retching   The involuntary, labored, spasmodic contractions of the abdominal and respiratory muscles without vomitus; "dry heaves"

rhinitis medicamentosa   Drug-induced congestion

rhinorrhea   Nasal discharge *(rhino* means *nose; rrhea* means *discharge)*; runny nose

route   How and where the drug enters the body

routine order   A drug given as prescribed until it is cancelled by the prescriber, or the prescribed number of doses has been given; scheduled medication

secondary infection   An infection caused by a microbe that follows the first infection caused by a different microbe

sedative   A drug that quiets the person; it gives a feeling of relaxation and rest

seizure   Violent and sudden contractions or tremors of muscle groups; convulsion

semi-synthetic   A natural substance that has been partially altered by chemicals

side effect   An unintended reaction to a drug given in a normal dosage

signs   See "objective data"

single order   A drug to be given at a certain time and only one time

slander   Making false statements orally

social distancing   Putting space (at least 6 feet) between yourself and others

soufflé cup   A small paper or plastic cup used for solid drug forms

spasm   An involuntary muscle contraction of sudden onset

spores   Bacterium protected by a hard shell

standard of care   Refers to the skills, care, and judgment required by nursing assistants under similar conditions

STAT order   The drug is to be given at once and only one time

sterile   The absence of all microbes

sterilization   The process of destroying all microbes

stomatitis   Inflammation *(itis)* of the mouth *(stomat)*

subcutaneous (subcut)   Beneath *(sub)* the skin *(cutaneous)*

subjective data   Things a person tells you about that you cannot observe through your own senses; symptoms

sublingual   Under *(sub)* the tongue *(lingual)*

suppository   A cone-shaped, solid drug that is inserted into a body opening; it melts at body temperature

surgical asepsis   The practice that keeps items free of all microbes; sterile technique

suspension   A liquid containing solid drug particles

symptoms   See "subjective data"

synapse   The junction between one neuron and the next

synthetic   A substance that is made rather than naturally occurring

syringe   A plastic measuring device with three parts—tip, barrel, and plunger

syrup   An oral dose form containing a drug dissolved in sugar

system   Organs that work together to perform special functions

systole   The working phase of the heartbeat; the heart contracts and pumps blood through the blood vessels

tablet   A dried, powdered drug compressed into a small disk

testosterone   The male hormone

therapeutic drug monitoring   The measurement of a drug's concentration in body fluids

thromboembolic diseases   Diseases associated with abnormal clotting within blood vessels

thrombosis   The process of clot formation

thrombus   A blood clot

thyroid replacement hormones   Drugs that replace thyroid hormones in the treatment of hypothyroidism

tissue   A group of cells with similar functions

topical   Refers to a surface of a part of the body

tort   A wrong committed against a person or the person's property

toxicity   Exposure to large amounts of a substance that should not cause problems in smaller amounts; the reaction when side effects are severe

tracheobronchial tree   The trachea, bronchi, and bronchioles

tranquilizers   Antianxiety drugs; anxiolytics

transdermal   Through *(trans)* the skin *(dermal)*

transdermal patch   A patch applied to the skin that provides continuous, gradual absorption of a drug through the skin and into the bloodstream; transdermal disk

triglycerides   Fatty compounds that come from animal and vegetable fats

troche   See "lozenge"

tumor   A new growth of abnormal cells; tumors are benign or malignant

ulcer   A shallow or deep crater-like sore of a mucous membrane

urethritis   Inflammation *(itis)* of the urethra *(urethr)*

urinary antimicrobial agents   Substances that have an antiseptic effect on urine and the urinary tract

urticaria   Raised, irregularly shaped patches on the skin with severe itching; hives

vaccination   Giving a vaccine to produce immunity against an infectious disease

vaccine   A preparation containing dead or weakened microbes

vasodilators   Drugs that widen blood vessels to increase blood flow

vasospasm   A sudden contraction of a blood vessel causing vasoconstriction

vein   A blood vessel that returns blood back to the heart

viruses   Microbes that grow in living cells

vital signs   Temperature, pulse, respirations, blood pressure, and pain

vomiting   Expelling stomach contents through the mouth; emesis

vomitus   The food and fluids expelled from the stomach through the mouth; emesis

vulnerable adult   A person 18 years old or older who has a disability or condition that puts them at risk to be wounded, attacked, or damaged

KEY ABBREVIATIONS

ACE Angiotensin-converting enzyme
ACTH Adrenocorticotropic hormone
AD Alzheimer's disease
ADE Adverse drug event
ADH Antidiuretic hormone
ADM Automated dispensing machine
ADME Absorption, distribution, metabolism, excretion
ADR Adverse drug reaction
AED Antiepileptic drug
AHA American Hospital Association
AIDS Acquired immunodeficiency syndrome
AIIR Airborne infection isolation room
ALR Assisted living residence
ARB Angiotensin II receptor blocker

BCMA Barcode medication administration
BP Blood pressure
BPH Benign prostatic hyperplasia

C Celsius; centigrade
C. diff Clostridium difficile
CAD Coronary artery disease
cAMP Cyclic adenosine monophosphate
CDC Centers for Disease Control and Prevention
CHF Congestive heart failure
CNA Certified nursing assistant
CNS Central nervous system
CO₂ Carbon dioxide
comt Catechol O-methyltransferase
COPD Chronic obstructive pulmonary disease
COVID-19 Novel Coronavirus (2019)
CPOE Computerized physician (or provider) order entry
CPR Cardiopulmonary resuscitation

DEA Drug Enforcement Administration
DNR Do not resuscitate
DVT Deep vein thrombosis

ECG Electrocardiogram
ED Erectile dysfunction
EHR Electronic health record
EMR Electronic medical record
EMT Emergency medical technician

F Fahrenheit
FDA Food and Drug Administration
ft Feet

g Gram
GED General education diploma
GERD Gastroesophageal reflux disease
GH Growth hormone
GI Gastrointestinal

h Hour
HAI Healthcare-associated infection
HBV Hepatitis B virus
HDL High-density lipoprotein
Hg Mercury
HIPAA Health Insurance Portability and Accountability Act of 1996
HIV Human immunodeficiency virus
HR Heart rate

IBD Inflammatory bowel disease
ID Identification
IM Intramuscular
in Inch
IOP Intraocular pressure
ISMP Institute for Safe Medication Practices
IV Intravenous; intravenously

kg Kilogram

lb Pound
LDL Low-density lipoprotein
LNA Licensed nursing assistant
LPN Licensed practical nurse
LVN Licensed vocational nurse

MA-C Medication assistant–certified
MAOI Monoamine oxidase inhibitor
MAR Medication administration record
mcg Microgram
MDI Metered-dose inhaler
MDRO Multidrug-resistant organisms
MDS Minimum data set
mg Milligram
MI Myocardial infarction
mL Milliliter
mm Millimeter
mm Hg Millimeters of mercury
MRSA Methicillin-resistant Staphylococcus aureus

NATCEP Nursing Assistant Training and Competency Evaluation Program
NCSBN National Council of State Boards of Nursing
NDC National Drug Code
NG Nasogastric
NSAID Nonsteroidal antiinflammatory drug

O₂ Oxygen
OAB Overactive bladder
OBRA Omnibus Budget Reconciliation Act of 1987
OCD Obsessive-compulsive disorder
ODT Orally disintegrating tablet
OPIM Other potentially infectious materials
OSHA Occupational Safety and Health Administration
OTC Over-the-counter

PDE-4 Phosphodiesterase-4
PDR Physicians' Desk Reference
PE Pulmonary embolism
PEG Percutaneous endoscopic gastrostomy
PG Prostaglandin
PO By mouth (per os); per os (orally)
POLST Physician Orders for Life-Sustaining Treatment
PPE Personal protective equipment
PPI Proton pump inhibitor
PRN, prn As needed, when necessary, when needed
PTSD Post-traumatic stress disorder
PUD Peptic ulcer disease
PVD Peripheral vascular disease

q Every
RBC Red blood cell
RN Registered nurse

RNA Registered nurse aide
RR Respiratory rate

SSRI Selective serotonin reuptake inhibitor
STAT Immediately; at once
STI Sexually transmitted disease
subcut Subcutaneous; subcutaneously

T₃ Tri-iodothyronine
T₄ Thyroxine
TB Tuberculosis
TCA Tricyclic antidepressant
TED hose Thromboembolic disease hose
TH Thyroid hormone; thyroxine
TIA Transient ischemic attack

TO Telephone order
TPN Total parenteral nutrition
TSH Thyroid-stimulating hormone
TURP Transurethral resection of the prostate
TZD Thiazolidinedione

UTI Urinary tract infection

VC Vomiting center
VO Verbal order
VRE Vancomycin-resistant Enterococcus

WBC White blood cell
WHO World Health Organization

INDEX

Page numbers followed by *f* indicate figures; *t,* tables; *b,* boxes.